HYSTERECTOMY

Edited by **Ayman Al-Hendy**
and **Mohamed Sabry**

Hysterectomy
Edited by Ayman Al-Hendy and Mohamed Sabry

Published by InTech
Janeza Trdine 9, 51000 Rijeka, Croatia

Publishing Process Manager Tajana Jevtic

Technical Editor Teodora Smiljanic

Cover Designer InTech Design Team

Additional hard copies can be obtained from orders@intechopen.com

Hysterectomy, Edited by Ayman Al-Hendy and Mohamed Sabry
p. cm.
ISBN 978-953-51-0434-6

For EU product safety concerns:
IN TECH d.o.o., Prolaz Marije Krucifikse Kozulić 3, 51000 Rijeka, Croatia,
info@intechopen.com or visit our website at intechopen.com.

Meet the editors

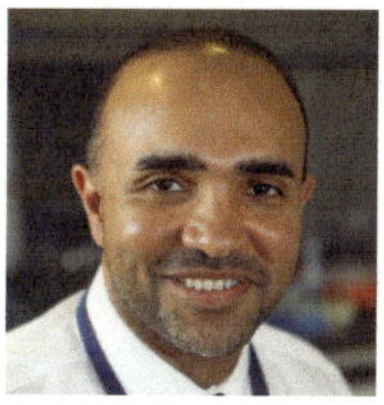

Dr Al-Hendy graduated from Zagazig University, Egypt in 1986. He earned his PhD from Turku University, Finland and gained additional postdoctoral training in gene therapy and clinical molecular genetics at McMaster and McGill Universities in Canada, clinical residency in OB/GYN at University of Saskatchewan, and fellowship training in laparoscopic surgery at Toronto University, Canada. In USA, Dr. Al-Hendy held various faculty positions at UTMB before moving to Tennessee, where he appointed as Professor and Vice Chair of the OB/GYN Department, Scientific Director of the CWHR at Meharry Medical College, Adj. professor at Vanderbilt University. In 2010 Dr. Al-Hendy's was awarded the ASRM Ira and Ester Rosenwaks Award for his significant contribution to the Reproductive Biology field.

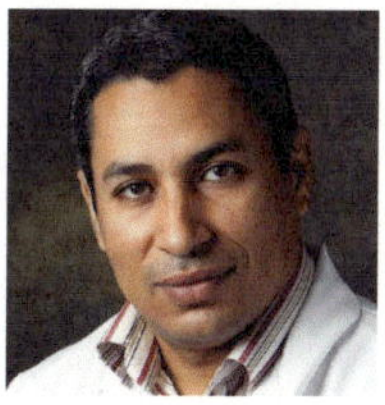

Dr Sabry is an assistant Lecturer of OB/GYN at Sohag University, Egypt. He earned his M.D. degree in 1999 from South Valley University, Egypt. After completing his residency training, he earned his Master degree in OB/GYN in 2007 from Sohag University, Egypt. Dr Sabry spent 3 years of fellowship training at Meharry Medical College, USA; during which he earned the Certificate of the American Registry of Diagnostic Medical Sonography, and shared through his publications and presentations in many national and international meetings focusing in the areas of ovarian biology, female infertility as well as developing novel medical treatment for uterine fibroids.

Contents

Preface

This book is intended for the general and family practitioners, as well as for gynecologists, specialists in gynecological surgery, general surgeons, urologists and all other surgical specialists that perform procedures in or around the female pelvis, in addition to intensives and all other specialities and health care professionals who care for women before, during or after hysterectomy. While removal of the uterus using newer techniques such as laparoscopic and robotic hysterectomy attract the most attention of both the patients as well as the practitioners, still, for most women, especially in low resources countries, the conventional hysterectomy, abdominal or vaginal, is considered the intervention of choice for removing the uterus. Such techniques have withstood the test of time and can be performed in almost any small or midsized surgical hospital without the need to travel to distant specialty hospitals.

It is the aim of this book to review the recent achievements of the research community regarding the field of gynecologic surgery and hysterectomy as well as highlight future directions and where this field is heading. While no single volume can adequately cover the diversity of issues and facets in relation to such a common and important procedure such as hysterectomy, this book will attempt to address the pivotal topics especially in regards to safety, risk management as well as pre- and post-operative care.

Finally, we dedicate this book to our wonderful prior, current and future patients for whom we strive for excellence and beyond, as we care for them with full and most respect and love as they are our daughters, sisters and mothers, all the time.

Ayman Al-Hendy, MD, PhD
Professor, Vice Chair and Scientific Director, Department of Obstetrics and Gynecology,
Center of Women Health Research, Meharry Medical College, Nashville, Tennessee,
Adjunct professor, Vanderbilt University and Vanderbilt University Medical Center,
Nashville, Tennessee,
USA

Mohamed Sabry, MD
Department of Obstetrics and Gynecology, Sohag University Hospitals, Sohag,
Egypt
Center for Women's Health Research, Department of Obstetrics and Gynecology,
Meharry Medical College, Nashville, Tennessee,
USA

Part 1

Types of Hysterectomy

1

Techniques of Hysterectomy

Nirmala Duhan
Department of Obstetrics and Gynecology,
Pt B D Sharma Post Graduate Institute of Medical Sciences, ROHTAK,
India

1. Introduction

Hysterectomy is the most common operation performed for gynecological disorders, second only to caesarean section. Annual medical costs related to hysterectomy exceed $ 5 billion in the US. Overall hysterectomy rates vary from 1.2 to 4.8 per 1000 women. Development of alternatives to hysterectomy like use of different energy sources for endometrial ablation and the availability of progestational intrauterine system for symptomatic uterine bleeding have led to a reduction in rates of hysterectomy in recent years. Besides, leiomyomas which have conventionally formed one of the important indications of hysterectomy in women in whom fertility conservation is not an issue, are now increasingly being managed by transcervical hysteroscopic resection (submucous myomas), transcatheter uterine artery embolization and magnetic resonance guided focussed ultrasound energy. These new, less invasive and safer management techniques coupled with the desire to avoid major surgery, have added to the reduction in hysterectomy rates.

1.1 Indications for hysterectomy

Even though alternatives to hysterectomy are being explored for benign conditions, hysterectomy continues to have a place in its definitiveness. Uterine myomas continue to form the indications for 40% of all abdominal hysterectomies, the others being endometriosis (12.8%), malignancy (12.6%), abnormal uterine bleeding (9.5%), pelvic inflammatory disease (3.7%) and uterine prolapse (3.0%). Prolapse forms the indication for 44% of all vaginal hysterectomies. In recent years, non - descent vaginal hysterectomy (NDVH) is being tried for most benign conditions and uteri of upto 12 weeks gestational size can be safely removed intact per vaginum. For moderate to large sized uteri with benign conditions, techniques like removal of wedge, bisection, coring and morcellation may be adopted in an attempt to reduce the uterine volume prior to removal. However, large leiomyomas, pelvic inflammatory disease, malignancy (invasive cervical cancer, endometrial carcinoma, ovarian and fallopian tube cancer and gestational trophoblastic tumors) and most suspicious adnexal masses may still be better approached abdominally.

1.2 Approaching the uterus: Abdominally or vaginally

The uterus may be removed abdominally or vaginally or by a combination of the two routes. Abdominal approach may further be categorized as open abdominal or laparoscopic.

Although abdominal approach continues to be the most common approach worldwide, uterine access by the vaginal route is associated with fewer complications, a shorter hospital stay, faster recovery and lower costs. Most patients with gynecologic malignancies are operated by open abdominal route, though laparoscopic and robotic surgical techniques are increasingly being used for endometrial and cervical cancer surgery. Significant uterine enlargement and/or fixity, adnexal fixation and obliteration of the Pouch of Douglas are some other factors suggesting preference for abdominal approach.

1.3 Preoperative counseling

The clinician needs to communicate clearly and in the patient's language, the indication for surgery, the treatment alternatives available, the reason(s) for preferring hysterectomy over them and the preferred approach. Besides, the risks, benefits and the adverse effects must be reviewed. The woman should also be encouraged to clarify her doubts, particularly regarding the type of anaesthesia preferred, tentative duration of surgery, the recuperative time, the management of normal ovaries at surgery and subsequent possible hormone replacement therapy and any impact on sexual function. The surgeon may also encourage the woman's partner / supportive family members during the preoperative discussions to express their opinions / concerns regarding the procedure. Emotional stress after hysterectomy, if it occurs, is usually short lasting and self limiting in most cases and only occasionally, psychiatric consultation and pharmacotherapy may be necessary.

1.4 Preoperative preparation

After a complete history, physical examination and a recent Pap test, haematological tests like estimation of hemoglobin, bleeding and clotting times, urea, and sugar are carried out. Preoperative electrocardiogram and chest x-rays are particularly important for women with cardiorespiratory disorders or malignancy. The uterus and other abdominal structures are evaluated by an ultrasonogram, however, a computed tomography scan of abdomen and pelvis or intravenous pyelogram are indicated only in women with cervical or large uterine / extrauterine masses. A good bowel preparation would help gain exposure and (especially for laparoscopic approach) avoid bowel trauma caused by packing and retraction. However, antibiotic bowel preparation is not routinely indicated but should be done when concomitant intestinal involvement / surgery is a possibility.

There is good level of evidence to support use of prophylactic parenteral antibiotics like cefoxitin (2 mg intravenous), cefazolin (1-2 intravenously) or metronidazole (1gm intravenously). Although studies have shown no benefit of continuing antibiotics postoperatively, a second shot may be given if the procedure lasts more than 3 hours. Povidone - iodine douches and antibiotic scrubs do not provide any additional benefit when perioperative parenteral antibiotics have been used.

The operative site should not be shaved prior to surgery as it has been shown to increase risk of wound infection as a result of folliculitis. The pubic hair may be clipped rather than shaved for the same reason.

2. Total abdominal hysterectomy

The surgeon should, on the day of surgery, preferably see the patient and her immediate family members to reinforce emotional support and reassurance.

The woman is placed in supine position. After she is anaesthetized, a self retaining catheter is inserted in the urinary bladder. The abdomen is scrubbed with antiseptic solution from xiphisternum to the mid thighs and sterile drapes are applied.

Most uteri of upto 14-16 weeks gestational size can be removed by a low transverse / Pfannensteil incision. Large uteri and/or malignancies should be approached through an extendable midline vertical incision.The pelvic pathology is carefully evaluated followed by palpation of the abdominal organs. A Trendlenberg tilt can aid packing of intestines and omentum into upper abdomen.

2.1 Technique

After opening the abdomen and packing the gut into upper abdomen, self retaining retractors are placed. Two long straight clamps are applied on the left round ligament about 1 cm apart and close to the uterine attachment. The intervening tissue is divided and that in the lateral clamps ligated. This is followed by similarly doubly clamping, cutting and ligating the ovarian ligament. The procedure is repeated on the opposite side. If the ovaries need to be removed, the infundibulopelvic ligament should be doubly clamped, cut and transfixed bilaterally instead of the ovarian ligaments. This pedicle should be doubly ligated as troublesome bleeding from it is common. The peritoneum, from the round ligament pedicle is divided upto the refection of the uterovesical pouch (anterior leaf of broad ligament) on both sides and the urinary bladder is pushed down with the help of a small sponge held on ring forceps. If prominent, the central vesicouterine ligament and the lateral bladder pillars should be divided with scissors before attempting to push the bladder. The posterior leaf of broad ligament is then divided vertically from the ovarian ligament (or infundibulopelvic ligament in case of removal of ovaries) downwards and then over the posterior cervix. The fascia over the uterine vessels may be incised to expose the vessels clearly. The fundus of the uterus should be pulled upwards to keep it in anatomic position before clamping the uterine vessels. A pair of curved clamps are used to clamp these vessels at the level of internal os close to the uterus and at right angles to longitudinal axis of the uterus. This would minimize the risk of injury to the ureter which is around 1 cm deep and lateral to the uterine artery. At this point, the uterine artery crosses the ureter from lateral to medial side. The Macenrodt and uterosacral ligaments should then be doubly clamped, cut and ligated to free the cervix. The procedure is repeated on the opposite side. The anterior vagina is then opened by a stab incision which is extended all around with the help of scissors keeping close to the cervix to remove the uterus. Fig. 1 shows the opening of vaginal vault in a case of hysterectomy for large cervical myoma. The angles of the vagina should be held with the help of straight clamps or Allis forceps. At this step, a betadine soaked sterile roller gauze may be put in the vagina to prevent vaginal contents (secretions / antiseptic tablets or solutions) from coming into the operative field. The vaginal angles are secured and the vagina closed by interrupted or continuous sutures. Continuous catgut sutures have been reported to pucker the vault causing dyspareunia but the author has not had any such case after using continuous vaginal suturing for more than 15 years. It is no longer considered necessary to reperitonize the pelvis. However, in the author's opinion, reperitonization should be done at least in cases where the vaginal vault is left open (after passing an encircling continuous interlocking suture on the vaginal margins) to avoid prolapse of fallopian tube stump or bowel through it. In an attempt to provide anchorage to the vault and consequently to avoid subsequent vault prolapse, the round ligament and uterosacral pedicles may be tied to the vaginal angle sutures. The abdomen is then closed after ensuring complete haemostasis and completing the instrument and sponge / gauze counts.

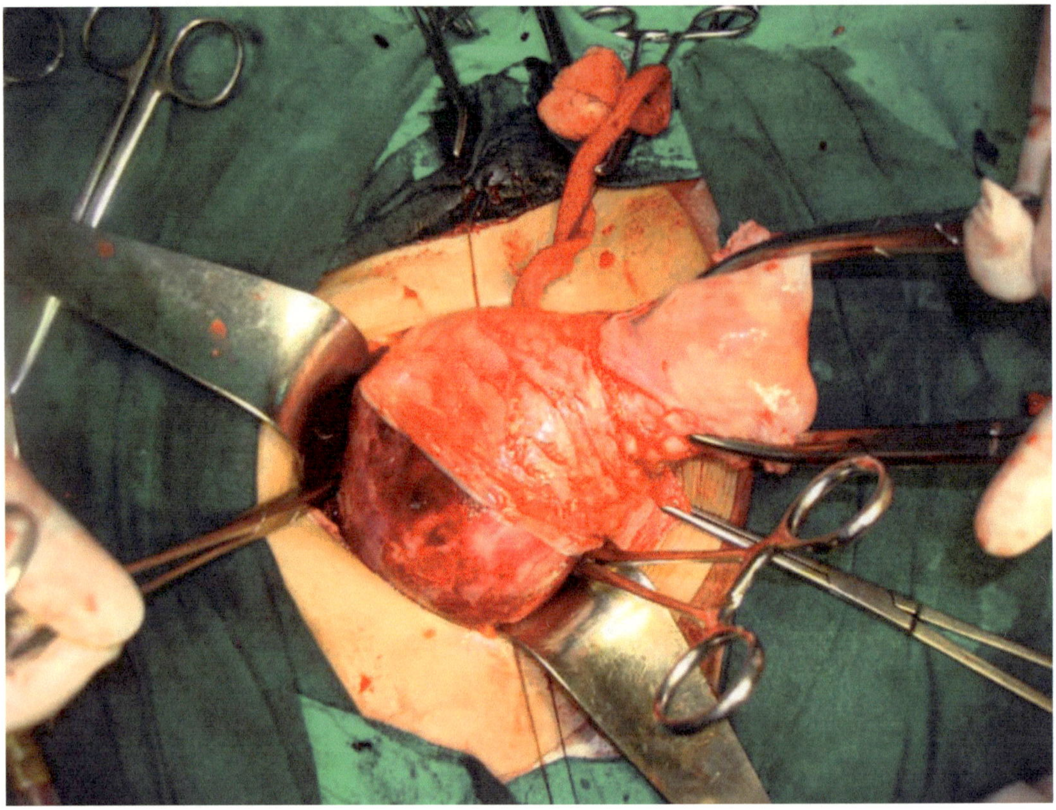

Fig. 1. Intraoperative picture showing a large cervical fibroid sitting atop a normal size body uterus at hysterectomy after opening the vagina.

2.2 Total versus subtotal hysterectomy

Total hysterectomy denotes the removal of body of uterus along with the cervix while subtotal procedure removes only the body of uterus. Subtotal hysterectomy is usually done in cases where removal of the cervix entails surgical difficulty due to dense adhesions and is a relatively quicker and technically easier procedure. Fig 2 is an intraoperative photograph of a total hysterectomy with bilateral salpingo-oophorectomy done for a clear cell carcinoma of the left ovary. Table 1 tabulates the differences between total and subtotal hysterectomy.

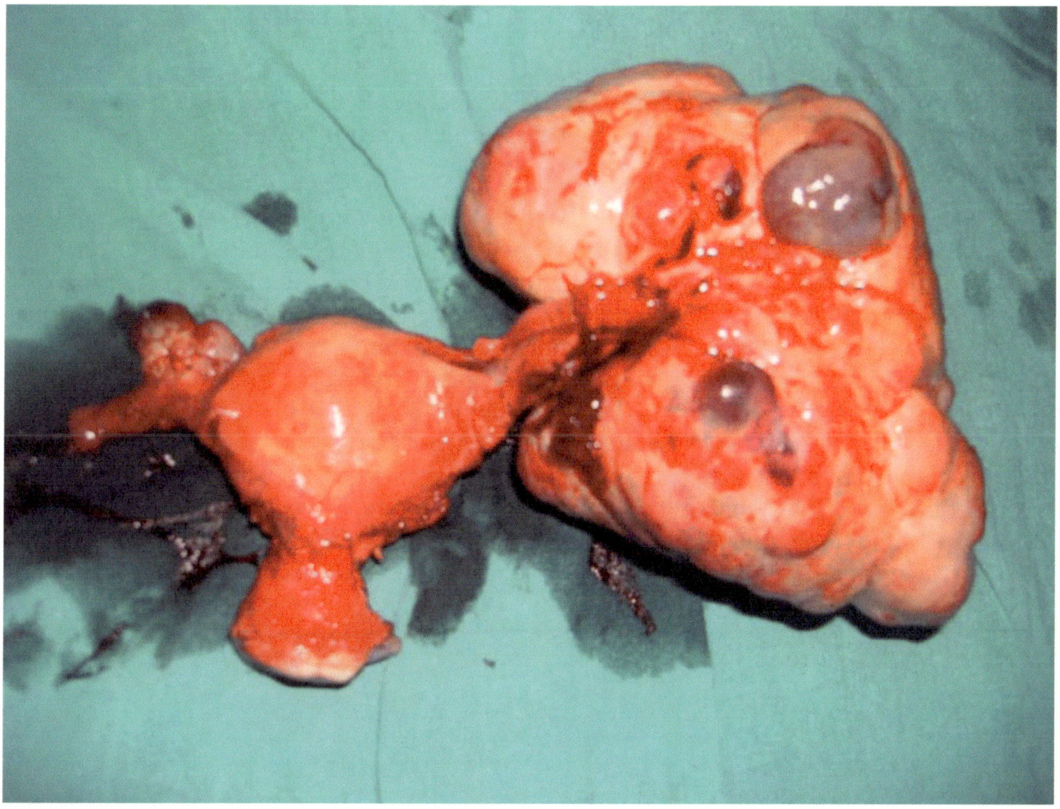

Fig. 2. A total hysterectomy specimen along with both tubes and ovaries for a left sided malignant ovarian tumor which later turned out to be a clear cell carcinoma.

Subtotal / supracervical hysterectomy	Total hysterectomy
1. Presence of cervix retains the uterine supports attached to it. Hence, vault prolapse is less common.	1. Division of Macenrodt's and uteroscral ligaments may predispose to vault prolapse
2. Easier and less morbid to urinary tract specially in the presence of dense endometriosis or chronic inflammation	2. Removal of cervix requires the urinary bladder to be well mobilized out of the field.
3. Coital function may be better retained in the presence of cervical secretions and roomy vagina.	3. Presence of sutures / chronic granulations may hamper coital function.
4. Requires comparatively less skill / experience on part of the surgeon	4. A skilled / experienced surgeon should be available.
5. Cancer of residual cervix occurs in 0.3% of all subtotal hysterectmies. Hence, cervical screening should be continued.	5. Cervical exfoliative cytology for cancer screening is no longer required.
6.Chronic cervicitis causing deep dyspareunia may persist in cervical stump.	6. No persistence of cervicitis or its sequelae.

Table 1. Comparison of total and subtotal hysterectomy

2.3 Special cases

1. Severe endometriosis : Extensive adhesion formation in this condition may prevent easy access to the uterus. The anterior wall of sigmoid colon is often adherent to the peritoneum on the posterior surface of the vagina and uterus and it must be mobilized before dividing the uterosacral ligament.

2. Cervical fibroids: The normal sized body of the uterus is commonly perched atop a large cervical myoma which is jammed inside the pelvis. These large fibroids tend to push the ureters high upwards so that they pass over the upper and lateral surface of the myoma. In these cases, the uterine vessels should be divided as high as possible, i.e. at the upper surface of the tumor and then drawn laterally by dissection from over the tumor surface. The ureters should then be identified at the upper and lateral tumor surface before proceeding to divide the peritoneum on the posterior surface of the tumor. Fig 3 shows a total hysterectomy specimen with a large cervical fibroid. Some surgeons prefer to carry out a myomectomy first (by a vertical central incision on the myoma capsule) and then proceed with hysterectomy. This debulking of the mass may also be achieved by sagittal hemisection of the small uterine body and shelling out of the cervical myoma. Removal of the myoma allows greater accessibility and eases the subsequent completion of hysterectomy.

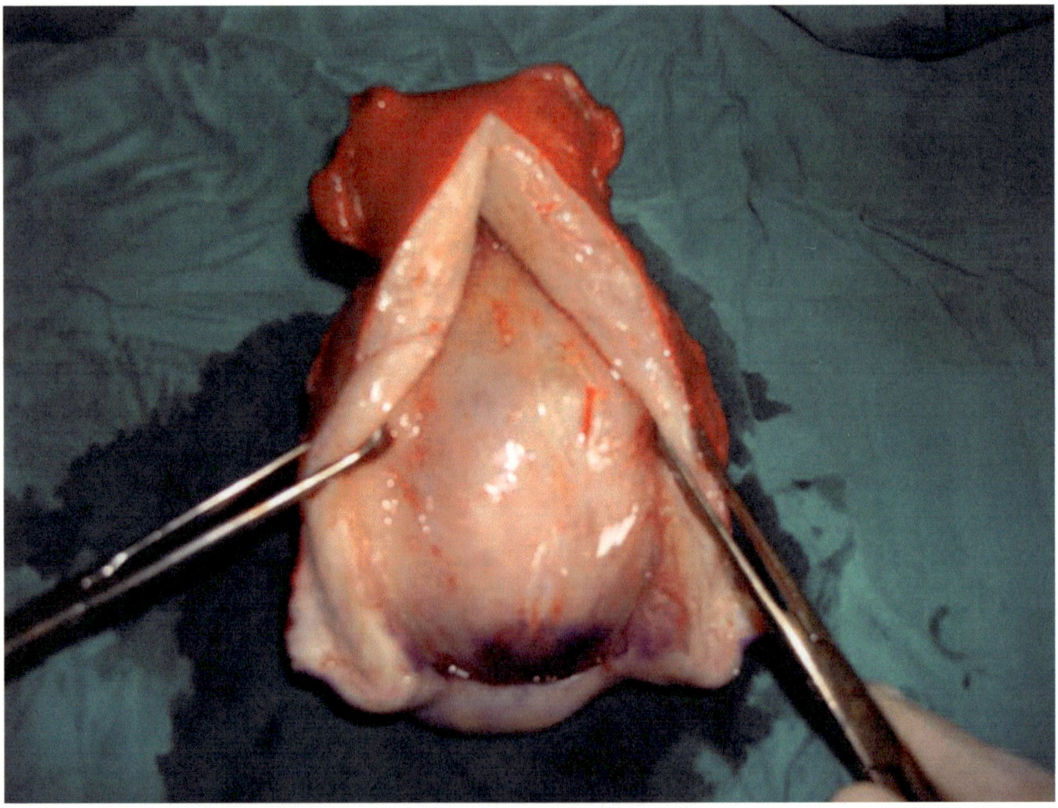

Fig. 3. A total hysterectomy specimen removed on account of a large cervical myoma causing urinary retention.

3. Isthmic fibroids

Fibroids arising from this region may present perplexing moments to the surgeon on the operating table and Fig 4 shows a large myoma arising from the anterior isthmus that had both intra abdominal and vaginal (coloured blue by methylene blue) extensions. Performance of hysterectomy in such a case would pose difficulty in assessing the anatomy of the pelvis and applying the lower clamps. Removal of myoma before proceeding with hysterectomy may be of immense help in such cases.

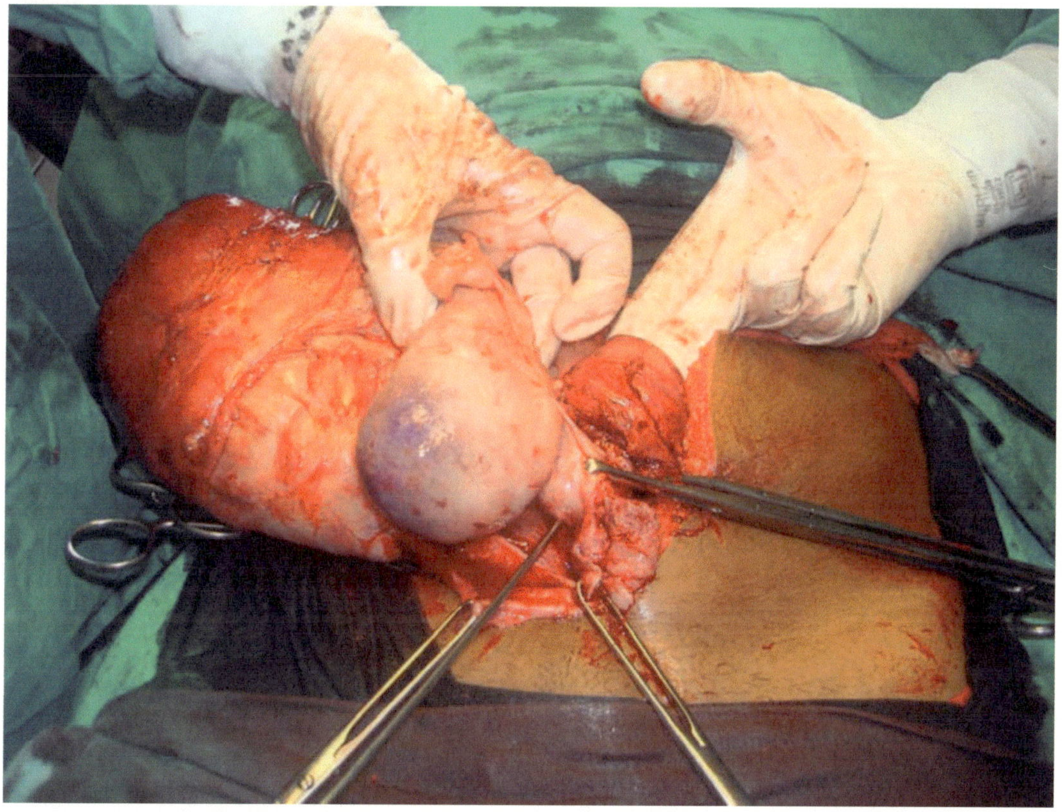

Fig. 4. An intraoperative picture of a large anterior isthmic myoma having a larger abdominal and a smaller vaginal extention.

4. Uterosacral tumors

Tumors (commonly myomas) arising from/near the uterosacral ligaments also predispose to ureteric injury if caution is not exercised. Fig 5 shows a hysterectomy in progress for a large myoma arising from one of the uterosacral ligaments.

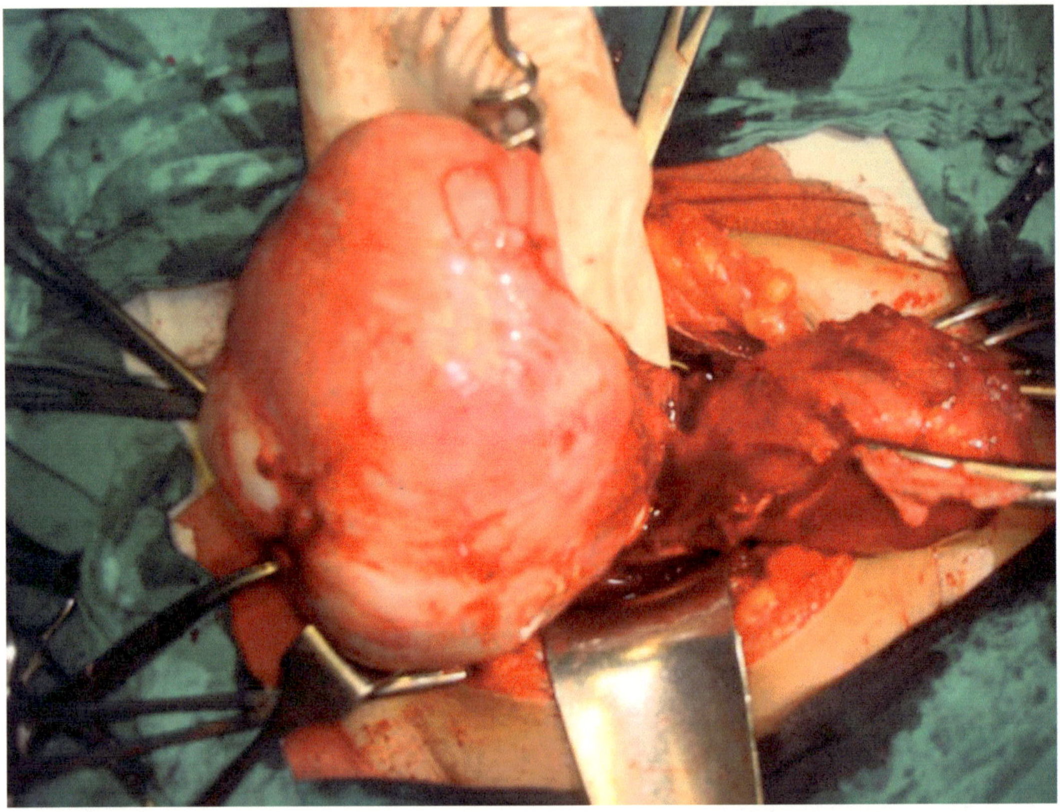

Fig. 5. Clinical operative photograph of abdominal hysterectomy for a large myoma arising from the right sided uterosacral ligament.

5. Broad ligament fibroids

Large broad ligaments fibroids may get impacted in the pelvis and may also distort the ureteric anatomy, depending on their site of origin (true or false broad ligament fibroids). It is important to identify the ureters tracing them from the pelvic origin downwards before clamping the uterine vessels in these cases.The ureter is usually medial to a true broad ligament myoma while it is lateral and superior to a false one. Fig 6 represents an intraoperative picture of a true broad ligament myoma in the process of being enucleated.

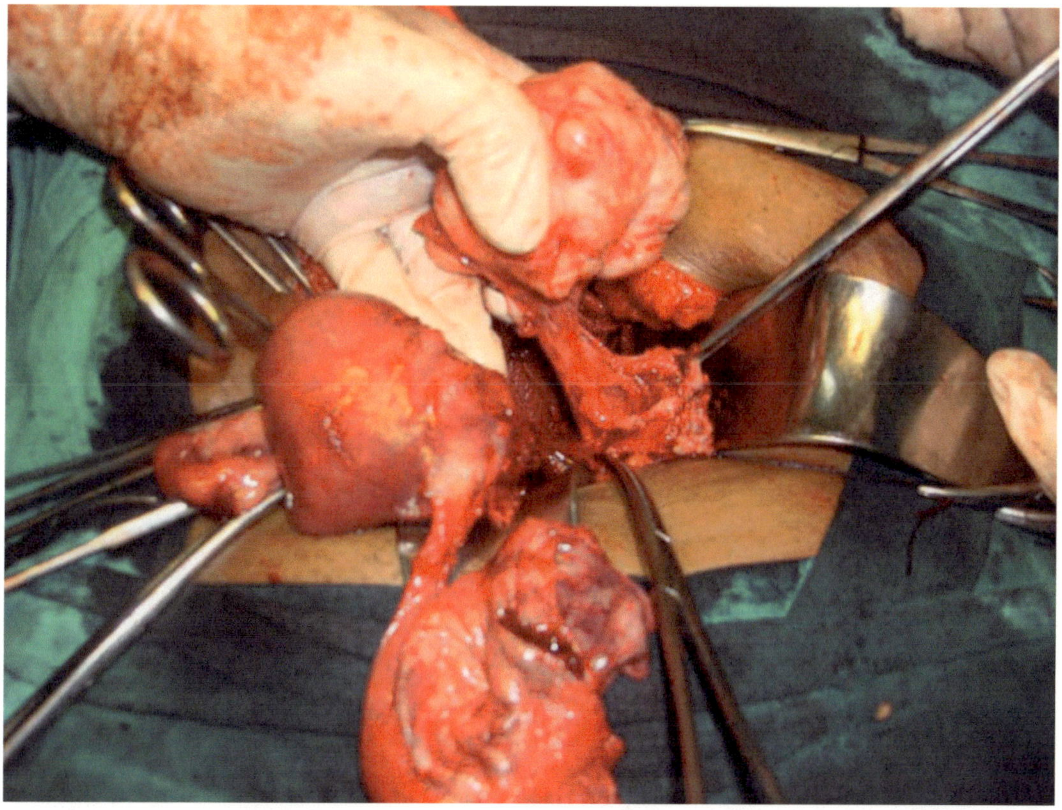

Fig. 6. Operative picture of enucleation of a true broad ligament myoma.

6. Pelvic inflammatory disease

Often the fallopian tube forms a hydrosalpinx and dense adhesions may bury the tube and ovary into the pouch of Douglas or bind it to posterior uterine surface. These must be mobilized before proceeding with hysterectomy. Adhesions between the sigmoid colon and posterior surface of uterus must also be divided. In cases of dense adnexal adhesions, conservation of ovaries may be more difficult than adnexal removal as the infundibulopelvic ligament is usually free of firm adhesions. In case of difficulty, sharp dissection and division of tuboovarian pedicle between two clamps is of help.

7. Anomalous uteri

Unilateral absence of the broad ligament in case of unicornuate uterus may make the development of retroperitoneal space impossible and the cervix may need to be cored by sharp dissection. A urorectal septum present between the two bodies of a didelphic uterus may need to be divided cautiously before proceeding further. Fig 7 shows a didelphic uterus with right horn enlarged by a myoma and the relatively smaller but hyperplastic left horn.

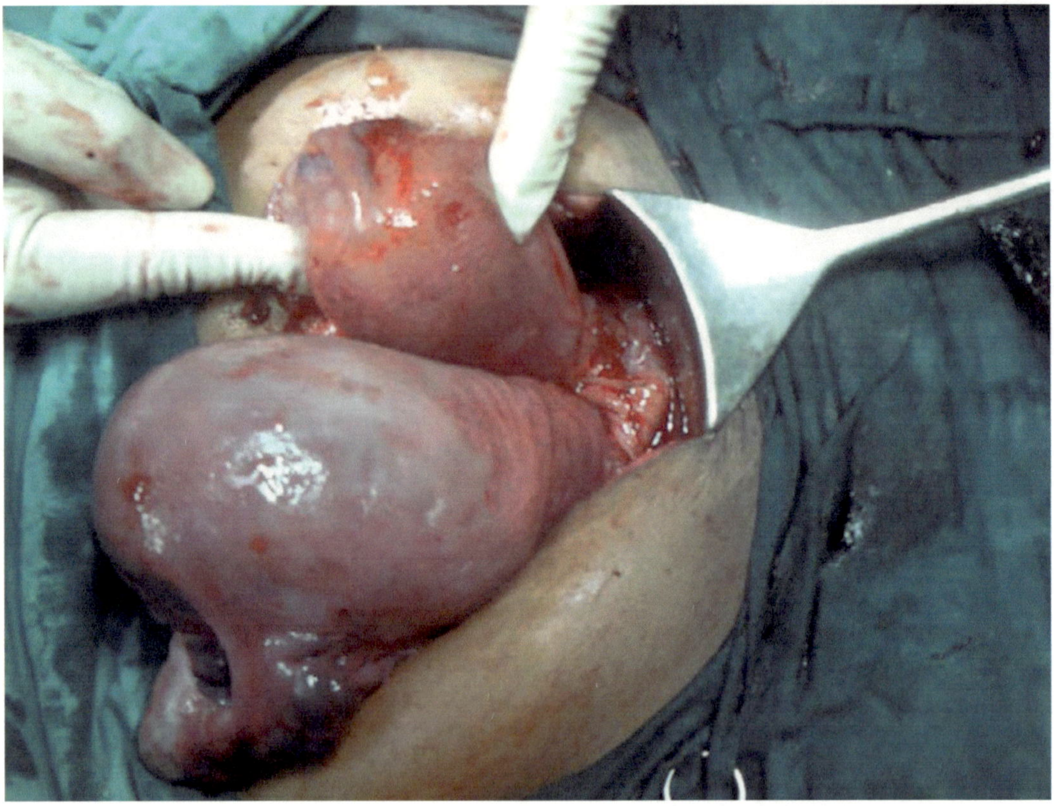

Fig. 7. Operative photograph of a didelphic uterus. The right horn is enlarged and congested as a result of a myoma while the left horn is relatively smaller.

8. Malignancy

Presence of uterine malignancy makes the uterus very soft, congested and friable. This could cause difficulty in application of clamps and passing/tying ligatures and these could easily cut through tissues and cause hemorrhage. Also the urinary tract is at greater risk of damage in such cases. Fig 8 shows a large leiomyosarcoma arising from the uterine body as seen at hysterectomy. A gentle handling of tissues, availability of blood and a multidisciplinary approach would be beneficial in such cases.

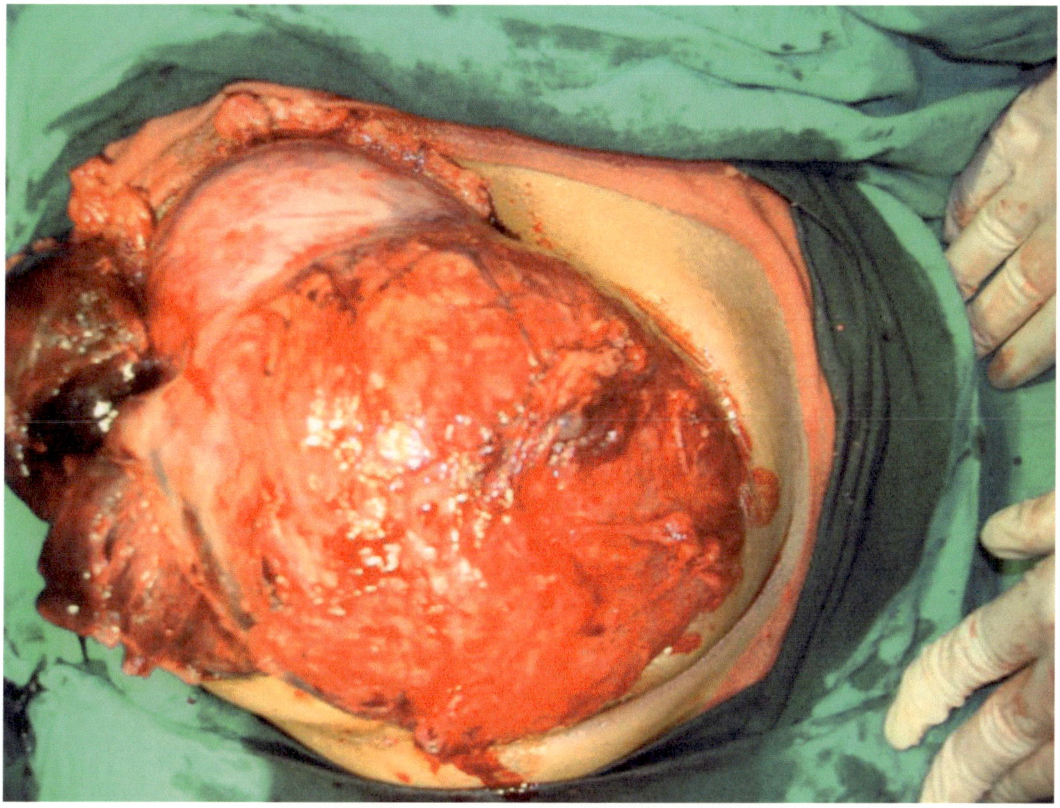

Fig. 8. A leiomyosarcomatous uterus at hysterectomy.

9. Complications of abdominal hysterectomy

9.1 Damage to the urinary tract

The urinary bladder may get damaged while pushing or dissecting it from over the cervix, particularly in cases of previous lower uterine surgery (Cesarean section commonly) or anterior myomectomy. The ureter may be injured near the infundibulopelvic ligament, near the uterine vessels or the anterior cervix. No pedicle should ever be clamped before defining both the ureters.

9.1.2 Injury to blood vessels

Ovarian or anastomotic vessels may be injured. All main vascular pedicles should be doubly secured to prevent slippage of ligatures..

9.1.3 Injury to bowel

Adherent bowel may be injured at dissection or clamping. For this, sharp dissection is usually better than blunt dissection. Use of electrocautery near adherent bowel may be avoided.

9.1.4 Infection of the wound, urinary tract, pneumonitis or thrombophlebitis

Infection of the wound, urinary tract or bronchopulmonary region usually responds to appropriate antibiotic therapy. Women at risk of thrombosis should be given thromboprophylaxis in the perioperative period in the form of heparin, apart from non-pharmacological measures like early ambulation, adequate hydration and stockings.

9.1.5 Psychological impact

Some women may develop depression after a hysterectomy procedure especially in the face of inadequate preoperative counseling.

9.2 Management of ovaries at the time of hysterectomy

Ovarian conservation should be discussed during preoperative counseling and patients wishes respected. Normal ovaries should not be removed if hysterectomy is being done for benign uterine disease irrespective of age. Rather, the only indications of concomitant bilateral oophorectomy in recent times are genital malignancies, extensive/ recurrent severe endometriosis, certain cases of breast carcinoma and women with familial predisposition to ovarian cancer. When ovarian removal is planned, the role of hormone replacement therapy must be discussed with the woman preoperatively.

10. Vaginal hysterectomy

A hysterectomy carried out by the vaginal route offers the advantages of fewer complications, shorter hospital stays and faster return to normal activities. Despite this, the abdominal approach continues to dominate the incidence charts world-over. The skill and experience of the surgeon plays a pivotal role in determining the approach route. The vaginal procedure has conventionally been done for women with uterine or pelvic prolapse. However, successful vaginal hysterectomies are being performed now in the absence of uterovaginal descent (called non descent vaginal hysterectomy - NDVH), often helped by uterine debulking techniques like coring, morcellation or bivalving. Laparoscopy is a useful aid for lymphadenectomy in cases of cervical or endometrial cancer, evaluating adnexal masses or endometriosis and aiding vaginal hysterectomy.

10.1 Preoperative preparation

The preoperative preparation continues to be the same as for the abdominal procedure with a few reinforcements. Bowel cleansing is very important for vaginal hysterectomy in order to evacuate solid stool from rectum, reduce the bacterial load of intestinal tract and to reduce the incidence of postoperative ileus and constipation. Prophylactic parenteral antibiotics, usually a cephalosporin, is administered an hour prior to the procedure after a test dose. Metronidazole is usually added in the postoperative period to take care of anaerobes. Betadine solution is used to clean the genitalia and vagina and alcohol based solutions should be avoided in the vagina. Sterile drapes are applied after positioning the patient.

10.2 Position

The patient, after anaesthesia administration is placed in lithotomy position, taking care to avoid neurovascular compression by the stirrups / leg holders. The buttocks should be brought to the edge of the table which is in zero horizontal position. The height of the stool / operating chair of the surgeon should bring the patient's pelvis at the level of the surgeon's eyes. The two assistants should stand within the stirrups, one on either side.

10.3 Technique

Two lateral sutures may be applied, one on either side, to retract the labia but are usually not essential in cases of prolapse.

The cervix is held with Valsellum forceps and the vagina is infiltrated with saline adrenaline solution (in strength of 1:200,000 to 1:400,000).

An inverted T-shaped incision is made on the anterior vaginal wall after holding the Fothergill's points on either side with Allis forceps. The horizontal limb of the T is placed at the cervicovaginal junction and the vertical limb extends from it to the level of neck of urinary bladder which may be made prominent by the bulb of a Foley's catheter placed in the bladder. The vaginal flaps are dissected on either side from urinary bladder keeping the fascia with the bladder. To free the bladder from the underlying cervix, the vesicocervical ligament is cut with scissors and the bladder is retracted with Landon's retractor to expose the uterovesical peritoneum which is incised transversely to expose the anterior uterine surface.

The cervix is now pulled forwards to expose the posterior vaginal wall. An inverted V-shaped incision is placed on the vaginal wall and peritoneum of Pouch of Douglas exposed and snipped to bring into view the posterior uterine wall.

The Macenrodt's and uterosacral ligaments are clamped between two long straight clamps, cut and ligated followed by the uterine vessels. It is important to remain close to the lateral uterine wall while applying the clamps. The uterine vessels should be doubly ligated bilaterally after cutting in between the clamps. The uppermost pedicle consisting of fallopian tube, ovarian and round ligaments is usually clamped with long curved clamps, cut and ligated. Each suture except that of uterine vessels should be transfixed. Before applying the upper most clamp, the fundus of the uterus should be delivered out usually through the pouch of douglas and the clamps applied under vision to avoid including omentum / gut loop in the tip of the clamp. Alternatively, the uterovesical pouch can also be used to deliver out the uterine fundus. The uterus is taken out along with the clamps. The anterior and posterior peritoneum may now closed with a continuous 00 chronic catgut suture, keeping the pedicles extraperitoneal. This would minimize chances of blood from any of the pedicles gaining entry into the pelvic cavity and would be revealed vaginally.

If an enterocele is present, the peritoneal sac of the enterocele may be excised and the posterior peritoneum closed as high as possible, preferably upto the level of yellow fat. This can be combined with a McCall culdoplasty which entails suturing of the uterosacral ligaments in the midline to obliterate the hiatus for enterocele.

The dissected anterior vaginal wall flaps may be excised. If a significant cystocele is present it may be repaired by passing multiple transverse polyglycolic acid (No. 2-0 or 3-0) sutures from the inner aspect of one vaginal flap to the other, including the fascia underneath the bladder (pubovesical fascia pillars). These are tied after all have been passed to support the bladder base with this fascia.

Alternatively, a purse string suture may be used to plicate this area, specially if cystocele is of minor degree. The vaginal incision is then closed vertically with interrupted or continuous chromic catgut sutures. A sterile betadine soaked gauze is used to pack the vagina for 24 hours. The self retaining catheter is left in place for 24-48 hours.

In the presence of a rectocele, the procedure may be combined with a posterior colpoperineorrhaphy.

10.4 Non Descent Vaginal Hysterectomy (NDVH)

The procedure is basically similar to that done for prolapsed uterus. However, in the absence of descent, the cervix and the pedicles tend to remain inside the vagina. Traction exposure plays an important role. Division of the lower ligaments (Macenrodt's and uterosacrals) provides the much needed mobility and the cervix is circumscribed at the cervicovaginal function followed by division of the vesicocervical ligament to expose the vesicocervical space. Fig 9 shows the descent of the cervix achieved after division of Macenrodt and uterosacral ligaments in a uterus with no preexisting descent. In the event of

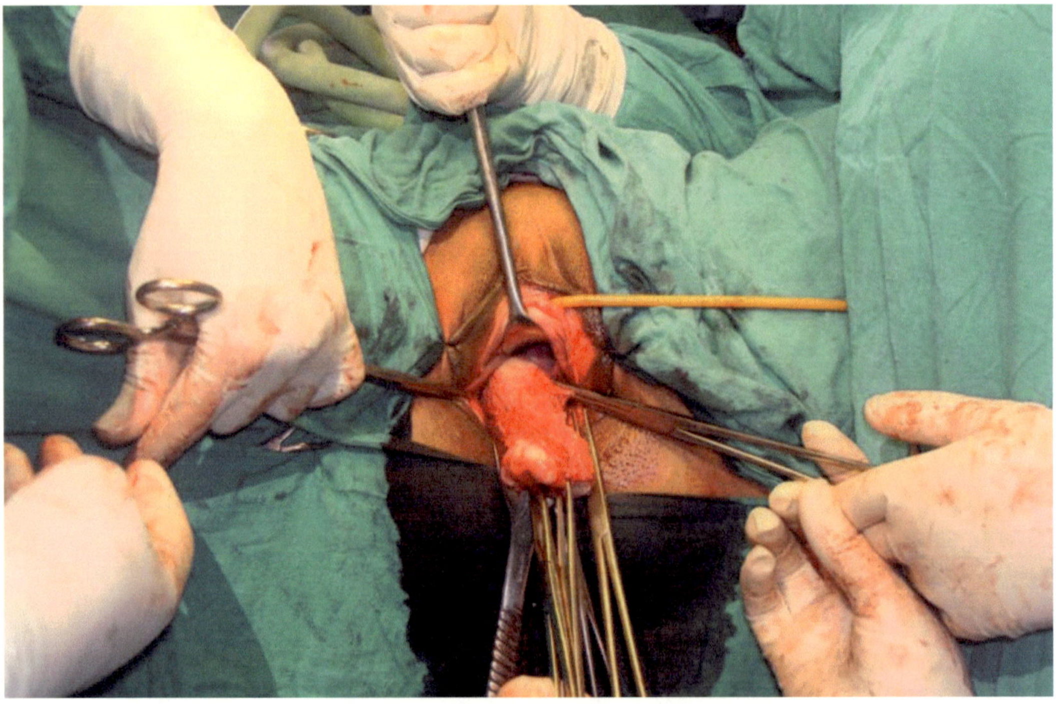

Fig. 9. A nondescent vaginal hysterectomy in progress. The lower pedicles have been clamped, cut and ligated to provide some mobility to the otherwise undescended uterus.

difficult in opening the uterovesical peritoneum, the pouch of Douglas may be opened early which helps in securing the uterosacral ligaments. This is followed by clamping, cutting and transfixing the Macenrodt's ligament on both sides. Some surgeons prefer to use an aneurysm needle to ligate the Macenrodt and uterine vessels. Removal of the cervix and lower uterus helps to facilitate grasp and traction on the remaining uterus but this may not be required in all cases. Fig 10 shows the excision of cervix and lower part of uterine body before proceeding with remaining hysterectomy. Delivery of the fundus of uterus is usually easier through the pouch of Douglas than through the uterovesical pouch as more space is available in the sacral curve. However, normal sized uterine fundi may be delivered by the anterior route without much difficulty. Fig 11 shows the delivery of enlarged uterine body during NDVH. The pedicles are then exteriorized and the peritoneum closed followed by transverse closure of the vaginal incision. The sutures of the Macenrodt and uterosacral pedicles may be brought out through the vaginal edge and tied at the end of the procedure, in order to suspend the vaginal vault.

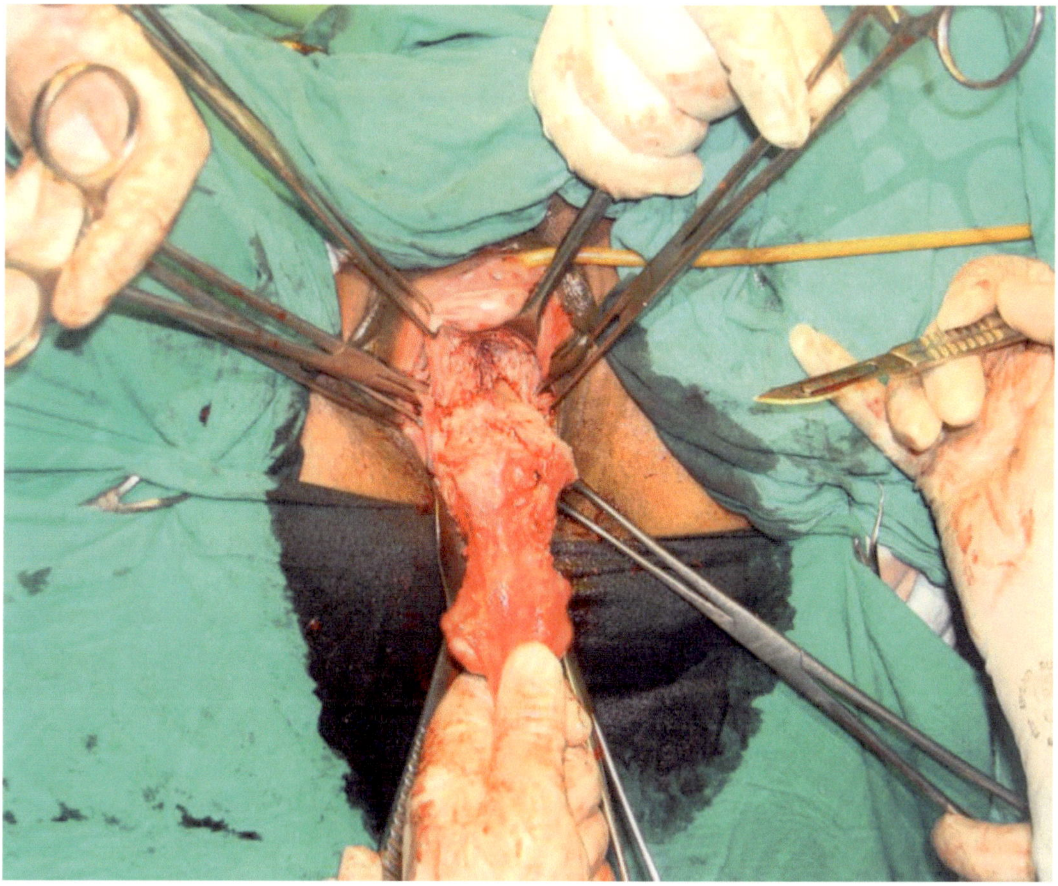

Fig. 10. Excision of the cervix in progress at NDVH to facilitate grasp on the body uterus.

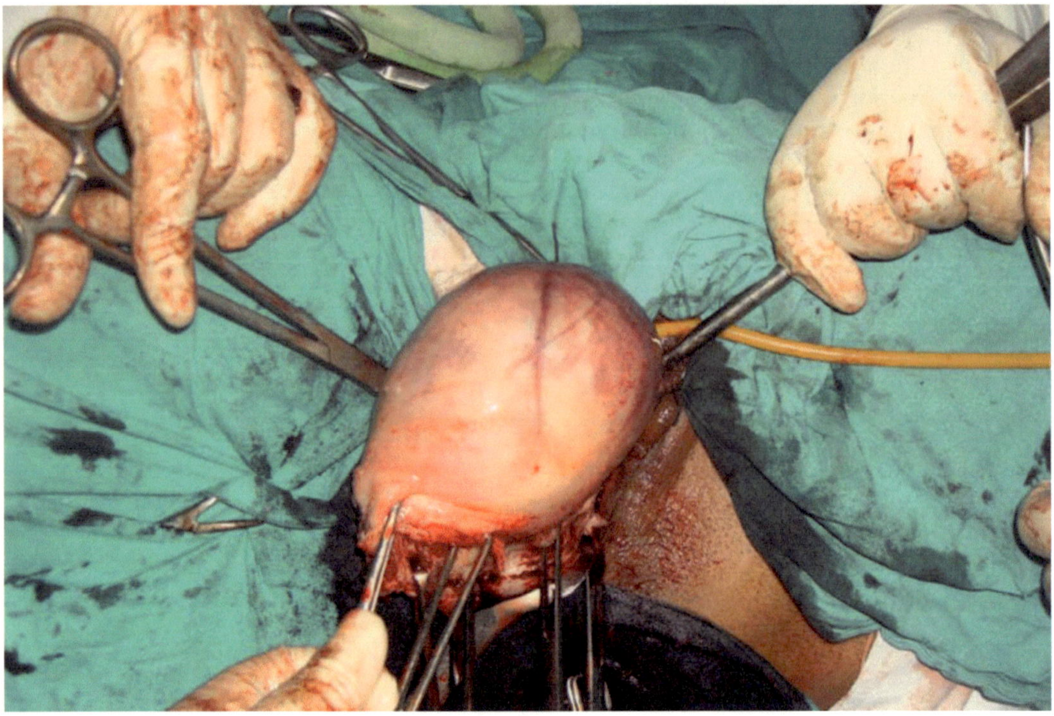

Fig. 11. Operative picture showing delivery of enlarged uterine body at NDVH.

10.5 Vaginal oophorectomy

Fear of restricted access to the ovaries and inadequate visibility of the adnexa at vaginal hysterectomy are responsible for avoidance of concomitant oophorectomy. Baden and Walker designed a classification for grading the degrees of ovarian descent after vaginal hysterectomy . Any ovary that is grade I or higher by this classification should be visible and accessible for transvaginal removal. Moreover, the use of laparoscope to perform an oophorectomy before a vaginal hysterectomy has been regarded as safe and easy.

11. Laparoscopic hysterectomy

Laparoscopy has been used to carry out Laparoscopic Assisted Vaginal Hysterectomy (LAVH), laparoscopic subtotal hysterectomy (LSH), total laparoscopic hysterectomy (TLH) and vaginally assisted laparoscopic hysterectomy (VALH). Raoul Palmer of France is credited with introducing operative laparocopy to gynecological practice in late 1950s. Reich et al published the first case of LAVH in 1989 and use of laparoscopy for hysterectomy has been rapidly growing since then.

11.1 Technique of LAVH

The patient, after administration of general anaesthesia, is placed in low lithotomy position. A bimanual vaginal examination is done to evaluate pelvic and vaginal dimensions and to assess the feasibility of removal of the uterus by this route. An intertuberous diameter of 9 cm or more, an obtuse pubic angle and a vaginal apex wider than 2 finger breadths is considered adequate for the procedure. A foleys's catheter is placed in the urinary bladder and the cervix is held with a Valsellum. An intrauterine manipulator is introduced to facilitate manipulation during the procedure. The laparoscope is inserted through an umbilical incision after creation of pneumoperitoneum (in lower lateral quadrants) with carbon dioxide. Two accessory ports (5 mm diameter) are used to insert operative instruments. A third accessory trocar may be placed on the primary surgeon's side 6 cm or more above the lower accessory trocar, to facilitate the surgeon to operate from one side.

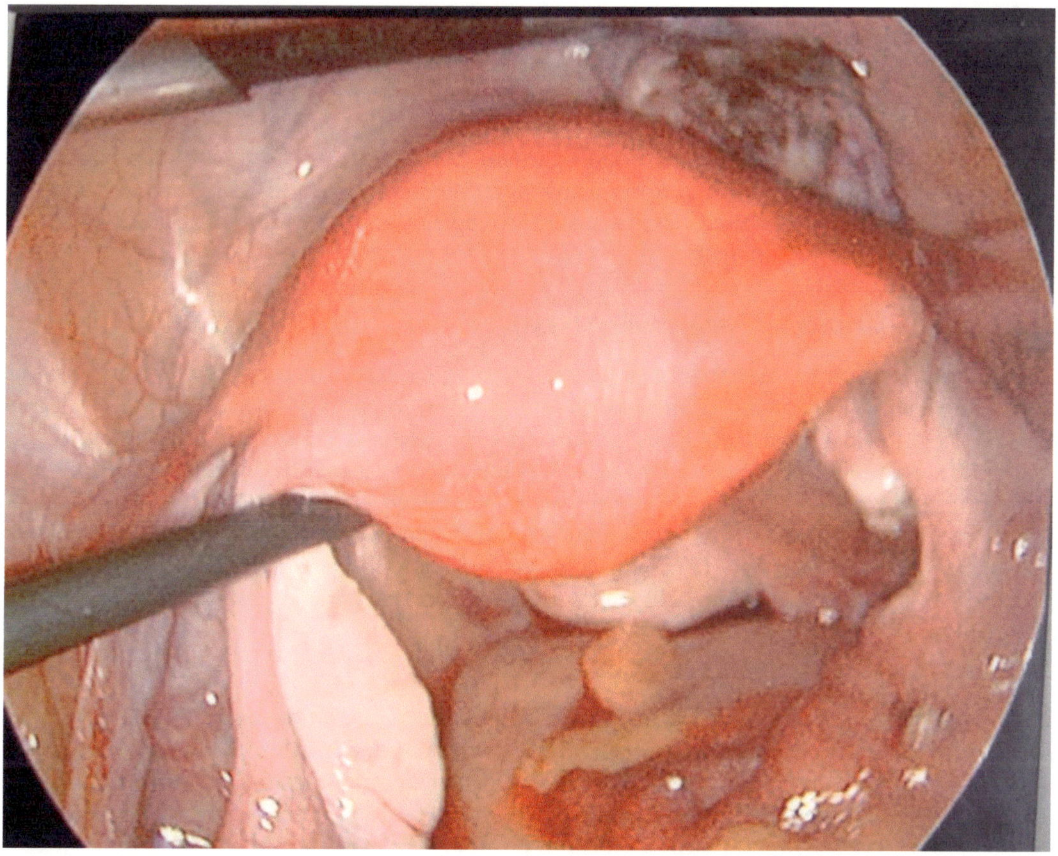

Fig. 12. Laparoscopic evaluation of pelvic organs at laparoscopic hysterectomy.

Fig12 shows the evaluation of uterus, adnexae and other pelvic structures at initiation of a laparoscopic hysterectomy. The uterine ligaments and vascular pedicles can be coagulated and cut by using bipolar electro coagulation (e.g. Valley lab Ligasure), ultrasonic energy (Ethicon Harmonic Scalpet) or mechanical energy (using stapler - cutter devices like Ethicon Endopath ETS). The uterus is deviated to one side with uterine manipulator and round ligament followed by tubo ovarian (or infundibulopelvic ligament in cases of ovarian removal) pedicle is coagulated and cut on both sides. The peritoneum of anterior broad ligament is cut infero-medially to meet the opposite side at bladder reflection. The retroperitoneal space is also opened to allow identification of both ureters, the left sided is visible less easily than the right due to presence of sigmoid colon on the left side. At this point, the laparoscopic procedure is completed and the remaining surgery (including ligation of the uterine vessels) is done vaginally in the same manner as for a standard vaginal hysterectomy. There is loss of pneumoperitoneum once the vagina is opened and the laparoscope can be used to check for haemostasis after closure of the vaginal vault. The procedure is completed with removal of all laparoscopic instruments.

11.2 Vaginally assisted laparoscopic hysterectomy

In this method, the uterine vessels are also coagulated and cut laparoscopically. This requires adequate mobilization of the bladder and filling it with 100 to 200ml saline could aid in the identification of the bladder extent. Uterine vessels are skeletonised by opening the anterior and posterior leaves of broad ligament, before they are coagulated and cut close to the uterus. Colpotomy is then done transvaginally followed by ligating and cutting the uterosacral ligaments to deliver the uterus. The vaginal and abdominal incisions are then closed after removing all instruments.

11.3 Total Laparoscopic Hysterectomy (TLH)

This is an extension of the laparoscopic technique to include the colpotomy incisions after adequate mobilization of the urinary bladder. Anterior colpotomy incision is usually made first as the anteversion of the uterus required for posterior colpotomy incision would help maintain the pneumo-peritoneum by occluding the anterior incision. Various colpotomy and vaginal occluding devices are available which may be used along with uterine manipulators (KOH colpotonizer system has a vaginal extender and a vaginal balloon for occlusion, McCartney tube). However, TLH can also be performed using simple and inexpensive instruments like laparoscopic tenaculum, uterine manipulator and Deaver's retractor.

11.4 Laparoscopic Subtotal Hysterectomy (LSH)

The procedure of LSH is similar to that VALH till the level of uterine arteries. After these are secured, the body of uterus is amputated from the cervix at the isthmus level. It is better to dissect the urinary bladder from the cervix to ensure adequate occlusion of uterine vessels and amputation at the level of isthmus. Removal of the body of uterus after amputation may be effected by a posterior colpotomy incision, an extension of the umbilical incision or use of electromagnetic morcellator.

11.5 Postoperative care

1. For open abdominal procedures, the patient is kept on parenteral fluids for 24 hours, following which a light diet is started and this is replaced by normal solid/ semisolid

diet after another 24 hours. Women who have undergone laparoscopic procedures are started on normal diet on the day of surgery itself.

2. Early ambulation is encouraged.
3. Self retaining urinary catheter is usually left in situ for 24 hours after open surgery but is not essential. Continuous bladder drainage is not required in post operative period after laparoscopic procedures.
4. Change of antiseptic abdominal dressing may be done after 5 to 6 days. If unabsorbable sutures have been placed in the skin, they are removed after a week of surgery.
5. If the wound gets infected, antibiotics are started, depending on the culture report.
6. Full physical activity is actually resumed by the end of 10-14 days post operatively.
7. Coital abstinence is advised for 6 weeks.

11.6 Complications of hysterectomy

1. Intraoperative: Anaesthetic (cardiorespiratory) and surgical problems like hemorrhage, injuries to surrounding viscera are avoided by appropriate preoperative evaluation and ensuring senior and multidisciplinary help.
2. Rarely, postoperative ileus and destruction.
3. Urinary tract infection.
4. Bleeding per vaginum may occur after a week of surgery due to the vaginal sutures falling off or infection.
5. Wound infection and inflammation.
6. Venous thromboembolism: Early ambulation, adequate hydration and leg stockings are some of the non pharmacological measures that help prevent thromboembolism.

12. References

[1] Jones III JA. Abdominal hysterectomy. In: Rock JA, Jones III JA (eds). Te Linde's Operative Gynecology 10th ed. Philadelphia: Lippincott Williams and Wilkins; 2003. p. 727-743.

[2] Kovac SR. Vaginal hysterectomy. In: Rock JA, Jones III JA (eds). Te Linde's Operative Gynecology 10th ed. Philadelphia: Lippincott Williams and Wilkins; 2003. p. 744-762.

[3] Howard FM. Laparoscopic hysterectomy. In: Rock JA, Jones III JA (eds). Te Linde's Operative Gynecology 10th ed. Philadelphia: Lippincott Williams and Wilkins; 2003. p. 763-773.

[4] Duhan N, Rajotia N, Duhan U, Sangwan N, Gulati N, Sirohiwal D. Isthmic Uterine Fibroids. The dynamics of growth. Arch Gynecol. Obstet. 2009;280:309-312

[5] Farquhar CM, Sterne' s CA. Hysterectomy rates in the United States 1990-1997, Obstet Gynecol 2002; 99: 229-234.

[6] American College of Obstetricians and Gynecologists. ACOG Practice Bulletin No. 74. Antibiotic prophylaxis for gynecologic procedures. Washington, DC: ACOG; 2006.

[7] Storm HH, Clemmenson IH, Manders T, Brinton LA. Supravaginal uterine amputation in Denmark 1978-1988 and risk of cancer. Gynecol Oncol 1992; 45: 198-201.

[8] Hudson CN, Settchell ME. Hysterectomy . In: Hudson CN, Setchell ME, Howkin's J (ed). Shaw's Textbook of Operative Gynaecology. 6th ed. New Delhi: Elsevier; 2001. p. 115-140.

2

Subtotal Versus Total Abdominal Hysterectomy for Benign Gynecological Conditions

Zouhair Amarin
Jordan University of Science and Technology, Jordan

1. Introduction

Abdominal hysterectomy is the most commonly performed major gynecologic operation for women (1). It is considered a safe procedure with a low mortality rate for benign indications (2). In addition, it is associated with higher rates of patient satisfaction than other treatments for dysfunctional uterine bleeding (3). However, operative morbidity can be high since hysterectomy disrupts the local nerve supply and anatomical relationships (4).

Until the late 1930s, the standard type of abdominal hysterectomy was subtotal, but this was gradually replaced by total abdominal hysterectomy, although the subtotal approach still remained popular (5). In the last few years there has been a major shift to less invasive means of treating benign gynaecological disorders. Total abdominal hysterectomy involves removing the body of the uterus and the cervix, whereas subtotal abdominal hysterectomy conserves the cervix. Although sometimes the indication for the operation necessitates removal of the cervix, the commonest conditions, menstrual disorders and fibroids, do not involve the cervix.

In the United Kingdom, according to the Department of Health and Social Security in 1985, 18600 hysterectomies were performed for menstrual disorders (6). In the series of Vessey et al. of 1992, 38.5% and 35.5% respectively were for fibroids and menstrual disorders, while 6.5% were for malignant disease. In this Oxford Family Planning Association study of 1985 hysterectomies, 87.2% were by the abdominal route, and only 0.7% were subtotal hysterectomies (7). The proportion of subtotal hysterectomies for benign diseases of the female genital organs in the USA in 1997–2005 was around 6% (8), much lower than that of 22% in Denmark in 1998 (9). Stang et al. reported that around 4% of the 305 015 hysterectomies carried out in Germany in the period 2005-2006 were subtotal abdominal procedures (10).

With the advent of laparoscopic hysterectomy, the popularity of laparoscopic subtotal hysterectomy started to rise during the 1990s as a new modality of treatment for abnormal uterine bleeding, with an increase in the overall number of subtotal hysterectomy procedures (5). However, there is a lack of well-designed randomized, controlled trials that compare laparoscopic subtotal hysterectomy with total abdominal hysterectomy, with attention to short- and long-term morbidity.

In a multi-centre retrospective cohort analysis to evaluate the peri- and postoperative outcomes in women undergoing laparoscopic subtotal hysterectomy versus laparoscopic total hysterectomy, the overall number of short-term and long-term complications was comparable for both procedures. Laparoscopic subtotal hysterectomy as compared with laparoscopic total hysterectomy and laparoscopically assisted vaginal hysterectomy was associated with more long-term postoperative complications, whereas laparoscopic total hysterectomy was associated with more short-term complications (11). The relatively large sample size may partially compensate for the major limitation of the retrospective nature of the design of this study.

Rate estimates of conversion from laparoscopic to open abdominal hysterectomy are sparse. Published conversion rates vary considerably and may depend on patient-related factors such as uterine size, pelvic and bowel adhesions, physician-related factors such as surgeons' competence, and intra-operative events such as viscous injuries and extensive bleeding (12-16). In a study from Germany the rates of conversion were highest for neoplastic disorders. The crude rates of conversion from laparoscopic to open abdominal hysterectomy for benign conditions were 10.5% (17).

Excising the uterine cervix at total abdominal hysterectomy is anatomically the most disruptive part of the operation. Subtotal abdominal hysterectomy requires less mobilization of the bladder and minimizes the risk of injury to the ureters. Subtotal hysterectomy is also associated with less anatomical disruption, and perhaps, it is associated with less adverse effects than total hysterectomy.

As residual amounts of endometrial tissue could result in vaginal bleeding after subtotal abdominal hysterectomy, the author routinely performs "reverse conization" of the cervix, followed by endocervical cautery to ablate the cervical epithelium down to the transformation zone. In the author's series of subtotal abdominal hysterectomy there have been no cases of cyclical vaginal bleeding in women whose ovaries were conserved, or in those who were prescribed hormone replacement therapy. Nevertheless, after subtotal abdominal hysterectomy, women need to have regular Papanicolau smears and a minority of women may experience slight cyclical bleeding (18).

The concern that cancer might develop in the cervical stump should not be considered a justification for routine use of total abdominal hysterectomy as continued screening would cover this concern, considering that the risk of cervical cancer after subtotal abdominal hysterectomy is less than 0.1 percent (19).

Subtotal abdominal hysterectomy is often combined with removal of the ovaries. There are inconsistencies in the prescription of hormone replacement therapy following subtotal abdominal hysterectomy, and evidence is lacking to guide hormone replacement prescription following subtotal abdominal hysterectomy and bilateral oophorectomy (20). Until such evidence become available, it is felt that women should be counseled prior to subtotal abdominal hysterectomy regarding hormone replacement therapy, which should include progesterone.

The main objectively measurable parameters in the comparison between subtotal and total abdominal hysterectomy are morbidity and mortality. The main short-term and long-term comparative events and complications of subtotal versus total hysterectomy for benign uterine diseases are listed in Table 1.

Intra-operative parameters
Anaesthesia-related complications Blood loss Blood loss requiring transfusion Technical problem Conversion Duration of operation
Post-operative parameters
Short term
Pain score
Pyrexia
Haemoglobin level
Blood transfusion
Urinary tract infection
Retention of urine
Vault hematoma
Wound hematoma
Ileus
Vaginal bleeding
Hospital stay
Long term
Re-Admission rate
Bowel obstruction
Vault granulation
Cyclical vaginal bleeding
Prolapse of vaginal vault or cervical stump
Dyspareunia
Ureter lesion
Urinary incontinence
Persistent pain
Bowel function
Quality of life (SF-36)/Psychological outcome
Overall
Mortality

Table 1. Short-term and long-term comparative events and complications of subtotal versus total abdominal hysterectomy for benign uterine diseases

Generally, the mortality rates for hysterectomy, standardized for age and race, are higher for procedures associated with pregnancy or cancer than for procedures not associated with these conditions. Although hysterectomies associated with pregnancy or cancer constitute around 10% of all hysterectomies, the majority of deaths occur in women with pregnancy or cancer related conditions (2). Mortality rate after abdominal hysterectomy for benign indications are low at 6 per 10,000 (2). As mortality at abdominal hysterectomy is such an infrequent event, there are no meaningful statistical comparisons comparing mortality of subtotal abdominal hysterectomy versus total abdominal hysterectomy.

In a study by the author to assess the standard of hysterectomy, so as to improve the quality of patient care and outcome, 134 patients undergoing hysterectomy for benign gynaecological conditions were included in a retrospective analytic study , 90 (67%) having total abdominal hysterectomies, and 44 (33%) having subtotal abdominal hysterectomies. Menorrhagia constituted the commonest indication for both types of procedure (89.5%). The majority of patients undergoing total abdominal hysterectomy (79%) were given prophylactic antibiotics, in contrast to only 32% of those undergoing subtotal abdominal hysterectomy.

The overall incidence of complications that included post-operative pyrexia, blood loss, hematoma formation, need for post-operative analgesia, low post-operative haemoglobin levels, blood transfusion, wound infection, wound re-suturing, urinary tract infection, presence of vaginal vault granulation tissue, duration of surgery, and length of hospital stay for subtotal abdominal hysterectomy were lower than those for total abdominal hysterectomy. In all, 75% of the subtotal abdominal hysterectomies were performed by trainees, while for total abdominal hysterectomy, all were performed by specialists, or had specialists as first assistants (21).

These finding are consistent with other studies which found that subtotal abdominal hysterectomy required less operative time and was associated with less blood loss, versus higher incidence of abscesses, wound infection with higher incidence of pyrexia and use of antibiotics and longer hospital stay in the total-hysterectomy group (22).

With regard to urological outcome, injury to the urinary tract is a frequent cause of litigation after total abdominal hysterectomy (23). It occurs in 0.5 to 3.0 percent of cases (24). Evidence regarding ureteric or bladder injuries following subtotal abdominal hysterectomy compared to total abdominal hysterectomy in randomized controlled trials is sparse.

Regarding urinary frequency, nocturia and incontinence, a systematic review on urinary function following subtotal abdominal hysterectomy and total abdominal hysterectomy identified five observational studies, three of which, in addition to one randomized, controlled trial showed an increased risk of incontinence after total abdominal hysterectomy (22, 25-27). The remaining two, in addition to one randomized controlled trial showed no difference (20,28,29).

In contrast, another randomised controlled trial showed that a significantly smaller proportion of women had urinary incontinence one year after total abdominal hysterectomy compared with subtotal abdominal hysterectomy (30). In addition, total and subtotal abdominal hysterectomy for benign indications have been compared in a meta-analysis performed to summarize the evidence from randomized clinical trials and observational studies, where less women suffered from urinary incontinence and prolapse after total than after subtotal hysterectomy (31).

In a review of evidence relating to the potential benefits of subtotal abdominal hysterectomy versus total abdominal hysterectomy for women considering hysterectomy for benign disease, the Cochrane Library, Medline, and Embase were searched for articles published in English from January 1950 to March 2008, where the results were restricted to systematic reviews, randomized control trials, controlled clinical trials, and observational studies, the recommendation was that subtotal abdominal hysterectomy should not be recommended as a superior technique to total abdominal hysterectomy for the prevention of postoperative lower urinary tract symptoms (32).

Although there are some studies on the effect of hysterectomies in general on bowel function, most have not addressed a possible difference between subtotal abdominal hysterectomy and total abdominal hysterectomy in relation to this variable (33-35), except for one randomized, controlled trial which found no difference in any of the measures of bowel function, namely constipation, hard stools, urgency, straining, need for laxatives, and incontinence of flatus, between the two groups before or after surgery or over time (22).

With regard to sexual outcome including coital frequency, desire, orgasm frequency, dyspareunia and overall sexual outcome, a systematic review of effect on sexual function following subtotal abdominal hysterectomy versus total abdominal hysterectomy identified four non-randomized studies, one of which showed that total abdominal hysterectomy had advantages over subtotal abdominal hysterectomy (20), two of which showed that subtotal abdominal hysterectomy had advantages over total abdominal hysterectomy with respect to sexual function (36, 37). The remaining one, in addition to five randomized controlled trials showed no difference (20,38-42).

Regarding psychological outcome, women show improvement following both total and subtotal hysterectomy, with no significant differences between them in the amount of anxiety, depression, and somatic symptoms or social dysfunction, between baseline and post-operative measurements (43).

In a survey regarding the attitudes and practice of gynecologists to total versus subtotal abdominal hysterectomy, nearly half of respondents stated that they always removed the cervix. The most common indication cited was to eliminate the risk of cervical cancer, and the most common reason for subtotal hysterectomy was surgical difficulty leading to an intraoperative conversion. Few counseled women regarding the advantages and disadvantages of both total and subtotal hysterectomy, the majority rarely or never did (44).

As probably would be expected, one randomised controlled trial showed that subtotal hysterectomy was faster to perform, had less intraoperative bleeding, and less intraoperative and postoperative complications (31).

In conclusion as inadequate study power is a major issue in most studies, to identify the advantages and disadvantages of subtotal abdominal hysterectomy and total abdominal hysterectomy, large randomized controlled studies are lacking. Until some further studies become available, and based on some of the known outcomes, it should be reasonable to discuss the advantages and drawbacks of both procedures, and consider patients' preferences. This might further improve satisfaction rates after hysterectomies performed for benign conditions.

2. References

[1] DeFrances CJ, Lucas CA, Buie VC, Golosinskiy A 2006 National Hospital Discharge Survey. Natl Health Stat Report. 2008;5:1–20.

[2] Wingo PA, Huezo CM, Rubin GL, Ory HW, Peterson HB. The mortality risk associated with hysterectomy. Am J Obstet Gynecol. 1985;152:803-808.

[3] Halmesmäki K, Hurskainen R, Teperi J, Grenman S, Kivelä A, Kujansuu E, Tuppurainen M, Yliskoski M, Vuorma S, Paavonen J. The effect of hysterectomy or levonorgestrel-releasing intrauterine system on sexual functioning among women with menorrhagia: a 5-year randomised controlled trial. BJOG: An International Journal of Obstetrics & Gynaecology. 2007;114:563-568.

[4] Dicker RC, Greenspan JR, Strauss LT, Cowart MR, Scally MJ, Peterson HB, DeStefano F, Rubin GL, Ory HW. Complications of abdominal and vaginal hysterectomy among women of reproductive age in the United States. The Collaborative Review of Sterilization. Am J Obstet Gynecol. 1982;144:841-848.

[5] Sutton C. Past, present, and future of hysterectomy. J Minim Invasive Gynecol. 2010;17:421-435.

[6] Department of Health and Social Security and Office of Population Censuses and Surveys. Hospital in-patient enquiry. DHSS:London,HMSO:1985.

[7] Vessey MP, Villard-Mackintosh L, McPherson K, Coulter A, Yeates D. The epidemiology of hysterectomy: findings in a large cohort study. Br J Obstet Gynaecol. 1992;99:402-407.

[8] Merrill RM. Hysterectomy surveillance in the United States, 1997 through 2005. Med Sci Monit. 2008;14:CR24–CR31.

[9] Gimbel H, Settnes A, Tabor A. Hysterectomy on benign indication in Denmark 1988-1998 A register based trend analysis. Acta Obstet Gynecol Scand. 2001;80:267–272.

[10] Stang A, Merrill RM, Kuss O. Hysterectomy in Germany: A DRG-Based Nationwide Analysis, 2005-2006.Dtsch Arztebl Int. 2011;108:508-514.

[11] van Evert JS, Smeenk JM, Dijkhuizen FP, de Kruif JH, Kluivers KB. Laparoscopic subtotal hysterectomy versus laparoscopic total hysterectomy: a decade of experience. Gynecol Surg. 2010;7:9-12.

[12] Leonard F, Chopin N, Borghese B, Fotso A, Foulot H, Coste J, et al. Total laparoscopic hysterectomy: preoperative risk factors for conversion to laparotomy. J Minim Invasive Gynecol. 2005;12:312–317.

[13] Ng CC, Chern BS, Siow AY. Retrospective study of the success rates and complications associated with total laparoscopic hysterectomy. J Obstet Gynaecol Res. 2007;33:512–518.

[14] Tohic AL, Dhainaut C, Yazbeck C, Hallais C, Levin I, Madelenat P. Hysterectomy for benign uterine pathology among women without previous vaginal delivery. Obstet Gynecol. 2008;111:829–837.

[15] Eisenkop SM. Total laparoscopic hysterectomy with pelvic/aortic lymph node dissection for endometrial cancer - a consecutive series without case selection and comparison to laparotomy. Gynecol Oncol. 2010;117:216–223.

[16] Tunitsky E, Citil A, Ayaz R, Esin S, Knee A, Harmanli O. Does surgical volume influence short-term outcomes of laparoscopic hysterectomy? Am J Obstet Gynecol. 2010;203:24–26.

[17] Stang A, Merrill RM, Kuss O. Nationwide rates of conversion from laparoscopic or vaginal hysterectomy to open abdominal hysterectomy in Germany. Eur J Epidemiol. 2011;26:125-133.

[18] Gimbel H, Zobbe V, Andersen BM, Gluud C, Ottesen BS, Tabor A; Danish Hysterectomy Group. Total versus subtotal hysterectomy: an observational study with one-year follow-up. Aust N Z J Obstet Gynaecol. 2005;45:64-67.

[19] Herbert A. Cervical screening in England and Wales: its effect has been underestimated. Cytopathology. 2000;11:471-479.

[20] Maina WC, Morris EP. Management of women requesting subtotal hysterectomy. Menopause Int. 2010;16:152-155.

[21] Jamal H, Amarin Z. Subtotal Versus Total Abdominal Hysterectomy. Bahrain Med Bull 2001;23:119-123.

[22] Thakar R, Ayers S, Clarkson P, Stanton S, Manyonda I. Outcomes after total versus subtotal abdominal hysterectomy. N Engl J Med 2002;347:1318-1325.

[23] Whitelaw JM. Hysterectomy: a medical-legal perspective, 1975 to 1985. Am J Obstet Gynecol. 1990;162:1451-1458.

[24] Hendry WF. Urinary tract injuries during gynaecological surgery. In: Studd J, ed. Progress in obstetrics and gynaecology. Vol. 5. Edinburgh, Scotland: Churchill Livingstone, 1985:362-377.

[25] Iosif CS, Bekassy Z, Rydhstrom H. Prevalence of urinary incontinence in middle-aged women. Int J Gynaecol Obstet. 1988;26:255-259.

[26] Kilkku P. Supravaginal uterine amputation versus hysterectomy with reference to subjective bladder symptoms and incontinence. Acta Obstet Gynecol Scand. 1985;64:375-379.

[27] Kilkku P, Hirvonen T, Gronroos M. Supra-vaginal uterine amputation vs. abdominal hysterectomy: the effects on urinary symptoms with special reference to pollakisuria, nocturia and dysuria. Maturitas. 1981;3:197-204

[28] Lalos O, Bjerle P. Bladder wall mechanics and micturition before and after subtotal and total hysterectomy. Eur J Obstet Gynecol Reprod Biol. 1986;21:143-150.

[29] Virtanen HS, Makinen JI, Tenho T, Kiiholma P, Pitkanen Y, Hirvonen T. Effects of abdominal hysterectomy on urinary and sexual symptoms. Br J Urol. 1993;72:868-872.

[30] Gimbel H, Zobbe V, Andersen BM, Filtenborg T, Gluud C, Tabor A. Randomised controlled trial of total compared with subtotal hysterectomy with one-year follow up results. BJOG. 2003;110:1088-1098.

[31] Gimbel H. Total or subtotal hysterectomy for benign uterine diseases? A meta-analysis. Acta Obstet Gynecol Scand. 2007;86:133-144.

[32] Kives S, Lefebvre G, Wolfman W, Leyland N, Allaire C, Awadalla A, Best C, Leroux N, Potestio F, Rittenberg D, Soucy R, Singh S. Supracervical hysterectomy. J Obstet Gynaecol Can. 2010;32:62-68.

[33] Taylor T, Smith AN, Fulton PM. Effect of hysterectomy on bowel function. BMJ. 1989;299:300-301.

[34] Prior A, Stanley K, Smith ARB, Read NW. Effect of hysterectomy on anorectal and urethrovesical physiology. Gut. 1992;33:264-267.

[35] Heaton KW, Parker D, Cripps H. Bowel function and irritable bowel symptoms after hysterectomy and cholecystectomy - a population based study. Gut. 1993;34:1108-1111.
[36] Kilkku P, Gronroos M, Hirvonen T, Rauramo L. Supravaginal uterine amputations vs. hysterectomy: effects on libido and orgasm. Acta Obstet Gynecol Scand. 1983;62:147-152.
[37] Kilkku P. Supravaginal uterine amputation vs. hysterectomy: effects on coital frequency and dyspareunia. Acta Obstet Gynecol Scand. 1983;62:141-145.
[38] Virtanen HS, Makinen JI, Tenho T, Kiiholma P, Pitkanen Y, Hirvonen T. Effects of abdominal hysterectomy on urinary and sexual symptoms. Br J Urol. 1993;72:868-872.
[39] Gorlero F, Lijoi D, Biamonti M, Lorenzi P, Pullè A, Dellacasa I, Ragni N. Hysterectomy and women satisfaction: total versus subtotal technique. Arch Gynecol Obstet. 2008;278:405-410.
[40] Flory N, Bissonnette F, Amsel RT, Binik YM. The psychosocial outcomes of total and subtotal hysterectomy: A randomized controlled trial. J Sex Med. 2006;3:483-491.
[41] Kuppermann M, Summitt RL Jr, Varner RE, McNeeley SG, Goodman-Gruen D, Learman LA, Ireland CC, Vittinghoff E, Lin F, Richter HE, Showstack J, Hulley SB, Washington AE. Sexual functioning after total compared with supracervical hysterectomy: a randomized trial. Obstet Gynecol. 2005;105:1309-1318.
[42] Zobbe V, Gimbel H, Andersen BM, Filtenborg T, Jakobsen K, Sørensen HC, Toftager-Larsen K, Sidenius K, Møller N, Madsen EM, Vejtorp M, Clausen H, Rosgaard A, Gluud C, Ottesen BS, Tabor A. Sexuality after total vs. subtotal hysterectomy. Acta Obstet Gynecol Scand. 2004;83:191-196.
[43] Thakar R, Ayers S, Georgakapolou A, Clarkson P, Stanton S, Manyonda I. Hysterectomy improves quality of life and decreases psychiatric symptoms: a prospective and randomised comparison of total versus subtotal hysterectomy. BJOG. 2004;111:1115-1120.
[44] Zekam N, Oyelese Y, Goodwin K, Colin C, Sinai I, Queenan JT. Total versus subtotal hysterectomy: a survey of gynecologists. Obstet Gynecol. 2003;102:301-305.

3

Robotic Surgery Versus Abdominal and Laparoscopic Radical Hysterectomy in Cervical Cancer

E. Ancuta[1], Codrina Ancuta[2] and L. Gutu[3]
[1]*Research Department, "Cuza-Voda" Hospital Iasi,*
[2]*"Gr.T.Popa" University of Medicine and Pharmacy Iasi,*
[3]*Institute of Oncology, Chisinau,*
[1,2]*Romania*
[3]*Moldova*

1. Introduction

The first abdominal radical hysterectomy has been performed by Ernst Wertheim, one of the most famous 19th century surgeons, and still remains the basis for many surgeons nowadays. The technique was then modified by Meigs in 1950s. Piver and colleagues have described five classes of surgery based on the estimated risk of cervical carcinoma involvement; moreover, a new classification has been recently proposed by Querleu (Jhingran & Levenback, 2007; Martinez & Ramirez, 2009).

First laparoscopic hysterectomy has been done in January 1988 and defined as the laparoscopic ligation of the major vessels supplying the uterus; it is considered the most efficacious way to perform a hysterectomy (Reich, 2011). Besides, laparoscopic radical hysterectomy has been performed by C. Nezhat in 1992. Every gynecologic oncologist must be familiar with this procedure because of its feasibility and safety for the patient.

Following a pilot study performed by the Gynecologic Oncology Group it has been shown that laparoscopic staging is feasible with acceptable complications and a superior quality of life as compared with the open approach (Magrina, 2008; Mendivil & Boggess, 2009).

The da Vinci Surgical Robotic System has been approved by Food and Drug Administration (FDA) in 2005, while robotic surgery designed for radical hysterectomies has been reported for the first time by Sert in 2006. Despite the fact, in an attempt to minimize morbidity and recovery time, gynecologists have increasingly utilized robotic surgery to treat gynecologic cancers since these procedures were first described in the early 1999s.

Potential benefits of robotic technology include 3-dimensional, high-definition, optics instrumentation that allows greater range of motion, precision, scaling and surgeon autonomy.

As we mentioned before, robotic surgery was utilized for gynecologic procedures, such as laparoscopic benign hysterectomy and sacral colpopexy, myomectomy and radical hysterectomy. In addition, robotic-assisted laparoscopic surgeries in gynecology include tubal re-anastomoses, lymph node dissection and sacro-colpopexies (Breda, 1991; Reich, 2011).

Well-designed prospective studies with well defined clinical long term outcomes including complications, costs, pain, return to normal activity and quality of life are needed to fully assess the value of this new technology.

The da Vinci Surgical System offers certain advantages over traditional laparoscopy and laparotomy like decreased blood loss, an increased lymph node yield and shorter length of stay (Basil & Pavelka, 2011). Average estimated blood loss for the da Vinci Surgical System is less than that seen in the laparotomy and laparoscopy (Leblanc, 2009).

An increase in the lymph node yield in the robotic surgery in gynecologic cancers when compared with the laparotomy and laparoscopic cohorts has also been reported (Basil & Pavelka, 2011).

Robotic assistance may make lymphadenectomy easier and more comprehensive by overcoming anatomic barriers to the process of stopping for uterine cancer, without increasing patient morbidity and may result in the increased use of minimally invasive treatment of uterine cancer (Reich, 2011; Sert & Abeler, 2007; Tang & Obermair, 2009).

Robotic technology would allow us to implement a program using robotic technology at our primary institution and to offer greater safety than conventional laparoscopic techniques.

Laparoscopic hysterectomy demonstrated a greater interest in the scientific community and was considered a substitute for abdominal hysterectomy but not for vaginal hysterectomy.

Additionally, hospitals may benefit because of the technique; advantages are multiple, including reduced duration of hospitalization and recovery, an extremely low rate of complication such as infection and ileus.

On the other hand, the surgeon must remember that if the patient is more comfortable with vaginal hysterectomy these should be done.

The purpose of this review is to compare abdominal radical hysterectomy, laparoscopic and robotic radical hysterectomy used in the management of gynecologic pathology, particularly in cancers.

2. Laparoscopic hysterectomy

2.1 Equipment

Trendelenburg's position (20-40^0) with shoulder braces and the arms at the patient's sides has been used in laparoscopic hysterectomy (Beste, 2005; Breda, 2001; Diaz-Arrastia, 2002; Reich, 2011).

A Valtchev uterine mobilizer is extremely valuable to delineate the posterior vagina and uterus can be moved from the horizontal in an arc between 45 and 120^0 (Diaz-Arrastia, 2002; Frumovitz, 2007; Reich, 2011).

For defining the rectovaginal space, an rectovaginal intraoperative examination is necessary. 5.5 mm diameter trocar and a 5 mm trocar sleeves with a retention screw grid around the external surface cannulas are adequate (Beste, 2005; Frumovitz, 2007; Meeks & Harris, 1997; Reich, 2011).

A little pneumoperitoneum is lost.

Vienna retractors are used for vaginal extractions of a large fibroid uterus (Beste, 2005; Frumovitz, 2007; Reich, 2011).

Monopolar cutting is used (Bipolar forceps) for coagulate vessels like uterine and ovarian arteries (Beste, 2005; Diaz-Arrastia, 2002; Reich, 2011).

Also the Kleppinger bipolar forceps is used for large vessel hemostasis (Beste, 2005; Frumovitz, 2007; Reich, 2011).

To maintain a fixed distance between the electrodes, for irrigation, and to identify bleeding sites microbipolar forceps are used (Beste, 2005; Frumovitz, 2007; Reich, 2011).

Richard Wolf Medical Instruments are used for evacuation of tissue. All laparoscopic surgical procedures are done by laparoscopic surgeon trained to hold the camera with the dominant hand, ambidexterity separates them from those trained traditionally (Beste, 2005; Diaz-Arrastia , 2002; Frumovitz, 2007; Reich, 2011).

The routine use of preoperatively antibiotics and general anesthesia are recommended in all cases.

Infections are very rare: less than 1% (Reich, 2011).

All incisions are closed with 4-0 Vicryl.

2.2 Indications and contraindications

The main indications are the following (Beste, 2005; Frumovitz, 2007; Meeks & Harris, 1997; Reich, 2011):

- *symptomatic uterine fibroids* (hypermenorrhea, pelvic pressure and, rarely, pain); all these cases can be performed laparoscopically after measurement of uterine size and weight;
- *benign pathology;*
- *endometriosis;* endometriosis can involve the posterior cervix and cause painful periods, pain all day or every day. Hysterectomy should be done only to remove possible deep intrauterine endometriosis (adenomyosis). In patients with stage IV endometriosis and extensive cul-de-sac obliteration hysterectomy lives the deep fibrotic endometriosis behind and is preferable to preserve the uterus. If the endometriosis is carefully removed, oophorectomy is no longer necessary;
- *stage I endometrial, ovarian and cervical cancer;*
- *abnormal uterine bleeding;* irregular uterine bleeding for more than eight days during more than a single cycle is defined as abnormal uterine bleeding;
- *pelvic reconstruction procedures;*
- *laparoscopic procedures* allowing cuff suspension, retropubic colpo-suspension and rectocele repair simultaneously;
- *obese woman;* the surgeon would be able to make an incision above the panniculus.

The main contraindications are represented by cases with a history of extensive abdominal adhesion should be referred to an expert laparoscopic surgeon because the medical status may prohibit surgery: anemia, diabetes, cardiac diseases, lung disorders and bleeding diathesis (Reich, 2011).

Both inexperience training of the surgeon and stage III ovarian cancer are also contraindications to the laparoscopic technique (Harris, 1997; Reich, 2011).

2.3 Surgical interventions

The laparascope is commonly used to a variety of operations, comprising:

- *Diagnostic laparoscopy with vaginal hysterectomy* to determine if vaginal hysterectomy is possible, if vaginal cuff and pedicle hemostasis is complete and to allow clot evacuation.
- *Laparoscopic assisted vaginal hysterectomy* used for vaginal hysterectomy after laparoscopic adhesiolysis and endometriosis excision.
- *Laparoscopic supracervical hysterectomy*, a less risky procedure than total hysterectomy. The uterus is removed with decreased risk of dissection of the ureter.
- *Total laparoscopic hysterectomy*. The laparoscopic dissection continues until the uterus is removed through the vagina and vaginal suture is done.
- *Laparoscopic hysterectomy*. This procedure may be performed when all surgical steps including ligation of the uterine vessels, anterior and posterior vaginal entry by transection cardinal and utero-sacral ligament division, uterine removal and vaginal closure have been done.
- *Hysterectomy*: partial, subtotal, fundectomy. If the cervix is left better names of hysterectomy would be partial hysterectomy, fundectomy or subtotal hysterectomy.
- *Laparoscopic pelvic reconstruction with vaginal hysterectomy*. This procedure is necessary when vaginal hysterectomy cannot repair the vaginal prolapse.

2.4 Total Laparoscopic Hysterectomy technique (TLH)

2.4.1 Incisions and vaginal preparation

Three laparoscopic puncture sites are typically used: one of 10 mm umbilical and two of 5 mm (left and right), in the lower quadrant. The uterus is removed in the anteverted position to delineate the posterior vagina for the laparoscopic hysterectomy. After the Voltchew uterine mobilizer is inserted and the endocervical canal is dilated, the cervix sits on a mide pedestal making the vagina visible (Beste, 2005; Cadiere, 2001; Reich, 2011; Tang & Obermair, 2009).

2.4.2 Exploration

After exploration of the upper abdomen and pelvis, if appendiceal pathology is present, appendectomy is done.

2.4.3 Ureteral dissection

Medial, superior and lateral approaches have been used for laparoscopic ureteric identification. The laparoscopic surgeon should skeletonize the ureterus during the performance of a laparoscopic hysterectomy. If the ureter is not dissected, cystoscopy should be done after vaginal closure to check for ureteral patency.

2.4.3.1 The medial approach (Reich)

The ureteral dissection is performed before the uterus is anteflexed and peristalsis is inhibited by surgical stress. This allows the peritoneum above the ureter to be incised and to grab the ureter and its peritoneum on the pelvic sidewall below. For safe division of the adnexal pedicle an atraumatic grasping forceps is classically used to grab the ureter on the pelvic sidewall below caudal to the ovary and lateral to the uterosacral ligament. Scissors are used to divide the ureter and the uterine vessels, allowing the safely ligation of the uterine artery at this time and diminishing bleeding from the upper pedicles (Beste, 2005; Cadiere, 2001; Reich, 2011; Tang & Obermair, 2009).

2.4.3.2 The superior approach

The superior approach is dissecting the infundibulo-pelvic ligament vessels from the roof of the broad ligament in order to identify the ureter

2.4.3.3 The lateral approach (Kadar)

The blunt dissection may be inserted alongside and lateral to the pelvic sidewall peritoneum into the loose areolar tissue, permitting the identification of both the uterine vessels and the uterus. The peritoneum recognized in the middle of the triangle formed by round ligament, external iliac artery and the infundibulo-pelvic ligament, is incised with scissors to expose the ureter at the place it crosses the common or external iliac artery (Beste, 2005; Cadiere, 2001; Reich, 2011; Tang & Obermair, 2009).

Consecutively, the operator explores for the ureter distal to the pelvic brim and lateral to the infundibulo-pelvic ligament. Thereafter, the dissection is carried bluntly underneath and caudal to the round ligament, until the obliterated hypogastric artery is visualized in the extraperitoneal space.

If any impediment is coming across, the artery if primarily identified intra-peritoneally (where it hangs from the anterior abdominal wall), traced proximally to (where it passes behind the round ligament), with both its intraperitoneal portion and the dissected space under the round ligament in view, the intra-peritoneal part of the ligament is moved back (Beste, 2005; Cadiere, 2001; Reich, 2011; Tang & Obermair, 2009).

Once the paravesical and pararectal spaces was opened uterine artery, cardinal ligament and the internal iliac artery on its lateral border became visible.

2.4.4 Retroperitoneal dissection

The laparoscopic surgeon makes an incision behind the round ligament for oophorectomy and in front of the round ligament for ovarian preservation. After that, the peritoneum is opened just to the retroperitonial space behind the uterus for oophorectomy and parallel to it for ovarian preservation (Beste, 2005; Cadiere, 2001; Reich, 2011; Tang & Obermair, 2009).

2.4.5 Bladder mobilization

The spoon electrode or scissors are used to make an incision in the round ligaments are their mid portion. The vezico-uterine peritoneum is opened at the left side and continuing across the midline to the right round ligament. Once the bladder is mobilized off, the uterus and the anterior vagina are identified with ring forceps (Beste, 2005; Cadiere, 2001; Reich, 2011; Tang & Obermair, 2009).

2.4.6 Upper uterine blood supply

If the ovary is to be preserved, the utero-ovarian ligament and fallopian tube may be suture-ligated to the uterus, using laparoscopic Metzenbaum type scissors and 2/0 - Vicryl.

If the ovarian preservation is not indicated, the anterior and posterior leaves of the broad ligament are opened to create a window. Through the windows thus created a free ligature is used. Two proximal and one distal suture are tied around the ovarian vessels, so that the ligament then divided (Beste, 2005; Cadiere, 2001; Reich, 2011; Tang & Obermair, 2009).

2.4.7 Uterine vessel ligation

The uterine artery is suture-ligated with 0-Vicryl at their origin each side; a single suture placed on the uterus or at the site where they cross the ureter is tied using a Clarke-Reich Knot pusher.

2.4.8 Division of cervico-vaginal attachments and circumferential culdotomy

The cardinal ligaments are incised using the spoon electrode and the utero-sacral ligaments are divided using the bipolar forceps. A vaginal delineator is placed in the vagina for preventing the loss of pneumoperitoneum (Beste, 2005; Cadiere, 2001; Reich, 2011; Tang & Obermair, 2009).

The operator then searches for the anterior cervico-vaginal junction and the lateral fornices to complete the culdotomy. Then the uterus can be morcellated and pulled out of the vagina.

2.4.9 Morcellation

If necessary, the uterus can be morcellated or not. The vaginal and laparoscopic morcellation is performed with the Steiner Electromechanical Morcellator. Laparoscopic vaginal vault closure and suspension is realized with McCall culdeplasty, vaginal closure being necessary for maintaining pneumoperitoneum. A 0-Vicryl suture on a CT-1 needle is placed through the left utero-sacral ligament and through the left cardinal ligament just below the uterine artery just along the vaginal cuff apex. This suture is used to fix the right side. The rest of the vagina is closed with two 0-Vicryl interrupted sutures. Once the vaginal cuff is closed the peritoneum is elevated and in most cases it is not closed (Beste, 2005; Cadiere, 2001; Reich, 2011; Tang & Obermair, 2009).

2.4.10 Cystoscopy

If the ureter is not dissected, the laparoscopic technique involves cystoscopy to check for ureteral pantency, ten minutes after indigo carmine dye administration.

2.4.11 Underwater examination

The peritoneal cavity is vigorously irrigated to detect bleeding. The operator then searches for any further bleeding from vessels and a microbipolar forceps is used to coagulate through the electrolyte solution.

2.5 Postperative considerations

In most cases patients return to their routine activities two weeks after the operation. Pelvic examination is usually indicated between 6-12 weeks, mainly are indicated for pain or pyrexia. Sexual activity may be allowed after six weeks.

2.6 Complications

Complications of laparoscopic hysterectomy include thromboembolic phenomenon, respiratory compromise, urinary retention, large vessel or ureters and bladder injury, trocar site incisions hernias, infections and subcutaneus emphysema (Reich, 2011).

2.6.1 Infection

Since the introduction of prophylactic antibiotics, febrile morbidity is less than half that of the abdominal hysterectomy (Jhingran & Levenback, 2007; Reich, 2011). Main complications of infections include cellulitis, vaginal cuff abscesses, adnexal abscesses, thrombophlebitis and septicemia. All patients with abscesses were responders to in hospital intravenous antibiotics and only few cases were treated by laparoscopic draenage, ultrasound guided aspiration and laparatomy draenage. To eliminate postoperative infection, the laparoscopic surgeon should do copious irrigation in the peritoneal cavity, to dilute the fibrin and to prevent prostaglandins arising from operated area.

2.6.2 Hemorrhage

Postoperative hemorrhage situations should be avoided by doing careful laparoscopic dissection during hysterectomy; moreover, if necessary blood transfusion should be performed for replacement of intra-operative blood loss.

2.6.3 Cuff dehiscence

Vaginal repair using chronic catgut is indicated when laparoscopic closure was accomplished by vaginal cuff dehiscence.

2.6.4 Urinary tract complications

Cistoscopy is done in all hysterectomy cases at the conclusion of the procedure to check for ureteral and bladder injuries. Potential complications include secondary ureteral stricture, ureteral ligation, bladder injury during uterine vessel ligation. Careful techniques of ureteral and bladder dissection are important to avoid urinary retention as a common complication. In patients who underwent general anesthesia, the Foley catheter should be removed postoperatively no longer than two hours, until the patient is awake. Signs of some injuries include: abdominal pain, fever or abdominal distention, low urine output relative to fluid intake, hematuria, hydronephrosis and ureteral colic. The treatment for vesico-vaginal fistula and uretero-vaginal fistula is based on Latsko surgical procedure and re-implantation or long term catheter placement, respectively. In most cases, ureteral injuries may occur during cutting severe pelvic adhesion by bipolar cautery. If the ureter is cut or coagulated, immediate reanastomosis is indicated by using a combined double J silicon catheter and laparoscopic end-to-end anastomosis with four extramucosal absorbable sutures. The Cook, Bard or Meditech stents can be removed six weeks later. Subsequently, the operator searches for the anastomosis patency; if necessary, uretero-neocystostomy should be done (Beste, 2005; Cadiere, 2001; Reich, 2011; Tang & Obermair, 2009).

2.6.5 Bladder injury

11Bladder injury may result from either a trocar puncture (if the bladder has not been drained of urine during dissection of it) or from an inflamed adnexa. If laceration is greater than 7 mm, it should be closed laparoscopically (Reich, 2011). Treatment consists of prophylactic antibiotics and placement an indwelling catheter for the next 7 to 10 days.

2.6.6 Bowel injury

Small bowel injuries are very uncommon during laparoscopic hysterectomy and should be closed with interrupted 3-0 Vicryl. If the defect involves more than 50% of the bowel circumference a segmental enterectomy is necessary in order to reduce the risk of stricture. Therefore, a side to side stapled anastomosis is constructed to avoid the risk of stricture, using a GIA60. An adequate umbilical incision to approximately 2.5 cm is necessary to permit extrusion and repair of the involved bowel. The bowel is than replaced to the abdominal cavity, while the pneumoperitoneum should also be re-established. Anastomotic inspection is made laparoscopically.

2.6.7 Peritonitis after unrecognized perforation

Peritonitis is the result of bowel perforation, after termal damage or Veress needle puncture that is not recognized during the laparoscopic hysterectomy. The laparoscopic surgeon inspects for some injury signs like abdominal pain, unexplained fever, abdominal distension and altered bowel function. Once verified, the patient should be investigated. Treatment consists of a transversally bowel resection of all necrotic area with end-to-end anastomosis, lavage and antibiotics. However, prompt recognition can prevent multiple surgical procedures. Also, mini-dose heparin therapy is used.

2.7 Complications unique to laparoscopy

2.7.1 Subcutaneous emphysema

After using laparoscopic techniques, subcutaneous emphysema should result from placement of the Veress needle into the extraperitoneal space or during prolonged procedures. Patient's companions should be told that during laparoscopic hysterectomy may secondarily occur subcutaneous emphysema as gas gains access through enlargement of the trocar incision in the parietal peritoneum and usually dissolves in 12-24 hours (Harris, 1997; Jhingran & Levenback, 2007; Kim, 2007; Li, 2007; Reich, 2011; Rhodes, 1999; Tang & Obermair, 2009).

2.7.2 Injury to abdominal wall vessels

The percentage of trocar-induced vascular damage to the abdominal wall is less than 2% (Reich, 2011). Rupture of superficial or deep vessels to the anterior abdominal wall can cause bleeding and hematoma. Therefore, this damage should be avoided by placement of the trocar with the laparoscopic visualization to the rectus muscles. Treatment depends on the location of the injury as well as the damage is arterial or venous. The greatest amount of clinical experience has been with use of a through-and-through loop of suture around the bleeding site (Harris, 1997; Jhingran & Levenback, 2007; Kim, 2007; Li, 2007; Reich, 2011; Rhodes, 1999; Tang & Obermair, 2009).

2.7.3 Injury to large vessels

The vascular surgeon must promptly repair vascular defects such as penetration to aorta, iliac vessels or vena cava that can occur on rare occasion during laparoscopic surgery. Thus, the laparoscopic surgeon and the vascular surgeon must perform direct laparatomy and repair the blood vessels.

2.7.4 Trocar site incisional hernias

If incisional hernia is suspected, symptoms usually occur within 10 days after surgery and laparoscopic reduction should be considered as therapeutic option.

2.7.5 Instrument failure

The incidence of these complications is low (Reich, 2011). If any instruments are faulty within the abdomen, it should be withdrawn from the abdomen laparoscopically in the majority of cases.

The indication for the role of laparoscopy in the future will be determined by the increased familiarity of gynecologic surgeons with these procedures.

3. Robotic hysterectomy. How the robotic system works?

There is no major difference between robotic-assisted hysterectomy and the laparoscopic hysterectomy regarding postoperative considerations and complications (Basil & Pavelka, 2011). Robotic surgery provides all the benefits of the laparoscopic technique with greater precision and effectiveness. However, we have to point out several considerations about the equipment and about how the robotic system works.

The robotic system, particularly the da Vinci System approved by the US Food and Drug Administration for gynecologic surgery since 2005 is superior to laparatomy and provides a shorter hospital stay, less morbidity than laparatomy and easier recovery (Beste, 2005; Carlson, 1994; Chitwood, 2000; Degueldre, 2000; Diaz-Arrastia, 2002; Reich, 2011; Tang & Obermair, 2009).

The da Vinci System allows gynecologists to performed hysterectomies more precise than conventional surgery. Robotic surgery is useful for the treatment of gynecologic cancers and other conditions such as fibroids, vaginal prolapsed (Beste, 2005; Reich, 2011; Stovall & Mann, 2011).

The technique may also be applied for several other therapeutic indications such as sacral colpopexy, tubal reanastomosis, endometriosis and pelvic pain (Cadiere, 2001; Basil & Pavelka, 2011; Reich, 2011; Stovall & Mann, 2011).

The variety and extent of surgery may be performed using a surgeon's console connected to three robotic arms with increased precision and effectiveness. Moreover, the variety of procedure is easier because of 3-dimensional visualization (Cadiere, 2001; Reich, 2011).

Robotic radical hysterectomy is typically indicated in the management of both cervical cancer (tumors more than 2 cm or tumors under 2 cm with lymphatic invasion up to stage IIA) and endometrial cancer with cervical stromal invasion. The da Vinci and Vinci S Robotic Systems are currently used (Cadiere, 2001; Chitwood; 2001; Reich, 2011; Stovall & Mann, 2011).

The robotic column is placed between the patient's lower extremities, at the feet level. Four main trocars are currently used including a 12 mm transumbilical trocar, two trocars of 8 mm placed at 10 cm to the right and left of the umbilical one, while the last trocar is positioned 10 cm lateral and 5 cm caudal to the right robotic trocar, respectively. The assistant trocar of 10 mm is located 3 cm cranial to the umbilical and left trocar. The instrumentation consists of an Endo Wrist PK grasper and an Endo Wrist monopolar that are used on the left and the right robotic arm, respectively; the Endo Wrist Prograsper that is used in the fourth robotic arm to assist with retraction, while an Endo Wrist needle holder is used to replace the monopolar spatula to suture the vaginal cuff; the Enseal device used for division of vascular pedicles. After removal of the specimen, a colpo-occluder balloon is placed in the vagina to maintain pneumoperitoneum (Chitwood; 2001; Reich, 2011; Scott, 1999; Stovall & Mann, 2011).

The robotic system is a technique that uses a remote control, two interactive mechanical arms and a 3D-image processing system, being considered the greatest advance in surgery in the past decades. The patient is placed in the same operating room as the unit. The motions of the surgeon are translated to the robotic arms by using the remote control unit, whereas the robotic arms hold interchangeable surgical instruments that can be moved in a specific manner. Although the robotic system has progressed from simple surgical tasks to more complicated surgery in the past decade, robotic surgery is still in stage of development (Cadiere, 2001; Degueldre, 2000; Diaz-Arrastia, 2002; Stovall & Mann, 2011).

Following the procedure, a second surgeon is positioned within the operation room, at the operating table to help with exchanging the instruments on the robotic "hands".

The da Vinci Robotic Surgical System uses 7 degrees of freedom of motion by the combination of the instruments wrists and the abdominal wall trocar positioned arms.

Robotically assisted gynecologic procedures are generally performed using a combination of remote control, foot pedals and hand controls. These include hand control for operating the instruments, one pedal which is capable to move camera resulting in precise orientation and focus on and a second pedal for repositioning and centering the hand controls. The surgeons first performed bilateral tubal ligations with robotic assistance before progressing to total hysterectomies using the system.

The da Vinci System offers some improvements over traditional laparoscopy: 3-dimensional images, hand tremors and dexterity limitations, but the additional costs, set-up time and limited tactile feedback are major boundaries. In some cases, adequate hemostasis is not advisable with ultrasonic energy; bipolar cautery should be used to assure hemostasis before dividing the entire cardinal ligament (Breda, 2001; Rhodes, 1999; Reich, 2011; Scott, 1999; Stovall & Mann, 2011).

The gynecologic surgeon should master the anatomy of female reproductive tract and the intricacy of lower urinary tract, large intestins and internal genital organs to avoid key surgical complication.

4. Abdominal hysterectomy

Abdominal hysterectomy is a surgical procedure in which the surgeon detaches the uterus from the ovaries, fallopian tubes and upper vagina, as well as from the blood vessels and connective tissue (Baggish & Schellhas, 2011; Beste, 2005; Carlson, 1994; Jhingran & Levenback, 2007; Scott, 1999).

The uterus is a hollow thick walled, muscular organ located in the lower abdomen and pelvis of the female. The lower portion of the uterus namely the cervix may be removed (total hysterectomy), but also may be left in place (partial or supracervical hysterectomy) (Baggish & Schellhas, 2011; Beste, 2005; Carlson, 1994; Jhingran & Levenback, 2007; Scott, 1999).

At its upper end, the uterus narrows into the fallopian tubes and end by curling around the ovary. At the time of the hysterectomy, ovaries and fallopian tubes may also be removed.

The decision concerning appropriate therapy and extent of the abdominal hysterectomy should be made by the woman in consultation with the surgeon for a number of conditions (Baggish. & Schellhas, 2011; Beste, 2005; Carlson, 1994; Jhingran & Levenback, 2007; Scott, 1999).

4.1 Reasons for abdominal hysterectomy

The main reasons for abdominal hysterectomy include abnormal uterine bleeding, fibroids or leiomyoma, pelvic organ prolapsed, cervical abnormalities, endometrial hyperplasia, cancers (uterus, cervix, ovary), severe bleeding after childbirth and chronic pelvic pain. Detailed presentation is presented below.

4.1.1 Abnormal uterine bleeding.

All women with any uterine bleeding before or after menopause should undergo evaluation (Jhingran & Levenback, 2007; Reich, 2011; Scott, 1999).

4.1.2 Fibroids or leiomyoma.

Fibroids produce symptoms of prolonged and excessive regular uterine bleeding; besides, fibroids may cause pelvic pain and excessive bleeding or pressure (Jhingran & Levenback, 2007; Reich, 2011; Scott, 1999).

4.1.3 Pelvic organ prolapsed

Pelvic organ prolapsed occurs due to failure of various anatomic structures to support the pelvic viscera. Pelvic muscles and ligaments are often weakened by vaginal childbirth and other pelvic trauma, life-style factors, chronic constipation and aging process. The patient should not undergo hysterectomy until all ulcers of cervix and vagina are healed. If necessary, vaginal or abdominal hysterectomy is performed carefully with a vaginal vault suspension (Jhingran & Levenback, 2007; Reich, 2011; Scott, 1999).

4.1.4 Cervical abnormalities.

An abdominal or vaginal hysterectomy is rarely needed (Jhingran & Levenback, 2007; Reich, 2011; Scott, 1999).

4.1.5 Endometrial hyperplasia.

Simple or complex hyperplasia without atypia can often be treated with medication. For older patients with complex atypical hyperplasia and those who fail progestin therapy, the risk of developing endometrial cancer is increased. Therefore hysterectomy is needed or preferred to medical therapy.

4.1.6 Cancer of the uterus, cervix or ovaries.

Classic or laparoscopic surgery is the primary treatment modality for carcinoma of uterus, cervix or ovaries. In addition, radiation therapy alone may be used in patients with significant medical comorbidities.

4.1.6.1 Endometrial carcinoma

It is important to realize a throughout inspection of the peritoneal cavity, peritoneal washing and staging biopsies in all cases of endometrial carcinoma. In addition, the surgeon should combine laparoscopic hysterectomy with laparoscopic lymphadenectomy. In patients with stage I grade 1 tumors an extrafascial total abdominal hysterectomy with bilateral salpingo-oophorectomy is always recommended. Furthermore, postoperative irradiation can be used if myometrial invasion to the outer third is diagnosed. In patients with stage I grades 2 and 3 tumors the use of paraaortic lymphadenectomy has gained popularity over the last years. Postoperative radiation is recommended for grade 2 or 3 tumors that invade the myometrium, full pelvic irradiation offering some benefit (Carlson, 1995; Jhingran & Levenback, 2007; Scott, 1999).

Patients with stage II endometrial carcinoma are treated with extrafascial hysterectomy and pelvic node dissection beam: a combination of external irradiation or brachytherapy followed by operation and simple hysterectomy followed by postoperative irradiation.

In stage III, tumor metastases has spread to the adnexa, serosa and/or positive cytology, but remains confined to the pelvis (exception of stage IIIc) in comparison to stage IV where disease spread outside the pelvis (Carlson, 1995; Jhingran & Levenback, 2007; Scott, 1999).

Therapeutic options may vary depending on the histologic type of endometrial carcinoma. Cytotoxic therapy may provide a potential benefit, while radiotherapy may be useful for patients who underwent operation as primary therapy. However, the patient should have a routine preoperative evaluation (Carlson, 1995; Jhingran & Levenback, 2007; Scott, 1999).

4.1.6.2 Cervical cancer

According to the FIGO staging system, radical hysterectomy and bilateral pelvic lymphadenectomy represent the standard technique in the management of patients with cervical cancer stage IB-IIA. Traditional radical hysterectomy includes removal of the uterus and cervix, one third of the vagina, the parametrial tissue at the pelvic sidewall and ligature of utero-sacrals (Carlson, 1995; Jhingran & Levenback, 2007; Reich, 2011; Scott, 1999; Stovall & Mann, 2011).

Recently, there has been a great interest in laparoscopic surgery regarding treatment in carcinoma of the cervix. These procedures permit a through exploration of the abdomen and the tumor itself. Pelvic and paraaortic lymphnodes can be removed through laparoscopic ports. Patients with gross adenopathy should be excluded from laparoscopic technique. CT and MRI provide information for identifying the extent of disease (enlarged nodes), to arrive at an accurate clinical staging. In considering the therapy of cervical carcinoma, patient suspected of having cervical carcinoma should first have biopsy of the tumor. The diagnosis of microinvasive cervical cancer cannot be established by biopsy of the tumor, therefore a cervical conisation must be performed. Occasionally, conisation can be used as safe therapy if the margins are free of tumor. If a decision is made to treat patients with stage IB and early stage IIA, radical hysterectomy and radiation therapy can be used. These are equally effective as treatments for minimal spread to the vagina (Carlson, 1995; Jhingran & Levenback, 2007; Reich, 2011; Scott, 1999; Stovall & Mann, 2011).

The five surgery classes proposed by Piver and colleagues according to the extent of the operation are the following (Jhingran & Levenback, 2007; Scott, 1999; Stovall & Mann, 2011):

- class I that completely removes the uterus and cervix, usually treating barrel-shaped cervix; the ureter is not dissected from its place;
- class II or modified radical hysterectomy in which the removal includes more tissue, but the ureters are not yet dissected; all cases are treated by radical hysterectomy and pelvic lymphadenectomy including utero-sacral ligaments ligature;
- class III operation involves uterine artery ligature at its origin from the hypogastric artery; the utero-sacrals are ligated to their distal attachments near to the rectum;
- class IV operation, the uterer being separated from its bed and the superior vesical artery divided at its origin.
- class V operation includes ureteroneocystostomy.

In fact, some investigators have reported that the carcinoma of the cervix is closely associated with endometrial cancer. Therefore, a brief review of methods of management is also presented.

It should be noted that patients with cervical carcinoma characteristically present symptoms such as bleeding, back pain, loss of appetite, weight loss and a history of not having had a cervical cytology (pap smear) for a long period. Several studies have shown there has been a great interest in molecular markers for prognosis and treatment in cervical cancer: the serum squamous cell carcinoma antigen, epidermal growth factor receptor, cyclooxygenase-2, DNA-ploidy, tumor vascularity and S-phase fraction.

4.1.6.3 Ovarian cancer

Despite numerous investigations currently used, ovarian cancer is the second cause of malignancy of the female genital tract and is characterized by advanced stage disease and high mortality. However, women with late menopause, a history of nulliparity and late childbearing appear to have an increase in risk for ovarian cancer (Carlson, 1995; Reich, 2011; Scott, 1999; Stovall & Mann, 2011).

Several screening modalities have been proposed for the diagnosis of malignancy in adnexal mass, such as physical examination, biomarkers (CA125), proteomics/genomics and ultrasonography (Jhingran & Levenback, 2007; Scott, 1999; Stovall & Mann, 2011).

In case of benign epithelial ovarian tumors like serous cystadenoma, hysterectomy and bilateral salpingo-oophorectomy are usually performed. As well, mucinous tumors can lead to the deposits in the peritoneal cavity by perforation and rupture. Adenofibromas are also treated by simple excision, while Brenner tumors are rare and almost benign, therefore oophorectomy is usually proposed. When these tumors occur in perimenopausal or postmenopausal period, hysterectomy and bilateral salpingooophorectomy offers the best treatment option. Most of the ovarian tumors can be approached surgically through a Phannenstiel incision or by laparoscopic excision. After the diagnosis of malignancy is established by histologic examination of tumor tissue excised at operation, a second procedure can be performed (Jhingran & Levenback, 2007; Scott, 1999; Stovall & Mann, 2011).

The most common borderline ovarian tumors tend to occur in young women aged between 38 and 45 years old (Markovska & Grabowski, 2009). Because several studies confirmed that the cells of these tumors do not invade the stroma of the ovary, it is desirable to ascertain the safety of conservative treatment for women with stage IA disease. Fertility sparing surgery with abdominal cavity inspection and biopsy of peritoneum and controlateral ovary is indicated (Markovska & Grabowski, 2009). Moreover, unilateral adnexectomy is performed. Mucinous borderline tumors are frequently associated with large amounts of mucinous material in the peritoneum; sometimes, an appendiceal adenoma or an appendiceal carcinoma which require appendectomy is identified. Based on these findings, surgery offers the best treatment for such tumors (Jhingran & Levenback, 2007; Scott, 1999; Stovall & Mann, 2011).

4.1.6.3.1 Invasive epithelial carcinomas

A total abdominal hysterectomy with bilateral salpingo-oophorectomy is performed once patient's abdomen is explored through laparatomy. Biopsy and cytologic evaluation is performed to obtained samples from the peritoneum or any suspicious nodules. Current evidence suggests that paraaortic and pelvic lymphnodes sampling is indicated (Benedetti, 2008; Benedetti, 2009). Additionally, surgical treatment may involve splenectomy, diaphragmatic stripping, posterior exenteration and bowel resection (Harris, 1997; Jhingran & Levenback, 2007; Scott, 1999; Stovall & Mann, 2011).

Criteria for preserving childbearing function in woman with stage IA include the following (Jhingran & Levenback, 2007; Scott, 1999; Stovall & Mann, 2011):

- tumor diagnosis confined to one ovary;
- tumor growth limited to one ovary; well differentiated tumor with no dissemination (capsule, lymphatics or mesoovarium);
- negative cytologic peritoneum samples;
- negative biopsy or preferable excision of omentum;
- younger women with stage IA diagnosis, for preserving future childbearing potential.

4.1.6.3.2 Stage I

The assessment of entire peritoneum, retroperitoneal paraaortic pelvic nodes and subdiafragmatic area is important before removal of the omentum, uterus, tubes and controlateral ovary (Jhingran & Levenback, 2007; Scott, 1999; Stovall & Mann, 2011).

4.1.6.3.3 Stage II

The primary treatment relays on removal of the uterus, tubes, ovaries and omentum. In addition, the pelvic and paraaortic nodes biopsies is currently performed (Jhingran & Levenback, 2007; Scott, 1999; Stovall & Mann, 2011). Postoperatively, three options are currently available in such cases: no postoperative treatment, postoperative radiation and postoperative chemotherapy.

4.1.6.3.4 Postoperative therapy for stage III and IV

Several randomized clinical trials using the taxane/platinum combination have been considered as the first line therapy for ovarian cancer. Neoadjuvant chemotherapy is performed as an alternative to extensive therapy. Moreover, certain studies have concluded that such therapy is able to improve the performance status. However, several other prospective and retrospective studies have suggested that many patients with negative second look operation develop recurrent disease. Therefore, some surgeons perform a second look procedure and they recommend such operation not to be done for patients who initially have stage I or II of disease (Jhingran & Levenback, 2007; Scott, 1999; Stovall & Mann, 2011).

4.1.7 Severe bleeding after childbirth

A few women with severe bleeding after childbirth should undergo hysterectomy too.

4.1.8 Chronic pelvic pain

Pelvic pain can be caused by many sources, including endometriosis, gastrointestinal and urinary systems. On the other hand, it is important for women with chronic pelvic pain to ask about the probability that her pain will improve after hysterectomy. Also, laparoscopic presacral neurectomy should be reserved for the patients with significant pain refractory to an adequate trial of conservative treatment.

4.2 Abdominal hysterectomy procedure

4.2.1 Pre-operative preparation

Before hysterectomy, preoperative testing may include a physical examination, ECG, chest X-ray and blood testing, depending upon medical condition and age. In addition, heart rate, blood pressure loss and respiration are closely observed before general or spinal anesthesia is given (Jhingran & Levenback, 2007; Reich, 2011; Scott, 1999).

4.2.2 Technique

Total hysterectomy requires the complete removal of the uterus, the fundus and the cervix, while partial hysterectomy will leave the cervical stump. There are several types of hysterectomy procedures and it is possible for a less invasive procedure to be performed, such as a laparoscopic hysterectomy or a vaginal hysterectomy. These procedures are not practical for complications; in such cases, therefore, the surgeon will made than likely have to revert to an abdominal hysterectomy.

Simple abdominal hysterectomy differs from radical hysterectomy with pelvic lymphadenectomy. The ureter should be identified and dissected after the peritoneum is entered by clamped, cut and sutured-ligated the round ligament. At this point, the peritoneum, the tissue containing lymphnodes and fat are all dissected and the psoas muscle, external iliac vessels and the ureter identified. The external iliac artery, external iliac vein and internal iliac artery are cleared of fat. The surgeon exposes the obturator fossa under the external iliac artery and vein. Second, the obturatory artery and nerve are cleaned of fat and lymphnodes (Baggish & Schellhas, 2011; Meeks and Harris, 1997; Reich, 2011; Rhodes, 1999; Scott, 1999; Stovall & Mann, 2011).

When the node dissection of the external iliac and of the obturator fossa is complete, the operator turns to the common iliac node dissection. Next, the uterine arteries are clamped, cut and suture-ligated distal to their origin from the hypogastric arteries. First, the ureter is dissected inferiorly. Also, at the place where the ureter penetrates the cardinal ligaments to the wall of the bladder, a right angle clamp should be inserted between the ureter and cardinal ligament. When the ureter is clearly free and mobile, the bladder pillars are clamped, cut and sutured. The ureters tunnel to the cardinal ligament must be cut. At that point, the vesico-uterine and retrouterine spaces should be dissected down-ward bellow the cervix and the utero-sacral ligaments are clamped, cut and suture-ligated (Baggish & Schellhas, 2011; Meeks and Harris, 1997; Reich, 2011; Rhodes, 1999; Scott, 1999; Stovall & Mann, 2011).

Then, the ureter is retracted to allow the operator to expose the lower cardinal ligament below the cervix and paravaginal fat. The vagina is clamped at 4 cm below the cervix. Now, the uterus and the attached parametria are removed and the anterior and posterior peritoneum is sutured with Vicryl. Finally, a catheter is placed retroperitoneally before the peritoneum is sutured. At the end the abdominal wall is closed (Baggish & Schellhas, 2011; Meeks and Harris, 1997; Reich, 2011; Rhodes, 1999; Scott, 1999; Stovall & Mann, 2011).

4.2.3 Recovery after abdominal hysterectomy

After operation, patients are transferred to post-anesthesia care unit where they will spend one or two nights. During this period, early recognition and management will preclude larger problems from developing. Thus, patients will resume to their normal daily activities as soon as possible. Pain drugs are given as needed and move from parental medication to oral drugs. Also, being active is important since it helps to prevent blood clots, pneumonia and gas pains (Frumovitz, 2007; Reich, 2011; Scott, 1999).

4.2.4 Complications

Several complications have been described (Jhingran & Levenback, 2007; Kim, 2007; Li, 2007; Reich, 2011; Scott, 1999).

4.2.4.1 Hemorrhage

The patient should return into the operation room to identify and stop the bleeding.

4.2.4.2 Infection

A high or persistent fever may be caused by infection. Finally, in less than 10% of patients, another surgical procedure is necessary. Most of the cases should be treated with intravenous antibiotics.

4.2.4.3 Constipation

Constipation occurs in most patients following operation, and can lie prevented with dietary fibers. Laxatives may be given to some women to control it.

4.2.4.4 Urinary retention

Urinary retention is more common in patients who underwent vaginal hysterectomy and can usually be controlled with a catheter within 24 to 48 hours.

4.2.4.5 Blood clots

The risk of developing blood clots is increased after hysterectomy. Medication such oral contraceptives or hormone replacement should be discontinued prior to surgery. Current guidelines recommend that hormone replacement therapy should be stopped for at least 30 days prior to surgery (Ardern, 2002).

4.2.4.6 Damage to adjacent organs

The urinary bladder, ureter and intestine injuries may occur during hysterectomy, but are usually detected and corrected during the time of surgery. If detected after hysterectomy, another intervention is commonly indicated.

4.2.4.7 Early menopause

Patients who have underwent hysterectomy with bilateral salpingo-oophorectomy may develop menopause earlier that the average age of menopause. Also, this may be related to an interruption in blood flow to the ovaries.

5. Conclusions

Total hysterectomy is currently indicated for a variety of gynecological conditions. Therefore, we haven't focus only on cervical cancer, but also we have made general consideration about hysterectomy in other gynecological cancers, taking into account both traditional and modern methods.

In "Cuza-Voda" Obstetrics and Gynecology Clinical Hospital, Iasi, Romania, most gynecologists are trained to perform abdominal hysterectomy. Unfortunately, they resort to the technique that they learned twenty-thirty years ago when they were residents. Large incisions result in more adhesions, pain and discomfort that if the intervention is done with a laparoscope.

Laparoscopic hysterectomy was introduced at the same time as laparoscopic cholecystectomy and represented a significant advance in clinical surgery. Patients require a shorter hospital stay, a more rapid convalescence and return to work and normal daily living.

Abdominal and vaginal hysterectomy techniques have become established as classic techniques. There is still no consensus between users and non-users. Unfortunately, after a century of experience, the gynecologists have no clear indications of the optimal method to be performed in different situations. Laparoscopic and abdominal hysterectomy has attracted very few comparative studies until the recent introduction of laparoscopic hysterectomy.

There has been a great interest in laparoscopic surgery regarding hospital stay, quicker recovery time, less blood loss, significant less pain and lower costs.

The goal of robotic and classic gynecologic surgery is to provide excellent patient's outcomes. The decision as to which technique is the best depend upon the risks, benefits of each types of surgery and the women's particular medical problems.

Well-designed case control studies are the most commonly used method to study each type of treatment. The goal of randomized clinical trials is to recruit as sufficient number of patients for providing adequate statistical power. But there are several problems including knowledge and surgeon experience with laparoscopic instrumentation in many countries.

Operative procedures should be performed depending on surgeon preference, available treatment options, patient's medical background, female pelvic condition, the average cost per case and other reasons. The reasons for the high costs are varied but frequently poor management systems are often found in many service areas, especially in operating rooms.

The provider who manages his funds for investment in equipments and new projects will be the winner in health care of the following years.

Also, a good communication system should effectively meet the needs of surgeons and patient's wishes. The training of residents and physician will be positively impacted as well.

Finally, the number of surgeons performing robotic surgery is growing as the technique has proven to be a far less difficult hysterectomy procedure than a traditional abdominal hysterectomy. This procedure does everything that a traditional abdominal hysterectomy would do but recovery time, hospital stay, complications and infection after a laparoscopic procedure are significantly reduced.

However, the robotic surgery allows the surgeon more precision, dexterity and control along with better view of the structures of the pelvis. Also, many of the risks have been eliminated by technological advances, therefore more women choosing robotic-assisted surgery instead of traditional "open" hysterectomy.

In contrast, the robotic system cannot make decisions nor can it performed any type of regulated and controlled movements without the surgeons input.

Finally, we can conclude that robotic surgery offers all the benefits of laparoscopic surgery along with increased precision and effectiveness, being more precise than conventional surgery, giving a reduced tissue trauma, a less use of pain medication and a quick return to normal activities for the patient.

6. References

Ardern, D.W.; Atkinson, R.D., Fenton, J.A. (2002), Perioperative use of estrogen continuing medications and deep vein thrombosis - a national survey, *N Z Med J*, vol 115 (1157): U26; ISSN: 1175-87-16

Basil, J. & Pavelka, J. (2011). Robotic gynecologic surgery, In: *3rd edition Atlas of Pelvic Anatomy and Gynecologic Surgery,* Baggish, M.S. & Karram, M.M. (Eds), Elsevier Saunders, pp.1327-1334, ISBN: 978-1-4160-5909-7.

Baggish, M.S. & Schellhas, H.F. (2011). Radical hysterectomy, In: *3rd edition Atlas of Pelvic Anatomy and Gynecologic Surgery,* Baggish M.S. & Karram, M.M., pp. 241-259, ISBN: 978-1-4160-5909-7.

Benedetti Panici, P.; Basile, S., Maneschi, F. (2008). Systematic pelvic lymphadenectomy vs no lymphadenectomy in early stage endometrial carcinoma: randomized clinical trial, *J Natl Cancer Inst*, Vol 100, 23, pp.1707-1716.

Benedetti Panici, P.; di Donato, V., Plotti, F., Basile, S., Bellati, F. (2009). Role of lympadenectomy in gynaecologic cancers, In: In: *Textbook of Gynaecological Oncology* Ayhan, A.; Gultekin, M. & Dursun, P. (Eds), Güneş Publishing, pp. 252-256, ISBN: 978-975-277-267-0.

Beste, T.M.; Nelson, K.H.; Daucher, J.A. (2005). Total Laparoscopic Hysterectomy Utilizing a Robotic Surgical System, *Journal of the Society of Laparoendoscopic Surgeons,* Vol. 9, pp. 13–15, ISSN 1086-8089.

Breda, G.; Nakada, S.Y.; Rassweiler, J.J. (2001). Future developments and perspectives in laparoscopy, *Eur Urol,* Vol. 40, No. 1, pp.84–91, ISSN: 0302-2838.

Cadiere, G.B.; Himpens, J.; Germay, O. (2001). Feasibility of robotic laparoscopic surgery: 146 cases, *World J Surg,* Vol. 25, No. 11, pp.1467–1477, ISSN (printed): 0364-2313. ISSN (electronic): 1432-2323.

Carlson, K.J.; Miller, B.A.; & Fowler, F.J. Jr. (1994). The Maine Women's Health Study: I. Outcomes of hysterectomy, *Obstet Gynecol,* Vol. 83, pp. 556, ISSN: 0368-2315.

Chitwood, W.R.; Nifong L.W.; Chapman W.H. (2001). Robotic surgical training in an academic institution, *Ann Surg,* Vol. 234, No. 4, pp. 475–484, ISSN: 0003-4932. Online ISSN: 1528-1140

Degueldre, M., Vandromme, J., Huong, P.T., Cadiere, G.B. (2000). Robotically assisted laparoscopic microsurgical tubal reanastomosis: a feasibility study, *Fertil Steril,* Vol. 4, No. 5, pp. 1020–1023, ISSN (printed): 0015-0282. ISSN (electronic): 1556-5653

Diaz-Arrastia, C.; Jurnalov, C.; Gomez, G.; Townsend, C. (2002). Laparoscopic hysterectomy using a computer-enhanced surgical robot, *Surg Endosc,* Vol. 16, No. 9, pp. 271–1273, ISSN 0930-2794

Frumovitz, M.; dos Reis, R., Sun, C.C. (2007). Comparison of total laparoscopic and abdominal radical hysterectomy for patients with early stage cervical cancer, *Obstet Gynecol,* Vol. 110, pp. 96-102., ISSN: 0368-2315.

Harris, WJ. (1997), Complications of hysterectomy. *Clin Obstet Gynecol,* 40, 928-938, ISSN: 0009-9201.

Jhingran, A. & Levenback, C. (2007). Malignant disease of the cervix. Microinvasive and invasive cancers, In: *5th Comprehensive gynecology,* Katz, V.L.; Lentz, G.M.; Lobo, R.A.; Gershenson, D.M., pp. 759-781, Mosby, Elsevier, ISBN: 978-0-323-02951-3. Philadelphia PA.

Kim,Y.T. (2007).Robotic radical hysterectomy with pelvic lymphadenectomy for cervical carcinoma: a pilot study, *Gynecol Oncol,* Vol. 105, pp. 176-180, ISSN: 0090-8258.

Leblanc, E.; Querleu, D., Narducci, F., Samouelian, V., Boulanger, L., Ferron, G. (2009). Laparoscopic surgeries in gynecological oncology, In: *Textbook of Gynaecological*

Oncology Ayhan, A.; Gultekin, M. & Dursun, P. (Eds), Güneş Publishing, pp. 270-277, ISBN: 978-975-277-267-0.

Li, G.; Yan, X.; Shang, H. (2007). A comparison of laparoscopic radical hysterectomy and pelvic lymphadenectomy and laparotomy in the treatment of Ib-IIa cervical cancer, *Gynecol Oncol* Vol. 105, pp. 176-180, ISSN: 0090-8258.

Magrina, J.J.; Kho, R.M., Weaver, A.L., Montero, R.P., Magtibay, P.M. (2008). Robotic radical hysterectomy: comparison with laparoscopy and laparotomy, *Gynecol Oncol,* Vol. 109, pp.86-91, ISSN: 0090-8258.

Markovska, J. & Grabowski, J. (2009). Borderline tumors of the ovary (ovarian tumors of low malignant potential) In: *Textbook of Gynaecological Oncology* Ayhan, A.; Gultekin, M. & Dursun, P. (Eds), Güneş Publishing, pp. 194-196, ISBN: 978-975-277-267-0.

Martinez, A. & Ramirez, T.P (2009). Techniques for abdominal radical hysterectomy, In: *Textbook of Gynaecological Oncology,* Ayhan, A.; Gultekin, M. & Dursun, P. (Eds), Güneş Publishing, pp. 286-289, ISBN: 978-975-277-267-0.

Meeks, G.R. & Harris, R.L. (1997). Surgical approach to hysterectomy: abdominal, laparoscopy-assisted, or vaginal, *Clin Obstet Gynecol,* Vol. 40, pp.886, ISSN: 0009-9201. Online ISSN: 1532-5520.

Mendivil, A. & Boggess, J.F. (2009). Robotic surgeries in gynaecologic oncology, In: *Textbook of Gynaecological Oncology,* Ayhan, A.; Gultekin, M. & Dursun, P. (Eds), Güneş Publishing, pp. 278-281, ISBN: 978-975-277-267-0.

Reich, H. (2011). Laparoscopic hysterectomy; www.adlap.com/PDF/hysto.pdf.

Rhodes, J.C.; Kjerulff, K.H.; Langenberg, P.W.; Guzinski, G.M. (1999). Hysterectomy and sexual functioning, *JAMA, V*ol. 282, pp.1934, Print ISSN: 0098-7484. Online ISSN: 1538-3598.

Scott, J.R.; di Saia, P.J.; Hammond, C.B. & Spellacy, N.J.N (Eds) (1999). In: *8th Danforth's Obstetrics and Gynecology,* Lippincott Williams Wilkins, ISBN: 0-7817-1206-8. Philadelphia PA.

Sert, B. & Abeler, V. (2007). Robotic radical hysterectomy in early stage cervical carcinoma patients, comparing results with total laparoscopic radical hysterectomy cases. The future is now? *Int J Med Robot,* 3 (3): 224-228.

Sharp, H.T. (1999). Endoscopic surgery, In: *Danforth's Obstetrics & Gynecology, 8th edition,* Scott, R.J., di Saia, J.P., Hammond, B.C., Spellacy, W.N. (Eds), Lippincott Williams & Wilkins, pp. 737-749 , ISBN: 07817-1206-8.

Stovall, T.G. & Mann, W.J. (2011). Patient information: Abdominal hysterectomy, In: *Up-to-date,* version 19.2

Tang, A. & Obermair, A. (2009). Technique of Laparoscopic Radical Hysterectomy and Comparison of Three Techniques: Laparotomy, Laparoscopy and Robotics, In: *Textbook of Gynaecological Oncology,* Ayhan, A.; Gultekin, M. & Dursun, P. (Eds), Güneş Publishing, pp. 293-295, ISBN: 978-975-277-267-0

4

The Role of Modified Radical Hysterectomy in Endometrial Carcinoma

Masamichi Hiura and Takayoshi Nogawa
Shikoku Cancer Center,
Japan

1. Introduction

Improvement of the treatment results in patients with endometrial carcinoma has been achieved by a multidisciplinary approach including surgery, chemotherapy and radiotherapy, similar to the case for many other carcinomas. Although total hysterectomy/bilateral salpingo-oophorectomy (TH/BSO), pelvic and para-aortic lymphadenectomy and peritoneal cytology are often required, cases with early carcinomas predominate among cases of endometrial carcinoma, and TH/BSO alone is sufficient to achieve a favorable prognosis in such cases. The recommended surgical procedure for the staging of a patient with endometrial carcinoma clinically confined to the fundal portion of the uterus includes peritoneal cytology and TH/BSO with pelvic and para-aortic lymphadenectomy (National Comprehensive Cancer Network, 2011). For operable patients with cervical involvement, peritoneal cytology and radical hysterectomy/bilateral salpingo-oophorectomy with pelvic and para-aortic lymphadenectomy should be considered. However, radical hysterectomy always has a major adverse effect with dysuria. Improvement of the treatment results and quality of life (QOL) can also be expected from modified radical hysterectomy performed in appropriately selected patients. One of the advantages of modified radical hysterectomy is that it can be switched from radical hysterectomy in high-risk patients in terms of the age, obesity and presence of medical complications. For operable patients with intra-abdominal disease, surgical procedure includes peritoneal cytology, TH/BSO with pelvic and para-aortic lymphadenectomy, and maximal debulking. The pathologic information obtained also provides an optimal basis for the selection of adjuvant therapy. Therefore, complete surgical staging including pathologic and prognostic data on which to base decisions regarding adjuvant therapy should be required for all patients who do not have medical or technical contraindication to lymphadenectomy.

There is no definitive data regarding the effectiveness of adjuvant chemotherapy in patients with uterine confined or intra-abdominal disease. The role of adjuvant chemotherapy in invasive high-grade tumor confined to the uterine body is the subject of current studies. Postoperative radiotherapy for patients with intermediate risk or high risk early stage endometrial carcinoma has been performed to prevent locoregional recurrence, however it did not increase overall survival (Creutzberg et al., 2000; Keys et al., 2004; Blake et al., 2008; Nout et al., 2010). Despite a traditional use of adjuvant radiotherapy, stage I/II patients with high risk factors may have a compromised survival due to extrapelvic metastatic disease, suggesting the need for effective systemic adjuvant therapy. Adjuvant chemotherapy may reduce the rate of distant recurrence in endometrial carcinoma. Therefore, it is reasonable to consider adjuvant chemotherapy for high risk endometrial carcinoma. Abdominal total hysterectomy is a basic gynecological surgical technique that beginners should try and master, and it is generally an extrafascial procedure. After obtaining full mastery over total hysterectomy, gynecologists in training should proceed to modified radical type II hysterectomy (Bidus & Elkas, 2007; Jones. 2008; Randall et al., 2009), a procedure positioned in between total hysterectomy and radical hysterectomy, with or without lymphadenectomy This form of surgery is indicated for stage Ia1-Ia2 uterine cervical carcinoma and stage Ib-Ic, IIa, and IIb (with slight infiltration of the cervical stroma) endometrial carcinoma. Complications of this procedure include bleeding and damage to the intestines, ureter and bladder. Due caution is necessary to avoid these complications or organ injuries, and it is important to extirpate the uterus together with the cardinal ligaments and to remove the vaginal wall with an extra 1.5-2.0 cm margin. There is uncertainty as to whether modified radical hysterectomy in high-risk endometrial carcinoma reduces locoregional recurrence. So, we performed modified radical type II hysterectomy including systematic pelvic and para-aortic lymphadenectomy in 284 stage I-IV endometrial carcinomas to prevent locoregional recurrence, patients with high risk factors (stages IC/II/III/IV) were treated by adjuvant chemotherapy.

The purpose of this study is to assess the role of modified radical hysterectomy in endometrial carcinoma, and identify the multivariate independent recurrence risk factors during past 10 years.

2. Modified radical hysterectomy (Hiura & Nogawa, 2011)

In our method of modified radical type II hysterectomy, the anterior procedure following development of the paravesical and pararectal spaces involves retraction of the ureter in a lateral direction after dissecting the anterior layer of the vesicouterine ligament. However, the posterior layer of the vesicouterine ligament is not seprated. As the posterior procedure, the cardinal ligament is clamped en bloc with the posterior layer of the vesicouterine ligament and the deep layer of the sacrouterine ligament after dissecting the sacrouterine ligament, and the vaginal wall is resected with an extra 1.5-2.0 cm margin. The uterus is resected by dividing as much as possible the anterior uterine support and vaginal wall from the cervix. Another characteristic of this technique is that more of the cardinal ligament is resected compared with that in a total hysterectomy.

2.1 Preoperative tests

1. Hemoglobin, blood type, irregular antibody screening, serum chemistry, tests for infections, blood coagulation profile, blood glucose, and urinalysis.
2. Electrocardiography, lung function testing, and plain chest radiography.
3. Cervical cytology and endometrial cytology.
4. Magnetic resonance imaging (MRI), Computed tomography (CT), and Positron emission tomography-computed tomography (PET-CT): Patients with endometrial carcinoma should be examined for muscular infiltration by contrast-enhanced MRI.

Contrast-enhanced CT is useful for evaluation of lymph node metastasis. PET-CT is also used for whole-body scanning when distant metastasis is suspected.

2.2 Informed consent

Informed consent is an extremely important element in establishing a trust relationship with the patient and her family. At our outpatient clinic, patients are provided with a full explanation at the time of their initial visits to the hospital, at the end of the examinations, and at the time of admission. Definitive written consent carrying the signature of the patient is obtained at the time of admission of the patient after following our institutional procedures in respect of giving information about the surgery and obtaining consent in the presence of the patient's family and a nurse. This is that part of a research protocol.

2.3 Practical features of modified radical hysterectomy

The operator basically stands on the left side, and the assistant on the right side of the patient. Intrapelvic procedures are easier from the left side for a right-handed operator. At laparotomy, the operator should wear a cotton glove on the left hand to avoid slippage when gently displacing and pulling the intestinal tract or the peritoneum. It is important for successful peritoneal procedures to obtain an adequate operative field, and incision of the abdominal wall allowing a 1-2 cm margin is an important point to this end. At our institution, in order to minimize postoperative pain, this surgery is performed under general anesthesia combined with epidural anesthesia, and an electric knife is used for every cutting procedure except for the hypogastric median skin incision. After laparotomy, the presence/absence of intraperitoneal lesions is examined by palpation and visual inspection, and the intraperitoneal site subject to surgical manipulation is observed carefully with the use of a lateral blades laparotomy retractor. With a full understanding of the positional relationships among the uterus, adnexa, intestinal tract and bladder, the operator elevates the small intestine from the minor pelvic cavity to the epigastric region, and compresses the left, right and central parts with gauze towels to prevent slippage of the small intestine. Then, a upper blade is set at the center to allow a sufficient operative field, and the surgical procedures are begun on the right side, proceeding thereafter to the left side. A flow-chart is given to illustrate the patient selection of modified radical hysterectomy for endometrial carcinoma (Fig. 1).

2.3.1 Holding the uterus

The uterus, adnexa and adjacent organs are palpated to confirm their positional relationships, and the degree of fixation and mobility. The round ligaments of the uterus, oviducts and ligaments of the ovary are clamped bilaterally with two long and straight Kocher forceps. The clamps are fixed firmly with gauze, and pulled to allow initiation of the manipulations from the right side.

2.3.2 Clamping, cutting and ligation of the infundibulopelvic ligament

To prevent ureteral injury, the infundibulopelvic ligament is clamped with two long and straight Kocher forceps after confirming the course of the ureter, while a short Kocher

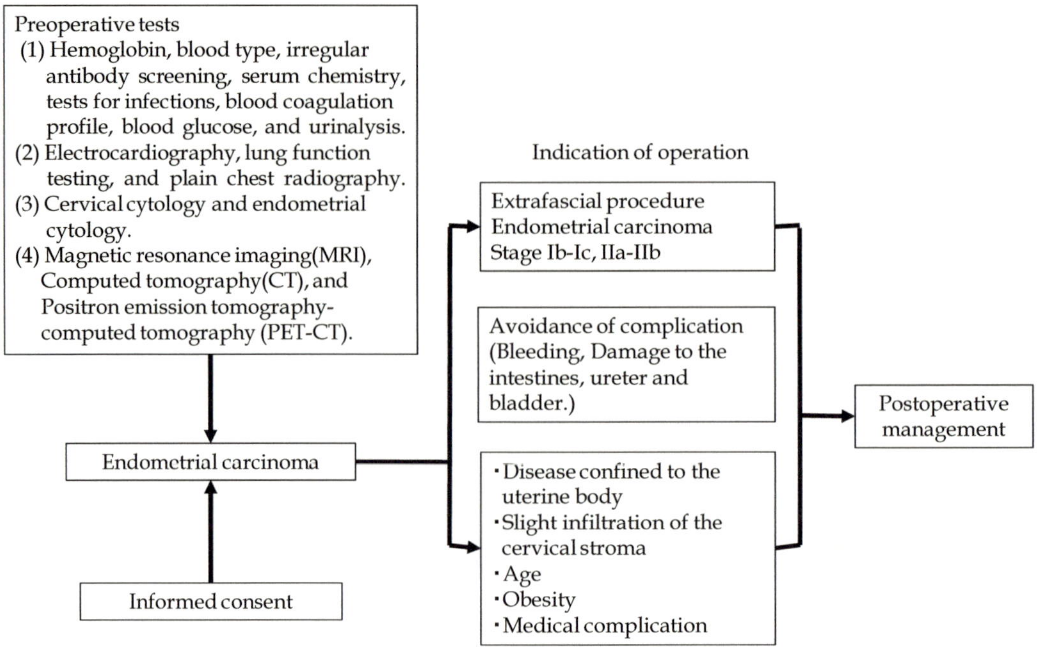

Fig. 1. Flow-chart of the patient selection for modified radical hysterectomy in endometrial carcinoma.

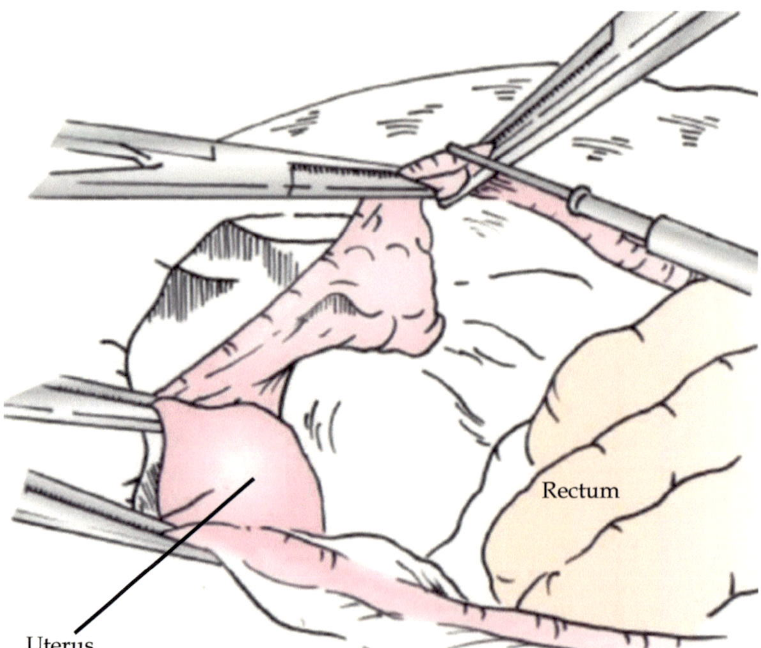

Fig. 2. Clamping, cutting and ligation of the infundibulopelvic ligament.

forceps is set for the infundibulopelvic ligament to be preserved in order to prevent slippage. The infundibulopelvic ligament is then cut and ligated with 1-0 silk suture to be held, and pulled (Fig. 2). At this point, ureteral injury can be avoided if the infundibulopelvic ligament is clamped with a long and straight Kocher forceps while elevating the infundibulopelvic ligament with forceps with some distance maintained from the ureter. Opening the broad ligament close to the round ligament of the uterus makes the subsequent processing of the round ligament easier. Because there is the possibility of hydrosalpinx and fallopian tube cancer, the mesosalpinx on the fallopian tube side should be coagulated, incised and resected with an electric knife.

2.3.3 Clamping, cutting and ligation of the round ligament of the uterus

The round ligament of the uterus is clamped, cut, ligated with 1-0 silk suture, and pulled, while setting two long and straight Kocher forceps at a position 2/3 lateral to the uterus (Fig. 3). The uterus is pulled upward, detached and incised with an electric knife from the anterior lobe of the broad ligament toward the peritoneum of the vesicouterine pouch. Because webby thin and sparse connective tissue appears on the inner side of the peritoneum, manipulation of the electric knife as though using Cooper scissors is necessary for the detachment procedure. When incising the bladder peritoneum, approximating too close to the bladder would cause bleeding, therefore, caution is required.

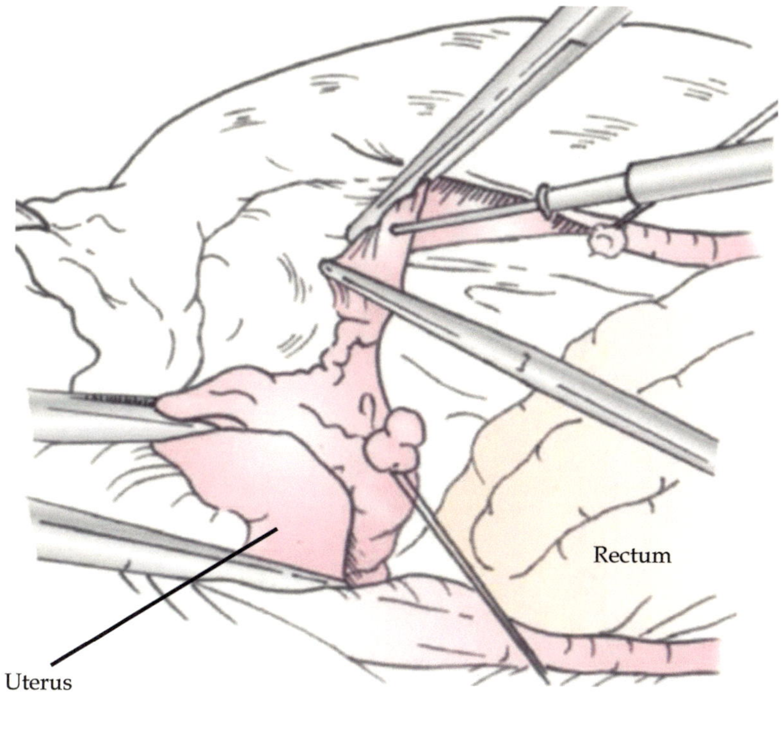

Fig. 3. Clamping, cutting and ligation of the round ligament of the uterus.

2.3.4 Development of the pararectal and paravesical spaces (in cases of pelvic lymphadenectomy)

While the uterus is pulled left anteriorly, the assistant clamps and pulls the posterior lobe of the broad ligament with the straight Pean forceps to confirm the course of the ureter. The pararectal space in the pelvic floor is displaced in a left inguinal direction with a side plate under the course of the ureter attached to the posterior lobe of the broad ligament, and simultaneously, the non-resistive sparse connective tissue is displaced in 1-2 installments with Cooper scissors toward 180-degree opposite side. By this procedure, the pararectal space can be developed easily (Fig. 4). If there is resistance, the internal iliac artery may be compressed, and forced development may cause bleeding. Beginners should be particularly cautious about this point. Next, when the curved Pean forceps set for the bladder peritoneum are pulled, a funicular structure can be found in the connective tissue running toward the paravesical space. This structure is the paraumbilical ligament. When non-resistive sparse connective tissue is expanded with a side plate and Cooper scissors on the right and left side of the paraumbilical ligament, the paravesical space appears (Fig. 5). If a vascular tape is set for the paraumbilical ligament and fixed with a short Kocher forceps, subsequent manipulations become easier. Development of the pararectal and paravesical spaces should be done by a side plate and Cooper scissors. Displacing non-resistive sparse connective tissue in 1-2 installments would allow easy development. If there is resistance, the direction may be wrong, and should therefore be rechecked. The procedural steps for pelvic lymphadenectomy are skipped in this paper.

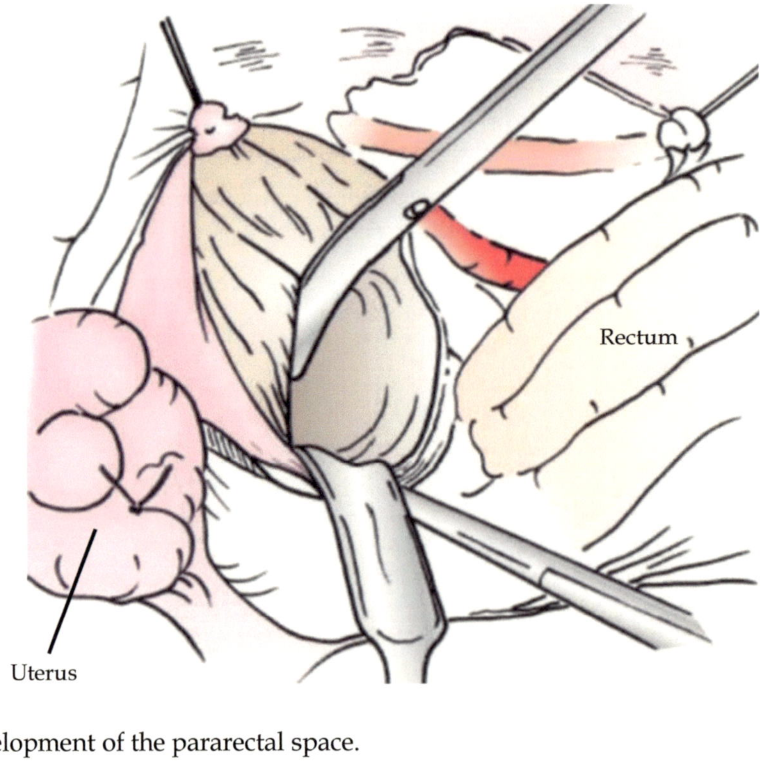

Fig. 4. Development of the pararectal space.

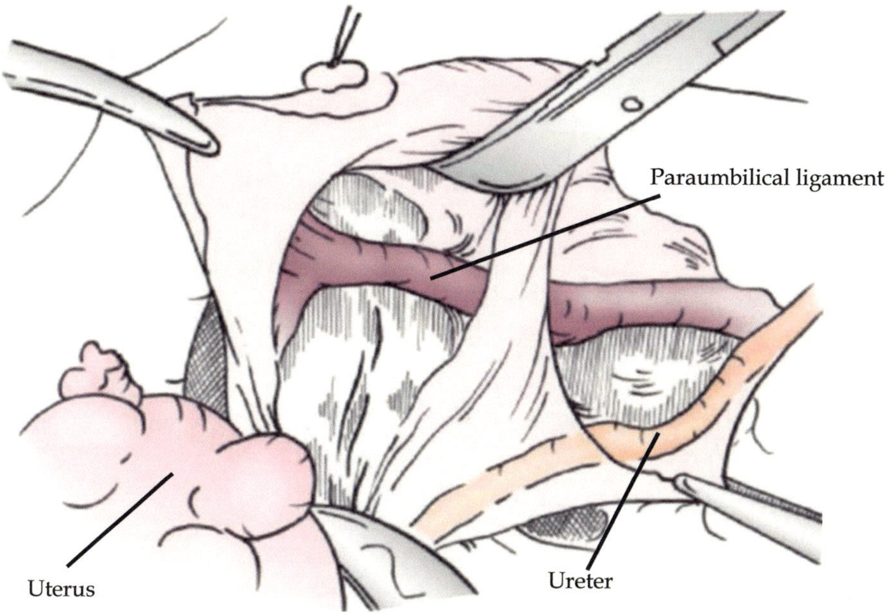

Fig. 5. Development of the paravesical space.

2.3.5 Detachment of the ureter and cutting of the posterior lobe of the broad ligament

After confirming the course of the ureter while pulling the posterior lobe of the broad ligament clamped with the straight Pean forceps, the ureter is isolated from the uterus by detaching it with Cooper scissors up to the vicinity of the right uterine artery. The knack for easier isolation of the ureter from the posterior lobe of the broad ligament involves detachment of the ureter with Cooper scissors first at an angle perpendicular to the course of the ureter and then along the course of the ureter (Fig. 6). Then, to separate the ureter from the uterus, the ureter is displaced laterally with a side plate, and the posterior lobe of the broad ligament is detached with an electric knife toward the vicinity of the sacrouterine ligament and the superficial layer, and then cut and developed. We commonly use a side plate because this surgical instrument is very useful for expansion of the operative field if the direction is properly determined on a side plate.

2.3.6 Cutting of the sacrouterine ligament and opening of the Douglas' pouch

While the assistant is pulling the uterus to make a 90-degree angle to the right sacrouterine ligament, the rectum and right pelvic peritoneum are tensed with the left hand, and the superficial layer of the right sacrouterine ligament is cut with an electric knife without ligation (Fig. 7).Then, while the assistant is pulling the uterus, the rectum is tensed with the left hand, and the Douglas' pouch is incised. After incising the thin funicular sparse

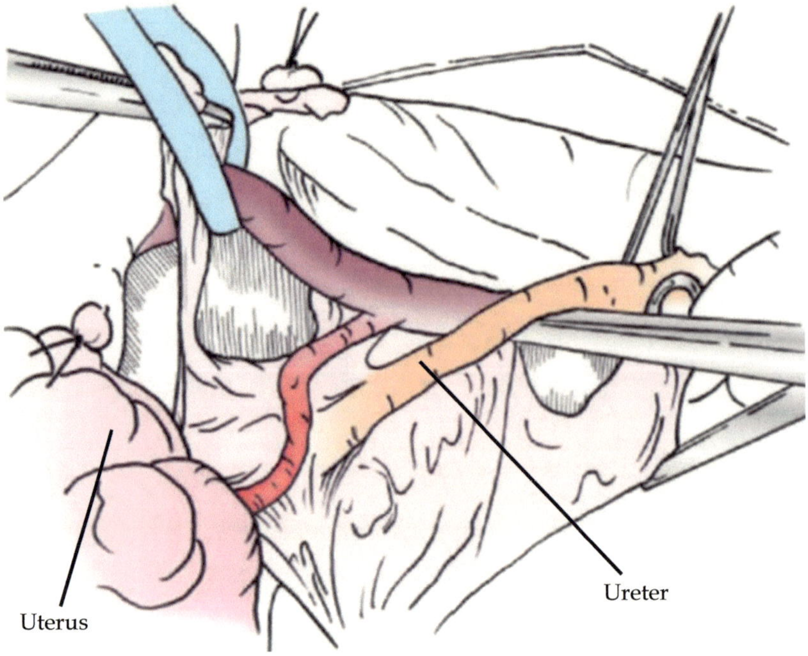

Fig. 6. Detachment of the ureter.

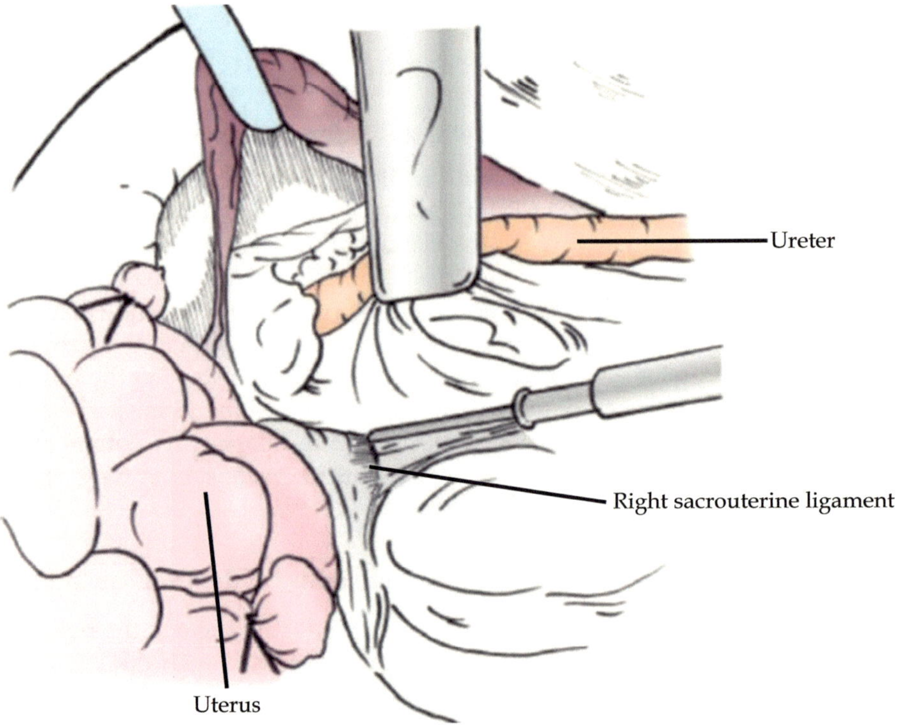

Fig. 7. Cutting of the sacrouterine ligament.

connective tissue with an electric knife, the pouch opens spontaneously (Fig. 8). While avoiding injury to the hypogastric nerve, the deep layer of the sacrouterine ligament is detached and cut. When gauze is placed between the rectum and the vaginal wall and displaced downward with the fingers, the rectum can be detached easily from the vaginal wall. At this time, for a better result, the superficial layer and the posterior layer of the thin and funicular sacrouterine ligament, firmly tensed with the hand wearing a cotton glove to avoid slippage of the rectum and right pelvic peritoneum, should be incised little by little.

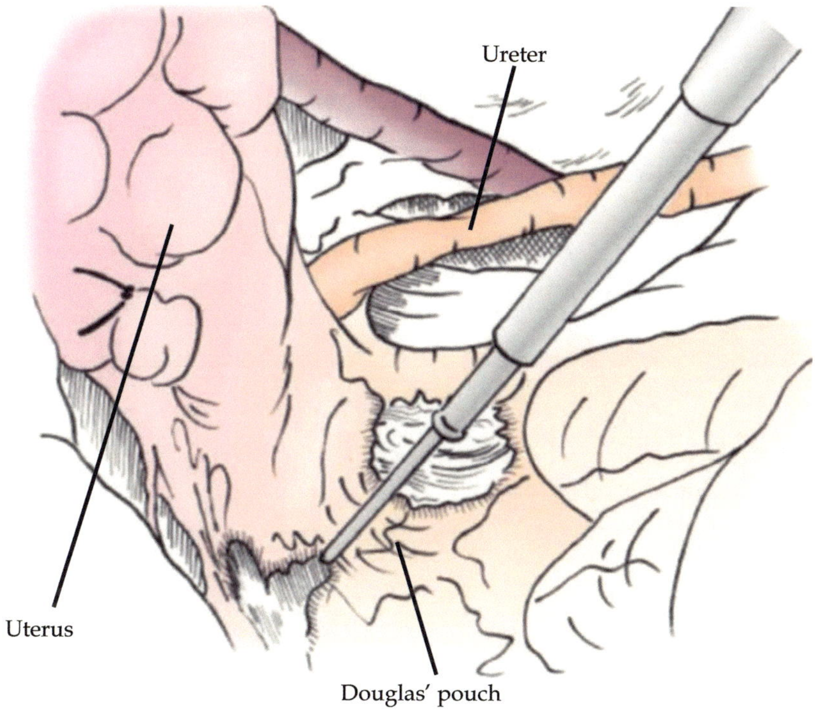

Fig. 8. Opening of the Douglas' pouch.

2.3.7 Detachment of the bladder

After similar manipulations on the left side, the operation proceeds to the process of detachment of the bladder. The uterus is elevated upward, and the positional relationship between the uterine cervix and the bladder is confirmed by palpation. Then, a small incision is made in the tensed vesicouterine pouch with an electric knife while the bladder peritoneum is elevated with the long and straight Pean forceps. This procedure causes the appearance of the bladder wall, the lustrous muscular layer of the uterine cervix, and the webby sparse connective tissue (Fig. 9).Gauze is placed in these structures, and the bladder is displaced and detached sufficiently with the gauze while manipulating it as though rolling it over downward with a side plate and Cooper scissors (Fig. 10). The bladder is detached and isolated at the center, and thereafter the sparse connective tissues on the left and right sides are detached with the Cooper scissors while pushing laterally. This procedure allows easy detachment of the bladder with scarcely any bleeding. If the sparse connective tissue on the lateral side of the uterus is sufficiently cut with an electric knife up

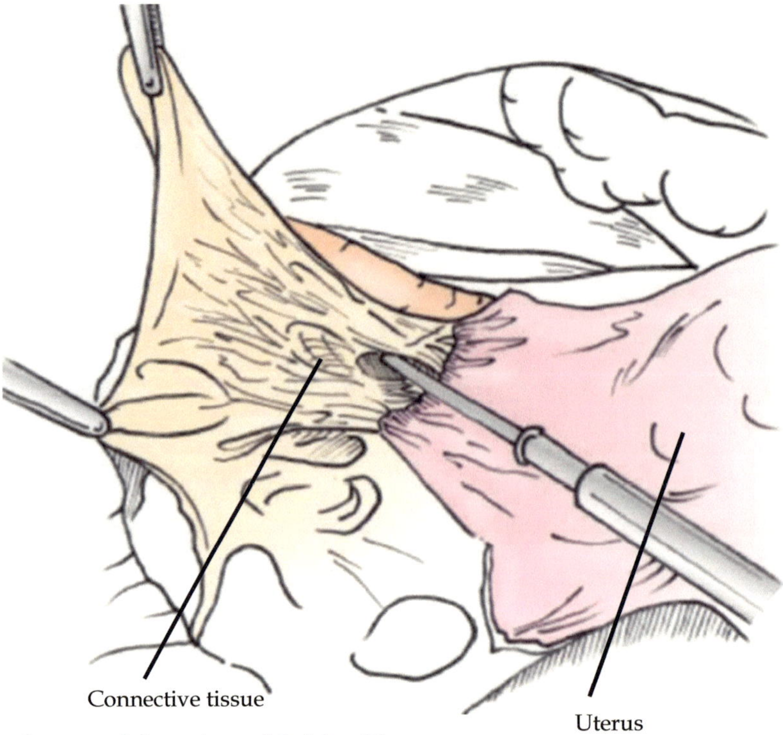

Fig. 9. Detachment of the urinary bladder (1)

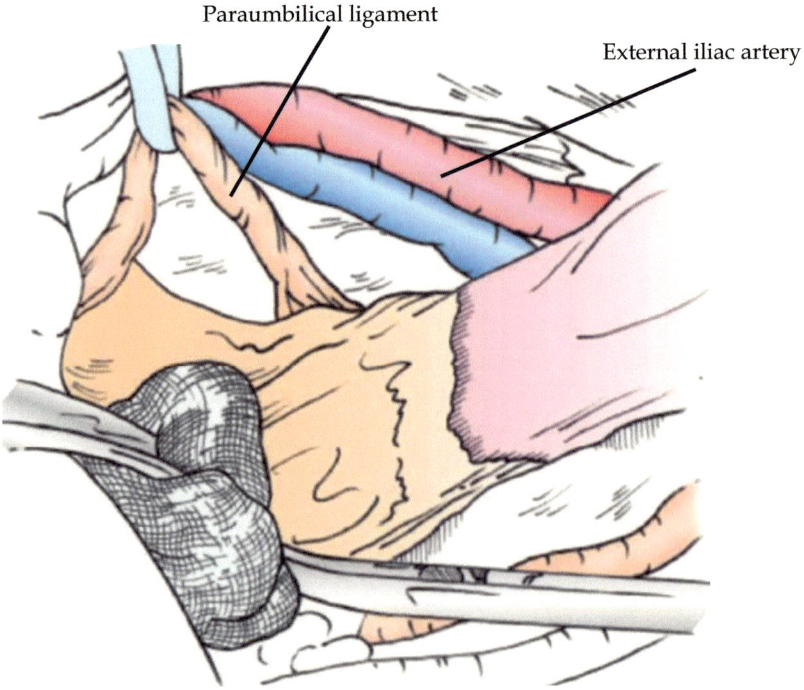

Fig. 10. Detachment of the urinary bladder

to the vicinity of the uterine artery when detaching the bladder, it will facilitate the subsequent procedure involving the anterior layer of the vesicouterine ligament. Bleeding occurring during detachment of the bladder disturbs localization of the vesicouterine pouch, often resulting in injury to the muscular layer of the uterine cervix or the muscular layer of the bladder. Detachment of the uterus from the bladder is extremely important and requires good manipulation of the non-resistive part with gauze, a side plate, and Cooper scissors. The injured muscular layer of the bladder, if any, should be sutured with Surgisorb 3.0.

2.3.8 Clamping, cutting, and ligation of the uterine artery

When adipose tissue in the periphery of the paraumbilical ligament is removed, the vesical artery, and then the uterine artery, become visible. The uterine artery bifurcates into the ascending and descending branches after going beyond the ureter and entering the uterus. To preserve the feeding vessels distributed over the ureter, the main trunk of the uterine artery before the bifurcation beyond the ureter should be cut (Fig. 11).

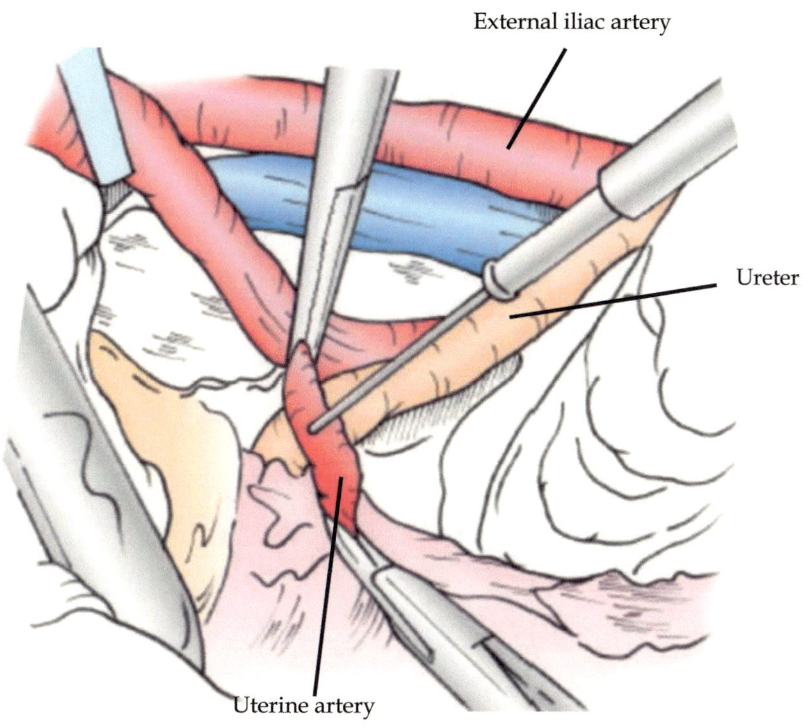

Fig. 11. Clamping, cutting, and ligation of the uterine artery

2.3.9 Dissection of the anterior layer of the vesicouterine ligament

While pulling the ureter with a ureteral retractor, the orifice portion of the ureter is displaced laterally with Cooper scissors. Then, a ureteral tunnel is formed by further lateral manipulation of Cooper scissors 2-3 times in a direction parallel to the course of the ureter while clamping the anterior layer of the vesicouterine ligament with forceps (Fig. 12).

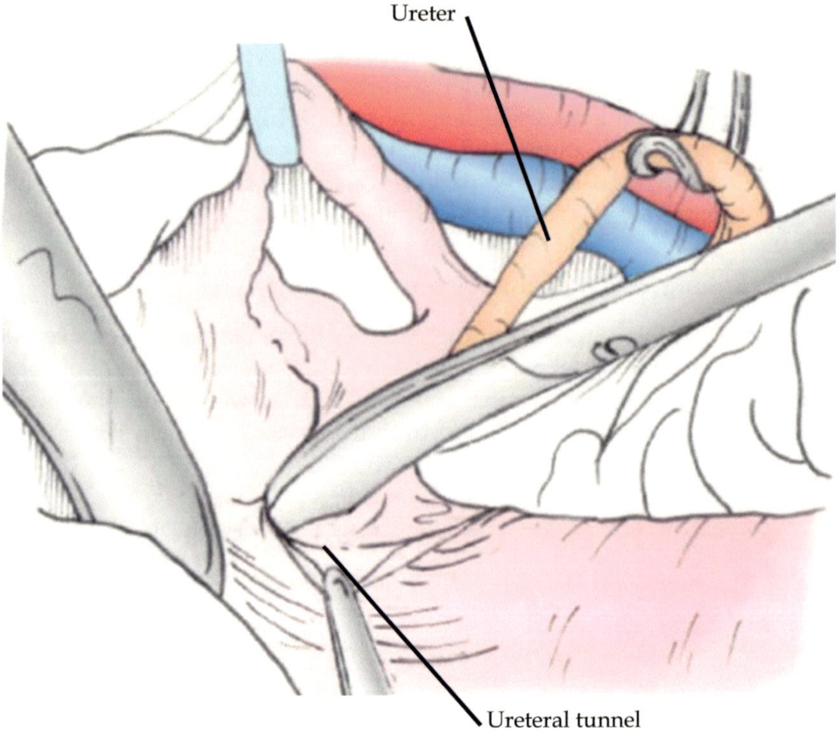

Fig. 12. Formation of a ureter tunnel.

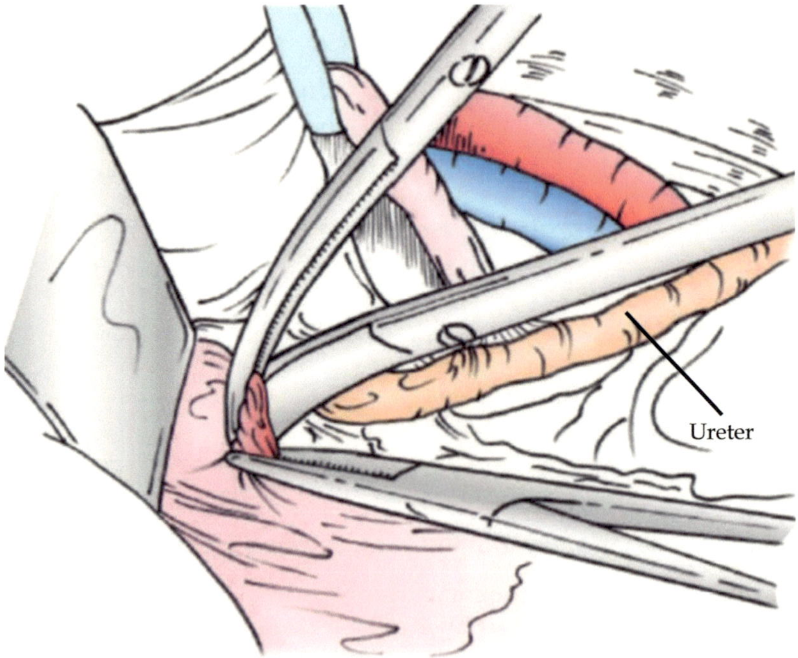

Fig. 13. Clamping, cutting and ligation of the anterior layer of the vesicouterine ligament.

Formation of a ureteral tunnel is smooth if the ureter is displaced laterally in parallel to the course of the ureter with Cooper scissors, making use of the small space made by elevation of the anterior layer of the vesicouterine ligament with tweezers. Then, while holding the laterally displaced ureter in the ureteral tunnel with Cooper scissors, the anterior layer of the vesicouterine ligament is clamped with Kelly forceps necessarily set perpendicular to the uterine axis (Fig. 13). Then, the anterior layer of the vesicouterine ligament on the uterine side is clamped with a short and straight Kocher forceps. At this time, it is necessary to exercise caution against clamping of the ureter. Then, the anterior layer of the vesicouterine ligament on the uterine side is clamped with a short and Kocher forceps and cut with an electric knife. A single procedure is usually adequate, but two divided procedures of cutting the anterior layer may be employed if the dissection of the anterior layer is difficult.

2.3.10 Detachment of the ureter in the posterior layer of the vesicouterine ligament

Although the ureter running in the posterior layer of the bladder is exposed, the lower portion of the ureter is adherent to the posterior layer of the vesicouterine ligament with sparse connective tissue. Therefore, the ureter in the posterior layer can be easily isolated from the uterine side if the ureter is displaced laterally with Cooper scissors from above with rolled gauze set in place (Fig. 14). No processing of the posterior layer of the vesicouterine ligament is necessary.

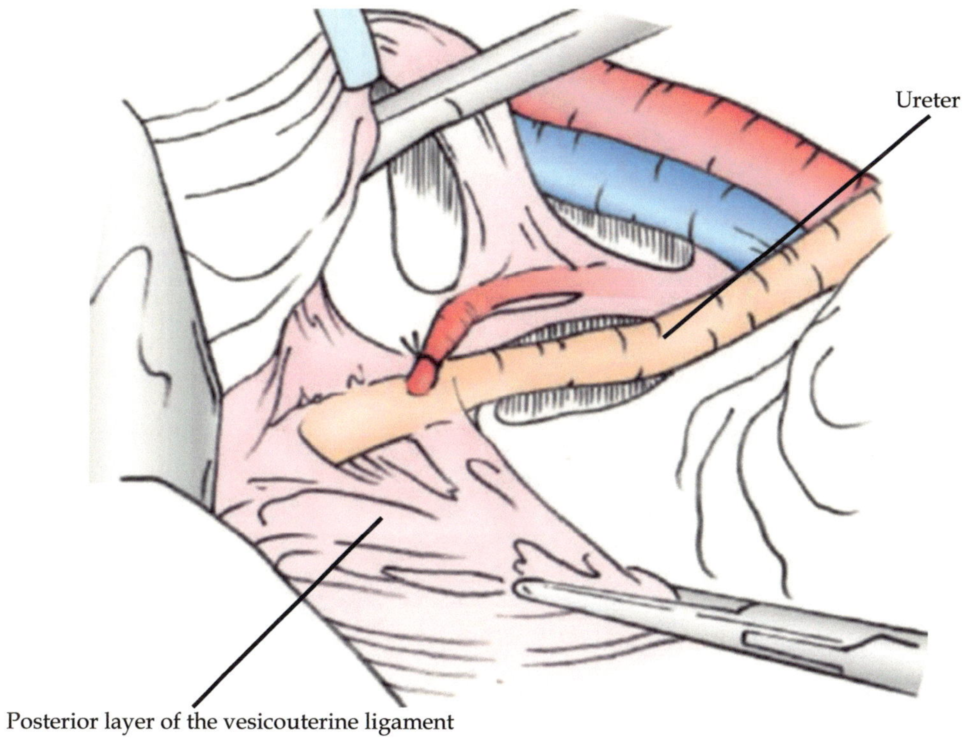

Fig. 14. Detachment of the ureter in the posterior layer of the vesicouterine ligament.

2.3.11 En bloc clamping, cutting and ligation of the posterior layer of the vesicouterine ligament, cardinal ligament and deep layer of the sacrouterine ligament

When the bladder is displaced downward with a bladder retractor, and the uterus is adequately pulled upward, the ureter can be confirmed in a far lower location. After the positional relation among the muscular layer of the uterine cervix, bladder, vaginal wall and the course of the ureter is confirmed by palpation, the posterior layer of the vesicouterine ligament, the cardinal ligament and the deep layer of the sacrouterine ligament are clamped en bloc with the versatile forceps, and a short and straight Kocher forceps is also used on the uterine side to prevent backflow of blood (Fig. 15). To prevent bleeding, the tissues are cut with an electric knife at a site slightly beyond the portion clamped with the versatile forceps to allow a safe margin, and sutured with a needle and #1 silk thread. At this time, the clamping area should be palpated before clamping to ensure that the muscular layer of the uterine cervix is not held with the versatile forceps. Because the ureter is detached sufficiently from the uterine side, a single clamping procedure is adequate to avoid injury to the ureter.

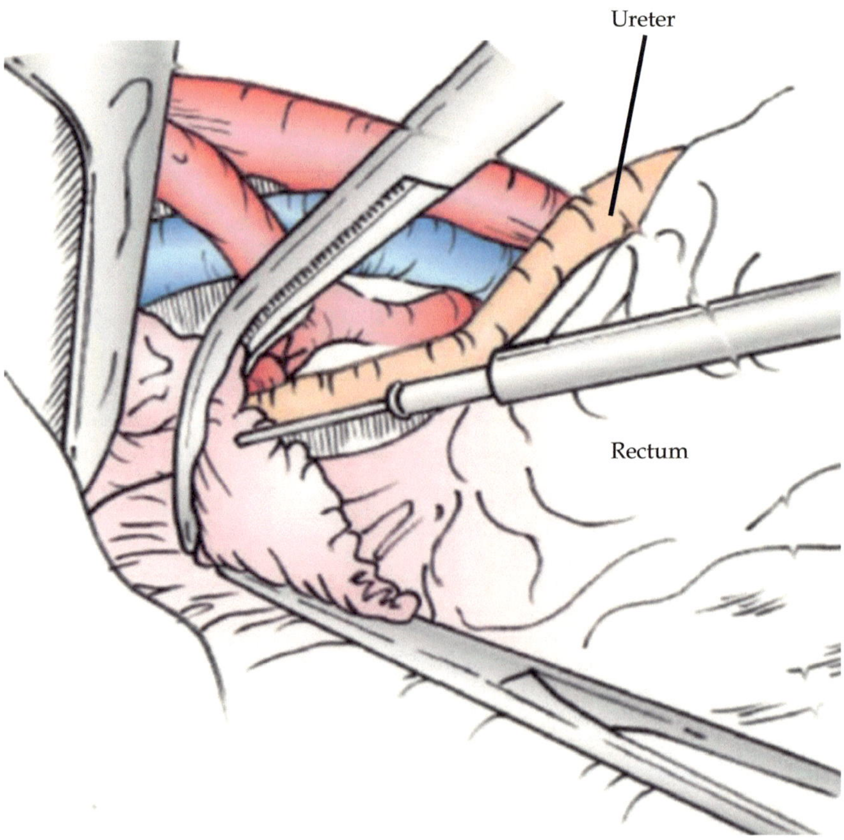

Fig. 15. En bloc clamping, cutting and ligation of the posterior layer of the vesicouterine ligament, cardinal ligament and deep layer of the sacrouterine ligament.

2.3.12 Clamping, cutting, and ligation of the paravaginal connective tissue

Then, the remaining paravaginal connective tissue is clamped with the versatile forceps and cut, while setting the short and straight Kocher forceps on the uterine side. By this procedure, the vaginal canal is completely isolated to allow sufficient resection of the vaginal wall.

2.3.13 Cutting of the vaginal canal and removal of the uterus

After clamping the bilateral cut ends of the vaginal wall with the curved Kocher forceps to avoid slippage, a towel gauze is placed in the Douglas' pouch, and the bladder is displaced downward sufficiently with a bladder retractor. The uterus is then elevated, and the cutting site is confirmed by palpation to avoid cutting into the uterine cervix, and the vaginal wall is clamped with the large and curved Kocher forceps to prevent any escape of endometrial carcinoma tissue (Fig. 16). The vaginal wall in the vaginal convexity is cut with an electric knife, and the inside of the vagina is disinfected with an Isodine cotton swab. After gauze is inserted into the vagina to prevent leakage of intravaginal secretory fluid, the vaginal wall is clamped, held, and pulled with the long and straight Kocher forceps while incising the vaginal wall.

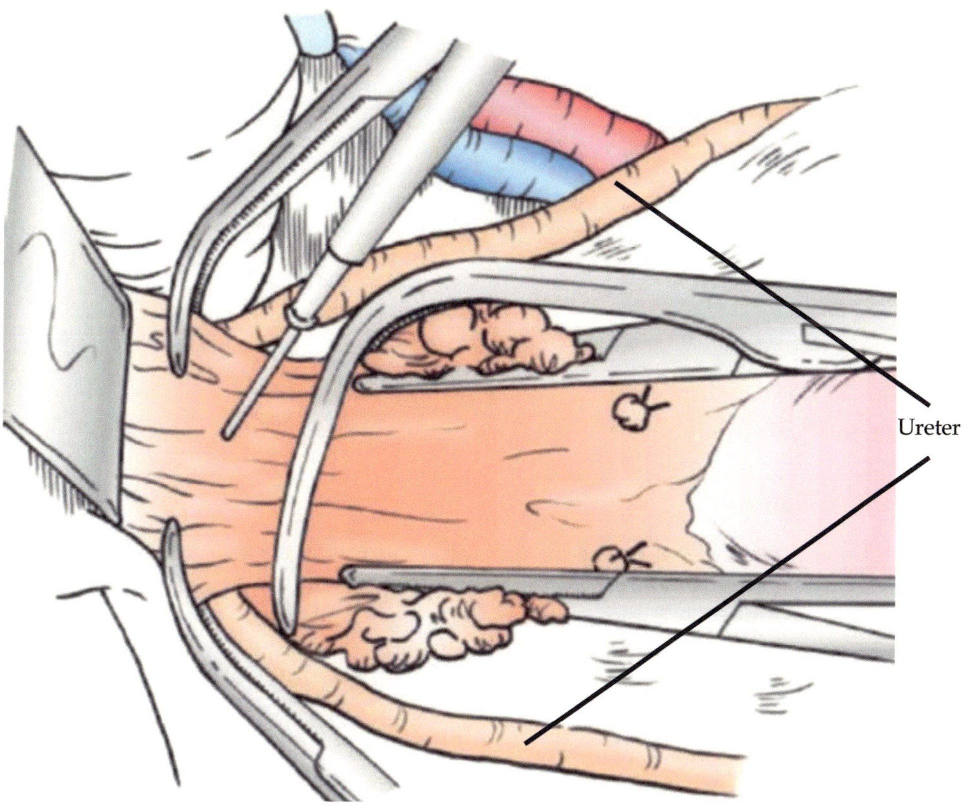

Fig. 16. Cutting of the vaginal canal and removal of the uterus.

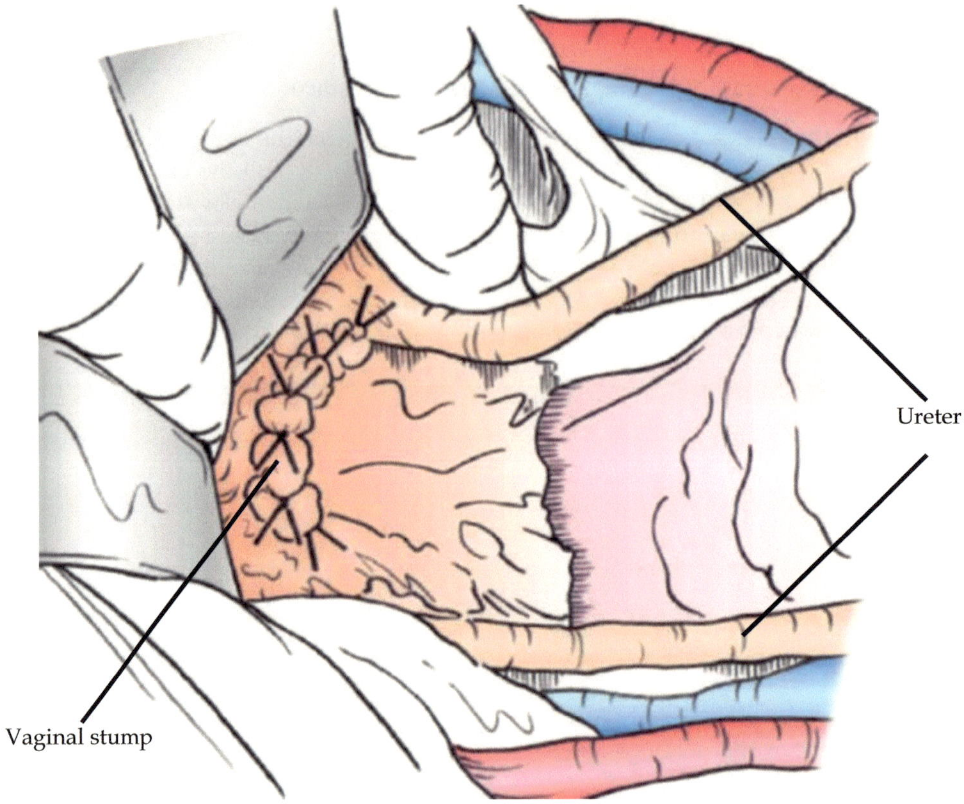

Fig. 17. Vaginal wall suture.

2.3.14 Vaginal wall suture

First, the bilateral vaginal wall cut ends are subjected to simple suture ligation with a blunt needle, 1-0 control release Vicryl, and cut, and the anterior and posterior portions of the vaginal wall are sutured by Z suture and pulled (Fig. 17). Because bleeding is likely to occur from the bilateral cut ends of the vaginal wall, particular caution is required. Taking into consideration prevention of shortening of the vaginal canal and the patient's QOL, including the postoperative sex life in individual cases, the cut ends of the vaginal wall are opened and sutured in a continuous fashion to keep the length of the vagina. When lymphadenectomy is performed, the retroperitoneum should not be sutured to allow for smooth drainage of lymph, and a closed-end drain should be inserted through the abdominal wall and retained in the pelvic floor.

2.3.15 Confirmation of hemostasis and abdominal wall suture

After arrest of bleeding from the posterior aspect of the detached bladder, the cut end suture site on the vaginal wall, en bloc cut ends of the vesicouterine ligament, cardinal ligament, and deep layer of the sacrouterine ligament, the cut end of the sacrouterine ligament, inside the pelvic cavity, and the cut sites is confirmed, double ligation of the bilateral infundibulopelvic ligament and round ligament of the uterus is performed. In cases of bleeding from the connective tissue, Z sutures with 3-0 silk thread are employed, and the simple suture thread of the vaginal cut ends is cut off. The pelvic peritoneum is opened, and Seprafilm® is attached to the bilateral retroperitoneal spaces for preventing adhesion. After putting the rectum back in its original position, the laparotomy incision is closed. The gauze count, including towel gauze, is confirmed by the doctors and nurses before closure of the incision. For closure of the laparotomy incision, the peritoneum is sutured continuously with a 2-0 Surgisorb cutting needle, and the cut ends of the fascia are sutured at 2 or 3 sites by a simple ligation suture with #1 Surgilon. The fascia should be sutured continuously with a #1 Polysorb blunt needle, while simple ligation is carried out at 2 or 3 sites to prevent abdominal wall hernia. The skin is closed by simple ligation suture by the mattress suture technique with 1-0 nylon thread, with the skin edges between the ligations are approximated with a Steri-strip. Finally, the vaginal wall is retracted with a vaginal speculum to remove gauze, and absence of bleeding from the vaginal wall cut ends is confirmed. The operation is ended after the absence of any remaining gauze is confirmed on a plain radiograph taken just before the end of the surgical procedure.

3. Materials and methods

Between December 1987 and December 2002 we performed modified radical type II hysterectomy with bilateral salpingo-oophorectomy including systematic pelvic and para-aortic lymphadenectomy, and peritoneal cytology in 284 endometrial carcinoma patients according to the classification of the International Federation of Gynecology and Obstetrics (stage IA, n=66; stage IB, n=96; stage IC, n=33; stage IIA, n=5; stage IIB, n=20; stage IIIA, n=28; stage IIIC, n=28; and stage IV, n=8, Announcements FIGO stage, 1989) who gave informed consents at our institute. Systematic pelvic and para-aortic lymphadenectomy included complete dissection of lymph nodes from the femoral ring caudally to the lower margin of the renal vessels. No patients had intraabdominal residual lesions after surgery. Other inclusion criteria were as follows: Eastern Cooperative Oncology Group (ECOG) performance status of 0 to 2, age 75 years or younger, normal bone marrow, renal, liver, and cardiac function. The mean age (range) was 56 (26-75) years, with the median follow-up being 70 (24-189) months, and there were 88 and 196 pre- and postmenopausal patients, respectively. Histological examination showed 257 endometrioid adenocarcinomas (grade 1, n=129; grade 2, n=101, grade 3, n=27), 16 adenosqamous carcinomas, 8 serous adenocarcinomas and 3 clear cell adenocarcinomas. The patients with a tumor confined to the uterus (stage IC and II) for intermediate group were treated by 3 courses of CEP (cyclophosphamide 750mg/m^2, epirubicin 50mg/m^2, and cisplatin 75mg/m^2) regimen 3-4 weeks apart and patients with intrapelvic lesions involving adnexa and/or pelvic lymph node (PLN) for high risk group were treated by 5 courses. In addition, 10 courses were given in the patients with extrapelvic lesions involving para-aortic lymph node (PAN) for high risk group. We have no indication for adjuvant radiotherapy in patients with endometrial carcinoma in this protocol. These anti-cancer agents were administered intravenously on Day 1. Univariate analysis for recurrence risk factors was performed by the X^2 test. Recurrence risk factors for endometrial carcinoma ware analyzed for multivariate logistic regression using StatView (SAS Institute Inc.) Version 5.0. P-values of less than 0.05 were considered to be statistically significant.

4. Results and discussion

The overall incidence of retroperitoneal lymph node (RLN) metastasis assessed by systematic pelvic and para-aortic lymphadenectomy was 12.0% (34/284) in Stage I-IV endometrial carcinoma, and incidences of PLN and PAN metastasis were 9.2% (26/284) and 7.4 % (21/284), respectively. However, PAN metastasis rate is 50% (13/26) in patients with PLN metastasis. Thirteen patients (4.6%) had lymph node metastasis in the pelvic region alone, 8 (2.8%) in the para-aortic region alone and 13 (4.6%) in both regions. This low incidence of isolated PAN metastasis was possibly considered due to many early stage I diseases, and para-aortic lymphadenectomy should be performed in high risk patients with intrapelvic extention, for example, PLN metastasis or ovarian metastasis. We are now performing systematic pelvic lymphadenectomy and resect in clinically suspicious PAN metastasis for high risk patients. The incidence of RLN metastasis by histological examination was 6.2% (8/129) in grade 1, 12.0% (12/101) in grade 2, 18.5% (5/27) in grade 3, 25.0% (4/16) in adenosquamous carcinoma, 50.0% (4/8) in serous adenocarcinoma and 33.3% (1/3) in clear cell adenocarcinoma. The incidence of lymph node metastasis was lower in endometrioid adenocarcinoma grade 1 than in endometrioid adenocarcinoma grade 2/3, and there was also a high incidence of lymph node metastasis in the histological subtypes, so-called adenosquamous carcinoma, serous carcinoma, and clear cell adenocarcinoma. The average number (range) of dissected nodes was 24.7 (10-62) for PLN and 10.1 (5-47) for PAN. We had more of operating time as well as blood loss for this operation, but this is clinically within permissible limits because there was no need to give a blood transfusion to the patients . Operating time and blood loss (mean average ± standard deviation: SD), in modified radical hysterectomy including systematic pelvic and para-aortic lymphadenectomy, were 222±61.6 min and 545±301 ml, respectively. There was no severe lymphedema associated with systematic lymphadenectomy.

One of the main postoperative adjuvant treatments is radiation and vaginal brachytherapy, however, there are few papers dealing with long-term survival in patients with systematic retroperitoneal lymphadenectomy followed by postoperative adjuvant chemotherapy. PAC (cisplatin, doxorubicin and cyclophosphamide) is one of the most commonly used regimens in endometrial carcinoma, and the less cardiotoxic analog epirubicin seemed to have the same activity as doxorubicin. Gadducci et al., (1999) described that the combination of cisplatin, epirubicin, and cyclophosphamide had good activity in advanced or recurrent endometrial carcinoma. Therefore, we examined recurrence risk factors over the past 10 years in patients with surgically staged endometrial carcinoma followed by postoperative CEP regimen. Postoperative adjuvant CEP chemotherapy was performed in 58 patients with a tumor confined to the uterus (Stages IC and II) in 3 courses 3-4 weeks apart and in 43 patients with extrauterine lesions involving adnexa and/or PLN in 5 courses, and also in 21 patients with PAN metastasis in 10 courses. No patient required major modification of the treatment modality of the postoperative adjuvant chemotherapy because of acute myelosuppression or gastrointestinal disorder (Hiura et al., 2010). Gynecologic Oncology Group (GOG) randomized trial (Randall et al., 2006) showed that AP (doxorubicin and cisplatin) chemotherapy significantly improved progression-free and overall survival compared with WAI (whole-abdominal irradiation) in patients with Stages III or IV endometrial carcinoma with a maximum of 2cm of postoperative residual disease. Paclitaxel (Lissoni et al., 1996) is active in patients with endometrial cancer pretreated with PAC, and also carboplatin (Burke et al., 1993) has definite activity in endometrial carcinoma and offers a well-tolerated palliative therapeutic alternative. Phase III randomized study of doxorubicin, cisplatin, paclitaxel, and filgrastim (G-CSF) versus carboplatin and paclitaxel in patients with stage III or IV or recurrent endometrial cancer (GOG 209) is now analyzing (National Cancer Institute, 2011).

Recurrence was detected in 20 (7.0%) cases (vaginal stump: 2, pelvic cavity: 2, external lymph node: 1, pelvic cavity + vaginal stump: 1, lung: 7, pleura: 1, PAN: 2, liver + abdominal cavity: 1, bone: 1, ascites: 1, pelvic cavity + abdominal cavity: 1) with a median

Stage	Local	Distant	Local + Distant
I/II (5)	Vaginal stump (1)	Lung (2) Pleura(1) PAN (1)	
III/ IV (15)	Vaginal stump (1) Pelvic cavity (2) External LN (1) Pelvic cavity + Vaginal stump(1)	Lung (5) Liver + Abdominal cavity (1) PAN (1) Bone (1) Ascites (1)	Pelvic cavity + Abdominal cavity (1)

Recurrence rate :7%(20/284) , PAN:Para-aortic lymph node, LN: Lymph node

Table 1. Sites of recurrence in endometrial carcinoma

CR (4) + PR (5)	CR; Lung (1), PAN (1), Vaginal stump (1) Pelvic cavity + Vaginal stump (1) PR: Pelvic cavity (2), External LN (1), PAN(1), Liver + Abdominal (1)
SD (4) + PD (2)	SD: Lung (1), Pleura (1), Pelvic cavity + Abdominal cavity (1) Vaginal stump (1) PD: Lung (2)

Response rate: 9/15 (60%), PAN: Para-aortic lymph node, LN: Lymph node,
CR: Complete response, PR: Partial response, SD: Stable disease, PD: Progressive disease

Table 2. Response rate in recurrent endometrial carcinoma

disease-free interval from initial surgery of 689 days. One vaginal stump recurrence (0.5%) in stage I/II and six cases of locoregional recurrence (vaginal stump: 1, pelvic cavity: 2, external lymph node: 1, pelvic cavity + vaginal stump: 1, pelvic cavity + abdominal cavity: 1, 9.4%) in stage III/IV were recognized (Table. 1). There were four cases of distant recurrence (1.8%) in stage I/ II. The incidence of local recurrence in stage I/II was extremely lower more than expected. The response rate to chemotherapy or radiotherapy for recurrent diseases was 60.0 (9/15) % (Table. 2). Six cases of locoregional recurrence and nine cases of distant recurrence were treated by radiotherapy and chemotherapy, respectively. Disease control rate (complete response: CR/particular response: PR/stable disease: SD) showed 86.7% (13/15). The response rate to chemotherapy or radiotherapy for recurrence disease was comparatively good. The incidence of recurrence by histological examination was 2.3% (3/129) in grade I, 8.9% (9/101) in grade II, 7.4% (2/27) in grade III, 12.5% (2/16) in adenosqamous carcinoma, 37.5% (3/8) in serous adenocarcinoma and 33.3% (1/3) in clear cell adenocarcinoma (Table 3). The incidence of recurrence was more lower in endometrioid adenocarcinoma grade I than in endometrioid grade 2/3, and there was a high incidence of recurrence in the histological subtypes, adenosquamous carcinoma, serous adenocarcinoma, and clear cell adenocarcinoma. Recurrence risk factors by univariate analysis were menopause (p=0.0099), histology (p=0.005), FIGO stage (p<0.0001), myometrial invasion (p<0.0001), adnexal metastasis (p=0.0009), lymphvascular space invasion (p<0.0006), tumor diameter (p=0.0076), peritoneal cytology (p=0.039), and RLN metastasis (p=0.0009) (Table 4). Cervical involvement (p=0.3092) was not recognized as a recurrence risk factor. A multivariate analysis showed that menopause (p=0.029) and FIGO stage (p=0.0369) were the most significant predictors of recurrence (Table 5). The careful follow-up is always required in endometrial carcinoma with the independent risk factors including menopause and FIGO stage III/IV.

Histological type	No. of Patients	Incidence
Endometrial adenocarcinomas		
Grade I	129	3 (2.3)
Grade II	101	9 (8.9)
Grade III	27	2 (7.4)
Adenosquamous carcinomas	16	2 (12.5)
Serous adenocarcinoma	8	3 (37.5)
Clean cell adenocarcinoma	3	1 (33.3)

Table 3. Incidences of recurrence by histological examination

	No. of Patients Total (N)	Recurrence (%)	p-value
Menopause			
Premenopause	87	1 (1.5)	0.0099
Postmenopause	197	19 (9.6)	
Histology			
G1	129	3 (2.3)	0.005
G2, 3 and others	155	17 (10.9)	
Cervical involvement			
Negative	247	16 (6.5)	0.3092
Positive	37	4 (10.8)	
FIGO stage			
I / II	220	5 (2.3)	<0.0001
III/ IV	64	15 (23.4)	
Myometrial invation			
≦1/2	201	5 (2.5)	<0.0001
>1/2	83	15 (18.1)	
Adenexal metastasis			
Negative	265	14 (5.3)	0.0009
Positive	19	6 (31.6)	
Lymph vascular space invasion			
Negative	166	4 (2.4)	<0.0006
Positive	118	16 (13.6)	
Tumor diameter			
≦4cm	171	6 (3.5)	0.0076
>4cm	113	14 (12.4)	
Peritoneal cytology			
Negative	251	13 (5.2)	0.039
Positive	33	7 (21.2)	
RLN metastasis			
Negative	258	14 (5.4)	0.0009
Positive	26	6 (31.6)	

RLN: Retroperitoneal lymph node

Table 4. Recurrence risk factors by univariate analysis in endometrial carcinoma

	p-value	Odd ratio	95%CI
Menopause			
Premenopause/ Postmenopause	0.029	9.553	1.295-72.449
Histology			
G1/G2, 3 and others	0.0663	3.253	0.923-11.460
FIGO stage			
I, II/III, IV	0.0369	4.017	1.088-14.830
Myometrial invasion			
≦ 1/2 / >1/2	0.2452	1.945	0.633-5.974
Lymph vascular space invasion			
Negative / Positive	0.2128	2.079	0.657-6.576
Tumor diameter			
≦ 4cm / >4cm	0.1629	2.025	0.751-5.458
RLN metastasis			
Negative / Positive	0.1773	2.245	0.671-7.265

CI: Confidence interval, RLN: Retroperitoneal lymph node.

Table 5. Recurrence risk factors by multivariate analysis in endometrial carcinoma

5. Conclusion

In modified radical hysterectomy, the uterus should be extirpated with the cardinal ligament allowing an extra 1.5-2.0 cm margin of the vaginal wall. The key point of the technique is formation of a ureteral tunnel during the dissection of the anterior layer of the vesicouterine ligament, while lightly pulling the ureter with tweezers, Cooper scissors and ureteral retractors. Modified radical hysterectomy has a broad range of applications, being positioned in between total hysterectomy and radical hysterectomy. This surgical technique has the advantage that postoperative urinary disturbances and other complications are minimized if the surgical candidates are selected appropriately. This surgical procedure could contribute to reduce locoregional recurrence, especially vaginal stump in stage I/II. It is suggested that management of endometrial carcinoma with risk factors by appropriate surgery and adjuvant chemotherapy is very important for preventing both locoregional and distant recurrence. Thus, further application of this technique is expected.

6. Acknowledgments

This study was supported by a grant from the Japanese Organization of the Ministry of Health, Labor and Welfare (2010).

7. References

Announcements FIGO stages - 1988 revision (1989). *Gynecol Oncol*. Vol.35, Issue 1, (Oct 1989), pp125-127.

Bidus, MA. & Elkas JC. (2007). Cervical and Vaginal Cancer, In: *Berek & Novak's Gynecology*, I.S. Berek (Ed), pp.1403-1456, ISBN: 978-0781768054, Philadelphia, USA

Blake, P. Swart, AM. & Orton, J. et al. (2008). Adjuvant external beam radiotherapy in the treatment of endometrial cancer (MRC ASTEC and NCIC CTG EN.5 randomised trials): pooled trial results, systematic review, and meta-analysis. *Lancet*, pp. 137-46, ISSN 0140-6736

Burke, TW. Munkarah, A & Kavanagh, JJ. et al. (1993). Treatment of advanced or recurrent endometrial carcinoma with single-agent carboplatin. *Gynecol Oncol.* Vol. 51, (Dec 1993), pp.397-400, ISSN: 0090-8258

Creutzberg, CL.; van Putten, WL. & Koper, PC. et al. (2000). Surgery and Postoperative Radiotherapy Versus Surgery Alone for Patients with Stage-1 Endometrial Carcinoma: Multicentre Randomised Trial. *Lancet*, Vol. 355, (April 2000), pp.1404-1411, ISSN 2078- 6891

Gadducci, A.; Romanini, A. & Cosio, S. et al. (1999). Combination of cisplatin, epirubicin, and cyclophosphamide (PEC regimen) in advanced or recurrent endometrial cancer: a retrospective clinical study. *Anticancer Res*, Vol. 19, (May 1999), pp.2253-2256, ISSN:0250-7005

Hiura, M.; Nogawa, T. & Matsumoto T. et al. (2010).Long-term Survival in Patients with Para-aortic Lymph Node Metastasis with Systematic Retroperitoneal Lymphadenectomy Followed by Adjuvant Chemotherapy in Endometrial Carcinoma. *International Journal of Gynecological Cancer*, Vol. 20, Issue 6, (August 2010), pp. 1000-1005, ISSN 1048-891X

Hiura, M.; Nogawa, T. (2011). Modified Radical Hystractomy in Endometrial carcinoma, In: *Obstetric and Gynecologic Surgery NOW No.6*. I. Konishi (Ed), 34-45, ISBN:978-4-7583-1205-9 C3347, Tokyo, Japan.

Jones Ⅲ, HW (2008). Cervical Cancer Precursor and Their Management, In: *Te Linde's Operative Gynecology*, I.S. J.A. Rock & H.W. Jones Ⅲ(Eds), 1208-1290, ISBN: 978-0781772341, Philadelphia, USA

Keys, HM.; Roberts, JA.& Brunetto VL. et al. (2004).A phase III trial of surgery with or without adjunctive external pelvic radiation therapy in intermediate risk endometrial adenocarcinoma: a Gynecologic Oncology Group study. *Gynecologic Oncology*, Vol. 92, Issue 3, (March 2004), pp.744-751, ISSN 0090-8258

Lissoni, A, Zaneta, G & Losa, G. et al. (1996). Phase II study of paclitaxel as salvage treatment in advanced endometrial cancer. *Ann Oncol.* Vol. 7, Issue 8, (Oct 1996), pp.861-863, ISSN: 0923-7534

National Cancer Institute. Phase III randomized study of doxorubicin, cisplatin, paclitaxel, and fligrastim (G-CSF) versus carboplatin snd paclitaxel in patients with stage III or VI or recurrent endometrial cancer.
http://www.cancer.gov/clinicaltrials/search/view?cdrid=305940&version=HealthProfessional

National Comprehensive Cancer Network® (2011). NCCN Clinical Practice Guideline Oncology ™ Uterine Neoplasms V.I. Available from
http://www.nccn.org/professionals/physician_gls/f_guidelines.asp

Nout, RA.; Smit, VT. & Putter, H. et al. (2010). Vaginal Brachytherapy versus Pelvic External Beam Radiotherapy for Patients with Endometrial Cancer of High-intermediate Risk (PORTEC-2): An Open-label, Non-inferiority, Randomised Trial. *Lancet*, Vol.375, Issue 9717, (March 2010), pp. 816-823, ISSN 0140-6736

Randall, ME.; Filiaci, VL. & Muss, H. et al. (2006). Randomized phase III trial of whole-abdominal irradiation versus doxorubicin and cisplatin chemotherapy in advanced endometrial carcinoma: a Gynecologic Oncology Group Study. *J Clin Oncol*, Vol. 24, (Jan 2006), pp.36-44, ISSN:0732-183X

Randall, ME.; Michael, H. Long III, H. & Tedjanati, S. (2009). Uterine Cervix, In: *Principles and Practice of Gynecologic Oncology*, R.R.Barakat,, M. Markman & M.E. Randall (Eds), 623-681, ISBN: 978-0781778459, Philadelphia, USA

5

New Approaches to Hysterectomy by Minimal Invasive Surgery (MIS)

Shanti Raju-Kankipati and Omer Devaja
University of London,
United Kingdom

1. Introduction

The most significant advancement in in reducing surgical morbidity in gynaecology over the last two decades has been an increased application of minimal invasive surgical techniques for both benign and malignant gynaecological disease requiring a subtotal, simple, or radical hysterectomy. [1,2,3,4,5,6].

Many variations of the procedures of laparoscopic assisted hysterectomy have been described, that vary principally by the extent of surgery performed via the laparoscopic route. The training and skill of the surgeon and equipment available may influence the extent of surgery performed via the laparoscope. This in turn has the potential impact on the clinical outcomes, such as perioperative complication rate and resource utilization outcomes such as readmission rate and post-surgical care.

Several attempts have been made to standardize the extent of surgery by minimal access approach by using a system of classification [7,8]. Unfortunately the clinical results published on this topic, in the literature seldom adhere to these classifications when describing their outcomes. The reluctance to adhere to these classifications may be due to the complexity of the classifications, with numerous subgroups in each type of the main four Types described by AAGL. Besides, this classification does not extend to more radical hysterectomies required for malignant conditions such as endometrial and cervical cancers.

Simplifying the classification described by AAGL for both subtotal and total hysterectomies by MIS and extending the classification to include pelvic and Para aortic lymphadenectomy and Piver's [9] classification of radical hysterectomy may be more useful to standardize and compare surgical outcomes by MIS in future. It is essential that surgeons have advanced laparoscopic skill recognised by their national or international governing body for training, before undertaking these procedures in the interest of their patients. The National Institute for Health and Clinical Excellence (NICE) of U.K. has recently issued the guidance on laparoscopic radical hysterectomy for early cervical cancer and emphasised the importance of adequate higher training in MIS for surgeons undertaking these procedures. (2010)[10].

2. Laparoscopic assisted hysterectomy for benign gynaecological disease

In the past two decades there has been a vast number of publications on laparoscopic hysterectomy: prospective, retrospective, randomised studies and met-analysis evaluating the complications, benefits to patients, cost to health services and quality of life. There are equal numbers of proponents of this surgical technique as there are for conventional hysterectomy by laparotomy and vaginal hysterectomy. The complication rates reported in earlier multicentre studies showed a higher complication rate [2, 11,12, 13] similar rates [3, 14], and lower complications with laparoscopic approach [15].

3. Laparoscopic hysterectomy with pelvic lymphadenectomy

Childers and Surwit proposed laparoscopic staging as an alternative for early endometrial cancer [16]. Several studies since have shown that this approach is associated with a shorter hospitalisation, faster recovery, lower complications when compared to open surgery. [5, 17, 18]. Meta analysis of 17 prospective and retrospective studies showed that laparoscopic approach to surgical treatment for women with endometrial cancer had lower complications and no significant difference in recurrent rates or disease free survival [19,20.]

4. Laparoscopic radical hysterectomy with pelvic lymphadenectomy

Over a thousand laparoscopic radical hysterectomies have been performed to-date, [21,22,23,24]. However, laparoscopic surgery has not gained popularity amongst gynaecological oncologists. Many gynaecologists have been slow to adopt laparoscopic approach to radical hysterectomy largely due to prolonged learning curve, complexity of the procedure, technical challenges leading to prolonged operating time and surgeon's fatigue. The disadvantages of the laparoscopic approach which includes, two dimensional view, decreased range of movements, reduced degree of freedom of instruments and dependents on the skill of assistants. Wattiez et al [25] in a series of 1,647 cases showed the learning curve for total laparoscopic hysterectomy is prolonged and the technique requires a high level of expertise and training as recommended by NICE [10]. The complications with laparoscopic hysterectomy have been reported to be higher when performed by less experienced surgeons. Although patients treated with laparoscopic approach have been shown to experience less intraoperative blood loss, less post-operative pain and ileus, and short hospital stay than those who had conventional open hysterectomy [26], minimal invasive surgery (MIS) is still an exception and not the rule in most gynaecologist practice.

5. Surgical robot – de Vinci surgical system (intuitive surgical inc.) (Fig 1.)

This robotic system was introduced in 1999 which is comprised of three components, the patient side surgical cart, the vision system, and the surgical console (fig 2). The surgeon's console is located remotely from the patient. The surgeon is seated at the console to control the robotic arms which hold the instruments within the patient's abdomen. With the aid of stereoscopic viewer, hand manipulators and foot pedals, the surgeon is able to conduct the surgery with greater precision and ease. The second component is the de Vinci 3D optics which consists of a sophisticated stereoscopic digital camera through a 12 mm endoscope (fig 3).

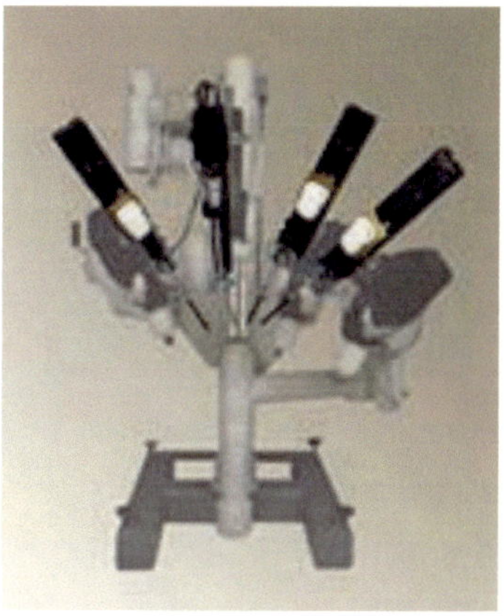

Fig. 1. da Vinci robot

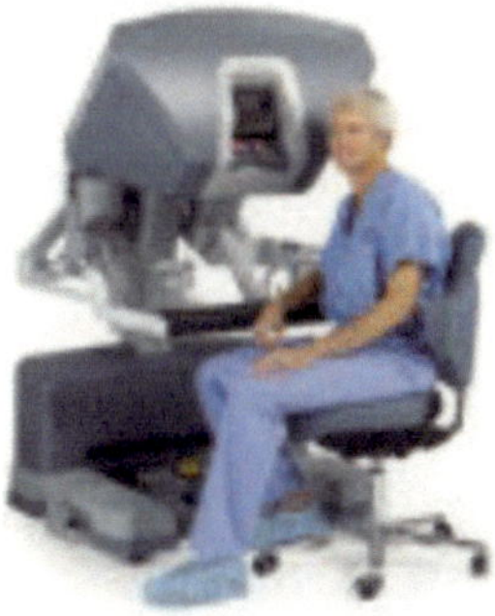

Fig. 2. Console

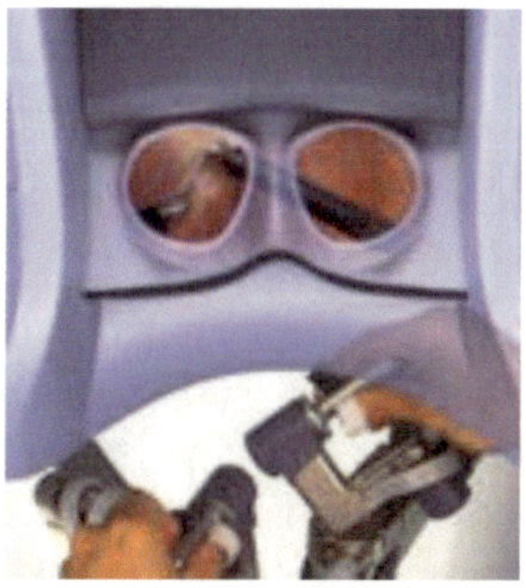

Fig. 3. 3D optics

The camera consists of two high definition units which recreate a true 3D colour image which is viewed by the surgeon at the console. The camera allows for up to 12 x magnification of the operating field, opening up the possibility of performing microsurgical procedures as well as spotting and managing small blood vessels to reduce bleeding and performing nerve sparing surgical dissection (fig 4). Three cameras are available for use on the de Vinci system, one straight and two angled cameras (up and down pointed), which allows the surgeon the options of viewing all nooks and corners of the pelvis and abdomen.

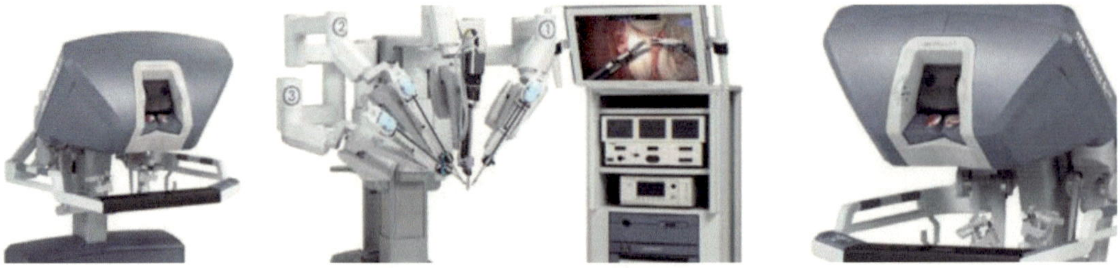

Fig. 4. Products

The third component is the surgical cart which is composed of three to four arms for controlling the 3D camera and two to three surgical instruments. The robotic instruments are "wristed", thereby providing 7 degrees of freedom (*df*) compared with 4 *df* with traditional laparoscopy (fig 5). The robotic instruments are controlled by the principal surgeon who sits away from the patient at the surgical console via two "masters". The movements of the surgeon's arms and legs are translating in real time to the robotic instruments inside the patient's abdomen and are processed and scaled to reduce any tremor and thus enhance precision of movements and avoid tissue trauma.

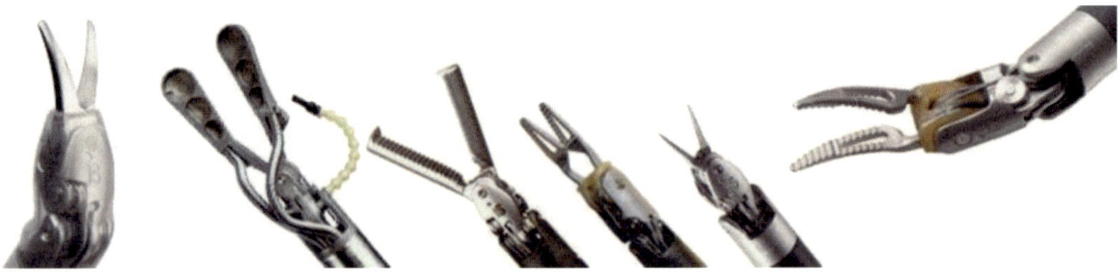

Fig. 5. Instruments

The surgical instruments and a stereoscopic video camera all work in unison during surgery. The hand-like surgical instruments move with 7 (df) and two degrees of axial rotation (fig 5). The surgical masters are placed in line with the surgeon's field of vision in order to restore a more intuitive eye-hand coordination than that experienced with traditional laparoscopy. The foot controlled pedals on the surgical console enable the surgeon to control and zoom the camera which gives complete control over the surgical field, unlike the traditional laparoscopy where the surgeon relies on the assistant to control the camera.

6. Robotic-assisted total hysterectomy technique

The steps of surgical technique are similar to those in an open or laparoscopic surgical approach, which include careful preparation of the vascular pedicles prior to ligation by bipolar, mono-polar energy sources or other energy sources (Harmonic scalpel, En seal,

Ligasure) for vessel sealing as described earlier [27]. There has been an increase in the use of robotic assisted technique over laparoscopic approach for minimal invasive surgery and hysterectomy in the past five years in the United states . This popularity of robotic approach may be attributed to greater degrees of freedom of movement, 3D viewing and ease of intra-corporal suturing and less steep learning curve when compared to laparoscopic approach. Laparoscopic hysterectomy has been shown to have a longer operative time compared to robotic surgery, with comparable blood loss, length of hospital stay and post-operative complications [28]. Others have shown that robotic surgery has a lower operating time when compared to laparoscopic surgery and decreased hospital stay, less blood loss and lower conversion to open surgery [29].

7. Robotic assisted hysterectomy & radical hysterectomy with pelvic +/- para-aortic lymphadenectomy in gynaecological oncology

Patients with endometrial cancer often are obese, elderly with increased incidents of medical comorbidities including diabetes and cardiovascular disease. The advantages of laparoscopic minimal invasive surgery in women with endometrial cancer have been shown by several studies, in the reduction of hospital stay, quicker recovery, lower incidents of thromboembolic complications and post-operative infections [5,30,31,32,33].

Since 2005 the use of robotic assisted MIS has gained popularity in gynaecological oncology. Robotic assisted surgery offers 3D, high definition visualisation in a stable field, more intuitive instrument control, better ergonomics and increased dexterity [4,34,35].

Unlike laparoscopic technique, once the patient is docked to the robot, the Trendelenburg position cannot be reversed without undocking the patient. At 30 degrees steep Trendelenburg position, there is a hypothetical risk of higher inspiratory pressure due to reduced ventilatory compliance which may compromise the advantages of MIS in obese and elderly women, which is frequently to co-morbidity in women with endometrial cancer. However, studies this far have not shown any increased risk using robotic assisted surgery in these high risk women with endometrial cancer, when compared to laparoscopic or open surgery. Table 1 shows comparison between open laparoscopic and robotic surgery in women with endometrial cancer [36, 39,40,41]. The rate of conversion to laparotomy has been reported between 3% to 16%, [36, 37, 38]. Older women had lower risk of surgical complications with laparoscopic vaginal approach [43, 44] yet implementation of laparoscopic surgery in these patients is low. In a prospective study Vakin et al showed that using robotic assisted technique in elderly patients with endometrial cancer had similar overall outcomes when compared with younger patients with endometrial cancer, despite having significantly more co-morbidities and more advanced disease [38]. Quality of life and patient satisfaction have shown to be superior with robotic assisted approach [38], which could be due to lower post-operative pain hence reduce intake of narcotic analgesics.

In 2006 Sert et al [45] described the first robotic assisted radical hysterectomy for early stage cervical cancer (stage IB1). They performed type III robotic assisted radical hysterectomy with estimated blood loss of 200 ml with no intra-operative or post-operative complications. The patient was discharged home four days later. Over the past five years several reports have been published on the robotic assisted radical hysterectomy [46,47,48,49,50]. Table II shows

Author	Cardenas et al	Jung et al	Bell et al	Boggess et al
Year	(2010)	(2010)	(2008)	(2008)
No of patients	(N=257)	(N=109)	(N=110)	(N=322)
Operating Time	R > L	R=L=A	R=L>A	A<R<L
Blood Loss	R < L	R=L<A	R=L<A	R< L or A
LN Yield	R = L	R=A>L	R=L=A	R> L or A
Hospital Stay	-	R=L<A	R=L<A	R< L or A
Complication rate	R = L	R=L<A	R<A<L	R<L (Conversion: R=L)

(R = robotic, L = laparoscopic, A = abdominal surgery, LN = Lymph nodes)

Table 1. Outcomes of robotics hysterectomy and pelvic lymphadenectomy

Study	No of cases	Op. Time	Blood loss (ml)	Lymph node(mean)	Hosp. Stay (days)	Complications
Maggioni	40	272	78	20.4	3.7	Nerve injury (2) Bowel injury (1) Transfusion (3) Vaginal dehiscence (3) Hernia (1) Recurrence (5) DOD (1)
Lowe	42	215 (median)	50 (median)	25 (median)	1 (median)	Conversion (1) Ureteric injury (1) Bladder injury (1) Infection (3) DVT (1)
Persson	64	262	150	26 (median)	-	Vaginal dehiscence (5) Pelvic abscess (7) Lymphoedema (13) Ureteric stenosis (1) Nerve injury (9) Hernia (3) DVT (2)
Canterell	63	213 (median)	50 (median)	29 (median)	1 (median)	Vaginal dehiscence (1) Nodal metastases (5) Positive margins (1) Recurrence (1)

Table 2. Outcomes of Robotic Radical Hysterectomy

some of the reported series with their outcomes. Although the recurrence rates seem to be equivalent to those after laparotomy and laparoscopic hysterectomies, long term follow up is still necessary. The intra-operative and post-operative morbidity of robotic assisted total hysterectomy are similar or sometimes less than those reported following open and laparoscopic hysterectomies.

To date, there are no randomised trials comparing the robotic assisted approach to radical hysterectomy, laparoscopy and laparotomy. There is an on-going phase III randomised clinical trial comparing the three techniques of radical hysterectomy in women with early stage cervical cancer, developed and designed by the Gynaecology Oncology Committee from American Association of Gynaecologic Laparoscopists [51]. The outcome of this trial may shed more light on the future approach to radical hysterectomy.

The potential for robotic assisted surgical devices to revolutionize complex surgery by reducing surgical morbidity, improving quality of life, minimising hospital stay which in turn reduced costs to the Health Service, is a high possibility in the near future.

8. Conclusions

Minimal invasive surgery ,both laparoscopic and roboticassissted surgery are alternative techniques to conventional open hysterectomy. However the training required to use these techniques, is an important factor to minimize complications during surgery. The reduced hospital stay., quicker recovery and increased patient satisfaction with these new approaches makes minimal invasive surgery certainly a viable challenge to conventional hysterectomy.

9. References

[1] Raju KS, Auld BJ, A randomised prospective study of laparoscopic vaginal hysterectomy versus abdominal hysterectomy each with, bilateral Salpingo oophorectomy. Brit. Jour. Obtet. Gynae. (1994) 101: 1068-1071.

[2] Garry R, Fountain. J. Mason. S, Hawe . J, Napp. V. et al . The eVALuate study: two parallel randomised trials, one comparing laparoscopic with abdominal hysterectomy, the other comparing laparoscopic with vaginal hysterectomy. BMJ (2004), 328: 1229-1236.

[3] Donnez O, Donnez J. A series of 400 laparoscopic hysterectomies for benign disease: a single centre, single surgeon prospective study of complications confirming previous retrospective study. Brit. Jour. Obstet. Gynaecol (2010), 117 (6). 752-755.

[4] Boggess JF. Robotic surgery in gynaecologic oncology: evolution of a new surgical paradigm. J. Robotic Surg. (2007) 1: 31-37.

[5] Devaja. O., Samara I., Papadopoulos AJ. Laparoscopically assisted vaginal hysterectomy (LAVH) versus Total abdominal hysterectomy (TAH) in Endometrial carcinoma: Prospective cohort study. Int. J. Gynae. Cancer (2010) 20, 4, 570-575

[6] Raju-Kankipati. S, Papadopoulos. AJ.,Khan. MS.,Dasgupta. P. A pilot study to assess the feasibility, safety and cost of robotic assisted total hysterectomy and bilateral Salpingo- oophorectomy. J. Robotic Surg. (2010) 4: 41-44.

[7] Munro mg, Parker WH . Classification of laparoscopic hysterectomy . Obtet. Gynecol. (1993) 82, 624-629.

[8] Olive. DL, Parker WH, Cooper JM., Levine RL. The AAGL Classification System for Laparoscopic Hysterectomy. Jour. Amer. Assoc. Gynecol. Lap. (2000) 7 (1), 9-15.
[9] Piver Classification for Radical Hysterectomy (1974) PMID 4417035.
[10] National Institute of Health and Clinical Excellence. Laparoscopic radical hysterectomy for early cervical cancer. (2010). Interventional procedure guidance. 24.
[11] Johnson N., Barlow D., Lethaby. A., Tavender E., Curr l., Garry R. Methods of hysterectomy systematic review and met-analysis of randomised controlled trials BMJ. (2005) 330; 1478
[12] Johnson N.,Barlow D., Lethaby A., Tavender E., Curr l., Garry R. Surgical approach to hysterectomy for benign gynaecological disease. Cochrane Database Sys. Rev. (2006) 2: CD 00 3677.
[13] Maresh MJ., Metcalfe MA., McPherson K. et al. The Value national hysterectomy study description of the patients and their surgery . Brit. Jour. Obstet. Gynae. (2002) 109: 302-312.
[14] Donnez O., Jadoul P., Squifflet J., Donnez J. A series of 3190 laparoscopic hysterectomies for benign disease from 1990 to 2006: evaluation of complications compared with vaginal and abdominal procedures. Brit. Jour. Obstet . Gynae. (2009) 116; 492-500.
[15] Karaman Y., Bingol M., Gunenc Z. Prevention of complications in laparoscopic hysterectomy: experience with 1120 cases performed by a single surgeon. J. Minim. Inv. Gynecol. (2007) 14: 78-84.
[16] Childers JM., Surwit EA. Combined laparoscopic and vaginal surgery for the management of two cases of Stage I endometrial cancer. Gynecol. Oncol (1992) 45: 46-51.
[17] Kim. DY., Kim MU., Kim JH., Suh DS. et. al. Laparoscopic assisted vaginal hysterectomy versus abdominal hysterectomy in patients with Stage I and II endometrial cancer Int. J. Gynecol. Cancer. (2005) 15: 932-937.
[18] Eltabbakh GH., Shamanki MI., Garafano LL. Laparoscopy as the primary modality of treatment of women with endometrial cancer. Cancer (2001) 91: 378-387.
[19] Palombo S., Falbo A., Mocciaro R., Russo T., Zulla F. Laparoscopic treatment for endometrial cancer: a meta- analysis of randomised controlled trials (RCT s) Gynecol. Oncol. (2009) 112: 415-421.
[20] Ju W., Myung SK., Kim Y., Choi HJ., Kim SC. Comparison of laparoscopy and laparotomy for management of endometrial carcinoma ; a meta- analysis. Int. J. Gynecol Cancer. (2009) 19 ; 400-406.
[21] Canis M., Mage G ., Wattiez A. Pouly JL. et.al. Does endoscopic surgery have a role in radical surgery of cancer of cervix uteri? J. Gynecol Obstet. Biol. Reprod. (Paris) (1990) 19 (7) 921.
[22] Nezhat CR., Burrell MO., Nezhat FR., Benigno BB. Welander CE. Laparoscopc radical hysterectomy with para-aortic and pelvic node dissection. Am. J. Obstet. Gynecol (1992) 166 (3) 864-865.
[23] Frumovitz M. dos Reis R., Sun CC., Milam MR. et.al. Comparison of total laparoscopic and abdominal radical hysterectomy for patients with early-stage cervical cancer. Obstet. Gynecol. (2007) 110 (10 96-102.

[24] Malzoni M., Tinelli R., Cosentino F., Fusco A., Malzoni C. Total laparoscopic radical hysterectomy versus abdominal radical hysterectomy with lymphadenectomy in patients with early cervical cancer: our experience. Ann. Surg. Oncol. (2009) 16 (5) 1316-1323.

[25] Wattiez A., Soriano D., Cohen SB., Nervo P., Canis M. et.al. The learning curve of total laparoscopic hysterectomy comparative analysis of 1647 cases. J. Am. Assoc. Gynecol. Lap. (2002) 9: 339-345.

[26] Aboud L., Boggess J. Current application of laparoscopy in gynaecologic oncology: a literature review . Womens Oncol. Rev. (2005) 5 (4) 193-201.

[27] Dasgupta p. (ED). U ROLOGIC ROBOTIC SURGERY IN CLINICAL PRACTICE. Springer. London pp. 159-180.

[28] Nezhat C. Lavie O., Lemyre M., Gemer O., Bhagan L., Nezhat C . L aparoscopic hysterectomy with and without a robot: Stanford experience. J.Soc. Laparo endosc. Surg. (2009) 13 (2) 125-128.

[29] Payne TN., Dauterive FR. A comparison of total laparoscopic hysterectomy to robotically assisted hysterectomy: surgical outcomes in a communitypractice. J. Minim. Inv.Gynecol. (2008) 15 (3) 286-291.

[30] Kalegiannidis I., Lambrechts S., Amout F., Neven P., Van Gorp T., Vergote I. Laparoscopy assisted vaginal hysterectomy compared with abdominal hysterectomy in clinical Stage I endometrial cancer: safety,recurrence and long-term outcome. AM. J. Obstet. Gynecol . (2007) 196- e8

[31] Malzoni M., Tinelli R., Cosentino F., Perone C., Raste M. et.al. Total laparoscopic hysterectomy versus abdominal hysterectomy with lymphadenectomy for early stage endometrial cancer: a prospective study. Gynecol. Oncol. (2009) 112, 126-13.

[32] Zullo F., Palombo S., Falbo A., Russo T., Mocciaro R. et al. Laparoscopic surgery vs laparotomy for early stage endometrial cancer: long term data of randomised controlled trials. Am J. Obstet. Gynecol.(2009) 200: 296-e9.

[33] Cho YH., Kim DY., Kim JH., Kim YM., Kim YT., Nam JH. Laparoscopic management of early uterine cancer: 10 year experience in Asan Medical Centre Gynecol. Oncol. (2007) 106: 585-590.

[34] Reynolds RK., Burke WM., Advincula AP. Preliminary experience with robot-assisted laparoscopic staging of gynaecological malignancies. J.S.L.S. (2005) 9:149-158.

[35] Field JB., Benoit MF., Dinh TA et. Al. Computer-enhanced robotic surgery in gynaecologic oncology . Surg. Endsc. (2007) 2444-246.

[36] Boggess JF., Gehrig PA., Cantrell L et.al. A comparative study of 3 surgical methods for hysterectomy with staging for endometrial cancer: robotic assistance, laparoscopiy. Laparotomy. Am. J. Obstet.Gynecol. (2008) 199: 360 el-360 e9.

[37] Seamon LG., Cohen DE., Henretta MS. et.al. Minimally invasive comprehensive surgical staging for endometrial cancer. Robotics or laparoscopy ? Gynecol. Oncol. (2009) 113: 36-41.

[38] Vaknin Z., Perri T., Lau S., Deland C., Drummond N. et.al. Outcome and Quality of life in a prospective cohort of the first 100 robotic surgery for endometrial cancer, with focus on elderly patients. Int. J. Gynecol. Cancer. (2010) 20: 1367-1373.

[39] Cardenas- GOICOECHEA J., Adams S., Bhat SB., Randall TC. Surgical outcomes of robotic-assisted surgical staging for endometrial cancer are equivalent to traditional

laparoscopic assisted staging at a minimal invasive surgical centre. Gynecol. Oncol. (2010) 117: 224-228.

[40] Jung YW., Lee WD., Kim SW., Nam EJ., Kim JH. Et.al Robotic assisted staging using three arms for endometrial cancer: comparison to laparoscopy and laparotomy at a single institution. Jour. Surg. Oncol. (2010) 101 (2) 116-121.

[41] Bell MC., Torgerson J., Seshadri-Kreaden U., Suttle a., Hunt.s. Comparison of outcomes and cost for endometrial cancer staging via traditional laparotomy. standard laparoscopy and robotic techniques. Gynecol. Oncol. (2008) 111 93) 407-411.

[42] Lowe MP., Johnson PR., Kamelle SA, et al. A multinational experience with roboti assisted hysterectomy with staging for endometrial cancer. Obstet.Gynecol. (2009) 114: 236-243.

[43] Scribner DR. Jr. Walker JL., Johnson GA, et.al. Surgical management of early stage endometrial cancer in the elderly: is laparoscopy feasible? Gynecol. Oncol. (2001) 83: 563-568.

[44] O'Hanlan KA., Huang GS., Lopez L. et al. Total laparoscopic hysterectomy for oncological indications with outcomes stratified by age. Gynecol. Oncol. (20004) 95; 196-203.

[45] Sert BM., Abeler VM . Robotic assisted laparoscopic radical hysterectomy (Piver type III) with pelvic node dissection- case report. Eur. J . Gynae. Oncol. (2006) 27 (5) 531-533.

[46] Sert B. Abeler V. Robotic radical hysterectomy in early stage cervical carcinoma patients, comparing results with total laparoscopic radical hysterectomy cases. The future is now? Int. J. Med. Robot. (2007) 3 (3) 224-228.

[47] Persson J. Reynisson P., Borgfeldt C. et.al. Robot assisted laparoscopic radical hysterectomy and pelvic lymphadenectomy with short and long term morbidity data. Gynecol. Oncol (2009) 113 (2) 185-190.

[48] Cantrell LA., Mendivil A., Gehrig PA., Boggess JF. Survival outcomes for women undergoing type III robotic radical hysterectomy for cervical cancer: a 3-year experience . Gynecol.Oncol.(2010) 117 (2) 260-265.

[49] Maggioni a . Minig L., Zanagnolo V., Peiretti M. et. Al. Robotic approach for cervical cancer, comparison with laparotomy: a case control study. Gynecol. Oncol.(2009) 115 (1) 60-64.

[50] Lowe MP., Chamberlain DH., Kamelle SA., Johnson PR., Tillmanns TD. A multi-institutional experience with robotic-sisted radical hysterectomy for early cervical cance, Gynecol.Oncol. (2009) 113 920 191-194.

[51] http://clinicaltrials.gov/archive/NCT00614211

6

Emergency Peripartum Hysterectomy

Abiodun Omole-Ohonsi
Department of Obstetrics and Gynaecology,
Bayero University/Aminu Kano Teaching Hospital, Kano,
Nigeria

1. Introduction

The most common indication for emergency peripartum hysterectomy is severe uterine hemorrhage, which cannot be controlled by conservative measures. Such hemorrhage may be due to abnormal placentation (eg, placenta praevia and placenta praevia accreta), uterine atony, uterine rupture, leiomyomas, coagulopathy, over distension of the uterus (multiple pregnancy, polyhdramnios), or laceration of the uterine vessel(s), which is not treatable by conservative measures. The relative frequency of these conditions varies among series, and is dependent upon the patient's population and practice patterns. Emergency peripartum hysterectomy is a life saving surgical procedure, which is usually carried out for postpartum haemorrhage, after a sequence of interventions are not successful. Advent of newer medical /conservative surgical methods of controlling postpartum haemorrhage, have reduced the incidence and indications of emergency peripartum hysterectomy. Sophistication in obstetric care and blood transfusion services has improved the outcome, especially in developed countries.

1.1 Emergency Peripartum Hysterectomy

Emergency hysterectomy refers to the surgical removal of the uterus, following an unexpected and sudden event that must be dealt with urgently by carrying out the procedure. When it is carried out on a pregnant uterus within 24 hours after delivery, it is termed emergency peripartum hysterectomy. This life saving obstetric procedure has been in use for more than 200 years, but it was in 1876 that Edward Porro published the first successful case report of this procedure, in which the mother and baby survived.

In developing countries, a variable incidence of 2 to 6 per 1000 births has been reported, compared to 0.2 to 2.7 per 1000 births from developed countries. In Nigeria, the incidence of emergency peripartum hysterectomy ranges from 1.8 to 5.4 per 1000 births. In Pakistan, an incidence of 5.6 per 1000 births was reported, in India 2.6 per 1000 births, and in the United States of America (USA) 1.2 to 2.7 per 1000 births. Lower incidence was reported in European countries like Norway, where 0.2 per 1000 births was reported, in Ireland and Netherlands 0.3 per 1000 births was reported from both countries.

The increasing incidence of the procedure in developed countries like USA and Canada, despite proper utilization of effective antenatal and delivery facilities, has been attributed to the increasing caesarean section rate, which predisposes to placenta praevia and placenta praevia accreta, which are now the leading indications for emergency peripartum hysterectomy in developed countries. Placenta praevia predisposes to primary postpartum haemorrhage, because of inefficient contraction and retraction of the lower uterine segment, following delivery of the baby or the placenta, while in addition, placenta praevia accreta may predispose to partial separation of the placenta, and with partial separation of the placenta, emergency peripartum hysterectomy is usually required to control haemorrhage. This may explain why placenta praevia accreta, is presently the commonest indication for emergency peripartum hysterectomy in developed countries, because most of their patients are booked and deliver in health facilities, assisted by skilled providers, which may have reduced the incidence of ruptured uterus in their obstetric practice, and uterine atony among the indications for emergency peripartum hysterectomy.

The preeminence of placenta praevia/placenta praevia accreta, as an indication for emergency peripartum hysterectomy, has been reported globally. This may be because of the increasing caesarean section rate worldwide, and the concomitant rise in the incidence of placenta praevia and placenta praevia accreta. In developed countries like The United States of America, the caesarean section rate is at a record high of 31.1% of all births, representing an increase of 30% in the past decade, probably because litigation and request caesareans are becoming commoner. In Aminu Kano Teaching Hospital, Kano, Nigeria, there has been an increase of 12% in the caesarean section rate over the past decade, because of increasing awareness by the obstetricians, about reduction in maternal and perinatal morbidity, in order to ensure good quality of life.

The association between placenta praevia/placenta praevia accreta and previous caesarean delivery has been reported. Placenta praevia was recorded in 4.4 per 1000 second-birth singletons, whose first births were delivered by caesarean section, and 2.7 per 1000 second-birth singletons, whose first births were delivered vaginally. In The United States of America, caesarean section for live birth is associated with a 47% increased risk of placenta praevia, in second pregnancy with a singleton. Placenta praevia accreta occurs in up to 15% of women with placenta praevia, and more in cases with previous lower segment caesarean section scar, because of decidual deficiency.

The higher incidence of emergency peripartum hysterectomy, in developing countries compared to developed countries, is because of the higher prevalence of risk factors of primary postpartum haemorrhage like, uterine fibroids in pregnancy, multiple pregnancy, grandmultiparity, cephalo-pelvic disproportion and prolonged obstructed labour/uterine rupture, previous caesarean section/myomectomy scar, and placenta praevia in developing countries, where majority of the maternity patients are unbooked, and deliver outside the health facilities unsupervised or poorly supervised.

Essential obstetric care facilities are poorly developed in developing countries. Most of the rural public hospitals and health centres are not functional 24 hours of the day, coupled with poor road network and transportation systems to the cities, which result in delay in getting appropriate care in labour, with the result that 70% of deliveries are conducted outside the hospitals, by unskilled birth attendants or quacks, Traditional Birth Attendants (TBAs), Traditional Priests, Herbalists or Prophets. In Nigeria 16.9% of women delivered on their own without assistance from anyone. In Pakistan 89% of women deliver at home, of these 80% are delivered by TBAs.

The high prevalence of unbooked patients, who labour and deliver outside the health facility poorly supervised in developing countries, has been attributed to socio-cultural barriers and aversion to western oriented programs like antenatal care and hospital delivery, as well as low literacy levels, female socioeconomic disadvantage from male gender dominance, poverty, poor access to available health facilities that are not free or subsidized, and upsurge in the use of spiritual homes as maternity centres, because of the belief that pregnancy complications are a result of spiritual attacks.

The likelihood that mothers will consult a health professional for antenatal care, increase as the mother's educational level rises, increasing from 44% among women with no education, to 97% among those with college education, while the proportion of births that took place in health facilities, varies from 6% among uneducated women, to 73% among women with college education.

The high prevalence of low adult literacy levels in developing countries, may account for the high prevalence of unbooked patients, who labour and deliver outside the health facility poorly supervised. Adult literacy rate, which is the share of literate persons in the population aged 15 years and older, is 57.1% in Nigeria, in a Demographic and Health Survey 2005-2008. This may explain why in Nigeria, 58% of the pregnant women received antenatal care from a skilled provider, 39% of births are assisted by a skilled provider, and 35% of births are delivered in a health facility. This calls for increasing female education and socioeconomic empowerment, if utilization of available antenatal care and delivery facilities is to improve, and the incidence of emergency peripartum hysterectomy is to reduce in developing countries.

In developed countries, where the adult literacy levels approach 100%, 9 out of 10 patients (91%) are booked, and deliver in adequately equipped health facilities, with the assistance of a skilled provider. This, in addition to the higher sophistication of their populace, socioeconomic empowerment of the women, provision of adequate essential obstetric care facilities, high contraceptive prevalence rate and desire for small family size, may explain the lower incidence of emergency peripartum hysterectomy in developed countries.

The amalgamation of closely related risk factors of emergency peripartum hysterectomy, that contributes significantly to the high maternal mortality in developing countries, like grandmultiparity, low socioeconomic class and unbooked status, is because grandmultiparity is associated with low socioeconomic class and unbooked status. The protective effect of primigravidity, may be because, risk factors of emergency peripartum hysterectomy like uterine rupture, uterine atony and placenta praevia/placenta praevia accreta are less common among them, and where primary postpartum haemorrhage occur, obstetricians will prefer the application of other techniques, that can be both life saving and uterus preserving to arrest haemorrhage.

The high prevalence of grandmultiparity in developing countries is attributed to early girl marriage/childbearing, male gender dominance, low literacy level, poverty and low contraceptive prevalence rate. Early girl marriage/childbearing refers to adolescents less than 18 years at first marriage/pregnancy. In Nigeria, the median age at first marriage is 18.3 years, and 23% of women age 15-19 years are mothers or presently pregnant.

Contraceptive prevalence rate (CPR), which refers to the percentage of women of reproductive age (15 to 49 years), married or in a stable union, currently using, or whose partner is using any method of contraception at a given point in time, is low in developing countries, because the contraceptive prevalence in a community, has direct correlation with level of education.

In Nigeria, where the adult literacy level is 57.1%, 15% of married women aged 15—49 years use any form of family planning, and 10% use modern methods of family planning, the mean ideal number of children for women age 15 to 49 is 6.1. In the Philippines, where 98.8% of the populace is exposed to one level of education, with 78.9% having secondary or tertiary education, the number of women using the modern methods increased from 28% in 1998 to 34% in 2008, the family size is 3.3 per women. In most European countries, where literacy level approach 100%, the contraceptive prevalence rate approximate the optimal level of 80 to 85%, which corresponds to a family size of 2 children per women, which is the replacement level (i.e. replacement of the couples). This may explain the desire for small family size, and the low prevalence of grandmultiparity in developed countries.

The leading indications for emergency peripartum hysterectomy in developing countries are uterine rupture and placenta praevia accreta, because grandmultiparity, uterine fibroids and previous myomectomy scar, contracted pelvis and previous caesarean section scars are common, and most of the women deliver outside the health facilities poorly supervised, with high incidence of mismanaged labour. This may be because uterine rupture and placenta praevia accreta, tend to be relatively less amenable to medical and conservative surgical treatments, and sometimes necessitate radical surgical intervention, such as hysterectomy. Uterine rupture being a rare feature of their practice in developed countries, may explain why placenta praevia/placenta praevia accreta, is the leading indication for emergency peripartum hysterectomy in developed countries, despite the sophistication of their populace and obstetric practice.

The prominence of uterine rupture, which is a reflection of poor level of obstetric care and/or utilization in any community, and placenta praevia/placenta praevia accreta, in which complications are usually secondary to mismanagement of the third stage of labour, as the leading indications for emergency peripartum hysterectomy in developing countries, may be because majority of the women labour/deliver without the assistance of a skilled provider. Studies from developing countries have shown that 74.7% of case referrals to tertiary centres were mismanaged, and such mismanagement contributed significantly to mortality and long term morbidity.

Booked status and delivery that is assisted by a skilled provider in a health facility, and efficient transfer system from peripheral to specialist hospital, will ensure that avoidable risk factors like ruptured uterus remain avoidable, and where they accidentally occur, it will take place in the hospital, with better chance of success of conservative treatments, as there will be no delay in instituting appropriate management. In Conakry, Guinea, there was a decrease in the prevalence of uterine rupture from 0.20% to 0.12%, and associated maternal mortality from 28% to 21%, after 6 months of implementation of a program of consultation, feedback and integration (effective transfer system) between peripheral delivery units and two hospitals. This shows that building relationships with the various levels of health facilities, can promote early and prompt referral, and reduce the prevalence of uterine rupture and emergency peripartum hysterectomy.

Uterine atony, which accounts for the highest incidence of primary postpartum haemorrhge in most communities of world, is responsible for 75 to 90% of the cases. In developing countries, this may be explained by the high prevalence of grandmultiparity, uterine fibroids in pregnancy, multiple pregnancies, unbooked status and prolonged labour from poorly supervised labour/deliveries. Uterine atony is less prominent as an indication for emergency peripartum hysterectomy worldwide, because, recent advances in the of sequence of medical and conservative surgical measures to control primary postpartum haemorrhage, like rectal misoprostol, intramyometrial prostaglandins, carboprost, manual compression of the uterus, uterine packing with catheters, internal iliac/uterine artery ligation, uterine artery embolism and insertion of B- lynch suture, in addition to oxytocin and ergometrine, will control most cases of primary postpartum haemorrhage from uterine atony.

Studies have shown that over 80% of the patients who had emergency peripartum hysterectomy had blood transfusion, which shows the importance of efficient blood transfusion services, in the management of primary postpartum haemorrhage and emergency peripartum hysterectomy. Involvement of governmental and non-governmental agencies like Safe Blood for Africa (SBFA) is needed, especially in developing countries, where the health budget is poor, and there is aversion to free blood donations.

SBFA, whose strategies are to ensure a safe, adequate and accessible supply of blood and blood products continent-wide, is recognized and approved by international organizations and agencies. In conjunction with the Federal Government of Nigeria, SBFA commissioned the Nigerian National Blood Transfusion Services (NNBTS) in Abuja, Nigeria, in 2005, a program which is administered by SBFA, has expanded to the current 12 zonal blood centres, with additional centres to become operational soon. SBFA has been providing technical assistance to the Botswana National Blood Transfusion Service since 2000, and has assisted with increasing the quality and quantity of safe blood in Botswana, by providing the required training. Since SBFA came into Botswana, the blood supply has increased by over 100%, and the Human Immunodeficiency Virus infection rate among donors has decreased from 9% to less than 2%.

In the management of primary postpartum haemorrhage, a sequence of conservative measures to control uterine hemorrhage, should be attempted before resorting to more radical surgical procedures. If an intervention does not succeed, the next treatment in the sequence should be swiftly instituted. Hysterectomy should not be performed too early or too late. The skills that are necessary for its performance are best acquired, under an experienced mentor during scheduled non-emergency cases.

Timing is critical to an optimal outcome. The obstetrician will have to strike a balance, between spending excessive time on alternative techniques that are proving ineffective, and moving to the definitive and life saving hysterectomy, because delay will lead to further haemorrhage, and probably disseminated intravascular coagulation. The moribund state of the patients at the time of hysterectomy, rather than the operative procedure, is said to be responsible for the high maternal mortality, because delay in instituting therapy, is associated with the likelihood that the hysterectomy will be seriously complicated by coagulopathy, severe hypovolaemia, tissue hypoxia, hypothermia, and acidosis, which further compromise the patient's status.

This calls for not only campaign for utilization of adequately equipped antenatal care, and hospital delivery facilities that is supervised by a skilled provider, but also, proper training and retraining of the health workers on the management of obstetric emergencies, in-order to improve not only the skill, but also the art of obstetric judgments during these circumstances, and avoid delay in instituting appropriate treatment, so as to ensure consistent near perfect performance, because consistency is the key to sustained success.

The high maternal mortality rate, that is associated with emergency peripartum hysterectomy, is usually attributed to delay in carrying out the life saving hysterectomy. Delay, is the inability of the patient to get treatment in time, in the event of an obstetric emergency. Type I delay, is delay in making decision to seek care, when experiencing an obstetric complication. Type II, is delay in reaching an appropriate health facility, once the decision has been made to go, and Type III, is delay in receiving adequate and appropriate care, once the facility has been reached. In studies from Nigeria, 77.8% of maternal deaths were attributed to Types I and III delay.

The importance of avoiding delay, can be appreciated in developing countries, where primary postpartum haemorrhage remain one of the leading causes of maternal deaths, because of delay in getting appropriate treatment, while in developed countries, because of proper utilization of high quality maternity services, which has eliminated delay in getting appropriate treatment in the United Kingdom over the past 50 years, the number of maternal deaths from haemorrhage has fallen from 40 to 3 per annum. This has resulted in the emergence of the concept of *severe adverse maternal morbidity* (SAMM), as a sensitive marker of the quality of obstetric care, as maternal death from postpartum haemorrhage is becoming too rare for adequate surveillance of services.

The high perinatal mortality rate, among patients who had emergency peripartum hysterectomy in studies from developing countries, is probably because uterine rupture, which occurred among women who laboured outside the hospital poorly supervised, is one of the leading indications for emergency peripartum hysterectomy. With uterine rupture, immediate laparotomy is necessary in order to salvage the fetus, which is not usually feasible among patients who laboured outside the hospital.

Wound sepsis, post-operative pyrexia, anaemia and urinary tract infection, are usually the commonest morbidities following emergency peripartum hysterectomy, especially in developing countries. This may be because uterine rupture is a leading indication for emergency peripartum hysterectomy, and the combination of trauma, sepsis from aseptic techniques of traditional midwives, anaemia from primary postpartum haemorrhage, and urethral catheterization for 14 days post delivery to prevent vesico-vaginal fistula formation, may predispose to these morbidities. Also, some of the manipulations and conservative procedures, which were carried out before resorting to emergency peripartum hysterectomy, may carry the risk of intrauterine infections, besides being associated with delay and further bleeding, with worsening anaemia.

Subtotal hysterectomy is more commonly performed, compared to total abdominal hysterectomy, in the management of emergency peripartum hysterectomy, because the patients are usually not fit for surgery and anaesthesia. This is because hysterectomy is usually resorted to after failure of conservative management, and the cervix and paracolpos are usually not involved as the source of haemorrhage, which make subtotal hysterectomy to be adequate to achieve haemostasis. It is safer, faster and easier to perform than total hysterectomy, especially in the hands of Senior Resident Doctors, who encounter most of the cases during call hours. The future risk of cervical stump carcinoma which is 0.1% - 0.15% is low, and can be prevented by regular cytological screening.

2. Conclusion and recommendations

The incidence of emergency peripartum hysterectomy is increasing globally, and fetomaternal outcome is poor, especially in developing countries. Improvement in literacy level and socioeconomic status of the women, as well as contraceptive acceptance, utilization of antenatal care and hospital delivery that is supervised by skilled providers, provision of adequate facilities and trained manpower to carry out medical/conservative surgical treatments of primary postpartum haemorrhage, and efficient blood transfusion services are urgently needed, especially in developing countries, in order to reduce the incidence of emergency peripartum hysterectomy, and improve the outcome. Women who are high risk for primary postpartum haemorrhage, should book for antenatal care and deliver in specialized health facilities. Governmental interventions that will improve the utilization of antennal care, and hospital delivery that is supervised by skilled providers, like the recent launching of the National Health Insurance Scheme in Nigeria, is needed, especially in developing countries, where health budget is poor and governmental policies are erratic.

3. References

[1] Nasima S., Asifa G., Shazia J.,Tehmina A. Emergency obstetric hysterectomy (EOH): A life saving procedure in obstetrics. Pakistan J. Surg. 2007; 23(3):217-9.
[2] Rossi AC, Lee RH, Chmait RH. Emergency Postpartum Hysterectomy for Uncontrolled Postpartum Bleeding: A systematic Review. Obstet Gynaecol. 2010; 115(3):637-44.
[3] Anita K., Kavita W.W. Emergency Obstetric hysterectomy. J. Obstet Gynaecol India. 2005; 55(2): 132-4.
[4] Akinbiyi A.A., Olatunbosun O.A. Emergency obstetric hysterectomy, A 28 years experience in Saskatoan. J. Gynaecol. Surg. 2004; 31:81-7
[5] Onwuudiegwu U, Okonofua F. Emergency obstetric hysterectomy in a semi-urban hospital. Niger. Med. J. 1993,2(2):54-7
[6] Udoma E, John M, Etuk S, Ekanem A. Mortality following emergency obstetric hysterectomy in Calabar, Nigeria. Niger. Med. Pract. 2003,66:52-5.
[7] Giwa-Osagie D, Uguru V, Akinla O. Mortality and morbidity of emergency obstetric hysterectomy. J. Obstet. Gynaecol. 1983;4:94-6
[8] Kastner E.S, Figueroa R, Garry D, Naulik D. Emergency peripartum hysterectomy; Experience at a Community Teaching Hospital. Obstet Gynaecol. 2002;99:971-5.
[9] Stance L.M, Schrimmer O.B, Paul R.M, Mishell DR. Emergency peripartum hysterectomy and associated risk factors. Am. J. Obstet Gynaecol. 1993; 168:879-83.
[10] Engelson I.B, Albrechsen S, Iversen O.F. Peripartum hysterectomy- incidence and maternal morbidity. Acta Obstet Gynaecol Scand. 2001; 80:409-12.
[11] Langdana M., Geary W., Haw D., Kean F. Peripartum hysterectomy in the 1990's; any new lesson?. J Obstet Gynaecol. 2001; 21:121-3.
[12]Kwee A., Bots M., Visser G., Bruinse H. Emergency peripartum hysterectomy: A prospective study in the Netherlands. Euro. J. Obstet Gynaecol. Repro, Biol. 2005; 124(2):187-92.
[13] Miller DA, Chollet JA, Godwin TM. Clinical Risk Factors for Placenta Praevia-Placenta Accreta. Am J Obstet Gynaecol. 1997; 177: 210-14.
[14] Adesiyun A.G., Eseiegbe E., Ameh C.A. Inevitable peripartum hysterectomy in a tropical hospital: Indications and maternofetal outcome. Pakistan Journal of Medical Sciences. 2008; 24(1):122-6.
[15] 2008 Nigeria Demographic and Health survey (NDHS)
[16] Omole-Ohonsi A., Ashimi O.A. Ruptured Uterus in Kano, Nigeria- Study of Risk Factors. Niger. Hosp. Pract. 2008;2(3):65-9.
[17] Shellhas CS, Gilbert S, Landon MB, Verner MW, Leveno KJ, Hauth JC et al. The frequency and complication rates of hysterectomy accompanying caesarean delivery. Obstet Gynaecol. 2009; 114:224.
[18] Zwart JJ, Dijk PD, van Roosmalen J. Peripartum Hysterectomy and arterial embolization for major obstetric haemorrhage: a 2 year cohort study in the Netherlands. Am J Obstet Gynaecol. 2010; 202: 150.

[19] Rachaga S, Sivanesaratnam. Caesarean hysterectomy- a review of 21 cases in the University Hospital, Kuala Lumpur. Reprod. Biol. 1984;16:321-6
[20] Singh R., Nagrat A. Emergency obstetric hysterectomy- a retrospective study of 51 cases over a period of 5 years. J. obstet Gynaecol. India. 2005;55(5):428-30.
[21] The SOGON National Partnership Plan for Sustainable Reduction in Maternal and Newborn Deaths. 2008
[22] National Study on Essential Obstetric Care Facilities in Nigeria. Federal Ministry Health, Nigeria. 2003. 21.
[23] Ezechi OC, Kalu BKE, Njokanma FO, Nwokoro CA, Okeke GCE. Emergency Peripartum Hysterectomy in a Nigerian Hospital: A 20-Year Review. Journal of Obstetrics and Gynaecology, 2004 Jun; 24(4): 372-373.
[24] Ozumba BC, Mbagwu SC. Emergency Obstetrics Hysterectomy in Eastern Nigeria. Int Surg 1991; 76:109–11.
[25] Mackenzie H. , Drahota A. , Pallikadavath S., Stones W., Dean T. What is the Impact of Contraceptive Methods and Mixes of Contraceptive Methods on Contraceptive Prevalence, Unmet Need for Family Planning, and, Unwanted and Unintended Pregnancies? An Overview of Systematic Reviews. Available at www.dfid,gov.uk/...FINAL-Q35-Contraceptive-Mix-Overview-of-Reviews... Retrieved on 12th February 2010.
[26] 2008 Philippines Demographic and Health survey. Preliminary report.
[27] Stons w, Lim W, Al-Azzawi F. An investigation of maternal morbidity with identification of life threatening 'near-miss episodes'. Health Trends. 1991; 23: 13-15.
[28] Kuti O, Dare FO, Ogunniyi SO. The role of referring centres in the tragedy of unbooked patients. Trop J Obstet Gynaecol. 2001; 18 (1): 24-26.
[29] Balde MD, Bastert G. Decrease in uterine rupture in Conakry, Guinea by improvements in transfer management. Int. J. Gynecol. Obstet. 1990;31(1):21-24.
[30] Yang Q., Wen S.W., Oppenheimer L., Chen S.K, Black D., Gao J., Walker MC. Association of caesarean delivery for first birth with placenta praevia and placental abruption in second pregnancy. BJOG. 2007; 114: 609-13.
[31] Omole-Ohonsi A, Attah R.A. Outcome of Caesarean Delivery at Aminu Kano Teaching Hospital. Kanem Journal of Medical Sciences. 2009, 3(2): 36-39.
[32] Baskett TF. Peripartum Hysterectomy. A Textbook of Postpartum Haemorrhage. B-Lynch C, Keith LG, Lalonde AB, Karoshi M (eds). Sapiens publishing. 2006. 312-315.
[33]Why does the National U.S. Caesarean Section Rate Keep Going Up. Available at www.childbirthconnection.org/article.asp?ck=10456. Retrieved on 10th February 2010.
[34] Declercq E, Menacker F, MacDorman M. Maternal risk profiles and the primary caesarean rate in the United States, 1991-2002. Am J Public Health. 2006b; 96: 867-72.
[35] Nigeria Successfully Implementing A National Blood Safety Program Led By Safe Blood for Africa Foundation(TM) to Fight the Spread of HIV/AIDS.ABUJA, Nigeria, 2005. Available at www.prnewswire.co.uk/cgi/news/release?id=159570. Retrieved on 10th February 2010.
[36] Safe Blood Programs - Safe Blood for Africa. Available at www.safebloodforafrica.org/programs.htm. Retrieved on 10th February 2010.
[37] Hall M. Haemorrhage. In Department of Health, Welsh Office, Scotland Office Department of Health and social services, Northern Island, Why Mothers Die. Report on Confidential Enquiries into Maternal Deaths in the United Kingdom 2000-2002. London: Her Majesty's Stationery Office, 2004.

7

Peripartum Hysterectomy

Chisara C. Umezurike[1] and Charles A. Adisa[2]
[1]*Department of Obstetrics and Gynecology, Nigerian Christian Hospital Aba,*
[2]*Department of Surgery, Abia State University, Uturu*
Nigeria

1. Introduction

Peripartum or obstetric hysterectomy is the removal of the corpus uteri alone or with the cervix at the time of a cesarean section, or shortly after a vaginal delivery. It is a challenging but life-saving obstetric procedure. The removal of the uterus at cesarean section is referred to as cesarean hysterectomy while the removal after vaginal birth is called postpartum hysterectomy [1]. Peripartum hysterectomy is reserved for situations in which severe obstetric hemorrhage fails to respond to conservative treatment [2,3]. It is therefore unplanned and must be performed expeditiously usually in patients that are generally in less than ideal condition to withstand anesthesia and trauma of surgery. It has been described as one of the riskiest and most dramatic operations in modern obstetrics[2,4,5]. It is therefore associated with significant maternal morbidity and mortality.

2. Evolution of peripartum hysterectomy

Cesarean hysterectomy was originally proposed in 1768 by Joseph Cavallini in animal experiments[6].

The first documented hysterectomy on a patient at Caesarean section was performed in United States by Horatio Storer in 1869. Although the uterus was removed successfully, the patient died in 68 hours after surgery[6,7,8]. James Blundell in 1823 based his opinion approving post-cesarean hysterectomy on work done with rabbits.[6]

In 1876, Eduardo Porro of Milan described the first cesarean hysterectomy in which both mother and baby survived. His patient was a primiparous dwarf, Julia Cavallani, who was 25 years of age and was only 144cm in height. In his procedure, the uterus was opened in situ and the child was removed alive. After removal of the placenta, an instrument called a cintrat's constrictor was passed over the neck of the uterus and the wire was sufficiently tightened to control hemorrhage and the uterus was then cut away. The stump was brought out through the abdominal wound which was closed with sutures of silver wire[7].

After Porro's report more cases were reported with various modifications of the Porro's technique. Notable among these modifications were those of Godson in 1884 and Lawson tait in 1890[7,8]

Originally the indications for periparturm hysterectomy included uterine sepsis (amnionitis) after prolonged labour, atonia uteri or uncontrollable hemorrhage from placenta site, cancer of the cervix, extensive atresia of the vagina, preventing discharge of lochia, cases of ruptured uterus where suturing would be unsafe, uterine fibroids and tuberculosis[7].

By the 1950s it was carried out as elective procedure for indications such as sterilization, uterine fibroids and cervical dysplasia. By the 1970s elective cesarean hysterectomy for such procedures fell into disrepute due to the association of the procedure with excessive blood loss and urological injury. Moreover, with the introduction of laparoscopic procedures in sterilization, the indications for peripartum hysterectomy have become almost exclusively emergent occurring complications [7,8].

3. Incidence and risk factors

The reported incidence of emergency peripartum hysterectomy varies between 0.2 and 5.4 in 1000 deliveries [5,9]. In general, the average incidence is put at 1 in 1000 deliveries, the higher incidence is being reported from the developing world while developed countries generally report lower rates[5,9]. The high incidence of peripatum hysterectomy in the developing world may be due to her phenomenon of unbooked emergencies and the earlier recourse to hysterectomy due to the lack of adequate cross matched blood and other blood products which limit the time available for examining the effectiveness of other conservative procedures [5,40]. Moreover, certain modern conservative procedures involving interventional radiology are not practicable in most developing world settings due to lack of human and material resources involved[5].

There is significant association between peripartum hysterectomy and previous caesarean section and placenta previa[10,11,12]. The combination of prior caesarean section and placenta previa is said to be an ominous risk factor for the life threatening hemorrhage and peripartum hysterectomy [11,12,25,30]. Owing to the rising cesarean section rate world wide and the concomitant rise in placenta previa and placenta previa accreta, the incidence of emergency peripartum hysterectomy is rising in many countries[5,11,12,25].

Compared to vaginal delivery, emergency peripartum and abdominal delivery are strongly associated [1,19].

The association of peripartum hysterectomy with abdominal delivery may be related to its indications such as placenta previa and previous caesarean sections[1,5,12,13]. It may also be related to the fact that the uterus is readily available for removal in abdominal delivery[19].

It has also been reported that the multiple pregnancy has a six fold increased risk of emergency peripartum hysterectomy[12,17]. Multiple pregnancies are associated with higher rates of premature labour requiring tocolysis and uterine distension with greater total fetal weight at delivery[12]. All these predispose to uterine atony that can lead to peripartum hysterectomy. The increase in multiple pregnancy rates associated with assisted reproductive technology may provide a further contribution to rising peripartum hysterectomy rates.

Other reported risk factors for peripartum hysterectomy include unbooked status, retained placenta, previous endometrial curettage, abruptio placentae and thrombocytopenia [5,14,15,18].

4. Indications

The most common indication for peripartum hysterectomy is hemorrhage but the underlying causes vary from series to series.

In the developing world, preventable factor such as uterine rupture or uterine atony is the most common indication for peripartum hysterectomy[5,9,13,14,22]. The common causes of uterine rupture in this part of the world include prolonged obstructed labour, rupture of a previous caesarean scar, injudicious use of oxytocics and trauma from instruments or manual removal. If the rupture is extensive and hemorrhage cannot be controlled by uterine repair, then hysterectomy may become necessary [22].

Non-utilization or unavailability of modern potent oxytocic agents may predispose the at risk women to uterine atony and peripartum hysterectomy. There are however cases in which the uterus is not responsive to such uterotonic agents.

Older studies from the developed countries also showed uterine rupture or uterine atony as the most common indication for peripartum hysterectomy. In these countries uterine rupture has been reduced to a rarity by large scale utilization of modern obstetric care while uterine atony has also been reduced by use of potent uterotonic agents[16,23,24,25].

With rising caesarean section rate and marked reduction in the incidence of uterine rupture and atony, recent studies from the developed world have shown that placenta accreta has replaced uterine rupture and atony as the most common indication for emergency peripartum hysterectomy [24,25,26,27,29]. This is due to the rising incidence of placenta previa or accreta associated with the increasing number of women with previous caesarean section [20,21,28,30,31,32,33].

The other indication for peripartum hysterectomy is sepsis. In this era of modern potent antibiotic, sepsis is not a common indicaton for peripartum hysterectomy. It may however be necessary in cases with extensive uterine sepsis with myometrial abcess formation, in which antibiotic fails to control the infection [12].

If an antenatal diagnosis or strong suspicion of placenta accreta is made, the patient should therefore be counseled about the likelihood of peripartum hysterectomy[28,31]. In addition a senior obstetrician with vast experience in obstetric hysterectomy should be present at surgery.

With the rising caesarean section rate also in the developing countries, placenta accreta is becoming superimposed on the prevalent preventable indication such as uterine rupture and atony[5,14]. Unfortunately placenta accreta is less amenable to conservative management when compared to uterine rupture and atony.

5. Subtotal or total hysterectomy

Peripartum hysterectomy may be either subtotal or total.A subtotal hysterectomy is thought to be technically easier and associated with shorter operating time, less blood loss, less urological injury and low morbidity [5, 13,22,37]. It is therefore preferred in situations where maternal instability mandates a more expeditious procedure [37]. Moreover in developing countries where homologous blood is often not available, pelvic pathologies are extensive and clinical presentation of patients is worse, subtotal hysterectomy may be preferred[22,40].

Subtotal hysterectomy may be associated with certain post-operative problems from the cervical stump such as cyclical bleeding, vaginal discharge and the need for regular cervical cytology. It may be associated with continued bleeding from the cervical branch of the uterine artery, which supplies the lower segment and the cervix[9,37].

Total hysterectomy is therefore recommended if the patient is in good condition and when there is placenta previa or placenta previa accreta involving the cervix[26,37]. In addition to increased complications associated with total hysterectomy, it is difficult to identify the lower extent of the cervix to enable total hysterectomy in laboring patients whose cervix is fully dilated[31,33,34].

It has therefore been recommended that the decision on the type of hysterectomy should be individualized. With the increasing rate of placenta previa accreta, the need to do total hysterectomy will be on the increase.

6. Difficulties associated with peripartum hysterectomy

Peripartum hysterectomy has been described as one of the catastrophes of modern obstetrics [2,4]. The difficulties associated with the procedure are not necessarily the surgical technique but the anatomical and physiological changes associated with late pregnancy and the indications for the surgery as well as the support for such ill patients[12,22].

These difficulties are more pronounced in developing countries where patients present very late and the facilities for intensive care are lacking.

Some of these features that pose the difficulties with obstetric hysterectomy include;

a. Often markedly enlarged and distended uterine and ovarian vessels. There is generally increased blood supply to the pelvic organs in pregnancy.
b. Pelvic tissues adjacent to the uterus are oedematous and friable.
c. Trauma of extensive uterine rupture gives rise to gross distortion of the anatomy and oedema of the area surrounding the site of rupture.
d. Placenta previa percreta may extend into the bladder and other pelvic organs.
e. Scarring from previous cesarean sections obliterates the utero-vesical space and makes the separation of the bladder from the uterus difficult and injury prone.
f. The ureters may be sectioned, clamped or stitched because often, heavy bleeding interferes with proper exposure.
g. Difficulty in identifying the vaginal angles or the cervix to complete a total hysterectomy in laboring patients where the cervix is fully dilated.
h. The decision to perform hysterectomy is difficult especially in nulliparous women as this brings an abrupt and unwelcome end to their reproductive career. However the delayed decision may cause more blood loss thereby increasing morbidity.

7. Complications

An emergency major surgery that is characterized by the above mentioned difficulties will understandably be associated with unavoidable complications.

7.1 Intraoperative complications

The most frequent complication of peripartum hysterectomy is excessive blood loss and need for transfusion. Only part of this blood loss is attributable to the procedure itself. The extensive blood loss is related mainly to the primary indications for hysterectomy and delay in deciding to carry out hysterectomy. Oedematous tissue, adhesions from previous surgery and the inherent risk for coagulopathy may contribute to blood loss [12,31,33,35].

Blood transfusion is therefore the most common adjunct therapy and therefore increases the risk of blood transmitted diseases such as Hepatitis B & C and HIV. The average number of units of blood transfused in cases of accreta is 6.6 units with some cases requiring over 20 units of blood [31,38]. At least 8-12 units of blood must be made available in suspected cases of accreta.

The next most frequently reported complication is urological injury which affects the bladder or the ureters.[9,31] The bladder is most frequently injured during the dissection from the lower segment in people with previous caesarean sections. The ureters can be clamped, sutured or stitched where they pass under the uterine vessels at the lateral aspects of the lower segment[31.35] The reported incidence of urological injuries with peripartum, hysterectomy is between 4.6% and 12.5%[5,9].

Less commonly reported complications include bowel injuries, laceration of the large pelvic vessels or infundibulo-pelvic ligaments [35].

7.2 Post-operative complications

The post operative morbidity of peripartum hysterectomy is high. The post operative complications include bleeding, wound sepsis/dehiscence, urinary tract infections, ileus, anemia, prolonged duration of hospital stay and/or injury after urinary tract infection. Occasionally pulmonary embolism occurs. Many complications such as bleeding, infections and fistula may require relaporotomy or reoperation for proper management [9,35].

Peripartum hysterectomy is associated with increased mortality. Maternal mortality associated with peripartum hysterectomy is decreasing in the developed world but it is high in the developing countries. Identifiable causes of mortality include persistent hemorrhage, disseminated intravascular coagulopathy renal failure and septicemia [5,9].

8. Important surgical techniques

8.1 Operative techniques that can reduce blood loss in peripartum hysterectomy

1. These include double clamping or back clamping of the pedicles followed by double ligature using an all encompassing tie followed by a transfixing suture.

2. Internal iliac artery ligation, balloon occlusion of the aorta and internal iliac vessels, intravenous administration of oxytocics and application of tourniquet around the uterine cervix can also reduce blood loss [33,41].
3. Moreover when planning delivery of a patient with predisposing factors for bleeding, a rapid or timely decision will prevent excessive blood loss.
4. When a decision has been made to carry out hysterectomy prior to the uterine incision in cases of placenta previa accreta (especially the percreta variant), the intact placenta should be left in situ following delivery of the fetus through a classical uterine incision.
5. If the cervix and paracolpos are not involved as the source of hemorrhage. Subtotal hysterectomy should be adequate to achieve hemostasis and is safer, faster and easier to perform than total hysterectomy. However if the lower segment and paracolpos are involved in the bleeding such as in cases of placenta previa accreta, total hysterectomy will be necessary to secure hemostasis [9,26].

8.2 Techniques that may reduce urologic complications

Such techniques include:

1. Careful sharp dissection of the bladder in the midline to mobilize the bladder flap in cases of previous cesarean section(s).
2. Placing clamps and sutures against side wall of the uterus and cervix,
3. Perioperative cystoscopy with ureteral stent placement, and checking the integrity of the bladder by filling with methylene blue solution.
4. In addition placing all clamps medial to those used to secure the uterine vessels and adopting the above mentioned measures to reduce bleeding in the operating field will ensure proper exposure and avoid clamping, sectioning or stitching of the ureters [33,35].

8.3 Other techniques

Measures that can help in identifying the lower extent of the cervix to enable total hysterectomy at full cervical dilatation include following the lower uterine segment between the thumb and forefinger, incising of the lower uterine segment and using a covering glove to explore the endocervical canal downwards and feel the external os of the cervix [31].

9. Alternatives to hysterectomy

The conservative treatment for massive obstetric hemorrhage has the advantage of preserving fertility and menstrual function, and reducing blood loss[36,39]. It is however only possible in the presence of a stable hemodynamic condition and adequate technical support. This treatment modality should be considered whenever feasible in the developing world where there is a strong desire for large family and aversion to hysterectomy [5]. Uterine rupture and atony are however more amenable to conservative treatment than placenta previa accreta. Conservative treatment may however be complicated by sepsis; secondary hemorrhage and treatment failure.

These alternatives to hysterectomy include effective and consistent use of oxytocics, packing of the uterus with gauze after removal of the placenta, uterine and internal arteries ligation, B-lynch uterine compression suture, balloon tamponade, uterine artery embolization, uterine repair for ruptured uterus, and argon beam coagulation of the placental site [36,39,41,42].

10. Practice points

- The combination of prior caesarean section and current placenta previa should alert the obstetrician that emergency peripartum hysterectomy may be needed and as such, adequate preparations should be made.
- A senior obstetrician with experience in peripartum hysterectomy must be present at surgery for suspected placenta accreta.
- If the personnel and material required for the management of diagnosed cases are lacking, referral to centers with such capacity should be made.
- Women undergoing caesarean section should not only be counseled about the short term complications but also the long term complications of placenta previa accreta and peripartum hysterectomy.

11. Research points

- There is need for a large multicenter trial comparing the conventional extirpative with conservative management. Although there are several case reports of successful conservative treatment, they cannot be used to evaluate benefits and disadvantages of each therapeutic strategy in a comparative manner.
- Even for the many alternative options to hysterectomy, there is need for randomized controlled trials to guide the choice of options.

12. Conclusions

The identification of the risk factors for placenta previa accreta and its antenatal diagnosis may represent a possibility for elective or semi elective peripartum hysterectomy in modern obstetrics.

In view of the rising incidence of placenta previa accreta, all over the world, the need for peripartum hysterectomy may be on the increase and as such residents in Obstetrics must be adequately trained to perform this difficult but life-saving procedure.

13. References

[1] Forna F, Miles A M, Jamieson DJ. Emergency Peripartum Hysterectomy: A comparison of Cesarean and post partum hysterectomy. Am J Obstet Gynecol 2004; 190:1440-4

[2] El-Jallad MF, Zayed F, Al-Rimawi HS. Emergency peripartum hysterectomy in Northern Jordan. Indications and Obstetric outcome (an 8-year review). Arch Gynecol Obstet 2004;270: 271-273

[3] Smith J, Nousa HA. Peripartum hysterectomy for primary post partum hemorrhage: Incidence and maternal Morbidity. J Obstet Gynecol 2007; 27 (1)44-47

[4] Yucel O, Ozdemir I, Yucel N, Somunkiran A. Emergency peripartum hysterectomy: A nine year review. Arch Gynecol Obstet 2006;274:84-87
[5] Umezurike CC, Feyi-Waboso PA, Adisa CA. Peripartum hysterectomy in Aba Southeastern Nigeria. Australian and New Zealand Journal of Obstetrics and Gynaecology 2008; 48:580-582.
[6] Chanrachakul B, Chaturachinda K, Phuapadit W, Rosingsipragarn R. Cesarean and post partum hysterectomy. Int J Gynecol Obstet 1996;54:109-113
[7] Durfee RB. Evolution of cesarean hysterectomy. Clin Obstet Gynecol 1969;12:575-579
[8] Mesleh R, Ayoub H, Alggwiser A, Kardic A. Emergency Peripartum hysterectomy. J Obstet Gynecol 1998;18(6): 533-537
[9] Zeteroglu S, Ustun Y, Engin-Ustun Y, Sahin G,Kamaci M. Peripartum hysterectomy in a teaching hospital in the Eastern region of Turkey. Eur J Obstet Gynecol Reprod Biol 2005; 120; 57-62.
[10] Whiteman MK, Kuklina E, Hills SD, Jamieson DJ, Miekle SF, Posner SF, MarchBanks PA. Incidence and determinants of peripartum hysterectomy. Obstet Gynecol 2006; 108:1486-1492.
[11] Turner MJ. Peripartum hysterectomy: An evolving picture. Int J Gynecol Obstet 2010; 109:9-11.
[12] Baskett TF; Peripartum Hysterectomy. In B-lynch C, Keith LG, Laloride AB, Karoshi M eds. A text book of Postpartum Hemorrhage. Dumfrieshire UK, Sapiens publishing 2006:312-315
[13] Ezechi OC, Kalu BKE, Njokanma FO, Nwokoro CA, Okeke GCE. Emergency peripartum hysterectomy in a Nigerian hospital: A 20 year review. J Obstet Gynaecol 2004;24:372-373
[14] Kwame-Aryee RA, Kwakye AK, Seffah JD. Peripartum hysterectomies at the Korle-Bu Teaching Hospital. A review of 182 consecutive cases. Ghana Medical Journal 2007;41(3):133-138
[15] Bodelon C, Bernabe-Oritiz A, Schiff MA, Reed SO. Factors associated with peripartum hysterectomy. Obstet Gynecol 2009; 114(1):115-123
[16] Zorlu CG, Turan C, Isik AZ, Danisman N, Murgan T, Gokman O. Emergency hysterectomy in modern obstetric practice changing clinical perspective in time. Acta Obstet Gynecol 1998;77:186-190
[17] Francois K, Ortiz J, Harris C, Foley MR, Elliot JP. Is peripartum hysterectomy more common in multiple gestations? Obstet Gynecol 2005;105:1369-1372
[18] Bai SW, Lee HJ, Cho JS, Park YW, Kim SK, Park KH. Peripartum hysterectomy and associated factors. Am J Reprod Med 2003;48:148-152
[19] Kacmar J, Bhimani Lisa, Boyd M, Shah-Hosseini R, Peipet JF. Route of Delivery as a Risk for emergent peripartum hysterectomy: A case control study. Obstet Gynecol 2003;102:141-145
[20] Yaegashi N, Cluba-Sekii, Okamura K. Emergency postpartum hysterectomy in women with placenta previa and prior cesarean section. Int J, Gynecol Obstet 2000;68:49-52
[21] Gielchinsky Y, Rojansky N, Fasouliotes SJ, Ezra Y. Placenta accreta- Summary of 10 years: A survey of 310 cases. Placenta 2002;23:210-214

[22] Okogbenin SA, Gharoro EP, Otoide VO, Okonta PI. Obstetric hysterectomy: Fifteen years experience in a Nigerian tertiary centre. J Obstet Gynaecol 2003;23:356-359
[23] Kastner ES, Figueroa R, Garry D, Maulik D. Emergency peripartum hysterectomy: Experience at a community teaching hospital. Obstet Gynecol 2002;99:971-975
[24] Kwee A, Bots ML, Visser GHA, Bruinse HW. Emergency peripartum hysterectomy: A prospective study in the Netherlands. Eur J Obstet Gynecol Reprod Biol 2006;124:187-192
[25] Zelop CM, Harlow BL, Frigolett FD, Safon LE, Saltzman DH. Emergency Peripartum hysterectomy. Am J Obstet Gynecol 1993:168:1443-1448.
[26] Engelsen IB, Albrechtsen S, Iverson OE. Peripartum Hysterectomy -incidence and maternal morbidity. Accta Obstet Gynecol Scand 2001; 80: 409-412.
[27] Yamani Zamzani TY. Indication of emergency peripartum hysterectomy. Arch Gynecol Obstet 2003; 268:131-135
[28] Umezurike CC. Placenta Percreta. A report of three cases and review of the literature. Journal of Medical investigations and practice 2009; 9:29-35.
[29] Chestnut DH, Eden RD, Gall SA, Parker RT. Peripartum hysterectomy: A review of cesarean and postpartum hysterectomy. Obstet Gynecol 1985; 65:367-370
[30] Clark SL, Koonongs PP, Phelan JP. Placenta praevia/accreta and prior cesarean section. Obstet Gynecol 1985;66: 89-92
[31] Eltabbakh GH, Watson JD: Postpartum hysterectomy. Int J Gynecol Obstet 1995;50: 257-262
[32] Stanco LM, Schrimmer DB, Paul RH, Mishell DR. Emergency peripartum hysterectomy and associated risk factors. Am J Obstet Gynecol 1993;168:879-883
[33] Wenham J, Matijevic R. Post partum hysterectomy : Revisited J Perinat Med 2001; 29: 260-265
[34] Lau WC, Fung HYM, Rogers MS. Ten years experience of cesarean and postpartum hysterectomy in a teaching hospital in Hong Kong. Eur J Obstet Gynecol 1997; 74:133-137
[35] Castaneda S, Karrison T, Cibils LA. Peripartum hysterectomy. J Perinat Med 2000; 28: 472-481
[36] Kayem G, Davy C, Goffinet F, Thomas C, Clement D, Carbol D. Conservative versus Extirpative management in cases of Placenta Accreta. Obstet Gynecol 2004; 104: 531-536
[37] Drife J. Management of Primary Postpartum hemorrhage. Br J. Obstet Gynecol 1997;104: 275-277
[38] Kuczkowski KM. Anaesthesia for repeat cesarean section in the parturients with abnormal placentation: What does an Obstetrician need to know? Arch Gynecol Obstet 2006;273:319-321
[39] Mechery J, Burch D. Alternative management of Placenta accreta. Gynecol surg 2006;3: 41-42
[40] Wake DG, Cutting WAM. Blood transfusion in developing countries; problems, priorities and practicalities. Trop Doct 1998; 28:4-8

[41] Ikeda T, Sameshima H, Kawagudi H, Yamuchi N, Ikenoue T. Tourniquet technique prevents profuse blood loss in Placenta accreta cesarean section. J Obstet Gynecol Res 2005;31:27-31
[42] Scarantino SE, Reilly JG, Moretti ML, Pitlari VT. Argon Beam Coagulation in the management of Placenta accreta. Obstet Gynecol 1999;94:825-827

8

Peripartum Hysterectomy Versus Non Obstetrical Hysterectomy

S. Masheer and N. Najmi
Aga Khan University Hospital, Karachi, Pakistan

1. Introduction

Hysterectomy is the surgical removal of the uterus. It is one of the commonest gynecological procedures performed all over the world. Most of the time it is done electively for common gynecological conditions like abnormal uterine bleeding, fibroid uterus, endometriosis, chronic pelvic pain and cervical dysplasia. In majority of these conditions, woman is peri menopausal or has already completed her family.

Cesarean hysterectomy is a unique entity where surgical removal of uterus is performed in order to save the patient's life. Although the basic steps of different types of hysterectomy are similar, yet according to their indications and pelvic anatomy, the technique can become more challenging leading to various outcomes in the post operative period.

2. Types of hysterectomy

Depending on the reason for doing hysterectomy, different types of hysterectomies are performed. These include:

1. Total abdominal hysterectomy
2. Supra cervical hysterectomy
3. Radical /Wertheim's Hysterectomy
4. Vaginal Hysterectomy
5. Laparoscopic assisted vaginal hysterectomy
6. Obstetric/Cesarean Hysterectomy

2.1 Total abdominal hysterectomy

This is, by far, one of the commonest gynaecological major operations. Abdominal hysterectomies are usually performed for large uterine fibroids, endometriosis and dysfunctional uterine bleeding etc. A further extension to total abdominal hysterectomy is the Radical hysterectomy which is reserved for carcinoma of the cervix or uterus.

For total abdominal hysterectomy, the patient is placed in dorsal position. Incision to the abdomen is made vertically or transversely according to the indication and size of the uterus. After opening the peritoneal cavity, abdominal sponges are used to pack the bowel and Balfour retractor is applied to have good access of the operating field. Uterus is grasped with medium sized clamps and pulled out of the incision to expose the anterior surface of the uterus.

The round ligament on each side is identified and clamped using firm grasping clamps like Kocher or Spencerville. Anterior fold of broad ligament is opened starting from the round ligament. After cutting and ligating the round ligament on each side, a window is created where peritoneum is thin with the index finger to clamp the infundibulo pelvic ligament which is then cut and transfixed. Urinary bladder is pushed down after opening the utero vesical fold completely. It is important to carefully identify the correct plane and reflect the bladder from the centre of the cervix as lateral reflection could lead to inadvertant bleeding. Next step is to clamp the uterine arteries at the level of internal cervical os with heavy clamps like Roberts or Mangots hugging on to the cervix and ligating them carefully. Then the cardinal ligament are clamped, cut and ligated, going medially towards the cervix to avoid injury to the ureters till the vagina is reached. The uterus is removed and the anterior and posterior walls of the cut vagina are grasped by Volsellum forceps. The vagina is closed with either figure of eight sutures or in button hole fashion in which vagina is left open.

2.2 Supra cervical hysterectomy

One of the commonest indications for performing supra cervical hysterectomy is Endometriosis where there is frozen pelvis and difficulty in accessing the area below the level of uterine arteries.

In supra cervical or subtotal hysterectomy, body of the uterus is removed in exactly the same fashion as the total abdominal hysterectomy until the level of ligation of uterine arteries. After this level, the uterine body is cut from the cervix and haemostatic sutures are taken on the cut edge of the left over cervix. Some surgeons also prefer to perform the conization of the endo cervix in order to reduce the chances of cervical cancer. Women undergoing supra cervical hysterectomy are advised to follow up with their Pap smear in the similar fashion as before the surgery.

2.3 Laparoscopic hysterectomy

Laparoscopic hysterectomies were introduced as a replacement of abdominal hysterectomy with the benefit of avoiding incision of the abdomen.

Patient should be placed in dorsal lithotomy position. Uterine manipulator is inserted according to the size of introitus and parity of the patient. Dilatation of cervix is rarely required to place the uterine manipulator. Foley catheter is inserted into the urinary bladder.

The best way to minimize laproscopic injuries is to insert primary Trocars with maximum care.

Most of the gynecologists prefer closed entry technique in which carbon dioxide is insufflated via Verses needle into the peritoneal cavity. Other method is open technique in which a small incision is made into the rectus sheath and has direct access to peritoneal cavity.

The incision for laparoscopy should be vertical from the base of the umbilicus as it is the thinnest part of the abdominal wall. The Verses needle should be sharp and its spring mechanism should be properly working. Lower abdominal wall should be stabilized by grasping and holding it upwards with one hand so that veress is inserted perpendicular to the skin with the other hand. Two audible clicks are usually heard when veress pierces the fascia and the peritoneum respectively. In case of difficult or failed attempts either the open method or the palmers point entry should be approached. For primary trocar insertion intra-abdominal gas pressure should be 20-25 mmHg which is later reduced to 12-15 mmHg for surgery.

The infunibulo pelvic ligament is desiccated with bipolar grasper. It is very important to stay close to the ovaries and transect them using Harmonic scalpel. During this step uterine manipulator should be pushed upwards and on opposite side to provide maximum visualization and good working space.

After this step, round ligament is transected in order to separate the leaves of broad ligament with Harmonic scalpel. This step differs from abdominal hysterectomy where round ligaments are transected as the first step of surgery. Identification of correct plane is vital.i.e.where peritoneum is loose and easily separable, uterovesical fold is opened anteriorly to mobilize the bladder down. It should be carefully done in patients with previous cesarean sections and uterine surgeries. Once the bladder is down, ureters are retracted laterally, so tha uterine arteries can be desiccated with bipolar grasper and transected with harmonic scalpel Two small incisions are made with Harmonic scalpel medial to uterine vessels so as to free the cervix from the transcervical ligaments. Vaginal fornices can be identified by pushing in upward direction with the uterine manipulator and Harmonic scalpel is used to cut the cervix from the vagina. Uterus is then removed and a glove with sponges is placed into the vagina to maintain pneumoperitoneum.

Vaginal cuff is closed in a running fashion, with almost one centimeter thickness including vaginal mucosa and pubocervical and rectovaginal fascia.

It is recommended to suture the rectus sheath of all non-midline port over 7mm and midline port greater than 10mm to avoid hernia formation.

2.4 Total vaginal hysterectomy

Patient is placed in dorsal lithotomy position with buttocks at the end of table. Two Jacobs's tenacula are used to grasp the anterior and posterior lip of cervix. Simple saline solution or adrenaline with the dilution of 1:100000 is injected into the vaginal mucosa at its junction with the cervix. After injecting the solution the Mucosa is incised with scalpel around the entire cervix.

Index finger is used to dissect the bladder up to the peritoneal vesico uterine fold. Alternatively, sharp dissection can also be done for this step. A right angle retractor is placed under the vaginal mucosa and bladder to elevate them and the peritoneal fold is incised with Mayo's scissors. Cervix is lifted up with Jacobs's tenacula and peritoneum of cul-de-sac is incised.

A curved Heaney clamp is placed in posterior cul de sac. The clamp is applied next to cervix and uterosacral ligaments are cut with mayo's scissors and ligated. This suture not only ligates the uterosacral ligament but plicates the pedicle to vaginal cuff.

The cardinal ligament is clamped adjacent to lower uterine segment and ligated.The uterine arteries are clamped, cut and ligated in the similar fashion close to the junction of lower uterine segment with internal cervical os. Uptil this step ligating and securing the pedicles is relatively easy as they are easily approachable surgically. The next step is clamping and ligating the tubo- ovarian ligaments. This step can be difficult sometimes especially if the uterus is enlarged. In such circumstances, either the fundus of the uterus can be delivered outside or uterus can be bisected longitudinally in the midline and each pedicle can then be secured separately.

Heaney clamps are applied to tubo- ovarian round ligament either directly or by following any of the above methods and uterus is then removed through the vagina.

Re-peritonealization is carried out with purse string sutures starting from anterior peritoneal edge and continued down through the uterosacral cardinal ligament pedicles and the vaginal mucosa.

Vaginal cuff is sutured with running locking stitch and is left open.

2.5 Radical hysterectomy

Patient selection is critical for radical hysterectomy. Young, thin patients with early stage carcinoma of cervix are usually the best candidates. Obesity is at times associated with carcinoma of the endometrium and is a relative contraindication. Preoperative preparation and informed consent are the prerequisite as in any other surgery.

Patient is placed in dorsal position. Abdominal incision is midline as it gives excellent access to pelvis and Para aortic lymph nodes are easily approachable when required. After opening the peritoneal cavity, peritoneal cytology is taken. Large sponges are used to pack the bowel and Balfour retractor is applied to have good view of the pelvis. If the patient is obese Book Walter retractor provides excellent access to the pelvis.

In radical hysterectomy round ligament is clamped on each side closed to the pelvic side wall and broad ligament is opened superiorly up to the paracolic gutter and the incision is extended inferiorly and medially to open the Utero-vesical fold. Laterally non toothed forceps can be used to freed the peritoneum from the adjacent soft tissue and reaches to the triangle bounded by urinary bladder medially, iliac vessels laterally and the pelvis inferiorly. If the ovaries are to be conserved the index finger is placed on the medial side of the ovary and then pierces the peritoneum through the thinnest part and clamp is applied and infundibulopelvic ligament is then cut. The same steps are repeated on the other side.

Uterine artery needs to be skeletonized so that it is completely separated from the ureters and obliterated hypogastric artery should be identified at this point. The uterine vessel should be accurately clamped with Meig's forceps close to its origin at the internal iliac artery. Now make sure that bladder is separated from the cervix. This can be easily done by pushing down the utero vesical fold with swab folded on the index finger.

Next important step is the identification and division of the roof of the ureters tunnel. Usually tissue forceps are placed medially to uterine arteries and canal roof is clamped and cut, exposing the ureters and this pedicle is tied. Next step is separation of ureters laterally from the upper vagina, this will expose cardinal ligament. Posteriorly peritoneum is opened just below the cervix, revealing soft tissue between vagina and the rectum. It is important to work under direct vision keeping an eye on the ureter. Make sure that uterosacral ligaments are free and away from the ureters and Zippelin forceps are applied and uterosacrals are cut. Another Zippelin clamp is applied on the cardinal ligament, it is cut and ligated and uterus is removed. Vault is closed with running suture or button hole fashion but caution must be applied on reviewing the ureters.

Radical hysterectomy is usually accompanied by dissection of pelvic lymph nodes. Some authorities prefer to do it before performing radical hysterectomy and some do it afterwards.

2.6 Obstetric/ peri partum hysterectomy

Obstetric hemorrhage is one of the leading causes of maternal mortality. The rise in mortality rate has been attributed to a number of factors, including increasing age at childbirth, increased numbers of multiple pregnancies and the rising caesarean section rate. Postpartum hemorrhage is one of the leading causes of maternal deaths and at times hysterectomy remains the life saving procedure in such cases. Almost all the literature on peri partum hysterectomy consists of analysis of retrospective cases in different hospitals all over the world.

2.6.1 Risk factors for obstetrics hysterectomy

Incidence of Peri partum hysterectomy in modern obstetrics is rising due to increase in rate of Cesarean section all over the world, leading to morbidly adherent placenta. Other reasons for peri partum hysterectomy are grand multi parity which can lead to uterine atony, uterine rupture and coagulopathy, presence of large leiomyomas, or bleeding from lacerated uterine vessel which is not treatable by more conservative measures. Hysterectomy also may be appropriate for women with postpartum uterine infection unresponsive to antibiotic therapy. In majority of the cases, peri partum hysterectomy is performed as an emergency procedure which leads to further morbidity to the patient.

Planned hysterectomy at the time of delivery is controversial because of increased morbidity related to surgery on the highly vascular pelvic organs. However, there are certain elective indications for peri partum hysterectomy. These include large or symptomatic leiomyomas and severe cervical dysplasia or carcinoma in situ.

2.6.2 Preparation

Most of the times, the obstetrician can anticipate the possible need for peri partum hysterectomy which helps in better preoperative preparation and management. Many of the litigations can be prevented by taking and documenting an informed consent for the procedure including the chances of all possible complications. This may not always be possible when one is dealing with acute emergency but it can be done electively prior to labor and delivery when there are risk factors present in the patient such as suspicion of morbidly adherent placenta.

Risk assessment of the pregnant woman should be routinely carried out at her first antenatal visit and then at 20weeks of gestation when anomalies scan can comment on placental localization. Follow-up imaging is required if the placenta covers or overlaps the cervical os at 20 weeks of gestation especially for women with previous cesarean scars where chances of acreta are higher. Antenatal sonographic imaging can be complemented by magnetic resonance imaging in equivocal cases to distinguish those women at special risk of placenta acreta.

Patients with high parity, major placenta previa and previous cesarean section should be vigilantly followed and delivered in well resourced settings where facilities of blood bank and multidisciplinary antenatal, intra partum and post operative care can be provided.

The National Patient Safety Agency (NPSA) in collaboration with the Royal College of Obstetricians and Gynaecologists (RCOG) and the Royal College of Midwives (RCM) developed a Care Bundle for placenta previa acreta. This Care Bundle has six elements of good care as follows:

- Consultant obstetrician planned and directly supervising delivery
- Consultant anaesthetist planned and directly supervising anaesthetic at delivery
- Blood and blood products available
- Multidisciplinary involvement in pre-op planning
- Discussion and consent includes possible interventions (such as hysterectomy, leaving the placenta in place, cell salvage and intervention radiology)
- Local availability of a level 2 critical care bed. Level 2 critical care bed are the high dependency area capable of providing service to meet the needs of patients who require more detailed observation or intervention ,short-term non-invasive ventilation and post- operative care.

The morbidities associated with placenta acreta/percreta can be reduced by following these six points of Care Bundle.

2.6.3 Technique

Women with placenta previa in the third trimester should be counselled about the risks of preterm delivery and obstetric haemorrhage, and their care should be tailored to their individual needs. This care plan should be documented in the antenatal folder so that if patient presents in an emergency situation, the procedures/prerequisites to follow are already present. Good communication among the team members is essential for successful outcome.

Prophylactic antibiotic is mandatory for such patients and majority of the times this is converted into therapeutic antibiotics depending upon the extent and nature of surgery. Similarly, thromboembolism prevention such as by using preoperative anti-embolism compression stockings and post operative physiotherapy are some universal steps which can lead to a better outcome.

Adequate exposure is important. Although Pfennenstiel incisions are mostly given in unanticipated cases, but midline skin incision can be considered if the morbidly adherent placenta is diagnosed or suspected. It will not only help in selection of uterine incision which may be classical but also will be valuable if proceeding for hysterectomy. In case of Pfennenstiel approach, incision can be extended in order to have good exposure of the surgical field. Semi Trendelenburg position of the patient and abdominal packing with large swabs will help in better exposure. Anterior abdominal wall retraction with Deaver is usually enough most of the time, Balfour retractor is not always necessary. As peri partum hysterectomy is associated with massive hemorrhage most of the time, therefore time constraints should be kept in mind. Both sided round ligament should be clamped with straight Heaney close to the uterus and double ligated with vicryl zero or one. Utero-vesical fold is already opened if proceeding to hysterectomy after the cesarean section. Otherwise this fold needs to be opened and bladder should be reflected down so that ureters move away from the infundibulo-pelvic ligament and uterine arteries. Posterior leaf of broad ligament is opened by blunt dissection with the help of index finger from posterior to anterior and with curved Heaney the utero-ovarian ligament and fallopian tube is clamped and transfixed with vicryl one. Ovaries are conserved in cases of peripartum hysterectomy. On the other hand, Round and infundibulo-pelvic ligaments can be taken together close to the fundus of the uterus in order to save time. Bladder should again be carefully reflected down further, both sided uterine arteries and veins are identified, clamped with curved Heaney, and ligated with vicryl one. By this point bleeding is usually controlled and body of uterus should be removed just below the ligation of uterine arteries and cervical stump can be closed with vicryl one. This subtotal hysterectomy is often the procedure of choice in obstetric hemorrhage.

If the bleeding is not controlled or morbidly adherent placenta is involving the lower uterine segment, then total hysterectomy should be performed which at times can be difficult. Lower margins of cervix can be felt with fingers when the scar is opened, it will roughly give an idea of cervical length and clamps should be applied medially to the secured uterine arteries close to the uterus. Once again bladder should be reflected down further before applying clamps. If uterus is not opened, clamps are applied in a similar way to the cardinal ligament, and the pedicle is ligated and transfixed. These steps are repeated till lateral vaginal fornix is reached. Just below the cervix curved clamps like Roberts are applied medially on both sides and uterus with cervix is removed. Cervix should be inspected for its complete removal. Both sided vaginal angle should be secured with figure of eight sutures. Vaginal vault can be closed with interrupted sutures using vicryl zero or one or can be left open with button hole sutures.

3. Complications of Peri partum hysterectomy Vs gynecological hysterectomy

The outcome of Peri partum hysterectomy depends upon its indication. In most cases, this is performed as an emergency procedure, thus the complications associated with it are definitely higher than non obstetrics hysterectomy. One of the most common complications encountered in Peri partum hysterectomies is the risk of hemorrhage. Massive post partum hemorrhage is encountered in almost all cases of peri partum hysterectomies. According to one study, the estimated blood loss ranged from 1-6 liters, leading to blood transfusion in 92% of patients, 20 % of whom also developed coagulopathy. Because of massive hemorrhage, hemostasis can be a challenging task and such patient may end up in having a repeat laparotomy for this reason. The percentage of patients undergoing repeat laparotomy could be as high as 16%. When compared with non obstetric hysterectomy, women who underwent a peri partum procedure are nearly eight times more likely to require surgical re-exploration and almost three times as likely to develop a wound complication.

Another complication commonly encountered is the risk of infection. It is one of the commonest reasons for prolonged hospital stay. Wound infections and puerperal sepsis can occur in up to 14-19% of cases.

Organ injury is more likely to occur in Peri partum hysterectomies especially those done for morbidly adherent placenta where bladder is injured. Similarly, ureters can also be injured in such emergency cases. Other organs like bowel are less commonly injured. According to one survey in UK, bladder damage was more likely to occur in cases of morbidly adherent placenta (23%) compared to uterine atony (8%, OR 3.41, 95% CI 1.55–7.48). Ureteric injury was similar in both cases (6%vs 4%). The percentage of organ injury is much higher when compared to prevalence of organ injuries in other benign gynecological reasons for hysterectomy (0.4%-2.5%).

When comparing peri partum hysterectomy to non obstetric benign hysterectomy, rates of postoperative hemorrhage (5% compared with 2%), wound complications (10% compared with 3%), and venous thromboembolism (1% compared with 0.7%) are all quoted to be higher in women who underwent peri partum hysterectomy. Similarly, peri operative cardiovascular, pulmonary, gastrointestinal, renal, and infections morbidities are all higher for Peri partum hysterectomy.

Because of the challenging nature of the surgery and the associated complications, the post operative stay in hospital, including the ICU stay, of such patients is much higher than those undergoing non obstetric hysterectomy. For the similar reasons, the chances of mortality of such patients are also higher compared to the other group. According to Wright et al, the mean length of stay for women who underwent peri partum hysterectomy was 8.7 days compared with 2.9 days for non obstetric hysterectomy. The peri operative mortality for peri partum hysterectomy was 1% compared with 0.04% for non obstetric hysterectomy. This study showed that the mortality in cases of peri partum hysterectomy was 14 times higher when compared to non obstetric hysterectomy.

4. Conclusion

Timely expert management in a well resourced centre is advocated. Hemorrhage is predictable in some situations when risk factors are present but severe uncontrollable hemorrhage can occur unexpectedly. It is in these situations that early decision making and the provision of adequate supplies of blood and blood products become extremely important. All obstetricians should be adequately trained in the performance of the B-lynch procedure, emergency hysterectomy and other complicated procedures such as ligation of the internal iliac arteries to control uterine hemorrhage. It is advisable that senior obstetrician must be involved in care of such patients. There must be national and local clear protocols and drills on the management of peri partum hemorrhage which may help reduce the incidence of peri partum hysterectomy.

All essential drugs for managing post partum hemorrhage should be available in the delivery unit all the time. Vigilant monitoring of laboring patients with previous scar can lead to timely decision of cesarean delivery which in turn leads to reduced chances of uterine rupture. On the other hand, increasing cesarean section rates leads to increased chances of morbidly adherent placenta which in turn leads to increased chances of peri partum hysterectomy. Therefore it is recommended that such cases should always be dealt in tertiary care with multi disciplinary team approach involving urologists, hematologist and intensive care experts. Despite advances in clinical practice, it is likely that peri partum hysterectomy will be more challenging for obstetricians in the future and therefore regular drills of these protocols can help reduce morbidity associated with it.

5. References

Cunningham FG, Leveno KJ, Bloom SL, Hauth JC, Rouse DJ, Spong CY .*Williams Obstetrics,* 23edition Section IV. Labor and Delivery Chapter 25. Cesarean Delivery and Peripartum Hysterectomy.The McGraw-Hill Companies.

Clifford R Wheel less, Marcelle L Roenneburg.Atlas of pelvic surgery, on line edition, October2011. http://www.atlasofpelvicsurgery.com/5Uterus/9TotalVaginalHysterectomy/chap5sec9.html

Drake MJ, Noble JG. Ureteric trauma in gynecologic surgery. *Int Urogynecol J Pelvic Floor Dysfunct.* 1998;9(2):108-17.

Jon I Einarasson, 2009.Total laproscopic Hystrectomy:10 steps toward a successful procedure, *Rev Obstet Gynaecol.*2(1): 57-64

Jacobs Allon. Peripartum hysterectomy. *UptoDate*: September 2010.

Jason D. Wright JD, Devine P, Shah M, et al.Morbidity and Mortality of Peripartum Hysterectomy. *Obstet Gynecol* 2010; 115:1187–93

K A Rabiu, F M Akinlusi and A A Adewunmi. Emergency peripartum hysterectomy in a tertiary hospital in Lagos, Nigeria: a five-year review. *Trop Doct* 2010; 40:1-4.

Knight M on behalf of UKOSS. Peripartum hysterectomy in the UK: management and outcomes of the associated haemorrhage. *BJOG* 2007;114:1380–1387.

Michael J. Turner; Peripartum hysterectomy: An evolving picture. *International Journal of Gynecology & Obstetrics* Vol 109, Issue 1, Pages 9-11, April 2010

RA Kwame-Aryee, AK Kwakye, and JD Seffah. Peripartum hysterectomies at the korle-bu teaching hospital: a review of 182 consecutive cases. *Ghana Med J.* 2007 September; 41(3): 133–138.

Paterson-Brown S, Singh C. Developing a care bundle for the management of suspected placenta accreta. *The Obstetrician & Gynaecologist* 2010;12:21–7.

RCOG Green-top Guideline No. 27. Placenta praevia, placenta praevia accreta and vasa praevia: diagnosis and management, January 2011

RCOG Green -top Guideline No. 49. Preventing Entry related Gynaecological Laproscopic injuries, May 2008

Tito Lopes et al 2010.Operations on the uterus, In:*Bonney's Gynaecological Surgery,* 105-120 Wiley- Blackwell, ISBN 9781405195652, UK

Tallab F, Helewa M.Peripartum hysterectomy: 10 years experience in two Manitoba tertiary centers. *Ann Saudi Med* 1998; 18 (5): 398-400.

William J Mann. Radical Hystrectomy, *Upto Date,* March 2011.

Yalinkaya A, Güzel A I, Kangal K. Emergency Peripartum Hysterectomy: A 16 years experience of a Medical Hospital. *J Chin Med Assoc* 2010;73(7):360–363.

Part 2

Alternatives to Hysterectomy

9

Medical Treatment of Fibroid to Decrease Rate of Hysterectomy

Mohamed Y. Abdel-Rahman[1],
Mohamed Sabry[1,2] and Ayman Al-Hendy[2]
[1]*Department of Obstetrics and Gynecology, Sohag University Hospitals, Sohag,*
[2]*Center for Women's Health Research, Department of Obstetrics and Gynecology,*
Meharry Medical College, Nashville, Tennessee,
[1]*Egypt*
[2]*USA*

1. Introduction

Uterine leiomyomas are the most common benign pelvic tumors in women [1, 2]. They are monoclonal tumors of the smooth muscle cells of the myometrium and consist of large amounts of extracellular matrix that contains collagen, fibronectin and proteoglycan [2, 3]. A thin pseudocapsule that is composed of areolar tissue and compressed muscle fibers usually surrounds the tumors [4]. Leiomyomas may enlarge to cause significant distortion of the uterine surface or cavity. Although they are benign, they commonly result in severe symptoms, such as heavy, irregular and prolonged menstrual bleeding as well as anemia. Uterine leiomyomas have also been associated with numerous other medical disorders, such as infertility, recurrent abortion and preterm labor [5]. These clinical complications negatively impact women's health. Uterine leiomyomas are the most cited indication for more than 600,000 hysterectomies performed in the US annually, and this major surgery is associated with morbidity and mortality as well as a huge economic impact on healthcare delivery systems that is estimated to be approximately $2.2 billion/year [6].

2. Current medical treatment options for uterine leiomyomas

Treatment options for leiomyoma vary. Treatment strategies are typically individualized based on the severity of the symptoms, the size and location of the leiomyoma lesions, the patient's age and their chronological proximity to menopause, and the patient's desire for future fertility. The usual goal of therapy is the relief of the symptoms (which include abnormal uterine bleeding, pain, and pressure). The treatment options range from the use of acupuncture (ancient Chinese method) to the total removal of the uterus and its myoma contents [7]. The gold standard of leiomyoma treatment is surgical intervention. Hysterectomy is the definitive surgical operation, but myomectomy is still commonly performed especially in women who desire future fertility. More recently developed techniques, which include uterine artery embolization (UAE), magnetic resonance-guided focused-ultrasound surgery (MRgFUS) and myolysis, are emerging as minimally invasive alternative procedures. To date, there is no definitive therapeutic agents for the treatment of uterine leiomyomas, which is a reflection of the dearth of randomized clinical trial data demonstrating the effectiveness and safety of medical therapies in the management of symptomatic leiomyomas [8]. This chapter will focus on medical treatment options for uterine leiomyoma as a promising tool to decrease the rate of hysterectomy with its burden to the health system as well as the patients.

2.1 COCs and progestins

Combined oral contraceptive hormones have been widely tried by physicians to reduce the blood loss associated with uterine fibroids. A large prospective study including more than 3000 patients with fibroids found a positive correlation between the early use of COCs (before 17 years) and the incidence of fibroid [9]. Other controlled trials showed no association between the use of COCs and the development of uterine fibroids [10, 11].

The effect of COcs and progestins in reducing the size of fibroids is not documented [12-14].

3. Levonorgestrel-releasing intrauterine system

The levonorgestrel-releasing intrauterine system (LNG) is one of the most effective treatments in reducing menorrhagia. In a small randomized trial; LNG decreased the blood loss significantly after 6 weeks of application in women with menorrhagia and fibroid [15]. However; it did not decrease the myoma size.

3.1 Promising GnRH antagonist (elagolix)

Elagolix is a second generation new non-peptide (GnRH) antagonist, highly potent antagonist orally active and rapidly bioavailable after administration that is being developed by Abbott Laboratories (Abbott) in collaboration with Neurocrine Biosciences [16, 17]. It Finalizing the Phase III for endometriosis and finalizing Phase II for uterine leiomyoma with opportunity to be its first and only approved oral treatment for uterine leiomyoma [18]. This promising compound inhibits gonadotropin releasing hormone (GnRh) receptors in the pituitary gland leading to a dose dependent suppression of LH, FSH and estradiol. Consequently, suppression of E2 is more prolonged at higher doses. Pituitary suppression is maintained for only a portion of the day, and baseline gonadotropin levels return by 24 hours [19].

These properties suggest that elagolix may enable dose-related pituitary and gonadal suppression in premenopausal women as part of treatment strategies for reproductive hormone-dependent disease states [19]. To date, elagolix has been studied in 18 clinical trials totaling more than 1,000 subjects.

Elagolix seems to be well tolerated for multiple-doses up to 200; rapidly absorbed after oral administration, with median time of maximum plasma concentration (Tmax) values ranging from 0.5–1 h, the primary metabolite (NBI-61962) appear in the serum rapidly after administration [19].

The therapeutic window of E2 levels for suppression of endometriosis using is attainable at a dose of 100-150mg/day with serum estradiol remained between 20 – 50 pg/ml [20]. This is supported by Barberi RL findings which showed that E2 levels between 30-50 pg/ml are effective in inducing endometrial atrophy [21]. The Elagolix therapeutic dose for management of uterine fibroid has yet to be determined.

4. Selective Estrogen Receptor Modulators (SERMS)

Selective estrogen receptor modulators (SERMs) are non-steroidal estrogen receptor ligands that display tissue-specific agonist–antagonist estrogenic actions. They are used frequently in the treatment and prevention of estrogen receptor-positive carcinoma of the breast in addition to their use as ovulation induction agents [22, 23]. Tamoxifen is one of the oldest known SERMs, but it may potentially cause endometrial carcinoma due to its partial agonistic effect on the endometrium [24]. There are no randomized controlled trials that have investigated the potential role of Tamoxifen in the treatment of uterine fibroids; however, a few case reports have suggested that it actually increases leiomyoma growth [22, 25]. Raloxifene is another SERM that can be theoretically considered to be a candidate therapeutic option for uterine fibroids. Raloxifene only slightly affected collagen biosynthesis in control myometrium cells; however, it significantly inhibited collagen biosynthesis in leiomyoma cells [26] and exerted its action at the transcriptional level [27]. A newly developed SERM, "Lasofoxifene", is currently awaiting FDA approval. However, the results of early trials suggest that there were no significant benefits compared to raloxifene for the skeleton, breast, heart, or reproductive tract [28, 29].

4.1 Mechanism of action

The most probable hypothesis that explain SERMs' mechanism of action is that they induce changes in estrogen receptors, which result in differential expression of specific estrogen-regulated genes in different tissues [30]. Every member of the SERM family has its own individual characteristics, which depend on its structure, the type of estrogen receptor they bind to, and the set of molecules that interact with its estrogen receptor/SERM complex in affected cells, and these characteristics result in either agonistic or antagonistic activity [31]. SERMS could potentially provide therapeutic benefits by having antagonistic effects at uterine myometrial level and by preventing ovarian stimulation which has been achieved in rat studies. The difference in activity of SERMS is based on the structure activity relationships (SAR) [32].

4.2 SERMs and treatment of uterine fibroids

All SERMs, with their estrogen blocking activity, would be theoretically expected to exert at least some therapeutic effect on uterine fibroids. Raloxifene has been showed to enhance the shrinkage of uterine fibroids in postmenopausal women [33, 34]. However, a recent report from Italy that addressed the effect of raloxifene on uterine leiomyoma showed that the leiomyoma size in premenopausal women who were administered daily 60-mg doses of raloxifene over a 2-year period exhibited no change in leiomyoma size [35].

4.3 Adverse events

Tamoxifen is not recommended for women with a prior history of deep venous thrombosis, pulmonary embolus, stroke, or transient ischemic attack because it increases the risk of ischemic stroke, particularly in women who are 50 years of age or older. Additionally, the risk of uterine/endometrial cancer was approximately doubled with tamoxifen use [36], and the risk of superficial thrombophlebitis was three times higher [24, 37]. Some of these side effects could be explained by the inhibition of cellular glutamine uptake, oxidative stress and the induction of apoptosis [38]. SERMs are seldom used for the treatment of uterine fibroids [26].

5. Aromatase inhibitors

Aromatase inhibitors (AI) significantly block both ovarian and peripheral estrogen production within 1 day of treatment [39]. Letrozole suppressed the production of estrogens, particularly estrone and estradiol, by 76-79% compared to their baseline levels [40]. The underlying mechanism is the inhibition of the aromatase enzyme, which is the enzyme that catalyzes the conversion of androgenic substances into estrogens [41]. Recent reports have suggested that aromatase is expressed to a greater extent in uterine leiomyoma tissues of African-American women compared to Caucasian women, which may contribute to the higher incidence of ULMs in African American women [42]. Aromatase inhibitors have been shown to be effective against fibroids in limited short term studies with dosing regimens that included 2.5 mg per day of letrozole and 1 mg per day of anastrozole [43]. One of the major concerns with the use of aromatase inhibitors is the reported bone loss with prolonged use, which necessitates the concomitant use of oral contraceptive pills or progesterone [44]. A recently published RCT compared the effects of three months of aromatase inhibitor (letrozole) to that of three months of gonadotropin-releasing hormone agonist (triptorelin) on uterine leiomyoma volume and hormonal status [45]. The results showed an advantage of the rapid onset of action of AIs in addition to the avoidance of the flare ups that initially occurs with GnRHa. Both treatment options induced significant shrinkage of the uterine fibroids and improvement in leiomyoma-associated symptoms [45]. The mean reduction of leiomyoma volume with 3 months use of anastrazole is 55.7% [46]. The authors suggested that aromatase inhibitors should be considered in women with fibroids on a short term basis or in women who want to avoid surgical intervention to preserve their potential fertility [47]. Another concern with the use of AIs as a treatment option for uterine leiomyoma is its off-label use, which mandates a thorough review with patients prior to the initiation of the therapy [44]. Several RCTs are underway that would hopefully add to our understanding of the potential promising role of AIs in the treatment of uterine leiomyomas [36].

6. Antiprogesterones

Estrogen has traditionally been considered to be the most important stimulus for leiomyoma growth and numerous studies that included cell culture and animal models supported this concept [48]. Surprisingly, recent findings suggest that volume maintenance and growth of human ULMs are also heavily progesterone-dependent, and hence anti-progesterone could reverse leiomyoma growth effects [16, 49]. One potential link between the effects of the two key steroid hormones on ULMs is that estradiol induced the expression of the progesterone receptor and supported progesterone action on leiomyoma tissue [48]. Clinical findings also support these laboratory observations; studies have involved the evaluation of mifepristone (RU 486) [50-52], azoprisnil [43, 49], and more recently, CDB-2914 and CDB-4124 (CDB: Contraceptive Development Branch) [53].

6.1 Mifepristone

Mifepristone (RU486), a well-known oral anti-progesterone compound, has been used for more than 20 years for multiple clinical indications [45, 54-56]. It has recently been evaluated as a potential therapeutic agent for uterine fibroids with a dose that ranges from 5 mg to 50 mg over a 3-month period [29, 57, 58]. Mifepristone reduced leiomyoma size (26% to 74%) and improved leiomyoma-related symptoms (63% to 100% induction of amenorrhea). Reported side effects included transient elevations in transaminases, which occurred in 4% of cases as well as endometrial hyperplasia and was detected in 28% of the women who were screened with endometrial biopsies [59]. However, these studies were mostly preliminary with limited numbers of subjects and therefore, larger randomized well-controlled trials that include thorough monitoring of liver function and endometrial histology are required to conclusively determine the safety and efficacy of this treatment modality.

6.2 Asoprisnil

Asoprisnil (J867, BAY86-5294) is an investigational selective progesterone receptor modulator (SPRM) that was developed for the treatment of progesterone-sensitive myomata. It induces unique morphological changes and is associated with inhibited proliferation of the endometrium and leiomyomata. These changes may lead to amenorrhea, which is usually encountered with its use [43, 60, 61]. Asoprisnil is a tissue selective molecule that binds to the progesterone receptors with a three-fold greater affinity than endogenous progesterone [57]. It reduces the uterine and leiomyoma volumes in a dose-dependent manner while achieving remarkable decreases in menorrhagia scores in women with menorrhagia [62]. Amenorrhea rates also increased as the dose of asoprisnil was increased [58, 60]. When asoprisnil was administered daily for longer than 3-4 months, significant endometrial thickening and unusual histological appearance of the endometrial glands occurred [29].

6.3 Telapristone acetate/ CDB-4124 (proposed trade names, proellex, progenta)

CDB-4124 is another SPRM, but it is a relatively pure progesterone antagonist. It was studied in recent years for the treatment of uterine fibroids and is still being evaluated to address its safety and dose parameters in premenopausal women [63]. Limited information or publications are currently available on the various clinical trials that have investigated CDB-4124; these studies have either been completed or were terminated due to adverse liver-related events according to the www.clinical trials.gov website. New clinical trials using lower doses of CDB-4124 have recently been approved by the FDA.

6.4 Ulipristal/CDB-2914 (VA 2914, ellaOne, ella)

Ulipristal is an FDA-approved selective progesterone receptor modulator (SPRM) that is indicated for emergency contraception. It is structurally similar to mifepristone and seems to be effective in the treatment of uterine fibroids. It is associated with a reduction in pain, bleeding and leiomyoma size between 17-24% [64], as well as an improvement in quality of life [65]. However, data on long-term treatment are lacking and similar to other SPRMs, ulipristal may be associated with endometrial thickening and endometrial hyperplasia [29, 39, 66]. Large randomized well-controlled clinical trials are needed to evaluate the utility of ulipristal for potential clinical treatment of uterine fibroids [39].

7. Somatostatin analogues

Increasing evidence has demonstrated a role for growth factors, such as insulin growth factor I (IGF-I) and IGF-II, in the initiation and progression of uterine fibroids [67-70]. Leiomyoma tissue expresses higher levels of IGF-I/IGF-II receptors compared to normal adjacent myometrium [62, 69]. Additionally, these tissues secrete their own IGF-1, probably for autocrine and paracrine use [70]. From a clinical perspective, it has been recently reported that patients with high levels of growth hormone (acromegalic patients) have a higher prevalence of uterine fibroids than the general population [71]. Lanreotide, which is a long-acting somatostatin analogue that has been shown to reduce growth hormone secretion, has also recently been evaluated in seven women with uterine fibroids in Italy [72]. Interestingly, lanreotide induced a 42% mean myoma volume reduction within a 3-month period. These results show that somatostatin analogues may potentially be a new therapy for uterine fibroids [73]. The treatment with somatostatin analogues for diseases other than leiomyoma appears to be safe and is usually well tolerated with some reports of gallstone formation [74, 75]. However, the lacking of clinical trials which test the long term use of somatostatin analogues along with the severe and adverse health implications such as decreased life expectancy due to accelerated heart disease which observed in adults with growth hormone deficiency may hinder its future use for leiomyoma treatment.

8. Cabergoline

Carbergoline is a well-known dopamine agonist that is effectively used in the treatment of prolactinoma and for the inhibition of lactation. A recent study [76] evaluated carbergoline as a therapeutic option for uterine fibroids. The rational for such an approach lies in its effect as an inhibitory agent on GnRH release. A group in Iran published a preliminary study in 2007 [76] that favored the use of carbergoline as a medical treatment of uterine fibroids on which they reported a volume reduction of about 50% with 6 weeks use [65]. The same group performed a subsequent study that compared carbergoline with diphereline, which is a gonadotropin-releasing hormone agonist [77]. They reported comparable results in terms of the shrinkage of the fibroids and the improvement in the sonographic, clinical, and intra-operative outcomes [77]. These findings warrant future larger controlled trials to clearly assess the potential use of carbergoline in the treatment of uterine fibroids.

9. Danazol

Danazol is a synthetic steroid that inhibits steroidogenesis through multi-enzymatic actions in addition to its suppressor effect on sex hormone binding globulin [78]. It reportedly induced a significant 24% volume reduction [79, 80]. However, a recent Cochrane study failed to identify any randomized controlled trials that compared danazol to placebo or any other medical therapy in women with uterine fibroids [81].

9.1 Gestrinone

Gestrinone is a steroid that possesses anti-estrogen receptor and anti-progesterone receptor properties in various tissues, including the endometrium [82]. A recent report from Italy evaluated the use of Gestrinone in the treatment of premenopausal women with uterine fibroids at a dose of 2.5 mg twice per week over a 6-month period [82]. The authors reported a 32% ± 10% reduction in uterine volume [82]. A subsequent study reported up to 60% leiomyoma shrinkage in size [83]. Gestrinone is a contraceptive agent and also exhibits several unfavorable side effects, such as mild androgenicity, weight gain, seborrhea, acne, hirsutism, and occasional hoarseness.

9.2 Vitamin D (VitD)

Data from our laboratory demonstrate that Vitamin D (VitD) is an antifibrotic factor and inhibits growth and induces apoptosis in cultured human leiomyoma cells through the down-regulation of PCNA, CDK1, and BCL-2 and suppresses COMT expression and activity in human leiomyoma cells [84-86]. We have also recently demonstrated similar effects in the Eker rat model of uterine fibroids [87]. Another group in Finland demonstrated that Vitamin D inhibit growth of both myometrial and leiomyoma cells in vitro [88] The growth inhibition was concentration dependent and the level of inhibition was statistically significant with the concentration of 1000 nM.

In a separate study from our group, the correlation between low serum levels of VitD and the increased risk of having symptomatic uterine fibroids were evaluated [89, 90]. We measured both the biologically active 1, 25 dihydroxyvitamin D3 and the precursor 25-hydroxyvitamin D3 in the serum from African American and white women with fibroids as well as normal healthy controls. Interestingly, then observed that 1, 25 dihydroxyvitamin D3 is significantly lower in women with fibroids compared to normal healthy controls; additionally, it has been detected that lower levels of total serum 25-hydroxyvitamin D3 in women with fibroids compared to healthy controls. These findings were observed both in African American women and in Caucasian women.

The aim of the study was to determine whether serum levels of VitD correlated with disease severity in women with symptomatic uterine fibroids. The study population consisted of 67 patients who had detailed repeated pelvic ultrasound evaluations over a 2-year period with specific measurements of the total uterine volume and the volume of the individual leiomyoma lesions. The patients also had detailed laboratory analysis including serum 25 hydroxy Vit D3 levels. As shown in (Fig I), a statistically significant negative correlation between the low serum Vit D levels and the total uterine leiomyoma volume ($P<.05$) as well as the number of leiomyoma lesions/uterus ($P<0.05$) was detected [63]. Taken together, our preliminary results suggest a strong dose-response correlation between lower serum Vit D levels and increased severity of uterine fibroids. This presents an opportunity for the potential use of Vit D or its potent analogues as novel treatment options or for the prevention of uterine fibroids.

To date there is no randomized controlled trials had been implemented to prospectively assess the efficacy of Vit D in the management of uterine fibroids.

10. Epigallocatechin Gallate (EGCG), green tea extract

Tea is one of the most widely consumed beverages all over the world. Both the green tea and the black tea are derived from the leaves of the plant 'Camellia sinensis' the most significant components of which are phytochemicals, of which Green tea is thoroughly studied for its health benefits.

A typical green tea beverage, prepared in a proportion of 1 g leaf to 100 ml water in a 3-min brew, usually contains 250–350mg tea solids, and catechins account for 30–42% of the dry weight of the solids [91]. It has been demonstrated that tea constituents exhibit various biological and pharmacological properties such anti-carcinogenic, antioxidative, anti-allergic, anti-virus, anti-hypertensive, anti-atherosclerosis, anti-cardiovascular disease and anti-hypercholesterolemic activities [92, 93].

The major green tea catechins are epigallocatechin-3-gallate (EGCG), epigallocatechin (EGC), epicatechin-3-gallate (ECG) and epicatechin. Catechines are a group of bioflavonoids that exhibit antioxidant and anti-inflammatory capacity. Chemically, catechines are polyhydroxylated with water-soluble characteristics [94]. Epigallocatechin gallate (EGCG), which is the principal catechin, comprises >40% of the total polyphenolic mixture of green tea catechins [95], Grapes also contain polyphenols and catechins such as EGCG [96]. Epigallocatechin gallate exhibits various biological activities including potent antioxidant and anti-inflammation capacity [97].

EGCG appears to block each stage of tumorgenesis by modulating signaling pathways involved in cell proliferation, transformation, inflammation, and oxidative stress, which are clearly involved in pathogenesis of various tumors including uterine fibroids [98].

In our laboratory, we studied the effect and potential mechanisms of EGCG action on human leiomyoma (HuLM) cells [99], as we assayed cell proliferation and apoptosis, the protein levels of PCNA, CDK4, BCL2, and BAX which examined by Western blot analysis, and we found that Epigallocatechin gallate inhibits the proliferation of HuLM cells and induces apoptosis. These results suggest that EGCG may be a potential anti-uterine fibroid agent acting through multiple signal transduction pathways [100]. Additional validation of these findings was achieved using orally administered EGCG to shrink pre-existing subcutaneous leiomyoma lesions in immune-compromised mice [99]. Previous studies have shown that EGCG inhibited the growth of various human cancer cells, such as epidermoid carcinoma cells [101], hepatoma cells [102], prostate carcinoma cells [103], and breast cancer cells [104]. Those findings motivated us to initiate a clinical trial to evaluate the promising clinical role of EGCG in women with symptomatic uterine fibroids.

11. References

[1] Stewart, E.A., *Uterine fibroids.* Lancet, 2001. 357(9252): p. 293-8.

[2] Sankaran, S. and I.T. Manyonda, *Medical management of fibroids.* Best Pract Res Clin Obstet Gynaecol, 2008. 22(4): p. 655-76.

[3] Parker, W.H., *Etiology, symptomatology, and diagnosis of uterine myomas.* Fertil Steril, 2007. 87(4): p. 725-36.

[4] Drinville Jamie S, M.S., *Benign Disorders of the Uterine Corpus" (Chapter),* in *CURRENT Diagnosis & Treatment Obstetrics & Gynecology, 10e,* N.L. DeCherney AH, Editor. 2010.

[5] Sunkara, S.K., et al., *The effect of intramural fibroids without uterine cavity involvement on the outcome of IVF treatment: a systematic review and meta-analysis.* Hum Reprod, 2010. 25(2): p. 418-29.

[6] Flynn, M., et al., *Health care resource use for uterine fibroid tumors in the United States.* Am J Obstet Gynecol, 2006. 195(4): p. 955-64.

[7] Zhang, Y., et al., *Acupuncture for uterine fibroids.* Cochrane Database Syst Rev, 2010(1): p. CD007221.

[8] Viswanathan, M., et al., *Management of uterine fibroids: an update of the evidence.* Evid Rep Technol Assess (Full Rep), 2007(154): p. 1-122.

[9] Marshall, L.M., et al., *A prospective study of reproductive factors and oral contraceptive use in relation to the risk of uterine leiomyomata.* Fertil Steril, 1998. 70(3): p. 432-9.

[10] Chiaffarino, F., et al., *Use of oral contraceptives and uterine fibroids: results from a case-control study.* Br J Obstet Gynaecol, 1999. 106(8): p. 857-60.

[11] Parazzini, F., et al., *Oral contraceptive use and risk of uterine fibroids.* Obstet Gynecol, 1992. 79(3): p. 430-3.

[12] Friedman, A.J., et al., *Long-term medical therapy for leiomyomata uteri: a prospective, randomized study of leuprolide acetate depot plus either oestrogen-progestin or progestin 'add-back' for 2 years.* Hum Reprod, 1994. 9(9): p. 1618-25.

[13] Orsini, G., L. Laricchia, and M. Fanelli, *[Low-dose combination oral contraceptives use in women with uterine leiomyomas].* Minerva Ginecol, 2002. 54(3): p. 253-61.

[14] Venkatachalam, S., J.S. Bagratee, and J. Moodley, *Medical management of uterine fibroids with medroxyprogesterone acetate (Depo Provera): a pilot study.* J Obstet Gynaecol, 2004. 24(7): p. 798-800.

[15] Murat Naki, M., et al., *Levonorgestrel-releasing intrauterine device insertion ameliorates leiomyoma-dependent menorrhagia among women of reproductive age without a significant regression in the uterine and leiomyoma volumes.* Fertil Steril. 94(1): p. 371-4.

[16] Yoshida, S., et al., *Cell-type specific actions of progesterone receptor modulators in the regulation of uterine leiomyoma growth.* Semin Reprod Med, 2010. 28(3): p. 260-73.

[17] Chen, C., et al., *Discovery of sodium R-(+)-4-{2-[5-(2-fluoro-3-methoxyphenyl)-3-(2-fluoro-6-[trifluoromethyl]be nzyl)-4-methyl-2,6-dioxo-3,6-dihydro-2H-pyrimidin-1-yl]-1-phenylethylamino }butyrate (elagolix), a potent and orally available nonpeptide antagonist of the human gonadotropin-releasing hormone receptor.* J Med Chem, 2008. 51(23): p. 7478-85.

[18] Abbott, *Future abbott pipeline* 2011.

[19] Struthers, R.S., et al., *Suppression of gonadotropins and estradiol in premenopausal women by oral administration of the nonpeptide gonadotropin-releasing hormone antagonist elagolix.* J Clin Endocrinol Metab, 2009. 94(2): p. 545-51.

[20] Dmowski, W., *Advances in the treatment of endometriosis – The potential of Elagolix.* US Obstetrics & Gynecology, 2008. 3(1): p. 21-23.

[21] Barbieri, R.L., *Hormone treatment of endometriosis: the estrogen threshold hypothesis.* Am J Obstet Gynecol, 1992. 166(2): p. 740-5.

[22] Lethaby, A.E. and B.J. Vollenhoven, *An evidence-based approach to hormonal therapies for premenopausal women with fibroids.* Best Pract Res Clin Obstet Gynaecol, 2008. 22(2): p. 307-31.

[23] Black, L.J., et al., *Raloxifene (LY139481 HCI) prevents bone loss and reduces serum cholesterol without causing uterine hypertrophy in ovariectomized rats.* J Clin Invest, 1994. 93(1): p. 63-9.

[24] Temin, S., *American Society of Clinical Oncology clinical practice guideline update on the use of pharmacologic interventions including tamoxifen, raloxifene, and aromatase inhibition for breast cancer risk reduction.* Gynecologic Oncology, 2009. 115(1): p. 132-134.

[25] Fisher, B., et al., *Endometrial cancer in tamoxifen-treated breast cancer patients: findings from the National Surgical Adjuvant Breast and Bowel Project (NSABP) B-14.* J Natl Cancer Inst, 1994. 86(7): p. 527-37.
[26] Wu, T., X. Chen, and L. Xie, *Selective estrogen receptor modulators (SERMs) for uterine leiomyomas.* Cochrane Database Syst Rev, 2007(4): p. CD005287.
[27] Zbucka, M., et al., *Mechanism of collagen biosynthesis up-regulation in cultured leiomyoma cells.* Folia Histochem Cytobiol, 2007. 45 Suppl 1: p. S181-5.
[28] Becker, C., *Another selective estrogen-receptor modulator for osteoporosis.* N Engl J Med, 2010. 362(8): p. 752-4.
[29] Spitz, I.M., *Clinical utility of progesterone receptor modulators and their effect on the endometrium.* Curr Opin Obstet Gynecol, 2009. 21(4): p. 318-24.
[30] Mitlak, B.H. and F.J. Cohen, *In search of optimal long-term female hormone replacement: the potential of selective estrogen receptor modulators.* Horm Res, 1997. 48(4): p. 155-63.
[31] Dutertre, M. and C.L. Smith, *Molecular mechanisms of selective estrogen receptor modulator (SERM) action.* J Pharmacol Exp Ther, 2000. 295(2): p. 431-7.
[32] Richardson, T.I., et al., *Structure-activity relationships of SERMs optimized for uterine antagonism and ovarian safety.* Bioorg Med Chem Lett, 2007. 17(13): p. 3544-9.
[33] Palomba, S., et al., *Effects of raloxifene treatment on uterine leiomyomas in postmenopausal women.* Fertil Steril, 2001. 76(1): p. 38-43.
[34] Palomba, S., et al., *Antiproliferative and proapoptotic effects of raloxifene on uterine leiomyomas in postmenopausal women.* Fertil Steril, 2005. 84(1): p. 154-61.
[35] Premkumar, A., et al., *Gynecologic and hormonal effects of raloxifene in premenopausal women.* Fertil Steril, 2007. 88(6): p. 1637-44.
[36] *Aromatase Inhibitors for Treatment of Uterine Leiomyomas.* Clinical Trials.gov 2010 July 28, 2009 [cited 2010 07-09-2010]; Available from: http://clinicaltrials.gov/ct2/show/NCT00945360?term=aromatase+inhibitors++fibroid&rank=1.
[37] Ettinger, B., et al., *Reduction of vertebral fracture risk in postmenopausal women with osteoporosis treated with raloxifene: results from a 3-year randomized clinical trial. Multiple Outcomes of Raloxifene Evaluation (MORE) Investigators.* JAMA, 1999. 282(7): p. 637-45.
[38] Todorova, V.K., et al., *Tamoxifen and raloxifene suppress the proliferation of estrogen receptor-negative cells through inhibition of glutamine uptake.* Cancer Chemother Pharmacol, 2010.
[39] Fiscella, K. and S. Eisinger, *CDB-2914 for uterine leiomyomata treatment: a randomized controlled trial.* Obstet Gynecol, 2008. 112(3): p. 707; author reply 707-8.
[40] Iveson, T.J., et al., *Phase I study of the oral nonsteroidal aromatase inhibitor CGS 20267 in healthy postmenopausal women.* J Clin Endocrinol Metab, 1993. 77(2): p. 324-31.
[41] Smith, I.E. and M. Dowsett, *Aromatase inhibitors in breast cancer.* N Engl J Med, 2003. 348(24): p. 2431-42.
[42] Ishikawa, H., et al., *High aromatase expression in uterine leiomyoma tissues of African-American women.* J Clin Endocrinol Metab, 2009. 94(5): p. 1752-6.
[43] Williams, A.R., et al., *The effects of the selective progesterone receptor modulator asoprisnil on the morphology of uterine tissues after 3 months treatment in patients with symptomatic uterine leiomyomata.* Hum Reprod, 2007. 22(6): p. 1696-704.

[44] Bedaiwy, M.A., Lui, J., *Long-term management of endometriosis: Medical therapy and treatment of infertility.* Sexuality, Reproduction and menopause, 2010. 8(3): p. 5.
[45] Baird, D.T., et al., *Mifepristone: a novel estrogen-free daily contraceptive pill.* Steroids, 2003. 68(10-13): p. 1099-105.
[46] Varelas, F.K., et al., *The effect of anastrazole on symptomatic uterine leiomyomata.* Obstet Gynecol, 2007. 110(3): p. 643-9.
[47] Parsanezhad, M.E., et al., *A randomized, controlled clinical trial comparing the effects of aromatase inhibitor (letrozole) and gonadotropin-releasing hormone agonist (triptorelin) on uterine leiomyoma volume and hormonal status.* Fertil Steril, 2010. 93(1): p. 192-8.
[48] Ishikawa, H., et al., *Progesterone is essential for maintenance and growth of uterine leiomyoma.* Endocrinology, 2010. 151(6): p. 2433-42.
[49] Wilkens, J., et al., *Effects of the selective progesterone receptor modulator asoprisnil on uterine artery blood flow, ovarian activity, and clinical symptoms in patients with uterine leiomyomata scheduled for hysterectomy.* J Clin Endocrinol Metab, 2008. 93(12): p. 4664-71.
[50] Carbonell Esteve, J.L., et al., *Mifepristone for the treatment of uterine leiomyomas: a randomized controlled trial.* Obstet Gynecol, 2008. 112(5): p. 1029-36.
[51] Fiscella, K., et al., *Effect of mifepristone for symptomatic leiomyomata on quality of life and uterine size: a randomized controlled trial.* Obstet Gynecol, 2006. 108(6): p. 1381-7.
[52] Engman, M., et al., *Mifepristone for treatment of uterine leiomyoma. A prospective randomized placebo controlled trial.* Hum Reprod, 2009. 24(8): p. 1870-9.
[53] Attardi, B.J., et al., *In vitro antiprogestational/antiglucocorticoid activity and progestin and glucocorticoid receptor binding of the putative metabolites and synthetic derivatives of CDB-2914, CDB-4124, and mifepristone.* J Steroid Biochem Mol Biol, 2004. 88(3): p. 277-88.
[54] Engman, M., et al., *The effect of mifepristone on breast cell proliferation in premenopausal women evaluated through fine needle aspiration cytology.* Hum Reprod, 2008. 23(9): p. 2072-9.
[55] Lalitkumar, P.G., et al., *Mifepristone, but not levonorgestrel, inhibits human blastocyst attachment to an in vitro endometrial three-dimensional cell culture model.* Hum Reprod, 2007. 22(11): p. 3031-7.
[56] Sharts-Engel, N.C., *The RU 486 story: the French experience.* MCN Am J Matern Child Nurs, 1992. 17(1): p. 56.
[57] Brahma, P.K., K.M. Martel, and G.M. Christman, *Future directions in myoma research.* Obstet Gynecol Clin North Am, 2006. 33(1): p. 199-224, xiii.
[58] Chwalisz, K., et al., *Role of nonhuman primate models in the discovery and clinical development of selective progesterone receptor modulators (SPRMs).* Reprod Biol Endocrinol, 2006. 4 Suppl 1: p. S8.
[59] Steinauer, J., et al., *Systematic review of mifepristone for the treatment of uterine leiomyomata.* Obstet Gynecol, 2004. 103(6): p. 1331-6.
[60] Chwalisz, K., et al., *A randomized, controlled trial of asoprisnil, a novel selective progesterone receptor modulator, in women with uterine leiomyomata.* Fertil Steril, 2007. 87(6): p. 1399-412.
[61] Chwalisz, K., et al., *The effects of 1-month administration of asoprisnil (J867), a selective progesterone receptor modulator, in healthy premenopausal women.* Hum Reprod, 2005. 20(4): p. 1090-9.

[62] Boehm, K.D., et al., *Expression of the insulin-like and platelet-derived growth factor genes in human uterine tissues.* Mol Reprod Dev, 1990. 27(2): p. 93-101.

[63] Abdelraheem, M.S. and A. Al-Hendy, *Serum vitamin D3 level inversely correlates with total fibroid tumor burden in women with symptomatic uterine fibroid.* Fertility and Sterility, 2010. 94(4): p. S74.

[64] Nieman, L.K., et al., *Efficacy and tolerability of CDB-2914 treatment for symptomatic uterine fibroids: a randomized, double-blind, placebo-controlled, phase IIb study.* Fertil Steril, 2011. 95(2): p. 767-72 e1-2.

[65] Melli, M.S., L. Farzadi, and E.O. Madarek, *Comparison of the effect of gonadotropin-releasing hormone analog (Diphereline) and Cabergoline (Dostinex) treatment on uterine myoma regression.* Saudi Med J, 2007. 28(3): p. 445-50.

[66] Levens, E.D., et al., *CDB-2914 for uterine leiomyomata treatment: a randomized controlled trial.* Obstet Gynecol, 2008. 111(5): p. 1129-36.

[67] Hoppener, J.W., et al., *Expression of insulin-like growth factor-I and -II genes in human smooth muscle tumours.* EMBO J, 1988. 7(5): p. 1379-85.

[68] Gloudemans, T., et al., *Insulin-like growth factor gene expression in human smooth muscle tumors.* Cancer Res, 1990. 50(20): p. 6689-95.

[69] Norstedt, G., A. Levinovitz, and H. Eriksson, *Regulation of uterine insulin-like growth factor I mRNA and insulin-like growth factor II mRNA by estrogen in the rat.* Acta Endocrinol (Copenh), 1989. 120(4): p. 466-72.

[70] Rein, M.S., et al., *The secretion of insulin-like growth factors I and II by explant cultures of fibroids and myometrium from women treated with a gonadotropin-releasing hormone agonist.* Obstet Gynecol, 1990. 76(3 Pt 1): p. 388-94.

[71] Cohen, O., B. Schindel, and R. Homburg, *Uterine leiomyomata--a feature of acromegaly.* Hum Reprod, 1998. 13(7): p. 1945-6.

[72] Nilsson, C.G., et al., *Intrauterine contraception with levonorgestrel: a comparative randomised clinical performance study.* Lancet, 1981. 1(8220 Pt 1): p. 577-80.

[73] De Leo, V., et al., *Administration of somatostatin analogue reduces uterine and myoma volume in women with uterine leiomyomata.* Fertil Steril, 2001. 75(3): p. 632-3.

[74] Feelders, R.A., et al., *Medical therapy of acromegaly: efficacy and safety of somatostatin analogues.* Drugs, 2009. 69(16): p. 2207-26.

[75] Davies, P.H., et al., *Long-term therapy with long-acting octreotide (Sandostatin-LAR®) for the management of acromegaly.* Clinical Endocrinology, 1998. 48(3): p. 311-316.

[76] Sivin, I. and J. Stern, *Health during prolonged use of levonorgestrel 20 micrograms/d and the copper TCu 380Ag intrauterine contraceptive devices: a multicenter study. International Committee for Contraception Research (ICCR).* Fertil Steril, 1994. 61(1): p. 70-7.

[77] Sayyah-Melli, M., et al., *Comparison of the effect of gonadotropin-releasing hormone agonist and dopamine receptor agonist on uterine myoma growth. Histologic, sonographic, and intra-operative changes.* Saudi Med J, 2009. 30(8): p. 1024-33.

[78] Steingold, K.A., et al., *Danazol inhibits steroidogenesis by the human ovary in vivo.* Fertil Steril, 1986. 45(5): p. 649-54.

[79] De Leo, V., A. la Marca, and G. Morgante, *Short-term treatment of uterine fibromyomas with danazol.* Gynecol Obstet Invest, 1999. 47(4): p. 258-62.

[80] La Marca, A., et al., *Hemodynamic effect of danazol therapy in women with uterine leiomyomata.* Fertil Steril, 2003. 79(5): p. 1240-2.

[81] Ke, L.Q., et al., *Danazol for uterine fibroids.* Cochrane Database Syst Rev, 2009(3): p. CD007692.

[82] La Marca, A., et al., *Gestrinone in the treatment of uterine leiomyomata: effects on uterine blood supply.* Fertil Steril, 2004. 82(6): p. 1694-6.

[83] Coutinho, E.M., *Treatment of large fibroids with high doses of gestrinone.* Gynecol Obstet Invest, 1990. 30(1): p. 44-7.

[84] Sharan, C., et al., *Vitamin D inhibits proliferation of human uterine leiomyoma cells via catechol-O-methyltransferase.* Fertility and Sterility. In Press, Corrected Proof.

[85] Halder, S.K., J.S. Goodwin, and A. Al-Hendy, *1,25-Dihydroxyvitamin D3 reduces TGF-beta3-induced fibrosis-related gene expression in human uterine leiomyoma cells.* J Clin Endocrinol Metab, 2011. 96(4): p. E754-62.

[86] Sharan, C., et al., *Vitamin D inhibits proliferation of human uterine leiomyoma cells via catechol-O-methyltransferase.* Fertil Steril, 2011. 95(1): p. 247-53.

[87] Halder, S.K., C. Sharan, and A. Al-Hendy, *Vitamin D treatment induces dramatic shrinkage of uterine leiomyomas growth in the Eker rat model.* Fertility and Sterility, 2010. 94(4): p. S75-S76.

[88] Blauer, M., et al., *Vitamin D inhibits myometrial and leiomyoma cell proliferation in vitro.* Fertil Steril, 2009. 91(5): p. 1919-25.

[89] Halder, S.K., S. Goodwin, and A. Al-Hendy, *Vitamin D exhibits antiestrogenic effects in human uterine leiomyoma cells.* Fertility and Sterility, 2010. 94(4): p. S219-S220.

[90] Halder, S.K., et al., *1, 25 dihydroxyvitamin D3 disorganizes actin fibers in human immortalized uterine leiomyoma cells.* Fertility and Sterility, 2009. 92(3): p. S127-S128.

[91] Khan, N. and H. Mukhtar, *Tea polyphenols for health promotion.* Life Sci, 2007. 81(7): p. 519-33.

[92] Kuriyama, S., et al., *Green tea consumption and mortality due to cardiovascular disease, cancer, and all causes in Japan: the Ohsaki study.* JAMA, 2006. 296(10): p. 1255-65.

[93] Lambert, J.D. and C.S. Yang, *Cancer chemopreventive activity and bioavailability of tea and tea polyphenols.* Mutat Res, 2003. 523-524: p. 201-8.

[94] Joo Eun, C., et al., *Amplification of antioxidant activity of catechin by polycondensation with acetaldehyde.* Biomacromolecules, 2004. 5(1): p. 113-8.

[95] Lin, J.-K., Y.-C. Liang, and S.-Y. Lin-Shiau, *Cancer chemoprevention by tea polyphenols through mitotic signal transduction blockade.* Biochemical Pharmacology, 1999. 58(6): p. 911-915.

[96] Zern, T.L., et al., *Grape polyphenols exert a cardioprotective effect in pre- and postmenopausal women by lowering plasma lipids and reducing oxidative stress.* J Nutr, 2005. 135(8): p. 1911-7.

[97] Mukhtar, H. and N. Ahmad, *Green tea in chemoprevention of cancer.* Toxicol Sci, 1999. 52(2 Suppl): p. 111-7.

[98] Khan, N., et al., *Targeting multiple signaling pathways by green tea polyphenol (-)-epigallocatechin-3-gallate.* Cancer Res, 2006. 66(5): p. 2500-5.

[99] Dong, Z., et al., *Antiproliferative and proapoptotic effects of epigallocatechin gallate on human leiomyoma cells.* Fertility and Sterility, 2010. 94(5): p. 1887-1893.

[100] Zhang, D., et al., *Antiproliferative and proapoptotic effects of epigallocatechin gallate on human leiomyoma cells.* Fertil Steril, 2010. 94(5): p. 1887-93.

[101] Ahmad, N., P. Cheng, and H. Mukhtar, *Cell Cycle Dysregulation by Green Tea Polyphenol Epigallocatechin-3-Gallate.* Biochemical and Biophysical Research Communications, 2000. 275(2): p. 328-334.

[102] Chen, C., et al., *Activation of antioxidant-response element (ARE), mitogen-activated protein kinases (MAPKs) and caspases by major green tea polyphenol components during cell survival and death.* Arch Pharm Res, 2000. 23(6): p. 605-12.

[103] Gupta, S., et al., *Growth Inhibition, Cell-Cycle Dysregulation, and Induction of Apoptosis by Green Tea Constituent (-)-Epigallocatechin-3-gallate in Androgen-Sensitive and Androgen-Insensitive Human Prostate Carcinoma Cells.* Toxicology and Applied Pharmacology, 2000. 164(1): p. 82-90.

[104] Tang, Y., et al., *Epigallocatechin-3 gallate induces growth inhibition and apoptosis in human breast cancer cells through survivin suppression.* Int J Oncol, 2007. 31(4): p. 705-11.

10

Hysteroscopic Surgery as an Alternative for Hysterectomy

Chang-Sheng Yin[1] and Fung-Wei Chang[2]
[1]*China Medical University Taipei Branch, Vice-Superintendent,*
National Defense Medical Center,
[2]*Reproductive Medicine Center,*
Department of Obstetric and Gynecology,
Tri-Service General Hospital, Taipei,
Taiwan

1. Introduction

Abnormal uterine bleeding (AUB) is a common complaint in reproductive age women. The World Health Organization reported that in developing countries, 8-27% of women suffered heavy menstrual bleeding. (1) Hysterectomy remains the gold-standard treatment, but can be associated with significant morbidity. In the past gynecologists will be criticized for performing hysterectomies for women with AUB but without any uterine pathology. Over the past two decades, several non-invasive or minimally invasive procedures have emerged as alternative treatment modalities. But do these new treatments remain effective over time? In the present chapter, I discuss first generation hysteroscopic ablation techniques (EA), as an alternative to hysterectomy, that have been extensively studied over the last 20 years but are actually underused. Because a great number of valuable papers and books have already been published on this topic, for the sake of simplicity references have been kept to a minimum. Also I will share my personal experiences as a hysteroscopist who has performed more than 1000 cases of operative hysteroscopic surgery in Taiwan over the last 15 years.

2. Indications for hysterectomy

A hysterectomy is an operation to remove a woman's uterus. Sometimes, the ovaries and fallopian tubes are also removed. Hysterectomies are very common - one in three women in the United States has had one by age 60.

The following benign diseases are the most common reasons for hysterectomy:

- Abnormal uterine bleeding (AUB) that persists despite treatment
- Uterine leiomyomata (fibroids)
- Adenomyosis not cured by medicine or conservative surgery
- Uterine prolapse - when the uterus drops into the vagina
- Chronic pelvic pain; intractable to medical treatments

Before a patient undergoes a hysterectomy, it is important to discuss alternative treatments with the patient. After hysterectomy her periods will stop, and she will no longer be able to get pregnant. If both ovaries are removed, a patient will enter menopause. Although hysterectomy is one of the most commonly used gynecological procedures, in recent years the number of patients undergoing hysterectomy has decreased in some area of the world. (2)

The possible reasons for this could be the availability of new emerging minimally invasive alternative procedures and the adverse effects after hysterectomy. (2,3) Current 'save the uterus ' attitude in the world has also become a support to narrow the range of indications of hysterectomy. Hysterectomy can alleviate all menstrual-related clinical symptoms, including dysmenorrhea and premenstrual symptoms, and the overall patient satisfaction rate with this approach is approximately 80%. However, it also has some disadvantages such as frequent peri-operative complications, prolonged operating time, delayed recovery, and high cost. Recent studies have shown that women below 50 years of age who undergo hysterectomy with or without oophorectomy are at a significantly higher risk of all-cause mortality and coronary heart diseases. (3, 4) Traditionally, hysterectomy has also been known to have a major psychological impact. Over the past 15-20 years, several non-invasive or minimally invasive procedures have emerged as alternative treatment modalities. Currently available alternative treatment modalities include insertion of levonorgestrel-intrauterine system (LNG-IUS), myomectomy, myolysis, uterine artery embolization, magnetic resonance imaging-focused ultrasonography, hysteroscopic endometrial ablation (EA), and second-generation global endometrial ablation.

3. Alternatives for hysterectomy

Avoiding unnecessary hysterectomy is a challenge. Abnormal uterine bleeding (AUB), defined as excessive or irregular bleeding, occurs in about 10–30% of women of reproductive age. Uterine leiomyomata (fibroids) is the most common benign gynecological tumor, occurring in about 30% of women. The 2002 report from Organization for Economic Co-operation and Development showed that rates ranged from a low of 114 per 100 000 women in Mexico to a high of 526 in Norway. In Taiwan, the incidence of hysterectomy was approximately 268 to 303 per100 000 women from 1996 to 2001. Fibroids are the most common indication for hysterectomy in Taiwan; a total of 22,000 hysterectomies are performed each year. (5) The overall cost of treating fibroids in US was estimated at $2.1 billion in 2000. More than 70% of those costs were directly related to hysterectomy.

Asymptomatic uterine leiomyomata may not require treatment, but in about 20–80% of cases, leiomyomata is accompanied by AUB and pelvic symptoms. AUB and leiomyomata are the main indications for hysterectomy. If AUB can be successfully treated with alternative modalities, then the need for hysterectomy may be reduced.

Recently, several non-invasive or minimally invasive procedures have emerged as alternative treatment modalities include insertion of levonorgestrel-intrauterine system (LNG-IUS), myomectomy, myolysis, uterine artery embolization, magnetic resonance imaging-focused Ultrasonography. While hysteroscopic endometrial ablation, and second-generation global endometrial ablation (EA), are to be choiced when menorrhagia is the primary indication and endometrial anatomy is appropriate. For patients requiring interventional treatment, selection among these procedures depends on the patient's age, symptoms, coexisting conditions, and reproductive plans.

EA is a suitable alternative for the treatment of AUB. Resectoscopic techniques are performed under hysteroscopic visualization, using resectoscopic instruments to ablate the endometrium or remove submucosal leiomyomata. Hysteroscopic EA and myomectomy have become increasingly popular treatment modalities for women with AUB. From 2003 to 2006, in England, EA was performed in 60% of cases of surgically treated AUB. (6)

The 2009 Cochrane Database meta-analysis of 21 randomized trials regarding resectoscopic ablation showed the following results: (a) the amenorrhea rate was 38% at 1 year and 48% at 2–5 years, (b) the patient satisfaction rate was 88% at 1 year and 87% at 2–5 years, and (c) the subsequent surgery rate was 25% for any surgery (including hysterectomy) and 19% for hysterectomy alone. (7) Since 1996, I have performed more than 1000 hysteroscopic EAs at 3 hospitals in Taiwan. The results were comparable to those in other medical literature, but had a lower subsequent surgery rate of approximately 5%. (8, 9) In my recent study, I followed up 334 women who were eligible for a follow-up after surgery; the follow-up duration ranged from 7 months to 109 months (mean, 48.7 months). Of the 334 women, 161 (48%) had normal flow, 33 (10%) had hypomenorrhea, 31 (9%) had heavy flow, and 82 (25%) continued to experience amenorrhea. Seventeen (5%) women were not satisfied with the results, and 7 (2%) underwent hysterectomy because of EA failure. Ten women (3%) underwent EA again. The subsequent surgery rate in my series was 5%. (8)

Although this procedure needs training and skills, it is less expansive and underused in many countries. Many insurance policies such as Taiwan's National Health Insurance do not cover second-generation endometrial ablation.

Most clinicians still perform hysterectomy as the first choice in treatment of women presenting intractable AUB.

The history and evolution of hysteroscopic endometrial ablation: In 1805, Bozzini described his simple instrument used to inspect the urethra of a living human but later was banned and censured for "undue curiosity."

In 1869, Pantaleoni took the first look inside the uterine cavity using a cystoscope to observe and cauterize uterine polyps in a 60-year-old woman.

In 1879, the first "modern" hysteroscope was designed and produced by Nitze by incorporating an interior light source with an optical system permitting magnification.

In 1925, Rubin introduced uterine distention with carbon dioxide .

The rod lens system designed by Harold H.Hopkins, (10) together with the fiber optic light transmission invented by Fourestiere in 1952, (11) has allowed extraordinary advances in operative hysteroscopy.

In 1869, Pantaleoni reported the first successful hysteroscopy (using cystoscopy), when he described a 60-year-old woman with postmenopausal bleeding and found an intrauterine polyp and cauterized it with silver nitrate. This was not only the first diagnostic hysteroscopy but also the first demonstration of intrauterine surgery.

Modern day operative hysteroscopy relies on two developments: the glass fiber optic for illumination and the uterine distention, and the hysteroscopic endometrial ablation developed from the occurrence of Asherman's syndrome that completes destruction of the endometrium will cause amenorrhea.

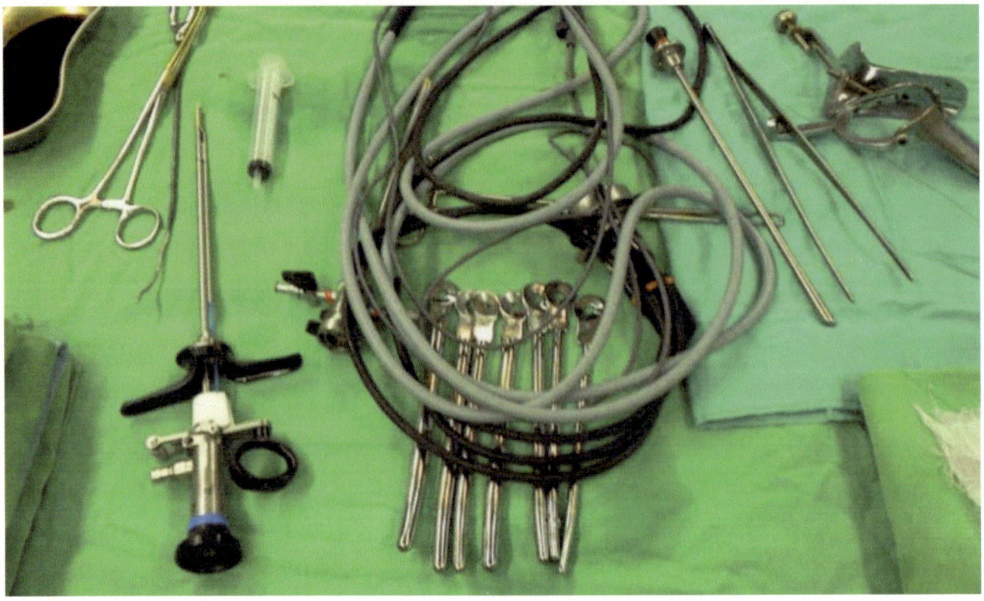

Fig. 1. instrumentation for hysteroscopic endometrial ablation include rigid resectoscope, cables, speculum, and dilators.

In 1976, Neuwirth & Amin used the urologic resectoscope to assist in the removal of a pedunculated submucous leimyomas in 5 cases. Two years later (1978) Neuwirth used a new hysteroscopic technique with a cutting loop and infusion distention fluid (32% dextran 70) system.

In 1979 Goldrath first performed hysteroscopic endometrial ablation by using the Nd:YAG laser.

In 1981 he reported on the successful treatment of intractable uterine bleeding in 21 of 22 cases.

4. The general assessment and management of AUB

The FIGO PALM-COEIN classification for abnormal uterine bleeding (AUB):

In 2011 a new classification system for abnormal uterine bleeding (AUB) was approved by the FIGO Executive Board. (12) AUB, can be classified as acute, chronic, intermenstrual or intermittent forms, which represents a common clinical problem facing the gynecologist.

Acute AUB was defined as an episode of heavy bleeding that is of sufficient quantity to require immediate intervention to prevent further blood loss.

Chronic AUB be defined as bleeding from the uterine corpus that is abnormal in volume, regularity, and/or timing, and has been present for the past 6 months. Chronic AUB would not require immediate intervention.

Intermenstrual or intermediate bleeding (IMB) occurs between clearly defined cyclic and predictable menses. Such bleeding may occur at random times or may manifest in a predictable fashion at the same day in each cycle.

The FIGO group recommended the word "metrorrhagia," and dysfunctional bleeding (DUB) should be abandoned.

Acute AUB may present in the context of existing chronic AUB or might occur without such a history. Although women of reproductive age with acute AUB require immediate intervention, their follow-up may be largely dependent upon whether they require investigation and ongoing care for an underlying chronic condition.

The prevalence of AUB, the difficulties in identifying its causes, and the cost of management argue for reliable diagnostic techniques and treatment strategies. An ideal approach would promptly identify patients with organic disease, facilitate patient comprehension and choice of treatment options, improve treatment efficacy, and reduce overall cost of care.

FIGO differentiates 9 categories and are arranged according to an acronym (PALM-COEIN) shown as below:

AUB-P: Polyps in the endometrium that are diagnosed by ultrasound or hysteroscopy. This classification system does not further categorize polyps on the basis of size, location, or number.

AUB-A: Adenomyosis which can be most accurately diagnosed on the basis of tissue analysis of a hysterectomy specimen, but in everyday clinical practice, MRI and ultrasound are both used to establish the diagnosis.

AUB-L: Leiomyomas, which can be solitary or multiple, can be located close to the cavity (submucosal), in the myometrium (intramural), close to the outer surface (subserosal), or independent of the uterus (parasitic). On the basis of these characteristics, further subcategories have been created.

AUB-M: Malignancy, including hyperplasia and endometrial cancer. The diagnosis requires the histologic analysis of a biopsy sample.

AUB-C: Coagulopathy, which in most cases is diagnosed in adolescents. Most abnormalities are the result of von Willebrand disease.

AUB-O: Ovulatory dysfunction, in which cycle length and volume of flow are unpredictable.

AUB-E: Endometrial problems, typically related to abnormal prostaglandin synthesis, but which could be the result of infection as well.

AUB-I: Iatrogenic causes, the result of exogenous hormone administration or anticoagulant therapy.

AUB-N: Nonclassified causes such as arteriovenous malformations and myometrial hypertrophy. Women with both acute and chronic AUB should be evaluated for anemia. In the absence of any other identifiable source, the clinician would proceed in a systematic fashion, designing the assessment to address each of the components of the FIGO classification system.

Current treatment for AUB is recommended only when symptoms such as pain, severe anemia, or hydronephrosis due to ureteral obstruction are present and unacceptable to patients. There is no evidence that women with no symptoms or with mild symptoms benefit from intervention. Medical therapy such as acetaminophen and non-steroidal anti-inflammatory drugs (NSAIDs) for pain relief is useful in some patients, but does not reduce uterine bleeding. A variety of hormonal therapies, mifepristone, and gonadotropin-releasing hormone agonists and antagonists have limited effects in reducing uterine volume and bleeding, but most of these treatments have not been evaluated in randomized trials.(11,12) Patients with ovulatory dysfunction (AUB-O) are best treated with oral contraceptives, NSAIDs (antiprostaglandins), or progestins or progestin-released IUD. Cyclic use of progestins and oral contraceptives reduce AUB, but ergot derivatives do not.

For patients requiring surgical alternatives, the current principal options include myomectomy, endometrial ablation, uterine fibroid embolization, and magnetic resonance-guided focused ultrasound (MR-g FUS). A thoughtful discussion of the options with patients is essential in choosing the most appropriate treatment for patients. Selection among these procedures depends on the patient's age, symptoms, and their preference.

A large study from the United Kingdom in 2005 observed that 16,100 out of 37,298 hysterectomies were performed as a result of AUB.

Wade et al. suggested that for women with AUB who were older than 40 years and did not desire pregnancy, the best treatment trial was with oral contraceptive pills (OCPs), followed by second generation endometrial ablation as the most cost-effective strategy. Unfortunately, currently in Taiwan the second generation endometrial ablation therapy is not covered by Taiwan National Health Insurance. Therefore, my personal experience and the experience of many other investigators have demonstrated that hysteroscopic endometrial ablation in patients with AUB is a reasonable alternative to classic hysterectomy. The advantages include no abdominal incision, less discomfort, very brief recovery period, no hysterectomy complications, fewer psychological problems and lower cost. Endometrial ablation is the hysteroscopic alternative to hysterectomy as treatment for women with AUB.

The pre-operative investigation procedure for women with AUB:

It is advised to begin a work-up when a patient complaining of AUB with a pictorial blood assessment chart scores (PBACS) above 150 or the patient's quality of life changes. A detailed clinical history and complete physical examination may reveal blood coagulation disorders, liver and renal disease. Laboratory studies include complete blood count (CBC), and monitoring of TSH, prolactin, and androgen levels if there are signs and symptoms of hypothyroidism, galactorrhea, hirsutism or acne. The gynecological examination with bimanual examination must be performed with specific attention given to the existence of possible lesions in the cervix, uterus, adnexa, urethra, bladder and rectum. Spe cial attention for the presence of endometrial cancer is also mandatory. It is mandatory to perform an office endometrial biopsy in all patients contemplating hysteroscopy surgery. A determination of uterine size is also useful because patients with uterine cavities greater than 10cm in length can expect less than optimal results.

Endometrial sampling directed by hysteroscopy may increase the accuracy in evaluating patients with abnormal intrauterine bleeding. Ultrasound and or saline infusion sonography

(SIS) may detect the presence of intrauterine lesions. The abdominal and or vaginal ultrasound evaluation of the pelvic organs is also very helpful for operation.

5. The procedure of the hysteroscopic endometrial ablation

The operation is always performed under spinal anesthesia in the proliferative phase of the menstrual cycle; if not, then a pre-operative thorough 3-min suction curettage is done.

Souter et al. conducted a meta-analysis about pre-operative administration of agents producing endometrial atrophy before surgery, and suggest it is associated with shortened operation times, greater rate of amenorrhea, and reduced dysmenorrhea. I prefer to pretreat the endometrium by trying to time the procedure in the early proliferative phase and using the suction curette to remove the rest of the endometrium.

Informed consent is obtained before the operation. Misoprostol (Cytotec) 200mcg # x2 per vagina is given the night before operation to ripen the cervix.

The patient is placed in the dorsal lithotomy position. A simultaneous laparoscopy is not performed.

The vulva area, vagina and cervix are cleaned with disinfecting solution. A bimanual examination should be performed to determine whether the position of the uterus is anteverted or retroverted. After placing a single valve speculum in the vagina, the cervix is grasped with a single-toothed tenaculum which allows for traction on the cervix. The cervix is then dilated to Hegar No:10,

A continuous fluid rigid hystero-resectoscope equipped with a 30 degree fore-oblique hysteroscope is slowly without force introduced into the uterine cavity. If there is any difficulty during insertion of the resectoscope, there is a risk of uterine perforation.

The 5% dextrose is an isotonic solution with sufficient optical quality, no electric conductivity, no allergic potential, and is the cheapest and most readily available in 500ml bottle form. It is safe for endometrial ablation but the danger of fluid overload and pulmonary edema still exists. The uterine cavity is distended with a solution of 5% dextrose under a gravity feed system with a 2-litre-bottle connected to the resectoscope by urologic tubing. Uterine distension is created by raising the bags to a suitable height, usually 1.0-1.5 m above the uterine cavity. Inspection of the input and output fluid volume is done every 5 minutes by the circulating nurse during the operation. The negative balance is limited to 2000 ml. After running distention fluid for about one minute, a clear field to see both uterine cornu and fundus is considered as the most important indicator that the operation can begin.

I prefer partial ablation to treat the posterior wall endometrium (depth < 3 mm), initially by the cutting loop electrode with the current set at 120 W of cutting current. From my right hand side to left, both lateral side of the endometrium are resected and ablated down next to the isthmus. The rest of the endometrium is then coagulated using the rollerball electrode, with the current set at 60 W of coagulation current.

The current total or global EA procedures cause significant intrauterine adhesion and contractures, and are associated with long-term adverse effects, which include painful central hematometra, cornual hematometra, and postablation tubal sterilization syndrome in patients with tubal ligation. Postablation tubal sterilization syndrome consists of painful hematosalinges, resulting from active endometrial tissue near the cornual region and endometrial scarring and contractures that prevent menstrual egress. A partial endometrial ablation procedure in which only one (anterior or posterior) wall is resected and ablated was proposed to prevent intrauterine scarring and contractures, and thus avoid such complications (16, 17). This approach allows the normal endometrial surface to oppose the injured exposed myometrial surface, so that adhesions and contractures do not occur. To date, there has been only one report of a pregnancy after partial EA. This pregnancy only proceeded to 28 weeks of gestation, and does not yet show potential benefits for women wishing to retain fertility (18).

After that any bleeding is coagulated using the roller ball electrode at a power of 40-60 W of coagulation current.

For women in whom uterine polyps or myomas are found, concomitant resections are done. Submucosal myoma resections are carried out using unipolar cutting-loop resection techniques.

All of the resected endometrial strips, myomatous fragments and polyps are sent for histological evaluation.

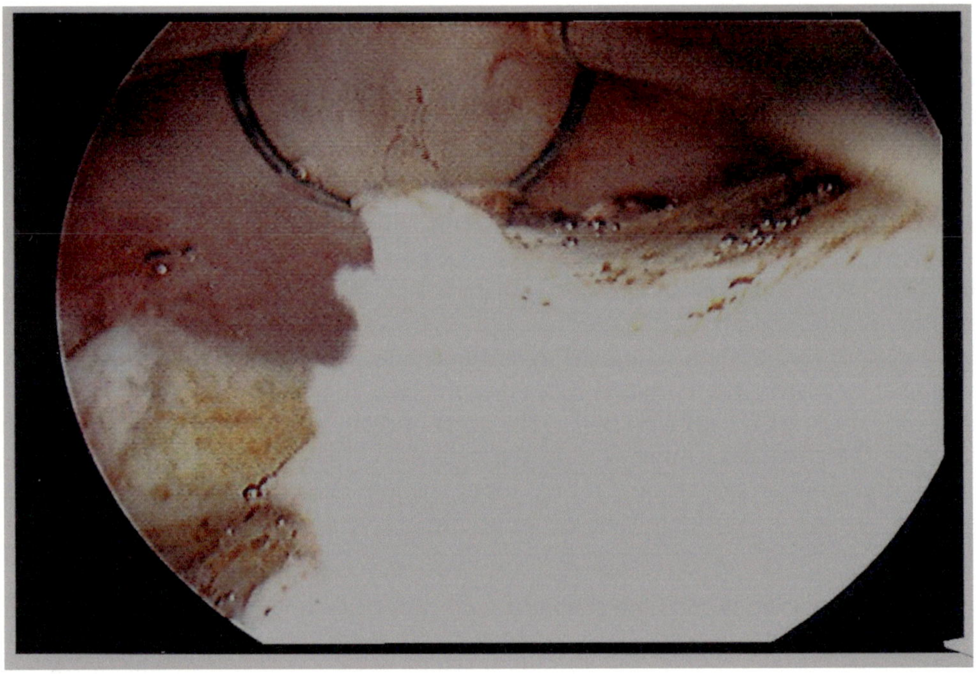

Fig. 2. Placement of the loop electrode behind this 4cm submucosal myoma in a 34 year old woman under direct vision

Most patients after endometrial resection will have a fairly light period for a few days, then become a watery pink discharge last for a week or two to three weeks.

The first post-operative office visit is scheduled for 1 week later, and 1 month after surgery, then followed up every 6 months by telephone, mail or at clinics.

Patient satisfaction is also important to assess the question "How satisfied or dissatisfied are you with the result of the surgery related to menstrual flow and dysmenorrhea?" Patients rate their overall satisfaction on a 4-points scale(1=very satisfied, 2=satisfied, 3=dissatisfied, 4=very dissatisfied). The need for repeat surgery or hysterectomy is also recorded. Patients with post-operative AUB may receive medical treatment, or if AUB, and dysmenorrhea are persistent, hysterectomy may be needed.

6. The safety of the procedure

Electrosurgical endometrial resection is not as easy as you think when watching an expert performing it. It is actually associated with more complications than any other procedure in the whole field of endoscopic surgery and performed only by obstetrician-gynecologists after thorough training. The most serious complications are fluid overload resulting in pulmonary edema and electrolytes imbalances. The first signs of pulmonary edema may perceived by the drop in oxygen saturation. Early and rapid treatment of furosemide and positive pressure ventilation may have a complete recovery. I used Dextrose 5% in water as the distention fluid because of its effective low-viscosity and electrolytically non-conductive and cheap. The most important factors predisposing to dilutional hyponatremia were nulliparity, type of preoperative endometrial preparation,increased uterine size and cavity length, concurrent myomectomy and duration of surgery. Fluid monitoring with input and output recording is essential during all operative hysteroscopic cases.

Uterine perforation may occur while removal of intrauterine chips, and can cause serious internal organs and vascular injury if unnoticed during resection.

There are several tips to avoiding uterine perforation complications ;

1. Learn the physics associated with electrosurgery and the hydrodynamics inherent in the fluid systems used.
2. Electrical energy should never be activated unless the surgeon can clearly see the operating field.
3. The roller-ball or wire loop must always be pulled towards the operator and never activated when it is pushed away from the surgeon. Most important is to avoid perforation; it can be surprisingly difficult to detect.
4. Always keep uterine "perforation" in mind, especially in cases with distorted uterine cavity and never activate the radiofrequency energy when bleeding blurs the field, as damage can occur to a wide variety of vessels and organs: the most dangerous complication is uterine perforation with electrical thermal injury and trauma.

Trauma to major blood vessels: aorta, inferior vena cava, mesenteric artery, sacral artery, iliac artery.

Trauma to bowel resulting in peritonitis and/or septicemia.

Trauma to bladder and/or ureter requiring laparotomy or ureteric stents.

Technique troubleshooting;

Poor vision may be due to bleeding and debris and bubbles.

Solution;

Bleeding – first make sure the instrument is in the uterine cavity then increase distention pressure and coagulate the bleeder.

Debris and bubbles - withdraw the scope running the distention fluid and rinse the perforations in the outer shaft.

- Hemorrhage requiring balloon tamponade, laparotomy or hysterectomy or blood loss leading to death.
- Distention medium overload.
- Other rare complications such as unintended pregnancy.
- Intrauterine adhesions and hematometra, burns.

Nearly all of my procedures have been completed safely; however, two women sustained uterine perforation and underwent hysterectomies. In a third woman, the procedure was abandoned because of suspected endometrial malignancy. None of my patients have showed any signs or symptoms of fluid overload or hyponatremia.

In my series over a 15-year-period, six pregnancies occurred after the procedure, and the mean age of these women was 36 years (range, 34–40 years). Because pregnancies have been reported after endometrial ablation, patients cannot be guaranteed that this is a sterilization procedure, and the risk potential for a subsequent pregnancy must be explained and sterilization or contraception offered. Tubal ligation does not reduce distention media absorption and therefore need not be a prerequisite.

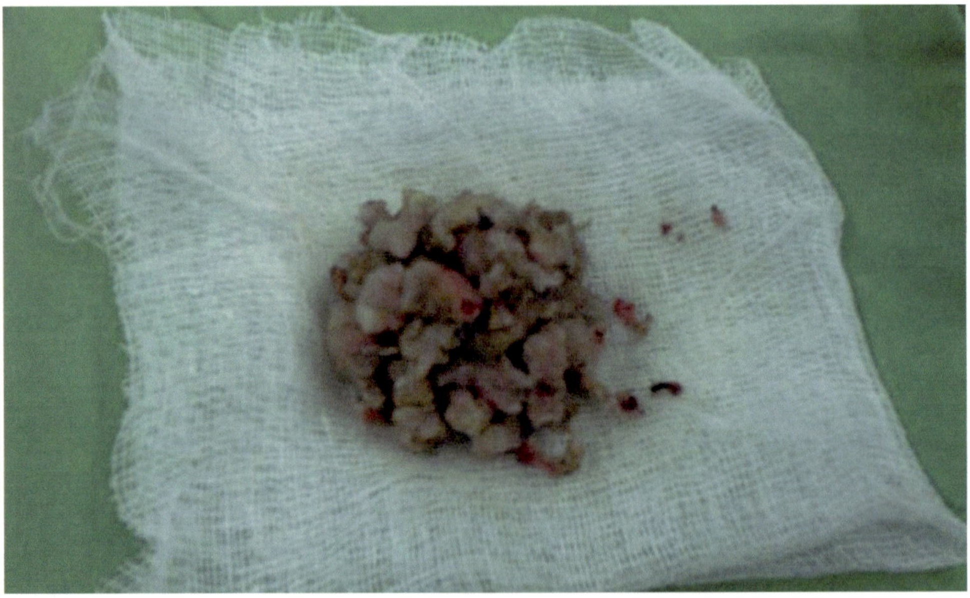

Fig. 3. Collection of myoma chips after resection.

Is endometrial ablation really decreased the hysterectomy rate?

An earlier report from England suggested that the increasing use of endometrial ablation did not reduce the rate of hysterectomy . (19) Despite initial optimism in the United States, two studies showed that the hysterectomy rate remained unchanged at 5.68 per thousand women between 1988 and 1997. (20,21) According to a 2010 population-based NHI database in Taiwan , demonstrated that there have been considerable changes in the surgical types of hysterectomy performed in Taiwan during the last 10 years, but the annual numbers of hysterectomies remained stationary. (5) This means that hysteroscopic endometrial ablation and other alternatives to hysterecotomy are still underused in Taiwan and many parts of the world. Many factors might influence the selection of treatment for uterine and menstrual disorders, some are surgeon, and others are patient-related. Widespread critical clinical skills and more educations about the alternatives to hysterectomy for surgeons and patients are needed.

7. Conclusion

Hysteroscopic endometrial ablation is the logic alternative choice for women with AUB after failed medical treatment.

Although hysteroscopic endometrial ablation offers many advantages, it is actually underused by gynecologist in the world. Every gynecologist must to learn the skill of diagnostic and operative hysteroscopy as their everyday routine practice. Even newer developments in 2nd generation global endometrial ablation, every gynecologist should retain their hysteroscopic operative skills whenever need.

8. References

[1] Harlow SD, Campbell OM. Epidemiology of menstrual disorders in developing countries: A systematic review. BJOG 2004;111:6-16.

[2] Babalola EO, Bharucha AE, Schleck CD, et al. Decreasing utilization of hysterectomy: a population-based study in Olmsted County, Minnesota, 1965-2002. Am J Obstet Gynecol. 2007;196:214.e1.

[3] Ingelsson E, Lundholm C, Johansson AL, et al. Hysterectomy and risk of cardiovascular disease: a population based cohort study. Eur Heart J. 2010 Dec 24. [Epub ahead of print].

[4] Parker WH, Broder MS, Chang E, et al. Ovarian conservation at the time of hysterectomy and long-term health outcomes in the nurses' health study. Obstet Gynecol. 2009;113:1027-1037.

[5] Wu MP, Haung KH, Long CY. et al. Trends in Various Types of Surgery for Hysterectomy and Distribution by Patient Age, Surgeon Age, and Hospital Accreditation: 10-Year Population-Based Study in Taiwan. Analysis on the causes and effects of hysterectomy in Taiwan. J Minim Invasive Gynecol. 2010, 17, 612–619

[6] Cromwell DA, Mahmood TA, Templeton A, et al. Surgery for menorrhagia within English regions: variation in rates of endometrial ablation and hysterectomy. BJOG. 2009;116:1373.

[7] Lethaby A, Hickey M, Garry R, et al. Endometrial resection/ablation techniques for heavy menstrual bleeding. Cochrane Database Syst Rev 2009; :CD001501.

[8] Yin CS, Wei RY, Chao TC, et al. Hysteroscopic endometrial ablation without endometrial preparation. Int J Gynaecol Obstet. 1998;62(2):167-72.
[9] Yin CS. Pregnancy after hysteroscopic endometrial ablation without endometrial preparation: A report of five cases and a literature review. Taiwan J Obstet Gynecol. 2010;49(3):311-319.
[10] Hamou JE, Historical background. In: Hamou J, ed. Hysteroscopy and microcolpolhysteroscopy. Text and Atlas. East Norwalk, CT: Appleton and Lange,1991:1-11.
[11] Goldrath MH, Fuller TA, Segal S. Laser photovaporization of endometrium for treatment of menorrhagia. Am J Obstet Gynecol 1981; 140:14-19. Bibliographic Links Library Holdings .
[12] FIGO classification system (PALM-COEIN) for causes of abnormal uterine bleeding in nongravid women of reproductive age. Malcolm G. Munroa, b, , , Hilary O.D. Critchleyc, Michael S. Broderd, Ian S. Frasere and for the FIGO Working Group on Menstrual Disorders. Int J Obstet Gynecol, vol.113, no.1 p3-13, April 2011
[13] Parker WH. Uterine myomas: management. Fertil Steril. 2007;88:255-71.
[14] Stewart EA. Uterine fibroids. Lancet 2001;357:293-8.
[15] Kjerulff KH, Erickson BA, Langenberg PW. Chronic gynecological conditions reported by US women: findings from the National Health Interview Survey, 1984 to 1992. Am J Public Health 1996;86:195-199.
[16] McCausland AM, McCausland VM. Partial rollerball endometrial ablation: a modification of total ablation totreat menorrhagia without causing complications from intrauterine adhesions. ***Am J Obstet Gynecol*** 1999;180:1512–21.
[17] McCausland AM, McCausland VM. Frequency of symptomatic corneal hematometra and postablation tubal sterilization syndrome after total rollerball endometrial ablation: a 10-year follow-up. *Am J Obstet Gynecol* 2002;186:1274–84.
[18] Maouris P. Pregnancy after planned partial endometrial resection. *Aust N Z J Obstet Gynaecol* 1994;34:122–3.
[19] Bridgeman SA. Trends in endometrial ablation and hysterectomy for dysfunctional uterine bleeding in the Mersey region. Gynecol Endosc. 1996;5:5–8.
[20] Wilcox LS, Koorin LS, Pokras R, Strauss LT, Xia Z, Petersen HB. Hysterectomy in the United States 1988–1990. Obstet Gynecol. 1994;83:549–555.
[21] Farquhar Steiner CA. Hysterectomy rates in the United States, 1990– 1997. Obstet Gynecol. 2002;99:229–234.

11

The LNG-IUS: The First Choice Alternative to Hysterectomy? Intrauterine Levonorgestrel-Releasing Systems for Effective Treatment and Contraception

D. Wildemeersch
Outpatient Gynaecological Clinic and IUD Training Center, Ghent, Belgium

1. Introduction

Hysterectomy (from Greek ὑστέρα *hystera* "womb" and εκτομία *ektomia* "a cutting out of") is the surgical removal of the uterus. Hysterectomy may be total (removing the body, fundus, and cervix of the uterus; often called "complete") or partial (removal of the uterine body while leaving the cervix intact; also called "supracervical"). It is the most commonly performed gynaecological surgical procedure although the incidence of hysterectomy varies widely across the world.[1] This is the case even when one considers only developed countries with comparable resources. In 2003, over 600,000 hysterectomies were performed in the United States alone, of which over 90% were performed for benign conditions.[2] In the USA a woman's life-time risk of hysterectomy is 25%, which compares to a much lower risk of 10.4% in Denmark.[3] In England and Wales the hysterectomy rate in NHS hospitals is estimated at 28 per 10,000 women per annum.[4] Even within each country, there are large regional variations.[5] Such rates being highest in the industrialized world has led to the major controversy that hysterectomies are being largely performed for unwarranted and unnecessary reasons.

Oophorectomy is frequently done together with hysterectomy to decrease the risk of ovarian cancer. However, recent studies have shown that prophylactic oophorectomy without an urgent medical indication has serious consequences.[6] Apart from the current occurrence of estrogen deficiency symptoms, women who are oophorectomized, particularly at an early age experience an increased risk of ischaemic heart disease as well as death from cardiovascular disease. Oophorectomy also leads to early loss of bone and an increased risk of osteoporotic fracture and may also be linked to impaired cognitive function. The impact on psychological health could also be substantial leading to long lasting anxiety, depression, loss of self-esteem and well-being and may also indirectly or directly give rise to problems of sexual function. This effect is not limited to pre-menopausal women; even women who have already entered menopause were shown to have experienced a decrease in long-term survivability post-oophorectomy.[7]

Hysterectomy and bilateral oophorectomy has surgical risks as well as long-term effects. So the surgery should normally be recommended only when other treatment options are not available. However, it is expected that the frequency of hysterectomies for non-malignant indications will fall as there are good alternatives in many cases.[8] As most of the hysterectomies are conducted for benign conditions, including fibroid disease, dysfunctional uterine bleeding, endometriosis, benign adnexal mass, pelvic relaxation/prolapse and chronic pelvic pain, many of these conditions can be effectively treated with alternative treatment modalities of which the LNG-IUS is probably the easiest, safest, most effective and most economical of the conservative alternatives of hysterectomy. In this chapter, a short review is given about these alternative treatments with special focus on current and future LNG-releasing systems.

2. Morbidity and mortality of hysterectomy

A multicenter study conducted in 102 hospitals in Canada evaluated the morbidity and mortality rates of laparoscopic, abdominal, and vaginal hysterectomy.[9] One thousand seven hundred ninety-two women underwent hysterectomy for benign, nonobstetric indications. The overall hysterectomy-related morbidity rate was 6.1%. The rate of morbidity was higher in the laparoscopic supracervical hysterectomy (LASH) group (9.4%) than in the abdominal hysterectomy (AH) group (5.2%, $p<0.01$), but no significant difference was noted between AH and vaginal hysterectomy (VH) (8.6%). The incidence of intraoperative bowel injury was 0.4% in the LASH group (a trocar injury in a patient) and 0.3% in the AH group. Bladder injury was encountered in two patients in the LASH group (0.9%) and in another two in the AH group (0.1%). Ureteral injury occurred in a patient in the AH group (0.07%). There were no cases of intraoperative vascular injury. Vaginal hysterectomy was associated with more urinary retention and hematoma formation than the other two groups. Discordant diagnosis was noted in four cases (two missed endometrial cancer, atonic and distended bladder mistaken for an ovarian cyst, and pelvic tuberculosis). The conversion rate to laparotomy was 1.7% in the LASH group and 0.4% in the VH group, and the incidence of reoperation was 0.4% in the AH group. It was concluded that besides the overall hysterectomy-related morbidity rate of 6.1%, compared with other types of hysterectomy, more urinary retention and hematoma formation occur after VH. LASH is associated with a higher morbidity rate than AH; mainly because of conversion to laparotomy and blood transfusion.

A review by Banu et al[10] on the health outcomes following hysterectomy reports that hysterectomy is highly effective, resulting in high satisfaction rates[11,12], improvements in health-related quality-of-life measures[13,14] and sexual functioning[15],and of course a complete resolution of the menstrual disturbance without the possibility of recurrence. However, hysterectomy is a major operation which causes discomfort and considerable disability in the weeks following surgery[16], has mortality rates in the range 0.38–1 per 1000[17,18], severe complications in 3% of women[9], and minor morbidity (mainly fever and infection) in up to 30% women.

Hysterectomy is also thought to be associated with urinary incontinence many years after the operation[19], and may cause early ovarian failure (and the consequences thereof).[20]

These issues, including the high surgery and hospital cost implications[21], have resulted in the search for effective alternatives.

3. Alternatives to hysterectomy in women with bleeding disorders and other gynaecological conditions

A Non-steroidal anti-inflammatory drugs

Mefenamic acid, and the antifibrinolytic agent tranexamic acid are effective treatments and are considered first-line treatment for menorrhagia.[22] The efficacy of these treatments has been demonstrated in several randomized trials and reported in systematic reviews.[23,24] Tranexamic acid reduces menstrual loss by about 50% and mefenamic acid by a third. Both drugs also relieve menstrual cramps.

B Systemically administered hormones

Cyclical progestogens given during the luteal phase of the cycle are ineffective, but are effective when given continuously for 21 days.[25] Side effects such as breakthrough bleeding, breast tenderness, weight gain, alteration in libido and depression reduce compliance. The additional contraceptive effect limits their use in women who wish to conceive. Where contraception is desired, the combined oral contraceptive pill appears to be a better choice for the treatment of menorrhagia. The hormones work by inhibiting the growth and development of the endometrium, thus significantly reducing blood loss.

C Locally administered hormones

The main focus of this section will be on the local administration of levonorgestrel (LNG) using an intrauterine drug delivery system (IUS) as LNG is a potent progestogen with many advantages.[26] The progesterone-releasing intrauterine device (IUD) will not be discussed as the Progestasert® IUD is not commercialized anymore. The natural hormone is much weaker than LNG and, therefore, less suitable for the treatment purposes described in this paper.

Our research group has been involved in the clinical development of frameless and framed LNG-releasing intrauterine systems since 1997. Another chapter in this book focuses on the effect of these systems on menstrual blood loss in women with and without heavy menstrual bleeding or menorrhagia. This section will mainly focus on the differences between these novel devices compared to the Mirena® LNG-IUS (BayerSchering AG, Berlin, Germany). In addition, the use of the LNG-IUS will be discussed for the treatment of precancerous lesions of the endometrium, including early endometrial cancer of the endometrium, conditions that usually are treated by hysterectomy.

In order to be successful as a method for intrauterine treatment, the prerequisite is that the following conditions are met. The method should:

1. be easy and safe to apply
2. be well-tolerated and fit in cavities of every size and shape
3. be well retained
4. release a sufficient amount of active substance per day
5. preferably release a high dosage during the first few weeks to establish fast and profound suppression of the endometrium
6. be long-acting
7. have few side effects and
8. be easy to remove

a. Comparison between Femilis® LNG-IUS and Mirena® LNG-IUS

Figure 1 depicts both intrauterine systems. The design of Femilis® is slimmer with shorter crossarms and thinner stem than Mirena®. Both release a similar amount of LNG (20 μg/day) except for the first weeks whereby comparative in vitro release studies showed that the release rate of Femilis® is approximately 2 to 3 times higher. Femilis® and Mirena® have a duration of action of at least 5 years.

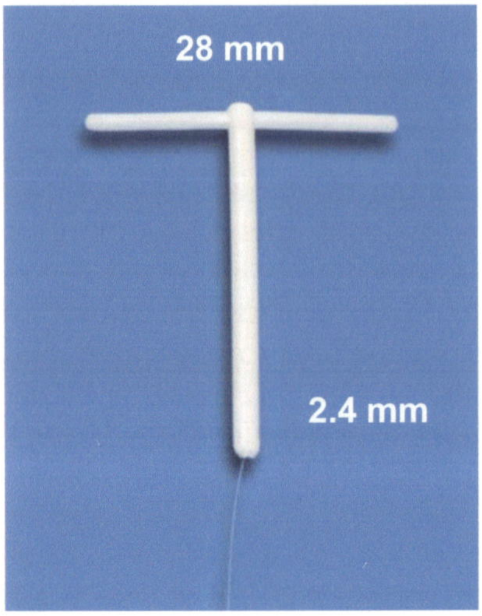

Fig. 1. Femilis® LNG-IUS.

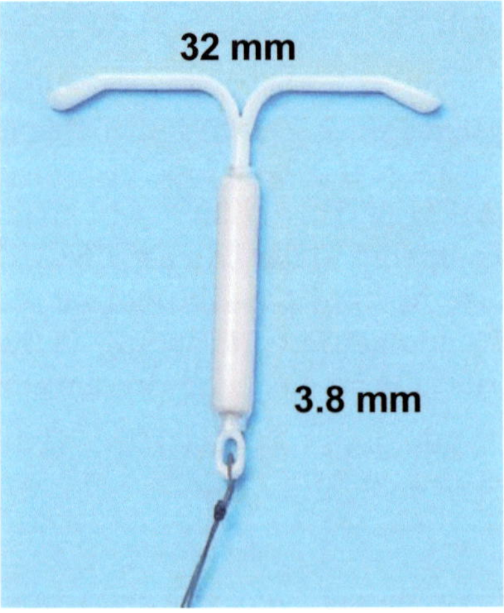

Fig. 2. Mirena® LNG-IUS

The difference in design is important as it has a bearing on the easiness and safety of the insertion procedure as well as on the acceptability and retention of the LNG-IUS.

As Femilis® is significantly smaller that Mirena®, it is suitable for parous as well as nulliparous women. Women with narrow, but not too narrow, uterine cavities tolerate the LNG-IUS. Figure 3 shows the blister package of Femilis® with uterine sound.

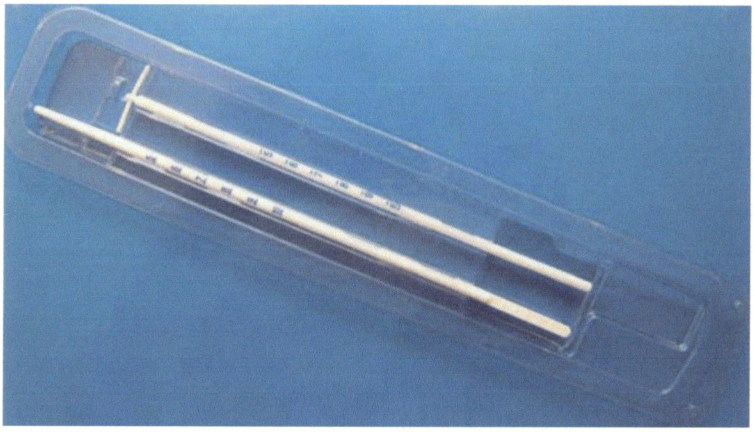

Fig. 3. Blister package with Femilis® inserter and uterine sound.

Figure 4 illustrates the insertion procedure of the Femilis® IUS and Figure 5 the insertion procedure of the Mirena® LNG-IUS.

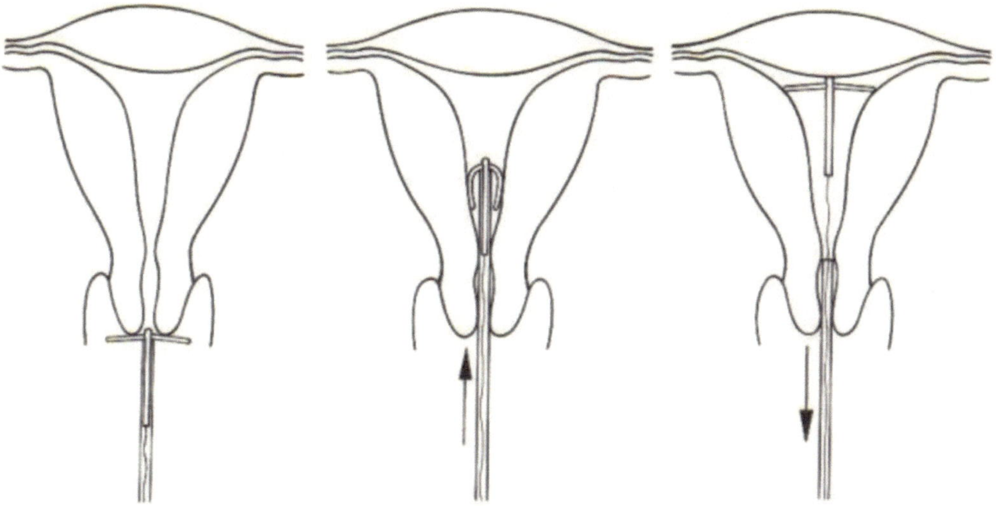

Fig. 4. Insertion of Femilis®. The applicator is positioned against the cervix (left) and pushed into the uterine cavity (middle) until its front end reaches the fundus (right). The inserter tube is then removed and the thread is trimmed at 2 cm from the cervix. Note: During insertion the sidearms unfold protecting against perforation.

Uterine cavities differ considerably in size and shape, and the uterus is subject to changes in size and volume during the menstrual cycle.[27,28] These changes are most pronounced at the time of menses. These individual variations in size and shape of the human uterus are probably greater than variations of the human foot (H.M. Hasson). Research has shown that if the width of the uterine cavity is too small, side effects and complications are likely to occur. The crossarms of standard T-shaped IUDs are frequently too long for a large number of uterine cavities, as the average transverse diameter of the uterine cavity in the majority of women is smaller than the span of the crossarms of the IUD. The average transverse

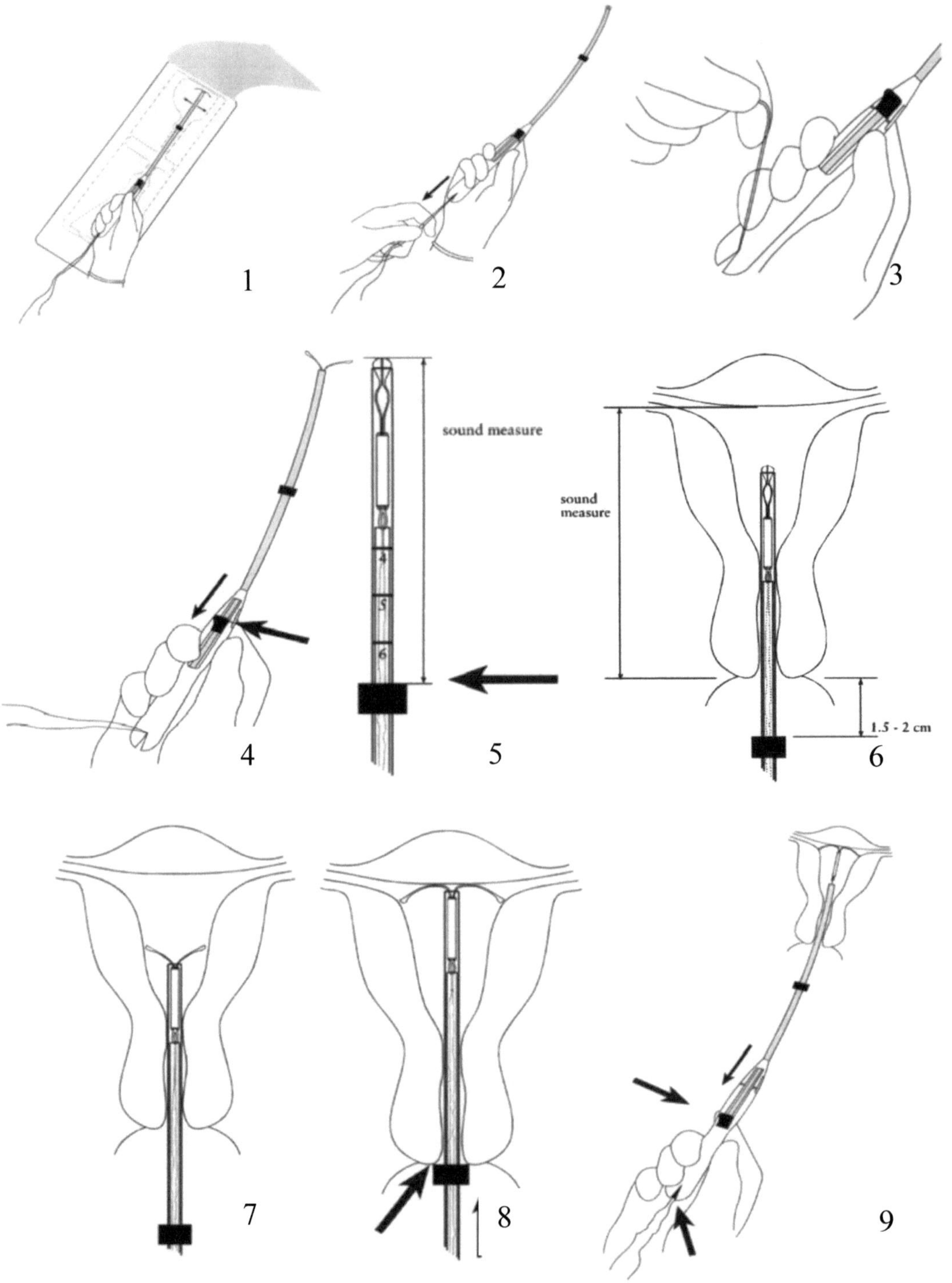

Fig. 5. Insertion of Mirena®: **1)** The package is opened and the shaft of the insertion instrument is grasped as shown. The arms of the IUS should be in horizontal position

(adjustment can be done on the sterile inner surface of the peel pack). **2)** The threads are now pulled until both knobs close the open end of the front end of the inserter. **3)** The thread is then fixed in the cleft at the end of the inserter. **4)** The sidearms of the IUS should be in the correct position as they should fold out horizontally. If not, open the arms by pulling the slider back to the raised mark on the shaft. Align the open arms on the sterile surface of the package and return the slider to its previous position. Check that the threads are still tight and that the arms have moved back into the inserter. **5)** Set the flange at a distance from the knobs corresponding to the uterine sound measure by using the scale marked on the insertion tube. Note that this measurement is from the end of the inserter to the top edge of the flange. **6)** Mirena® is now ready to be inserted. Hold the slider with the forefinger or thumb firmly in the most distal position. Move the inserter carefully through the cervical canal into the uterus until the flange is situated at a distance of about 1.5 - 2 cm from the cervix to give sufficient space for the arms to open. Do not force the inserter. **7)** While holding the inserter steady, release the arms of the IUS by pulling the slider back until it reaches the raised mark on the shaft. **8)** Holding the slider firmly, push the inserter gently inward until the flange touches the cervix. The IUS should now be at the fundus. **9)** Holding the inserter firmly in position, release the IUS by pulling the slider all the way back. Remove the inserter and cut the strings at 2 cm from the cervix.

diameter of the uterine cavity at the fundal level in nulliparous women between 15 and 34 years of age, as well as in many parous women, is much smaller than the length of the crossarms of most currently used T-shaped IUDs resulting in dimensional problems. The length of the crossarms of the Mirena® LNG-IUS is 32 mm. The average fundal transverse dimension in nulliparous as well as parous women is only around 25 to 27 mm. Recent 3-D sonography studies compared women with abnormally and those with normally located IUDs with respect to their indication for sonography and found that the proportion of patients whose principal indication for sonography was bleeding, pain or bleeding and pain were significantly greater in those with an abnormally located IUD, including imbedded IUDs, compared with those whose IUD was not located abnormally on 3-D sonography.[29,30] It should be noted that standard 2-D sonography is not able to detect many abnormally located IUDs particularly with regard to abnormal location of the sidearms of the IUD. Accurate location of the sidearms is only possible by hysteroscopy and with 3-D coronal sonography, as shown in Figure 6. Due to the shorter crossarms of the Femilis® LNG-IUS it has been demonstrated in clinical trials that the IUS fits better in uterine cavities with small transverse dimensions. This indicates that side effects (e.g., pain, bleeding and expulsion) due to incompatibility can be avoided by reducing the length of the crossarms. IUDs that do not fit well contribute to early discontinuation.[31] In addition, insertion of the Femilis® IUS is straightforward. Following uterine sounding, the IUS is simply pushed in the uterine cavity, up to the fundal wall. The ease and safety of this insertion technique was demonstrated in a multicenter clinical trial.[32,33]

b. Use of the LNG-IUS in women with precancerous or early cancer of the endometrium

The use of the LNG-IUS as an alternative to hysterectomy for treatment of heavy menstrual bleeding was covered in another chapter in this book. Other uterine pathologies such as precancerous changes of the endometrium and even early endometrial cancer of the uterus can effectively be treated by the LNG-IUS. Our group evaluated the effect on endometrial

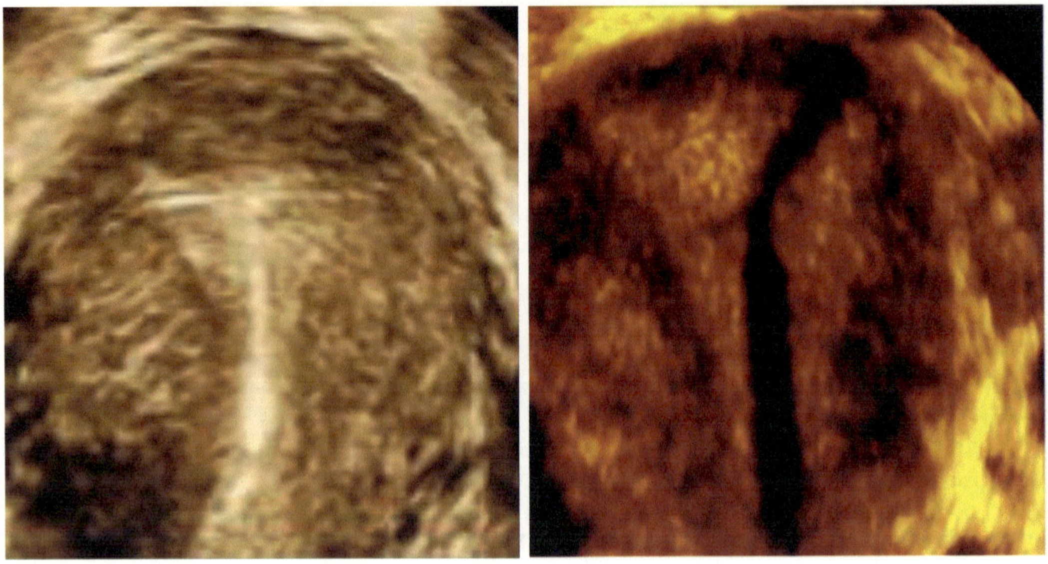

Fig. 6. Left: Femilis® fitting snugly in a small uterine cavity. Right: Mirena® showing unfolded and embedded crossarm due to incompatibility with the narrow uterine cavity.

non-atypical and atypical hyperplasia in 20 women. The aim of the study was to evaluate the long-term cure (remission) rate. All women in this small series developed a normal endometrium, except one asymptomatic woman with atypical hyperplasia who still had focal residual non-atypical hyperplasia at 3 years follow-up in the presence of a thin (<4 mm) endometrium. This patient is being followed-up on a regular basis. It was concluded that continuous intrauterine delivery of LNG appears to be a promising alternative to hysterectomy for the treatment of endometrial hyperplasia and could enhance the success rate when compared with other routes of progestogen administration as well as intrauterine progesterone delivery.[34] As many women with atypical hyperplasia harbour cancer cell, patients should be followed-up long-term and the endometrium should continuously kept suppressed with a LNG-IUS.

Two cases of early, respectively well- and moderately differentiated endometrial carcinoma were also effectively treated with the LNG-IUS. Below is the summarized report of one of these patients. The patient presented with minimal postmenopausal bleeding. An outpatient endometrial pipelle biopsy was performed which revealed a moderately differentiated adenocarcinoma (Figure 7) with minimal myometrial invasion (Clinical FIGO stage I).[35] An LNG-IUS (Femilis®) was inserted and advice was given to conduct a repeat biopsy within the next 3 to 6 months. Spotting continued for several weeks and then stopped. As the patient was completely free of symptoms 6 months after insertion of the LNG-IUS, a pelvic transvaginal ultrasound was performed, including a 3-D ultrasound. The uterus appeared completely normal, and there was no evidence of any pathology. The endometrium showed normal thickness, and there was no evidence of any endometrial abnormality or myometrial invasion. The LNG-IUS was identified in situ, as expected. Six months later, in order to ascertain complete remission, it was decided to remove the LNG-IUS and to perform a full D&C. The uterine sound length was 6 cm. The whole cavity was explored, and very scant tissue was removed. Histological examination of the specimen revealed a secretory

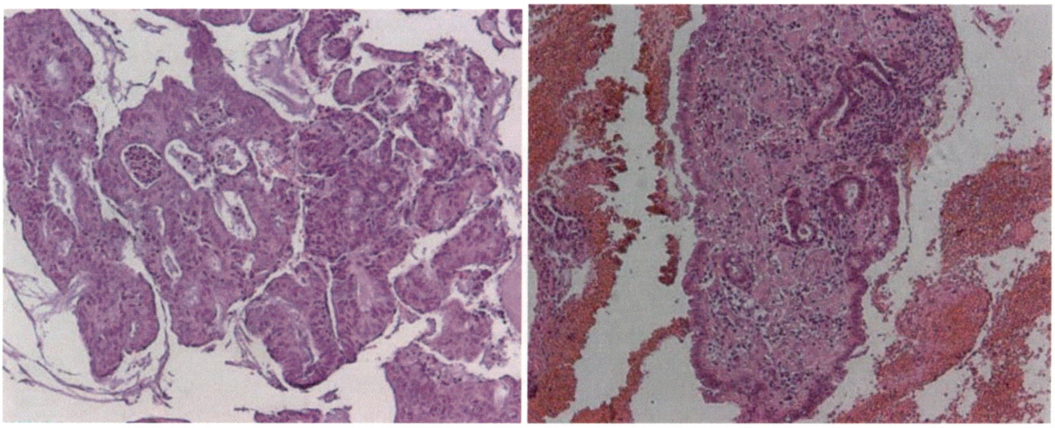

Fig. 7. Left: Endometrial curetting prior to therapy, irregular cribriform glands, and mild atypia: moderately-differentiated endometrioid carcinoma (H&E 100x). Right: Endometrial curetting post-therapy, small regular glands with tubal metaplasia, surrounded by decidualised stroma (H&E 100x).

endometrium without signs of hyperplasia or atypia (Figure 7). A new LNG-IUS was inserted as a precaution. The patient was again examined two years following initial treatment. She had no symptoms, and vaginal ultrasound showed a very thin endometrium and normal position of the LNG-IUS in the uterine cavity.

c. Use of the LNG-IUS in women with primary or secondary dysmenorrhea, endometriosis/adenomyosis and chronic pelvic pain

Our group evaluated the effect of a frameless LNG-IUS releasing 14 µg of LNG/d (Figure 8) on menstrual pain in women with primary and secondary dysmenorrhea.

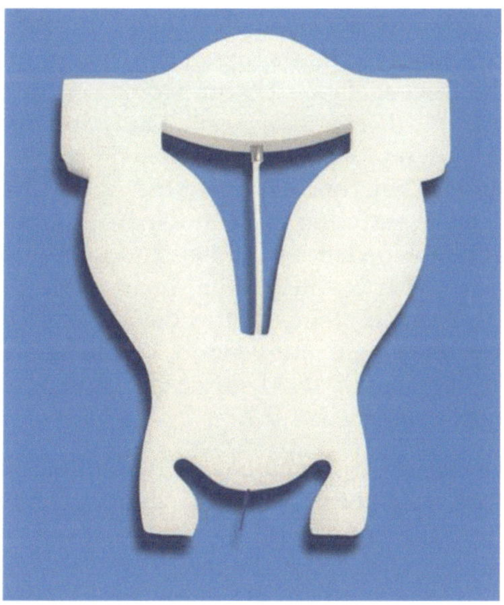

Fig. 8. The frameless FibroPlant® LNG-IUS

Eighteen insertions were performed in women between 16 and 52 years of age. Eight women were categorized as having primary and 10 having secondary dysmenorrhea. Twelve women complained of heavy bleeding. Two women had significant fibroids and three were suspected to have adenomyosis. All women, except one with significant fibroids, reported much reduced pain, no pain at all, or strongly reduced bleeding, which started as soon as one month after insertion of the frameless LNG-IUS. The results of this small study suggest that the LNG-IUS could be an effective method in women with primary or secondary dysmenorrhea, associated or not with excessive menstrual bleeding, and avoid surgery in many of them as both bleeding and pain are effectively treated with the LNG-IUS. An additional advantage is that the LNG-IUS is a potent contraceptive as well. The absence of a frame is particularly advantageous in these cases as it does not elicit uterine contractions.

Endometriosis affects almost 10–20% of women of reproductive age, while 70–90% of women with chronic pelvic pain (CPP), dysmenorrhea, dyspareunia, infertility and menstrual disturbances also have endometriosis, a disease that impairs patients' quality of life.[36] Many therapies are proposed. These include nonsteroidal anti-inflammatory drugs, antiestrogens, progestogens such as depot medroxyprogesterone acetate (DMPA), GnRH analogues to induce pseudo-menopause, androgen derivatives (danazol) and continuous combined oral contraceptives (COC) to induce pseudo-pregnancy. Medical treatments are based on the reduction of lesions or on ovarian estrogen suppression; however, adherence and long-term therapy continue to represent a challenge in the management of endometriosis. Because of the profound hypoestrogenism provoked by some of these drugs, bone mineral density is the principal concern that limits their use to 6 months, although longer treatment with add-back hormone therapy is possible. GnRH-a is also expensive and not readily available to women worldwide, especially in developing countries.

One of the options to treat these conditions, and alleviate the pain complaints, is the levonorgestrel-releasing intrauterine system. Bahamondes et al. recently reviewed the literature regarding the use of LNG-IUS (Mirena®) in women with endometriosis, adenomyosis, cyclic pelvic pain and dysmenorrhea.[37] They found that all studies reported an improvement in pelvic pain and dysmenorrhea, and a reduction in menstrual bleeding. One study found an improvement in the staging of the disease at 6 months of use, and the studies that evaluated the use of LNG-IUS in women with adenomyosis reported a reduction in uterine volume. Furthermore, the only study in which women were followed up for 3 years after insertion found improvement in pelvic pain at 12 months of use, but no improvement after that period. They concluded that the use of LNG-IUS is an alternative for the medical treatment of women suffering from endometriosis, adenomyosis, chronic pelvic pain or dysmenorrhea, but that experience is limited and long-term studies are necessary to reach definitive conclusions. Other authors came to the same conclusion.[38] However, for women who do not wish to become pregnant, this device offers the possibility of at least 5 years of treatment following one single intervention. It is to be expected that many of these women, without further fertility, could avoid surgical treatment which would be viewed as an enormous benefit for those concerned.

Given the above scientific evidence, it should be concluded that the LNG-IUS is effective for the treatment of the most frequently occurring gynaecological conditions for which gynaecologists are consulted. The use of local medical treatment has many advantages and should, therefore, be considered as the first line treatment before a surgical intervention.[39,40] In a randomized trial comparing the LNG-IUS with hysterectomy, 42% in the LNG-IUS group subsequently underwent hysterectomy, and, thus, surgery and the associated risks with surgery were avoided in 58% of the women. The number of hysterectomies for menorrhagia in England has fallen substantially to just over one third (36%) of the number of a decade ago (Figure 9).[41] This trend can be explained by an increase in medical treatment as well as by the more widespread use of endometrial resection or ablation.

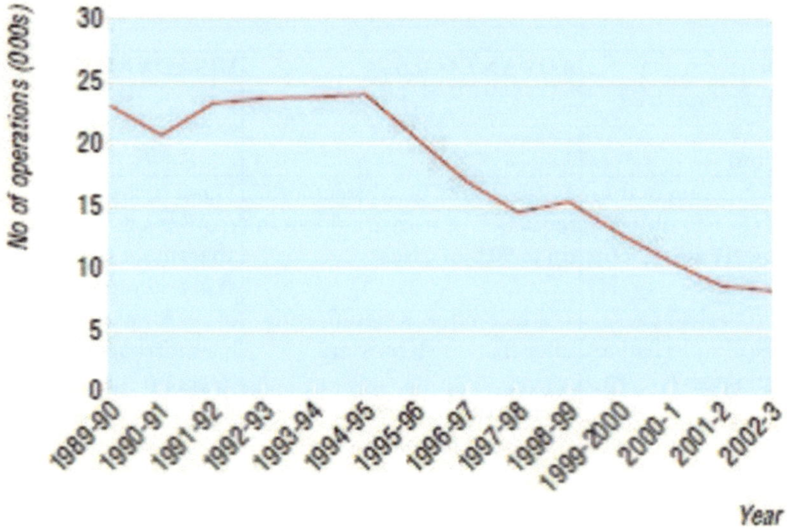

Fig. 9. Number of hysterectomies for menorrhagia from 1989-90 to 2002-3 in NHS trusts in England

Active education of good management of menorrhagia and promotion of effective medical management in primary care halves the number of referrals to secondary care. However, despite the strong evidence that medical treatments, in particular the LNG-IUS, are effective, many hysterectomies and endometrial ablations/resections are still performed annually without first evaluating medical treatment.[37]

d. Health-related quality of life and cost of the LNG-IUS vs. hysterectomy

Hurskainen et al. (Finland) compared outcomes, quality-of-life issues, and costs of the LNG-IUS vs. hysterectomy in the treatment of menorrhagia.[42] After 5 years of follow-up, 232 women (99%) were analyzed for the primary outcomes. The 2 groups did not differ substantially in terms of health-related quality of life (HRQL) or psychosocial well-being. Although 50 (42%) of the women assigned to the LNG-IUS group eventually underwent hysterectomy, the discounted direct and indirect costs in the LNG-IUS group ($2817 [95% confidence interval, $2222-$3530] per participant) remained substantially lower than in the hysterectomy group ($4660 [95% confidence interval, $4014-$5180]). Satisfaction with treatment was similar in both groups. Compared to other medications the LNG-IUS is much cheaper per menstrual cycle unless it is removed before 5 years. Long-term acceptability is therefore essential.[43]

D Endometrial ablative techniques

In recent years various surgical techniques have been developed to ablate the endometrium. An excellent review on these techniques was recently published.[10] The reader is therefore referred to this paper. It suffices to make some observations and conclusions.

The endometrial ablative techniques can be divided into two broad groups: the first-generation hysteroscopic endometrial ablation (HEA) procedures performed under direct vision, and the second-generation non-hysteroscopic endometrial ablation (NHEA) procedures which are largely 'blind'. These techniques are mainly used to treat women with excessive menstrual bleeding. They are summarized in Table 1.

TECHNIQUE	ADVANTAGES	DISADVANTAGES
Hysteroscopic endometrial ablation (first generation)		
Transcervical resection of the endometrium (TCRE) utilizes an electrosurgical cutting loop Transcervical rollerball uses an electrosurgical rollerball to coagulate the tissues Laser photo-vaporization uses a high-energy beam to destroy endometrial tissues	TCRE results in satisfactory reduction of menstrual loss in up to 90% of cases The technique is significantly safer than hysterectomy Rollerball endometrial ablation is the easiest technique to master and generally the quickest to perform. The risk of perforation is greatly diminished	These first-generation techniques require a general or regional anaesthetic, specialized surgical skill and often carry a small risk of perforation at the thin cornua, haemorrhage, fluid overload and infection Recurrence of menorrhagia or dysmenorrhoea and pelvic pain are principal reasons for further surgery The cost of the laser-photo-vaporization machine as well as the single-use laser fibre limits its more general application
Non-hysteroscopic endometrial ablation (NHEA) (second generation)		
Cavatherm device Hydrothermablation ThermaChoice MenoTreat System VestaBlate HydroThermAblator NovaSure GyneLase MEA	These second-generation 'less invasive' techniques are designed to ablate the full thickness of the endometrium by the controlled application of heat, cold, microwave or other forms of energy The techniques are simpler and quicker to perform than hysteroscopic methods, while satisfaction rates and reduction in menstrual blood loss are high (up to 90%)	Women choosing one of these options need to be aware that they are likely to continue to experience some degree of menstrual bleeding and that further surgery may be necessary for persistent heavy bleeding The data on the safety of all the second generation techniques are as yet incomplete, but all systems appear to be associated with minimal complication rates

Table 1. Endometrial ablative techniques.

Myomectomy (laparoscopic, robotic assisted laparoscopic, vaginal, laparoscopic assisted vaginal, laparotomy)	
Advantages	Disadvantages
-Overall results are 81% resolution of menorrhagia symptoms, with similar results for pelvic pressure symptoms -Laparoscopic approach to myomectomy is associated with a shorter postoperative recovery period, shorter hospital stay and cost-saving benefits -Robotic-assisted laparoscopic myomectomy could considerably reduce learning curve (Nisolle et al. 2011) -Vaginal myomectomy is only possible in selected cases -Combined approach renders haemostasis and uterine repair easier than by the laparoscopic approach alone	-Only a limited range of fibroids is amenable to the laparoscopic approach -Risk of conversion to open myomectomy is 2-8% -Rupture of the pregnant uterus has been reported after laparosopic myomectomy -Myomectomy performed via a laparotomy is associated with increased blood loss, operating time, pain, postoperative morbidity and longer hospital stay than hysterectomy, while an additional procedure (such as repeat myomectomy or hysterectomy) is necessary in 20–25% of women -Recurrence of fibroids following myomectomy occurs in up to 50% -Myomectomy carries a risk of postoperative pelvic adhesions
GnRH analogues in the management of uterine fibroids	
Advantages	Disadvantages
-GnRH analogues prior to either hysterectomy or myomectomy has shown that uterine volume and size, as well as fibroid volume, were all reduced, as were pelvic symptoms -Hysterectomy is rendered easier, with reduced operating time, and a greater proportion of hysterectomy patients were able to have a vaginal rather than an abdominal procedure -Blood loss and rate of vertical incision were reduced for both myomectomy and hysterectomy -Duration of hospital stay was reduced	-Disadvantages of GnRH analogues include cost, menopausal symptoms (but can be prevented by 'add-back' HRT) and, with prolonged therapy, bone demineralization -Some believe that benefits do not justify the costs -GnRH analogues render surgical planes less distinct, perhaps due to softening of the fibroids, which makes enucleation more difficult -Their use as primary therapy in younger women is questionable as fibroids re-grow to their original size within a few months of discontinuation of treatment

Uterine artery embolization (UAE)	
Advantages	Disadvantages
-Clinical success rates are good with good fibroid shrinkage rates (10–70%) and symptom improvement (70–94%) -UAE is now widely practiced in Western Europe and North America, and the National Institute for Clinical Excellence (NICE) in the UK has decreed that it can be routinely offered as a primary treatment for uterine fibroids, although it is recommended that all procedures are registered -However, the fact remains that UAE has never been compared with conventional treatments in a prospective randomized controlled trial (RCT), as either a pilot or a full study -There is also a lack of long-term data	-Complications secondary to arterial puncture, contrast injection, arterial catheterization and non-target-organ embolization are intrinsic to all embolization procedures, but are uncommon, and further minimized by operator experience and good technique -Chronic discharge is a frequent complication, affecting up to 7% of patients -Infections are also more common with larger fibroids -Fibroid extrusion occurs in about 10% of cases. Larger ones may necessitate a surgical procedure for removal, especially if impacted at the cervix -Clinical features of the so-called post-embolization syndrome include a flu-like illness, high temperature, high white cell count and a feeling of malaise, and may be due to release of cytokines and toxins from the ischaemic tissue. This might be difficult to differentiate from sepsis

Table 2. Summarizes these new approaches, their advantages and disadvantages (adapted from Banu et al.[10]).

A Cochrane review concluded that while short-term follow-up studies might indicate an advantage for endometrial ablation, longer-term studies show a narrowing of the gap, and hysterectomy appears to have consistently higher rates of satisfaction and better health-related quality-of-life outcomes.[44] A study conducted by Maia et al. is also worth mentioning in this respect.[45] They investigated 106 women with HMB. After endometrial resection, the women were randomized into two groups, 53 women in each. Women in the treatment group were fitted with Mirena®. In this group, amenorrhoea was achieved in 72% of cases after 3 months, in 89% after 6 months and in 100% after 1 year. In the resection-only group, the corresponding numbers were 19%, 17% and 9%, and in this group, 19% of the women underwent a second resection.

A second study by Maia et al. (CEPARH, Brazil) was recently reported at the World Congress on the Menopause (Abstract Book p. 74). Ninety-two perimenopausal women with menorrhagia, dysmenorrhea and premenstrual syndrome (PMS) were enrolled in this study. Sixty-two patients had adenomyosis and the remaining 30 had submucous and intramural myomas. The use of the LNG-IUS (Mirena®) following endometrial resection significantly increased amenorrhoea rates. The rate was 98% in the fifth year. Complete resolution of dysmenorrhea and PMS was reported by over 90% of patients. In historical controls submitted to endometrial resection, the amenorrhoea rate was only 20% with a failure rate of 40%. This study also showed an inhibition of the expression of aromatase in the ectopic glands in the myometrium of patients with adenomyosis, thereby contributing towards interrupting the progression of the disease. This may explain why the rates of amenorrhoea are far superior to those achieved with endometrial resection alone. It was concluded that endometrial resection with LNG-IUS is a viable alternative to hysterectomy in perimenopausal women.

E. Alternative therapies for the management of fibromyomas

Uterine myoma (leiomyoma, fibromyoma, fibroid) is a very common disease. They are more common in certain ethnic populations, especially the Afro-Caribbean.[46] Leiomyomas occur with an incidence of up to 77%.[47] Fibroids can cause menorrhagia, pelvic pain/discomfort, and bladder and bowel compression symptoms. They are often asymptomatic but some 25-50% of women will experience symptoms such as menorrhagia and pelvic discomfort. About 5% of the fibroids are intracavitary and submucosal and are most difficult to treat.[48,49] Hysterectomy is still the most commonly used procedure although medical treatments are preferable.[50,51] Uterine fibroids are responsible for 30% of hysterectomies. Notwithstanding the success of radical surgery, it is not always desirable particularly in the younger woman desiring fertility. Also psychological factors play a role as the uterus has been regarded as a sexual organ, a source of energy and vitality, and a maintainer of youth and attractiveness. Many women, therefore, might wish to avoid a hysterectomy, even when their families are complete.

Recently, new conservative treatment options have been developed such as the treatment with GnRH analogs and the levonorgestrel-releasing intrauterine system (LNG-IUS).[52,53] GnRH analogs, however, are only temporarily indicated before surgical intervention.

4. Conclusion

Because of its multiple health benefits, the LNG-IUS is likely to continue to conquer the worldwide markets to treat frequent gynaecological conditions and simultaneously provide contraception when needed. In addition, The LNG-IUS may also offer major benefits for the prevention of uterine pathologies and conditions, including endometrial polyps, endometrial hyperplasia, endometrial carcinoma in association or not with tamoxifen treatment of breast cancer, peri-menopausal menstrual disturbances, post-menopausal endometrial hyperplasia with hormone replacement therapy, endometrial hyperplasia and uterine myomas, endometriosis, adenomyosis, acute pelvic inflammatory disease and infertility.[27] Just as we are very conscious about the health benefits of estrogens in the prevention of osteoporotic fractures, the LNG-IUS and other hormone-releasing systems will be used mostly for the prevention of benign diseases in gynaecology. However, successful treatment of precancerous lesions and early cancer of the endometrium are within reach of the LNG-IUS.

The challenge also remains to promote novel LNG-IUSs who are easy to apply and are designed to fit in uterine cavities with different size and shape to improve tolerance and maximize continued use. Furthermore, new conservative approaches and minimally invasive techniques should be explored. Progesterone antagonists and progesterone receptor modulators may have a major role in the future to treat conditions such as fibroids and endometriosis conservatively. Endometriosis accounts for approximately 20% of the hysterectomies currently performed. There is no doubt that these new approaches will help reduce the number of hysterectomies further. However, hysterectomy will always remain the first choice for infiltrative cancer of the uterus and for most forms of pelvic relaxation although vaginal pessaries are increasingly used in older women. Currently, utero-vaginal prolapse is the indication for 15% of hysterectomies.

5. Conflict of interest

Dirk Wildemeersch, MD, PhD, is a Belgian gynaecologist and Medical Director of Contrel Drug Delivery Research, an organization which was established to manage clinical research and to develop and study innovative drug delivery technologies, aimed at finding improved methods for prevention and treatment of gynaecological conditions, improvements to birth control methods, and higher levels of safety, user acceptability, compliance and quality of life for women. Contrel is the manufacturer of GyneFix®, FibroPlant® and Femilis®. The research organization also provides insertion training for doctors. The funds generated are used for conducting further research and to participate in humanitarian projects.

6. References

[1] Vessey MP, Villard-Mackintosh L, McPherson K, Coulter A, Yeates D. The epidemiology of hysterectomy: findings in a large cohort study. Br J Obstet Gynaecol 1992;99:402-7.

[2] Wu JM, Wechter ME, Geller, EJ; Nguyen TV, Visco AG. Hysterectomy rates in the United States, 2003. Obstet Gynecol 2007;110:1091-5.

[3] Settnes A, Jorgensen T. Hysterectomy in a Danish Cohort. Prevalence, incidence and sociodemographic characteristics. Acta Obstetricia et Gynecologica Scandinavica 1996;75:274-80.

[4] Coulter A, McPherson K, Vessey M. Do British women undergo too many or too few hysterectomies? Soc Sci Med 1988;27:987-94.

[5] Bernstein SJ, McGlynn EA, Siu AL, Roth CP, Sherwood MJ, Keesey JW, Kosecoff J, Hicks NR, Brook RH. The appropriateness of hysterectomy: a comparison of care in seven health plans. JAMA 1993; 269: 2398-402.

[6] Shuster LT, Gostout BS, Grossardt BR, Rocca WA. Prophylactic oophorectomy in premenopausal women and long-term health. Menopause International 2008;14:111-6.

[7] Shoupe D, Parker WH, Broder MS, Liu Z, Farquhar C, Berek JS. Elective oophorectomy for benign gynecological disorders. Menopause 2007;14(Suppl. 1): 580-5.

[8] Bahamondes L, Bahamondes MV, Monteiro I. "Levonorgestrel-releasing intrauterine system: uses and controversies". Expert Review of Medical Devices 2008;5:437-45.

[9] Boyd ME, Groome PA. The morbidity of abdominal hysterectomy. Can J Surg. 1993;36:155-9.

[10] Banu NS, Manyonda IT. Alternative medical and surgical options to hysterectomy. Best Practice & Rese Clin Obstet Gynaecol. 2005;19:431-49.

[11] Dwyer N, Hutton J & Stirrat GM. Randomised controlled trial comparing endometrial resection with abdominal hysterectomy for the surgical treatment of menorrhagia. Br J Obstet Gynaecol 1993;100:237-43.

[12] Weber AM, Walters MD, Schover LR, Church JM, Piedmonte MR. Functional outcomes and satisfaction after abdominal hysterectomy. Am J Obstet Gynecol 1999;181:530-5.

[13] Thakar R, Ayers S, Georgakapolou A, Clarkson P, Stanton S, Manyonda I. Hysterectomy improves quality of life and decreases psychiatric symptoms: a prospective and randomised comparison of total versus subtotal hysterectomy. BJOG 2004;111:1115-20.

[14] Rannestad T, Eikeland O, Helland H & Quarnstrom U. The quality of life in women suffering from gynaecological disorders is improved by means of hysterectomy. Acta Obstet Gynecol Scand 2001;80:46–51.

[15] Rhodes JC, Kjerulff KH, Langenberg PW & Guzinski GM. Hysterectomy and sexual functioning. JAMA 1999;282:1934-41.

[16] Dicker RC, Greenspan JR, Strauss LT, Cowart MR, Scally MJ, Peterson HB, DeStefano F, Rubin GL, Ory HW. Complications of abdominal and vaginal hysterectomy among

women of reproductive age in the United States: the collaborative review of sterilization. Am J Obstet Gynecol 1982;144:841-8.
[17] McPherson K, Metcalfe MA, Herbert A, Maresh M, Casbard A, Hargreaves J, Bridgman S, Clarke A. Severe complications of hysterectomy: the value study. BJOG 2004;11:688–94.
[18] Wingo PA, Huezo CM, Rubin GL, Ory HW Peterson HB. The mortality risk associated with hysterectomy. Am J Obstet Gynecol 1985;152:803-8.
[19] van der Vaart CH, van der Bom JG, de Leeuw JR, Roovers JP, Heintz AP. The contribution of hysterectomy to the occurrence of urge and stress urinary incontinence symptoms. BJOG 2002;109:149-54.
[20] Riedel HH, Lehmann-Willenbrock E & Semm K. Ovarian failure phenomena after hysterectomy. J Reprod Med 1986;31:597-600.
[21] Carlson KJ, Miller BA & Fowler FJ. The Maine Women's Health Study: I. Outcomes of hysterectomy.Obstet Gynecol 1994;83:556-65.
[22] National Evidence-Based Clinical Guidelines. The Management of Menorrhagia in Secondary Care. Royal College of Obstetricians and Gynaecologists, London.
[23] Lethaby A., Augood C, Duckitt K. Nonsteroidal anti-inflammatory drugs for heavy menstrual bleeding. In: Cochrane Collaboration, ed. Cochrane Library, Issue 1. Update Software, Oxford; 1999.
[24] Cooke I, Lethaby A, Farquhar, C. Antifibrinolytics for heavy menstrual bleeding. Antifibrinolytics for heavy menstrual bleeding. In: Cochrane Collaboration, ed. Cochrane Library, Issue 1; 1999.
[25] Lethaby A, Irvine G, Cameron, I. Cyclical progestagens for heavy menstrual bleeding. In: Cochrane Collaboration, ed. Cochrane Library, Issue 1. Update Software. Oxford; 1999.
[26] Fraser IS. Non-contraceptive health benefits of intrauterine hormonal systems. Contraception 2010;82:396-403.
[27] Hasson HM. Clinical studies of the Wing Sound II metrology device. In: Zatuchni GI, Goldsmith A, Sciarra JJ (eds). Intrauterine Contraception: Advances and Future Prospects. Harper & Row, Philadelphia, 1984; 126-41.
[28] Kurz KH. Cavimeter uterine measurements and IUD clinical correlation. In: Zatuchni GI, Goldsmith A, Sciarra JJ (eds). Intrauterine Contraception: Advances and Future Prospects. Harper & Row, Philadelphia, 1984; 142–62.
[29] Benacerraf BR, Shipp TD, Bromly B. Three-dimentional ultrasound detection of abnormally located intrauterine contraceptive devices which are the source of pelvic pain and abnormal bleeding. Ultrasound Obstet Gynecol 2009;34:110-5.
[30] Shipp TD, Bromly B. Benacerraf BR. The width of the uterine cavity is narrower in patients with an embedded intrauterine device (IUD) compared to a normally positioned IUD. J Ultrasound Med 2010; 29: 1453-6.
[31] Wildemeersch D. Commentary. Intrauterine contraceptives that do not fit well contribute to early discontinuation. Eur J Contracept Reprod Health Care 2011;16:1-7.
[32] Wildemeersch D, Janssens D, Weyers S. Ease of insertion, contraceptive efficacy and safety of new T-shaped levonorgestrel-releasing intrauterine systems. Contraception 2005; 6:465-9.
[33] Wildemeersch D, Janssens D, Andrade A. The Femilis® LNG-IUS: Contraceptive performance- an interim analysis. Eur J Contracept Reprod Health Care 2009;14:1-8.
[34] Wildemeersch D, Pylyser K, De Wever N, Dhont M. Treatment of non-atypical and atypical endometrial hyperplasia with a levonorgestrel-releasing intrauterine system: longterm follow-up. Maturitas 2007;57:210-3.
[35] Wildemeersch D, Anderson E, Lambein K, Pauwels P, Dhont M. Successful Treatment of Early Endometrial Carcinoma by Local Delivery of Levonorgestrel: A Case

Report. Obstetrics and Gynecology International 2010, Article ID 431950, doi:10.1155/2010/431950.
[36] Marques AA, Bahamondes L, Aldrighi JM, Petta CA. Quality of life in Brazilian women with endometriosis assessed through a medical outcome questionnaire. J Reprod Med 2004;49:115-20.
[37] Bahamondes L, Petta CA, Fernandes A, Monteiro I. Use of the levonorgestrel-releasing intrauterine system in women with endometriosis, chronic pelvic pain and dysmenorrhea. Contraception 2007;75:S134-S9.
[38] Anpalagan A, Condous G. Is There a Role for Use of Levonorgestrel Intrauterine System in Women with Chronic Pelvic Pain? A review. J Minimally Invasive Gynecol 2008;15:663-6.
[39] Milsom I. The levonorgestrel-releasing intrauterine system as an alternative to hysterectomy in peri-menopausal women. Contraception 2007;75:S152-S4.
[40] Lähteenmäki P, Haukkamaa M, Puolakka J, Riikonen U, Sainio S, Suvisaari J, Nilsson CG. Open randomised study of use of levonorgestrel releasing intrauterine system as alternative to hysterectomy. BMJ 1998;316:1122-6.
[41] Reid PC, Mukri F. Trends in number of hysterectomies performed in England for menorrhagia: examination of health episode statistics, 1989 to 2002-3. BMJ 2005;330:938-9.
[42] Ritva Hurskainen R, Teper J, Rissanen P, Aalto AM,Grenman S, Kivela A, Kujansuu E, Vuorma S, Yliskoski M, Paavonen J, Outcomes and Costs With the Levonorgestrel-Releasing Intrauterine System or Hysterectomy for Treatment of Menorrhagia. Randomized Trial 5-Year Follow-up. JAMA 2004;291:1456-63.
[43] Lethaby AE, Cooke I & Rees M. Progesterone /progestagen releasing intrauterine system versus either placebo or any other medication for heavy menstrual bleeding. Cochrane Database Syst Rev22000:CD002126.
[44] Marjoribanks J, Lethaby A & Farquhar C. Surgery versus medical therapy for heavy menstrual bleeding. Cochrane Database Syst Rev22003:CD00385.
[45] Maia H Jr, Maltez A, Coelho G, Athayde C, Coutinho EM. Insertion of mirena after endometrial resection in patients with adenomyosis. J Am Assoc Gynecol Laparosc. 2003;10:512-6.
[46] Kjerulff K, Guzinski G & Langenberg P. Hysterectomy and race. Obstet Gynaecol 1993;82:757-64.
[47] Cramer SF, Patel A. The frequency of uterine leiomyomas. Am J Clin Pathol 1990;94:435-8.
[48] Buttram VC, Reiter RC. Uterine leiomyomas: etiology, symptomatology and management. Fert Steril 1981;36:433-45.
[49] Donnez J, Schindler AE, Wall weiner D, Audebert A. Fibroids: management and treatment. In: Lunenfeld B, Insler V, eds. GnRH analogues: The State of the Art 1996. Carnforth, UK: Parthenon Publishing, 1996:71-82.
[50] Vollenhoven BL, Lawrance AS, Healy DL. Uterine Fibroids: a clinical review. Br J Obstet Gynaecol 1990;97:285-98.
[51] Cramer SF, Hoiszny JA, Leppert P. Epidemiology of uterine leiomyomas. With an etiologic hypothesis. J Reprod Med 1995;40:595-600.
[52] Nisolle M and Donnez J. Medical management of uterine fibroids: short-term therapy with GnRH agonists. In: Brosens I, Lunenfeld B, Donnez J, eds. Pathogenesis and medical management of uterine fibroids. Carnforth, UK: Parthenon Publishing, 1999:113-119.
[53] Donnez J, Gillerot S, Squifflet J and Nisolle M. Progestogens and antiprogestogens. In: Brosens I, Lunenfeld B, Donnez J, eds. Pathogenesis and medical management of uterine fibroids. Carnforth, UK: Parthenon Publishing, 1999:121-128.

12

Menorrhagia and the Levonorgestrel Intrauterine System

Johnstone Shabaya Miheso
Crosshouse Hospital, Kilmarnock, UK

1. Introduction

1.1 Menorrhagia

Heavy menstrual bleeding can be defined as excessive blood loss which interferes with a woman's physical, emotional, social and material quality of life. It is a subjective complaint by a woman of heavy periods. Menorrhagia on the other hand is an objective diagnosis of blood loss over 80 millilitres over several consecutive cycles.

The average blood loss in a Caucasian female population is approximately 30-40 millilitres per menstrual flow (Cole et al. 1971; Hallberg et al. 1966), the majority of which is lost in the first forty eight hours. Menorrhagia is the commonest cause of iron deficiency anaemia in women in the developed world and occurs in sixty per cent of women with objective menorrhagia.

1.2 Significance

Only half of the women who present to clinicians with heavy menstrual loss have objective menorrhagia. However, it is the main reason for women requesting hysterectomy and 1 in 5 women have a hysterectomy in the United Kingdom for this reason by the age of fifty five. At histopathology, a vast majority of these uteri are found to be benign. With less invasive and effective alternatives to hysterectomy, women should be carefully counselled with regards to morbidity and mortality associated with this major operation.

Menstrual disorders are now more common than they were a century ago because modern career women are choosing to have smaller or no families and not breastfeeding. Menorrhagia affects about 1.5 million women in England and Wales and accounts for twenty per cent of all gynaecology referrals to the outpatient clinic (Census 2001.2002).

1.3 Pathophysiology

A majority of cases of menorrhagia have no identifiable cause and hence are described as 'dysfunctional'. Dysfunctional uterine bleeding is associated with anovulation and occurs in a fifth of women at extremes of their reproductive life.

Menorrhagia is also associated with uterine fibroids, endometrial polyps, adenomyosis, pelvic infection, bleeding diathesis, and rarely malignancies like endometrial cancer. Over a half of women with blood loss over 200 millilitres will have underlying fibroids.

The exact mechanism of menorrhagia is poorly understood. It is thought to result from increased activity of prostaglandins or the endometrial fibrinolytic activity. There is an elevation of prostaglandins (PGE2 and PGF2α) in the endometrium of women with menorrhagia, suggesting that menorrhagia may result from an increase in vasodilator PGE2 as compared to vasoconstrictor PGF2α prostaglandins (Smith et al. 1981).

The endometrium also contains a fibrinolytic system whose activity is increased in women with menorrhagia compared to those with normal menstrual loss.

1.4 Causes of menorrhagia

Although no cause can be found in most cases, other causes of menorrhagia such as uterine pathology and medical disorders (Table 1) should be actively sought and excluded.

Dysfunctional uterine bleeding (DUB)
Uterine pathology
Medical disorders including thyroid or bleeding disorders

Table 1. Causes of heavy periods

1.4.1 Dysfunctional uterine bleeding

Dysfunctional uterine bleeding is a diagnosis of exclusion, when no other cause of bleeding can be found. Some people further sub-classify it into ovulatory and anovulatory bleeding although this does not have much clinical relevance. Ovulatory or 'idiopathic' bleeding is where periods are regular while anovulatory bleeding tends to occur at the extremes of the reproductive age.

In ovulatory cycles, bleeding results from the withdrawal of progesterone. It is typically painful and characterized by a cramping sensation. Anovulatory bleeding is caused by excessive proliferation of endometrium due to unopposed oestrogen. The absence of prostaglandins in the endometrium, which is usually synthesized in response to progesterone, may explain the absence of pain/cramps.

1.4.2 Uterine abnormalities

Fibroids are benign whorls of smooth muscle and collagen. They usually present in multiples and can grow to enormous sizes. They occur in a fifth of women and are commoner in women of the Afro-Caribbean origin. They occur in the uterine body or cervix and can be submucosal, intramural or subserosal.

The clinical signs and symptoms depend on their site and size. Symptoms include heavy periods, infertility, miscarriage or dyspareunia. They may cause pain in pregnancy due to red degeneration. When large they can cause pressure effects on surrounding organs and may present with urinary frequency, hydronephrosis and recurrent urinary tract infections. Only less than 0.1% of fibroids undergo malignant change resulting in leiomyosarcoma.

Polyps are localized growths of the endometrium which comprise of fibrous tissue surrounded by columnar epithelium. It is thought that they arise from disordered apoptosis and regrowth of the endometrium. Malignant change is extremely rare.

1.4.3 Medical causes

In rare cases, menorrhagia can occur as a result of systemic diseases which result in hepatic and renal impairment although amenorrhea is common with end stage disease. Both hypo and hyperthyroidism can also cause heavy menstruation.

Bleeding disorders like von Willebrand's disease or platelet defects are associated with menorrhagia.

1.5 Diagnosis

1.5.1 History

The diagnosis of menorrhagia is often made on history alone. This will take into account the severity of the complaint as judged by the presence of clots or how frequently a woman changes pads or sanitary towels, or if a woman uses both as 'double protection'. Efforts should be made to find out the impact of the bleeding on the woman's quality of life including time taken off work, avoidance of usual activities, embarrassment as well as the effect of anaemic symptoms and treatment.

A full obstetric and gynaecological history should include the woman's general health, weight and height (body mass index), number of deliveries, pregnancy losses and cervical smears. The presence of other symptoms such as dyspareunia may point to a specific cause.

Drug history including tamoxifen use and a history of bleeding tendency are also important. Previous pelvic surgery and associated findings should be noted as well as past history of polycystic disease, hormonal usage, bowels or ovarian cancer.

1.5.2 Examination

This is aimed at assessing the general state, diagnosing anaemia and identifying possible causes of menorrhagia. It should therefore entail vital signs, inspection of mucous membranes, finger nails and abdominal palpation. A speculum assessment should be done to look for vaginal and cervical abnormalities. A bimanual pelvic examination will assess the size of the uterus, presence of adnexal mass and/or signs of a pelvic infection.

1.5.3 Investigations

A full blood count is useful to determine haemoglobin level and can be used to monitor treatment with haematinics. Thyroid function tests, coagulation defects, liver and kidney function tests should be done if clinically indicated.

An ultrasound scan of the pelvis and abdomen is a useful tool in diagnosis and for describing masses suspected or actually found on physical examination, especially in obese women where examination can be suboptimal. It is not usually required if uterine size is less than 10 weeks and there is no suspicion of other pathology. It is also justifiable after failure of medical treatment of heavy periods.

Cervical smear should be undertaken if screening is not up to date or where the cervix looks suspicious. Similarly an endometrial biopsy should be taken if a woman is over 40 or under 40 with particular risk factors like tamoxifen use, unopposed oestrogen or obesity.

1.6 Treatment of menorrhagia

1.6.1 Medical

Several medical options are available for treatment of women with heavy menstrual loss. Non-steroidal anti-inflammatory drugs act by inhibiting prostaglandin synthesis and reduce bleeding by about a quarter. The commonest used medication is mefenamic acid of which the main side effect is dyspepsia.

Tranexamic acid is an anti-fibrinolytic medication. It inhibits plasminogen activator and hence promotes clots formation in spiral arterioles and decreases bleeding by about a half. Side effects include nausea, vomiting, diarrhoea and rarely tinnitus and thromboembolic events. Hypotension may occur if given rapidly by the intravenous route.

The combined oral contraceptive pill makes periods regular and is associated with a fifty per cent reduction in blood loss. It is suitable for all age groups unless there are specific contraindications like family or personal thromboembolic disease, migraines with aura, hypertension, obesity and immobility.

Oral progesterones act by ovulation inhibition and directly suppressing the endometrium. Norethisterone 5mg three times a day from day 5 to 26 has been shown to reduce blood loss by eighty per cent. Depo-Provera may cause unpredictable bleeding initially but usually amenorrhea results. Common side effects include nausea, breast tenderness, bloatedness, weight gain, acne and voice changes.

Non-steroidal anti-inflammatory drugs e.g. Mefenamic acid
Anti-fibrinolytic drugs e.g. tranexamic acid
Hormones
Combined contraceptive pill
Synthetic progestogens (norethisterone, provera, medroxyprogeterone acetate)
Intrauterine progesterone (levornogetrel intrauterine system)
Danazol and gestrinone
Anti-oestrogen e.g. gestrinone
Gonadotrophin releasing hormone agonists

Table 2. Medical treatment of menorrhagia

Gonadotrophin releasing hormone analogues act by down-regulating the pituitary hence inhibiting ovarian activity. Women become hypo-oestrogenised and may have distressing vasomotor symptoms of hot flushes and night sweats as well as vaginal dryness. They also cause demineralization of bones. Add-back hormone replacement therapy as well as bone mineral density scans should be considered if treatment goes beyond six months.

Danazol was originally produced for treatment of endometriosis but was found to cause amenorrhea. It is a synthetic androgen which has both oestrogenic and progestrogenic effects. It works by inhibiting the pituitary and also suppressing the endometrium directly. It has debilitating androgenic effects which restrict its use including acne, deep voice, hirsutism, breast tenderness and weight gain.

Gestrinone on the other hand, is a synthetic derivative of 19-nortestosterone which has both oestrogenic and progestrogenic as well as androgenic effects. It is not commonly used for treatment of heavy periods. Its androgenic side effects are less that danazol but after cessation of use, bleeding can become heavy again.

The levonorgestrel intrauterine system is a medicated device that is inserted into the uterus and delivers progesterone which acts locally on the endometrium to cause thinning and amenorrhea. It is covered in more details in the second part of this chapter.

1.6.2 Surgical treatment

Endometrial destructive techniques can be divided into first and second generation. The former involve hysteroscopic destruction of the endometrium by rollerball, transcervical endometrial resection or laser ablation.

The cumulative hysterectomy rate after endometrial resection was found in one study to be 27.4 per cent after four years (Poorey et al., 1998).

Endometrial resection is associated with a long surgical learning curve and significant risks include uterine perforation and fluid overload resulting in hyponatremia. They have generally been superseded by second generation techniques which are quicker and safer.

First generation	Roller ball Trans-cervical resection Laser ablation
Second generation	Thermal balloon ablation Microwave ablation Novasure ablation
Hysterectomy	Total Subtotal

Table 3. Different modalities of surgical treatment

Second generation endometrial ablation techniques aim to destroy the endometrium with resultant amenorrhea. They do not involve direct visualization of the endometrium. Techniques include thermal balloon, microwave or novasure endometrial ablation.

In practice, although patient satisfaction rates are over 70 per cent, the amenorrhea rate is less than 30 per cent (Lethaby et al., 2001). These are more successful in women over 45. The procedure can be repeated in women with persistent heavy menstrual bleeding after assessing the cavity hysteroscopically.

Rare complications include uterine perforation and accidental organ injury. Effective contraception is essential following endometrial ablation.

Hysterectomy remains the only method of ensuring complete amenorrhea and is generally offered to women where all other methods have been unsuccessful. It can be undertaken laparoscopically, vaginally or abdominally. The choice depends on the size of uterus, degree of uterine descent, previous surgery, whether ovaries are to be conserved, patient preference and surgeon's skills.

1.6.3 Specific treatment

Organic causes of heavy bleeding should be addressed. These include fibroids which can be resected hysteroscopically or by laparotomy or a laparoscopic approach if a patient wants to preserve fertility. In these cases, women should be warned of the risk of significant intra-operative bleeding necessitating blood transfusion and the possibility of an emergency hysterectomy.

Polyps can be removed at out patient hysteroscopy or in theatre under a general anaesthetic. Where malignancy is suspected, appropriate biopsies and referral should be made to the multidisciplinary team.

2. Medicated Intrauterine system

2.1 Background

The levonorgestrel intrauterine system is a reversible long acting contraceptive device that is aseptically fitted into the uterine cavity. It has a hormone cylinder that contains 52 mg of levonorgestrel that is released at the rate of twenty micrograms per day.

The term intrauterine system (IUS) is used to differentiate it from the intrauterine contraceptive device (IUCD) in the United Kingdom.

It was primarily produced as a contraceptive device but has other non-contraceptive benefits. It can be beneficial in the management of chronic pelvic pain, endometriosis, anaemia, dysmenorrhoea, and endometrial protection in women on oestrogen hormone replacement therapy.

Over one hundred and fifty million women worldwide use the intrauterine system for contraception. It is easy to insert and remove and does not require high level of technical skills. It is licensed for contraception use for up to 5 years following which a replacement can be made.

It can be inserted at any time of the cycle and during caesarean section (Lopez-Farfan, MacIel-Martnez, Velez-Machorro, & Vazquez-Estrada, 2010). It is useful in the peri and postmenopausal woman for bleeding, contraception and hormone replacement therapy (Kirk & McFall, 2009).

It is also widely used for menorrhagia. Its therapeutic effect is achieved by endometrial atrophy with a subsequent reduction in the heaviness of menstrual loss of eighty per cent in the first 6 months and up to 90 per cent in a year (Irvine et al., 1999, Hallberg et al., 1966, Stewart, et al., 2001).

Studies show that it is highly acceptable with 40 % women choosing to have a second device inserted after five years (Lete et al., 2011).

2.2 Comparison with other treatments of menorrhagia

Its effect on heavy menstrual loss has been compared to alternatives in clinical practice. It has been found to be more successful than cyclical norethisterone (given from day 5-26 of the menstrual cycle) in treating women with dysfunctional uterine bleeding although it was associated with more side effects such as breast tenderness and intermenstrual bleeding (Lethaby et al., 2010).

In comparison with tranexamic acid and non-steroidal anti-inflammatory drugs, it has been found to be superior in reducing menstrual loss (Stewart et al., 2001).

The intrauterine system has been proved to be effective in over 85% of patients with simple endometrial hyperplasia although the authors recommend long term follow up with periodic biopsies for up to 2 years (Scarselli et al., 2011).

When compared with thermal balloon endometrial ablation, no difference was noted in the quality of life, number of women requesting alternative treatment, or satisfaction between the two groups (Busfield et al., 2006). Both groups however showed an improvement in quality of life although patients with the intrauterine system recorded lower PBAC (Pictorial Blood loss Assessment Chart) scores at 12 and 24 months.

Compared to trans-cervical resection of endometrial (TCRE), satisfaction rates were both 80% in one study (Gupta, 2006) although intrauterine system requires less skill with no operative hazards. Continuation rates at five years were high with reasons sited in one study being bleeding, pain and infection (Backman et al., 2001).

It can be used successfully in selected women with coexisting morbidities. These include leiomyomas, obesity and those on anticoagulation therapies. There has not been any deleterious difference in endothelial or vascular function in thromboembolic high risk women on intrauterine system (Brito et al., 2010) and it is therefore can be considered after assessing the risks and benefits.

In a prospective comparative trial of 132 perimenopausal patients who smoked, IUS was found to be superior in preventing anaemia to both medroxyprogesterone acetate and continuous oral progesterone (Kucuk et al., 2008).

Like all hormonal contraception, the World Health Organization recommends avoidance among women with present or past history of breast cancer although there has not been any known increase in risk compared to the copper intrauterine contraceptive device (Gemzell-Danielsson, 2010). It is safe and effective in Human Immunodeficiency Virus positive women and like in the healthy equivalent, causes a reduction in bleeding. It has no effect on ovarian function and is not associated with increased viral secretion from the cervical mucus (Heikinheimo, 2010).

Compared to hysterectomy, the intrauterine system was found to be more cost effective (Hurskainen et al., 2004). However, a recent study (Roberts et al., 2011) has shown that although hysterectomy is initially costly, it produces more quality assured life years compared to the other treatment modalities for menorrhagia and therefore more cost effective in the long run. It is therefore a reasonable option of initial primary treatment.

The use of the intrauterine system has reduced the rate of hysterectomy among women with adenomyosis by 70% by decreasing dysmenorrhoea and bleeding episodes (Kulshrestha, et al, 2011).

2.3 Contraindications

Intrauterine system is contraindicated in pregnancy, local or systemic infection, suspected malignancy of the cervix or uterus, weight gain and unexplained vaginal bleeding among others.

2.4 Complications

During fitting there is a risk of perforation of the uterus with potential damage to surrounding organs. There is also a risk of infection which can spread to the pelvis and rarely systemically.

The expulsion rate is 4 per cent and is most common in the first year after insertion. Risk factors include young age, nulliparity and immediately postpartum. The rate of expulsion is not related to the uterine cavity length (Bahamondes, et al, 2011)

2.5 Side effects

It has been associated with a change in pattern of bleeding, spotting, amenorrhea or irregular bleeding. Rarely it may cause abdominal/pelvic pain, breast tenderness, acne, bloatedness, weight gain, headaches, hair loss, migraines, ovarian cysts, mood changes, nausea and low sex drive.

3. Conclusion

The levonorgestrel intrauterine system is an acceptable and cost effective treatment of heavy menstrual loss. It has additional benefits that make it a preferred choice for management of a number of other gynaecologic conditions at the same time. More research is required in long term outcome and cost analysis taking into account clinician preferences of choice.

4. Acknowledgment

I am grateful to Dr David Rae and Dr Wael Agur for their substantial input.

5. References

Backman, T., Huhtala, S., Tuominen, J., Luoto, R., Erkkola, R., Blom, T., et al. (2001). Sixty thousand woman-years of experience on the levonorgestrel intrauterine system: An epidemiological survey in finland. European Journal of Contraception and Reproductive Health Care, 6(SUPPL. 1), 23-26.

Bahamondes, M. V., Monteiro, I., Canteiro, R., Fernandes, A. D. S., & Bahamondes, L. (2011). Length of the endometrial cavity and intrauterine contraceptive device expulsion. International Journal of Gynecology and Obstetrics, 113(1), 50-53.

Brito, M. B., Barboza, R. P., Martins, W. P., Oliveira, L. C. O., Ferriani, R. A., & Vieira, C. S. (2010). The levonorgestrel-intrauterine system was associated with no adverse effect in endothelial function in women with history of thrombosis or thrombophilia. European Journal of Contraception and Reproductive Health Care.Conference: 11th Congress of the European Society of Contraception and

Reproductive Health, ESC the Hague Netherlands.Conference Start: 20100519 Conference End: 20100522.Conference P(TRUNCATED), 15, 143-144.

Busfield, R.A, Farquhar, C. M, Sower, M. C et al: A randomised trial comparing the levonorgestrel intrauterine system and thermal balloon ablation for heavy menstrual bleeding. BJOG: 2006 113 (3) PP257-263.

Cole SK, Billewicz WZ, & Thomson AM (1971) Sources of variation in menstrual blood loss - a population study. J Obstet Gynecol Br Cmmwlth 78, 933-9

Gemzell-Danielsson, K. (2010). IUS in women with breast cancer. European Journal of Contraception and Reproductive Health Care.Conference: 11th Congress of the European Society of Contraception and Reproductive Health, ESC the Hague Netherlands.Conference Start: 20100519 Conference End: 20100522.Conference P(TRUNCATED), 15, 204.

Gupta, B., Mittal, S., Misra, R., et al. Levonorgestrel-releasing intrauterine system vs. transcervical resection of the endometrium for dysfunctional bleeding, International Journal of Gynaecology and Obstetrics 2006 95 (3) pp 261-266.

Hallberg L, Hogdahl AM, Nilsson L, Rybo G. Menstrual blood loss- a population study. Variation at different ages and attempts to define normality. Acta Obstet Gynecol Scand 1966; 45:320-351.

Heikinheimo, O. (2010). Levonorgestrel-releasing intrauterine system (LNG-IUS) in human immunodeficiency virus (HIV) infected women - A five-year follow-up study. Reproductive Sciences.Conference: 57th Annual Scientific Meeting of the Society for Gynecologic Investigation, SGI 2010 Orlando, FL United States.Conference Start: 20100324 Conference End: 20100327.Conference Publication: (Var.Pagings), 17(3 SUPPL. 1), 88A.

Hurskainen R, Teperi J, Rissanen P, Aalto AM, Grenman S, Kivale A, et al. Clinical outcomes and costs with the levonorgestrel-releasing intrauterine system or hysterectomy for the treatment of menorrhagia- randomized control trial 5-year follow-up. JAMA 2004;291:1456-63.

Irvine GA, Cameron IT. Medical management of dysfunctional uterine bleeding. Bailliere's Clin Obstet Gynecol 1999; 13(2):189-202

Kirk, K., & McFall, P. (2009). The use of the mirena intrauterine system in a regional menopause clinic. Maturitas.Conference: 8th European Congress on Menopause, EMAS London United Kingdom.Conference Start: 20090516 Conference End: 20090520 Sponsor: PANTARHEI BIOSCIENCE, FSDeducation.Eu.Conference Publication: (Var.Pagings), 63, S31-S32.

Kucuk, T. and Ertan , K. Continous oral or medroxyprogesterone acetate versus the levonorgestrel releasing intrauterine system in the treatment of perimenopausal menorrhagia: A randomized, prospective, controlled clinical trial in female smokers. Clinical and Experimental Obstetrics and Gynaecology 2008 35 (1) pp57-60.

Kulshrestha, V., Kriplani, A., Agarwal, N., & Bhatla, N. (2011). Role of levonorgestrel-intrauterine system in medical management of adenomyosis. Journal of Obstetrics and Gynaecology.Conference: 1st World Congress of Obstetrics, Gynaecology and Andrology: Psychosomatic and Biological Perspectives on Clinical Controversies, WCOGA 2011 London United Kingdom.Conference Start: 20110321 Confe(TRUNCATED), 31, 27.

Lete, I., Del Carme Cuesta, M, Marin, J M., et al> Acceptability of the levonorgestrel intrauterine system in the long term treatment of heavy menstrual bleeding: How many women choose to use a second device? European Journal of Obstetrics Gynaecology and Reproductive Biology 2011 154 (1) pp67-70.

Lethaby, A, Cook I, Rees, M: Progesterone or progesterone-releasing systems for heavy menstrual bleeding. Cochrane Database of systematic reviews. 11,2010

Lethaby A, Shepperd S, Cooke I, Farquhar C. Endometrial resection and ablation versus hysterectomy for heavy menstrual bleeding (Cochrane Review). In: The Cochrane library, Issue 4. Oxford: Update software, 2001.

Lopez-Farfan, J. A., MacIel-Martnez, M., Velez-Machorro, I. J., & Vazquez-Estrada, L. (2010). Application of mirenaan during caesarean section (CS). European Journal of Contraception and Reproductive Health Care.Conference: 11th Congress of the European Society of Contraception and Reproductive Health, ESC the Hague Netherlands.Conference Start: 20100519 Conference End: 20100522.Conference P(TRUNCATED), 15, 165-166.

National statistics Online. Census 2001.2002. www.statistics.gov.uk/census2001/pop2001/england_wales.asp.

Stewart A, Cummins C Gold L, Jordan R, Phillips W. The effectiveness of the levonorgestrel-releasing intrauterine system in menorrhagia: a systematic review. Br J Obstet Gynaecol 2001; 108:74-86.

Poorey AS, Ewen P, Sutton CJ. Does transcervical resection of the endometrium for menorrhagia really avoid hysterectomy? Life table analysis of a large series. J Am Assoc Gynecol Laparosc 1998; 5:229-35.

Roberts T E, Tsourapas A, Middleton L J, Champaneria R, Daniels J P, Cooper K G, Bhattachara S, Barton P M. Hysterectomy, endometrial ablation, and levonorgestrel intrauterine system (Mirena) for treatment of heavy menstrual bleeding: cost effectiveness analysis. BMJ 2011;342:d2202

Scarselli, G., Bargelli, G., Taddei, G. L., Marchionni, M., Peruzzi, E., Pieralli, A., et al. (2011). Levonorgestrel-releasing intrauterine system (LNG-IUS) as an effective treatment option for endometrial hyperplasia: A 15-year follow-up study. Fertility and Sterility, 95(1), 420-422.

Smith SK, Abel MH, Kelly RW & Baird DT (1981) Prostaglandin synthesis in the endometrium of women with ovular dysfunctional bleeding. Br J Obstet Gynecol 88, 434-42.

13

Is Embolization Equal to Hysterectomy in Treating Uterine Fibroids?

Tomislav Strinic
*Split University, School of Medicine,
University Hospital Split,
Croatia*

1. Introduction

It is important for women to ensure that they make their own individual decision about whether to have a hysterectomy. Making this decision can be a difficult and emotional process. It is important for women to be well informed about the procedure so they can confidently discuss all available options with their gynaecologist. Because a hysterectomy involves the removal of the uterus, it is important that women realise they will no longer menstruate or be able to conceive after the procedure. For some women the prospect of no more periods and the removal of the fear of pregnancy will bring relief. Other women may find the finality of the ending of their reproductive capability distressing.

In November 1843, Charles Clay performed the first hysterectomy in Manchester, England. The earliest hysterectomies were supracervical, or subtotal hysterectomies. The body of the uterus was removed while the cervix remained intact. In 1929, Richardson, performed the first total abdominal hysterectomy (TAH), in which the entire uterus and cervix were removed (Johns, 1997). Total abdominal hysterectomy involves removal of the uterus and cervix through an abdominal incision. A hysterectomy can be performed in three different ways: abdominal, vaginal and endoscopic. The method chosen will depend on the surgeon's skills, expertise and preference. Also taken into account is the reason for the hysterectomy and characteristics such as a woman's weight, pelvic surgery history and if they have had children.

2. Hysterectomy

Hysterectomy is the most common non-pregnancy-related major surgery performed on women worldwide. This surgical procedure involves removal of the uterus and cervix, and for some conditions, the fallopian tubes and ovaries. Reasons for choosing this operation are treatment of genital malignancy and various common noncancerous uterine conditions. Primary indication for benign hysterectomy are uterine leiomyoma, endometriosis, uterine prolapse/incontinence, and abnormal uterine bleeding. Although this procedure is highly successful in curing the disease of concern, it is a surgical alternative with the accompanying risks, morbidity, and mortality that an operative procedure carries and it leads to sterility in women who are premenopausal. The patient may be hospitalized for several days and may require 6-12 weeks of convalescence. Complications, such as excessive bleeding, infection, and injury to adjacent organs, also may occur (Jacobson et al.,2006; Gimbel, 2007).

Choosing the route of hysterectomy has been an important issue in gynecologic surgery for a number of years. In the past, many gynecologists believed that surgical indication determines the route of hysterectomy: abdominal, vaginal, laparoscopic or combined. However, suggests the factors may influence the route of hysterectomy for any surgical indication include uterine size, mobility, suspected adhesions, accessibility, and pathology confined to the uterus (ACOG Committee Opinion, 2009; Kovac et al., 2002). Physicians should take into consideration how the procedure may be performed safely and cost-effectively to fulfill the medical needs of the patient. However, analysis of recent surgical data shows that abdominal hysterectomy is performed in 66% of cases, vaginal hysterectomy in 22% of cases, and laparoscopic hysterectomy in 12% (ACOG Committee Opinion, 2009; Benassi et al., 2002; Kovac et al., 2002; Nieboer et al., 2009). Not all hysterectomies demand a specific operative approach; that is, some hysterectomies can be performed vaginally, laparoscopically, or abdominally for similar indications. For benign conditions requiring hysterectomy, surgeons should choose the approach depending on the feasibility of the procedure and the difficulties expected during surgery. These decisions would broadly comprise the traditional indications and contraindications for abdominal, laparoscopic, and vaginal hysterectomy. Surgical inexperience with vaginal hysterectomy should not be an indication for abdominal or laparoscopic hysterectomy. Technical feasibility may also mean that a surgeon is technically unable or unwilling to perform a vaginal hysterectomy because of his/her comfort, preference, training, capability, or experience with abdominal or laparoscopic methods. The most commonly reported indication for laparoscopic hysterectomy is menstrual disorders (ACOG Committee Opinion, 2009; Dodero et al., 2005). The most common indication for abdominal hysterectomy is leiomyoma. Because the majority of hysterectomies are safe and successful operations, and most patients recover well over time, surgical decision making is often only questioned when a complication occurs. Some authors also noted a 3 to 5 fold increase in subtotal hysterectomy worldwide (Johns, 1997; Benassi et al., 2002; Dodero et al., 2005; Nieboer et al., 2009). This change in preference is hard to explain, given the lack of evidence to support this practice. Most likely physician and patient perception of the merit of subtotal hysterectomy had a significant influence: women may believe subtotal hysterectomy may have less impact on sexuality, while physicians might consider the procedure less likely to effect bowel and bladder function and to have lower rates of infectious morbidity, be less likely to lead to prolapse, and have lower operative time and less blood loss than total abdominal hysterectomy. Given the lack of convincing evidence favoring this approach, the motivating reasons behind this change in practice pattern remain unclear (Johns, 1997; Benassi et al., 2002; Dodero et al., 2005; Nieboer et al., 2009).

Abdominal hysterectomy is the most invasive hysterectomy. Laparoscopic hysterectomy is moderately invasive. Vaginal hysterectomy is and has always been the most minimally invasive hysterectomy (ACOG Committee Opinion, 2009; Benassi et al., 2002; Dodero et al., 2007; Gimbel, 2005; Kovac et al., 2002; Nieboer et al., 2009). No amount of spin can deny this fact. It is time that proponents of laparoscopic hysterectomy are challenged about regarding laparoscopic hysterectomy, even performed robotically, as the minimally invasive hysterectomy (Holloway et al., 2009).

It is possible that increased use of laparoscopic and hysteroscopic procedures, development and acceptance of endometrial ablation devices, introduction of a progestin-based intrauterine device, and the emergence of uterine artery embolization have begun to substitute for hysterectomy in the general population (Farquhar & Steiner, 2002; Johns, 1997; Weber & Lee , 1996). The level of information available to patients on different treatment alternatives may also be greater among patients. Additionally, changes in patient preferences for hysterectomy or alternative treatments, as well as changes in provider preferences and counseling, could also contribute to decreasing hysterectomy rates (Benassi et al., 2002; Dodero et al., 2007; Farquhar & Steiner, 2002; Johns, 1997; Weber & Lee, 1996).

In recent years, there is an increasing need for conservative options to treat symptomatic uterine fibroids because of the wish to avoid major surgery, the desire to preserve fertility potential and the belief that the uterus plays a role in perceived sexual satisfaction. An ideal conservative treatment for uterine myomas should be safe, eliminate symptoms, decrease the size of myomas, preserve fertility and have long-term effects. Several procedures including endometrial ablation, uterine artery embolization, high-intensity focused ultrasound and myolysis have been suggested or developed as a conservative treatment to avoid hysterectomy or myomectomy (Guarnaccia & Rein, 2001; Myers et al., 2002).

3. Uterine fibroids

Uterine fibroids (also called myomas or leiomyomas) are the most common solid pelvic tumors in women and the leading indication for hysterectomy. Uterine fibroids may occur singly but most often are multiple and vary in size from an unnoticeable few millimetres to over 20 cm in diameter, significantly enlarging the abdominal cavity. They are named according to their location. Intramural fibroids lie wholly within the uterine walls, submucosal fibroids project into the uterine cavity and subserosal fibroids project from the outer surface of the uterus. They may also be pedunculated, where they are attached to the uterine wall by a stalk-like structure. Symptoms and treatment options are affected by the size, number, and location of the leiomyomas. Despite extensive research on the factors involved in the growth of leiomyomas, the precise causes of these tumors still remain unknown. Several predisposing factors have been identified, including age (late reproductive years), nulliparity, obesity, and African-American ethnicity. These tumors contain estrogen and progesterone receptors, and, typically develop in women at fertile age, increase with age, and shrink after the menopause. The growth of leiomyomas is ovarian hormones dependent. Growth factors with mitogenic activity also are elevated in leiomyomas, and, there is increasing evidence of genetic basis (Flake et al., 2003; Stewart, 2001). Although many women with uterine leiomyomas are asymptomatic and can be monitored without treatment, some will require more active measures. The two most common symptoms of uterine fibroids for which women seek treatment are abnormal uterine bleeding and pelvic pressure. The most common kind of abnormal uterine bleeding associated with leiomyomas is heavy or prolonged menstrual bleeding, which frequently results in iron deficiency anemia (Fraser et al., 2007). This heavy bleeding may result in significant disruption of a woman's daily activities. Some studies reporting leiomyomas in 70% of white women and more than 80% of black women by age 50 years (Day Baird et al.,

2003). Hysterectomy remains the most common surgical treatment for leiomyomas because it is the only definitive treatment and eliminates the possibility of recurrence. Many women seek an alternative to hysterectomy because they desire future childbearing or wish to retain their uteri even if they have completed childbearing. As alternatives to hysterectomy become increasingly available, the efficacies and risks of these treatments are important to delineate. The lack of a simple, inexpensive, and safe long-term medical treatment means that most symptomatic leiomyomas are still managed surgically.

4. Alternatives to hysterectomy in the management of leiomyomas

Although hysterectomy is often the definitive treatment for many pelvic pathologies, nonsurgical alternatives should always be attempted in elective cases. Hormonal therapy, gonadotropin-releasing hormone agonists and antagonists, progesterone-containing IUD, endometrial ablation, focused ultrasonographic surgery, and uterine artery embolization have been used with success. In choosing an alternative to hysterectomy, both safety and efficacy need to be considered for each treatment. It must be recognized that all alternatives to hysterectomy allow the possibility for new leiomyomas to form, and preexisting small or undetected leiomyomas may exhibit significant growth, necessitating another treatment. The risk of recurrence must be balanced against the potential benefits of uterine-sparing procedures, such as decreased rates of morbidity and continued fertility. However, procedural complications may rarely lead to an unanticipated hysterectomy (Manyonda et al., 2004). For example, gynecologists of United States of America perform approximately 250,000 surgeries for fibroids each year. According to a Wall Street Journal article (August 24, 2004), most women with symptomatic fibroids are not informed by their gynecologists that uterine artery embolization (UAE) is an option.

4.1 Medication

Although several small studies have shown a decrease in leiomyoma size during progestin therapy (Venkatachalam et al., 2004; Wallach & Vlahos, 2004), other studies using progestin therapy alone or in conjunction with a gonadotrophin-releasing hormone (GnRH) agonist identify an increase in uterine or leiomyoma volume (Friedman et al., 1992; Harrison-Woolrych & Robinson, 1995). Gonadotropin-releasing hormone agonists lead to amenorrhea in 70-80% of women and provide a 35–65% reduction in leiomyoma volume within 3 months of treatment. The effects of GnRH agonists are temporary, with gradual recurrent growth of leiomyomas to previous size within several months after cessation of treatment (Olive et al., 2004).

The levonorgestrel intrauterine system leads to minimal systemic effects, and the localized endometrial effect is beneficial for treatment of menorrhagia (Wallach & Vlahos, 2004). Small studies suggest that the levonorgestrel intrauterine system may be effective for treatment of heavy uterine bleeding in women with leiomyomas (Mercorio et al., 2003).

Several small studies and case reports have identified reductions in leiomyoma size and symptoms with the use of aromatase inhibitors (Attilakos & Fox 2005; Shozu et al., 2003; Varelas et al., 2007).

Antiprogesterone agents act at the level of the progesterone receptors found in high concentration in leiomyomatous uteri. Several studies of high-dose mifepristone have reported a reduction of leiomyoma volume of 26–74%. Leiomyomas appear to have a slower rate of recurrent growth after cessation of mifepristone treatment (Fiscella et al., 2006; Steinauer et al., 2004).

4.2 Myomectomy

Myomectomy may be an option for women who desire uterine preservation. This procedure is to remove the visible and accessible myomas and then reconstruct the uterus. Most myomectomies have been performed by laparotomy; however, endoscopic options increasingly are being used. However, women choosing myomectomy face the risk of recurrence of leiomyomas. Hysteroscopic myomectomy is an method for the management of abnormal uterine bleeding caused by submucous leiomyomas. Submucosal leiomyomas are estimated to be the cause of 5–10% of cases of abnormal uterine bleeding, pain, and subfertility and infertility (Guarnaccia & Rein, 2001; Narayan et al., 2010; Wallach & Vlahos, 2004). Laparoscopic myomectomy minimizes the size of the abdominal incision, resulting in a quicker postoperative recovery, a shorter time to hospital discharge, reduced analgesic requirements and less blood loss. Because of the complex nature of laparoscopic dissection and suturing, special surgical expertise typically is required (Altgassen et al., 2006; Sizzi et al., 2007). Robot-assisted laparoscopic surgery also has been used to perform myomectomy. It may have the advantage of improved optics, including a three-dimensional view, and enhanced surgeon dexterity. Disadvantages with robot-assisted surgery in general include diminished haptic (tactile) sensation, additional operating room time, and increased cost (Advincula et al., 2004).

4.3 Magnetic resonance imaging-guided focused ultrasound surgery

Since 2004 used a magnetic resonance imaging (MRI)-guided system for the localization and treatment of uterine leiomyomas with focused ultrasound therapy. This noninvasive approach uses high-intensity ultrasound waves directed into a focal volume of a leiomyoma. The ultrasound energy penetrates soft tissue and produces well defined regions of protein denaturation, irreversible cell damage, and coagulative necrosis. Whereas short-term studies show safety and efficacy, long-term studies are needed to discern whether the minimally invasive advantage of MRI-guided focused ultrasound surgery will lead to durable results (Fennessy et al., 2007; Morita et al., 2007; Stewart et al., 2006).

5. Uterine Artery Embolization (UAE)

UAE represents a relatively new, minimally invasive approach to the treatment of fibroids. It selectively blocks the feeding arteries that supply blood to the fibroids and causes ischemic necrosis and subsequent reduction, absorption or expulsion of leiomyoma (Franz et al., 2003). Unlike leiomyoma, the normal myometrium is supplied by multiple collateral arteries and it escapes the vascular deprivation resulting from UAE. Uterine fibroid embolization has several advantages over conventional hormone suppression (progestogens and GnRH analogues) and surgical procedures (myomectomy, hysterectomy), including avoidance of the side effects of drug therapy and postoperative complications resulting from surgery (Pelage et al., 2000). There is neither need for the blood transfusion nor the abdominal incision. Recovery is shorter than recovery from hysterectomy or open myomectomy (seven to 10 days versus six weeks), and UAE results in long-term clinical success with outcomes comparable or superior to those of abdominal myomectomy (Narayan et al., 2010; Worthington-Kirsch et al., 1998) and early menopause-like symptoms are rarely induced as a result of UAE, as are often seen with gonadotrophin releasing hormone (GnRh) therapy. All fibroids are treated at once, which is not the case with myomectomy. UAE recurrence rates appear to be lower than those of myomectomy (Michael et al., 2002). The ideal candidates are women who no longer desire fertility but wish to avoid surgery and/or retain their uterus or are poor surgical risks. Embolization is also an excellent option for patients who will not accept blood transfusions and for those who are severely anaemic and require immediate intervention.

5.1 History of procedure

Embolization of the uterine arteries has been the standard of care for management of acute bleeding after childbirth or after gynecologic surgeries since the late 1970s (Heaston et al., 1979; Oliver & Lance, 1979). In the late 1980s, Jacques Ravina, a French gynecologist, became interested in the possible utility of embolization as a pre-emptive measure before gynecologic surgeries such as myomectomy. He was familiar with the utility of embolization for postoperative bleeding and decided to investigate preoperative embolization, hoping that this would decrease intraoperative bleeding as well as decrease the risk for postoperative hemorrhage. Preoperative embolization of the uterine arteries did indeed prove to be useful to decrease perioperative bleeding complications (Ravina et al., 1995). In some cases, there was a delay between the embolization and the planned surgery of at least a few days and in some cases a few weeks. Many of these patients experienced relief of their fibroid-related symptoms from the embolization alone and refused to go on with the planned surgery. Ravina et al. (Ravina et al., 1995) published their initial experience in 1995, and have since continued their studies of uterine artery embolization (UAE) as a primary treatment for fibroids (Ravina et al., 1999). UAE for fibroids was first reported in the United States by Goodwin (Goodwin et al., 1997) from University of California Los Angeles (UCLA) Medical Center in 1996. Since then, there has been rapid spread of the procedure across the United States, Europe, and worldwide.

However its use for management of uterine fibroids was reported by Ravina from France (Ravina et al., 1995). In the beginning they offered embolization as palliative management in 16 women who presented with high operative risks i.e. thromboembolic accidents, severe obesity, diabetes, and AIDS. It was discovered that with a mean follow-up of 20 months, symptoms resolved in 11 patients while three patients improved partially. The blockage of the blood supply caused degeneration of the fibroids and this resulted in resolution of their symptoms. This led to the use of this technique as a stand-alone treatment for symptomatic fibroids. Recently, the same group presented their findings in 243 patients with follow-up care ranging from 6 months to 7 years and cited an 83% rate of improvement in abnormal bleeding after embolization (Ravina et al., 2000). Since then UAE has become increasingly accepted as a minimally invasive, uterine-sparing procedure, and more than 200,000 procedures have been performed worldwide during the past decade (Committee on

Gynecologic Practice, American College of Obstetricians and Gynecologists, 2004). The advantages of embolization, including a significant reduction in the length of the hospital stay and 24-hour pain level, and a more rapid return to usual activities, need to be weighed against the risk of treatment failure requiring a second intervention and the possibility, although infrequent, of major late adverse events.

5.2 Preprocedure testing

Before UAE is performed in a patient, it is typically required that she has been seen by a gynaecologists and an interventional radiologist. It is important to obtain a complete history. Careful pre-procedure evaluation is essential to exclude pregnancy and genital tract malignancy, especially suspected leiomyosarcoma. In addition to the gynaecologic examination, Pap smear is required, and women with irregular periods should undergo endometrial sampling before UAE to exclude endometrial carcinoma or endometrial hyperplasia as the cause of bleeding. Patients with a history of pelvic inflammatory disease should have high cervical swabs and cultures for gonorrhoea and Chlamydia trachomatis. If pregnancy cannot be excluded by patient history and gynaecologic examination, a pregnancy test should be performed. Other absolute contraindications include comorbidities that may increase the risk for infectious complications (e.g. pelvic inflammatory disease, or active genitourinary infection), the presence of an adnexal mass and conditions that contraindicate any endovascular procedure (e.g. reduced immune status, severe coagulopathy, severe contrast medium allergy, or impaired renal function). To proceed with UAE, a full blood count should be taken. It is especially important to screen for anemia in patients with menorrhagia to have a baseline status for follow-up. Other blood tests are serum creatinine level, blood urea nitrogen and coagulation parameters. Furthermore, relative contraindications are presence severe endometriosis, presence of pelvic adhesions which distorts vascular anatomy, history of previous pelvic irradiation or surgery, and peripheral vascular occlusive disease. The desire to avoid a hysterectomy under any circumstances is also an absolute contraindication to UAE. There are no restrictions to the size and number of fibroids that can be treated with UAE (Volkers et al., 2006). Anatomic exclusion criteria only include submucosal fibroids that may be effectively treated with hysteroscopic resection, and pedunculated subserosal fibroids with a narrow stalk because of the potential risk and complications from infarction of the stalk and subsequent fibroid detachment from the uterus (Paxton et al., 2006). Clinical examination should confirm the diagnosis of leiomyomata supplemented by ultrasound and MRI. Imaging of the uterus and adnexa is vital for patient selection for UAE, both to confirm the diagnosis and to assess the extent of symptomatic leiomyomas. The diagnostic work-up is depending on local practice patterns, availability, and patient insurance coverage. Pelvic ultrasonography has been commonly used prior to and following UAE. In the majority of cases, ultrasonography examination can provide sufficient detail to determine a patient's suitability for embolization and to identify relative contraindications such as pregnancy, uterine anomalies, endometriosis, adenomyosis, pelvic malignancy, and pedunculated fibroids. MRI is currently considered to be the most accurate imaging technique for detection and localization of fibroids (Ruuskanen et al., 2010). MRI is more sensitive than ultrasonography in the detection of fibroids. MRI may also accurately assess an enlarged fibroid uterus, which is not possible with ultrasound because of the limited field of view. The capability of

MRI to demonstrate the uterine zonal anatomy allows accurate classification of individual masses as submucosal, intramural, or subserosal (Ruuskanen et al., 2010). Contrast material-enhanced MR imaging exceeds ultrasound's technical limitations in precise fibroid mapping and characterization. Thus, MR imaging may result in a change in management. However, neither size, localization or MR signal intensity characteristics have shown to be useful predictive factors of clinical success. In addition, although some MR appearances may suggest uterine sarcoma, there is no accurate test available. The presence of other pathologies which are likely to have similar clinical profile such as adenomyosis should be ruled out as the role of UAE in such conditions is debatable. There is some evidence that ovarian devascularisation may follow UAE subsequently resulting in iatrogenic menopause though the reported incidence is less than 1% (Amato & Roberts, 2001; Chrisman et al., 2000; Hehenkamp et al., 2007; Rashid et al., 2010). Hence an assessment of follicle-stimulating hormone (FSH) on the third day of the cycle before the procedure is helpful in evaluating ovarian status before the procedure so that declining ovarian function is documented and patient would not attribute this to treatment per say. However there is no general consensus regarding the role of routine hormone assay in patients undergoing UAE.

The use of prophylactic antibiotics to reduce posttreatment infection is debatable. Theoretically there is a possibility of anaerobic and bacterial infection in the avascularised tissue. Likely causal organisms include Escherichia Coli, Streptococci, Staphylococci and Bacteroides. Published work suggests that the procedure is associated with a post-treatment infection rate of 2%, even though prophylactic antibiotic therapy has sometimes been used. Evidence from the use of prophylactic antibiotic therapy in association with vaginal hysterectomy suggests that single dose prophylactic antibiotic therapy is reasonable (Volkers et al., 2006). The ideal time for UAE in relation to menstrual cycle is not yet established. The fear is possibility of pregnancy if performed in postovulatory phase of menstrual cycle. However if the patient has taken adequate contraceptive precautions, embolization may be performed at any stage of the menstrual cycle. If adequate contraception has not been used, treatment should only be given in the early to mid-follicular phase of the cycle. Symptomatic or asymptomatic uterine fibroids in women 40 – 45 years old is an ideal case for this procedure. Though recently there are multiple case reports of successful pregnancy after UAE for fibroids, the existing evidence has not fully established its application in younger age as an alternative for medical or surgical therapy (myomectomy) (Michael et al., 2002). Patient education on possible complications and the possibility of amenorrhea occurring after the procedure is a must. UAE should not be contemplated on those who are desirous of childbearing because preservation of fertility can not be assured based on current available evidence. The presence of any conditions mentioned below should deter the interventional physician in performing UAE.

5.3 Main procedure

An interventional radiologist is responsible for all aspects of the procedure; initial evaluation, conducting the embolization, and follow-up care. UAE should only be carried out in a specialist angiographic suite having digital subtraction angiography with measures to minimize X-ray dosage (Nikolic et al., 2000). The procedure is usually done in the hospital with an overnight stay after the procedure. To ensure an optimal therapeutic outcome and patient satisfaction, it is advisable to inform the patient during the initial consultation for UAE about the concept behind the treatment, potential side effects and the medication given alongside the procedure and offer time for questions. It is recommended to explain briefly the environment of an angio suite to the patient. The patient should then be informed about the level of mental awareness she can expect during the procedure combined with the offer to sedate her, if preferred. The preparation for the procedure including insertion of a Foley catheter, shaving, draping etc. and administration of local anesthesia are explained. The time course, duration, and severity of the postprocedural pain, the components of the postembolization syndrome and the corresponding medications that will be administered to relieve these temporary effects of UAE should be discussed. Certainly postembolization symptoms and potential complications have to be discussed. Most centers use conscious sedation to assure patient comfort during the embolization procedure, although some operators prefer epidural or spinal analgesia. General anesthesia is neither required nor recommended. Prior to the procedure, intravenous cannulation is established, allowing intravenous sedation and analgesia to be given during the procedure and patient-controlled analgesia instituted at the end of the procedure. Thirty to sixty minutes before the procedure each women was given analgesia with diclofenac or ketorolac by intramuscular injection. During the procedure patient controlled analgesia with use of intravenous opioids morphine, meperidine, hydrocodone, or fentanyl. Most radiologists prefer standard percutaneous transfemoral approach, invariably via the right side, whereas some find it easier to catheterise both arteries using a bilateral approach. The choice of an access site should be made by the operator based on his or her personal preference and the vascular anatomy of the patient. An awareness of the uterine artery normal variants is important for the radiologists. The uterine artery arises from the anterior division of the internal iliac artery. When fibroids are present, however, the uterine artery dilates and takes on a readily identifiable configuration. In most cases, the paired uterine arteries are the dominant source of blood flow to uterine fibroids. Variant anatomy has been described, including ovarian artery collaterals (26%), multiple uterine arteries (2%) and partial uterine artery replacement (2%) (Nikolic et al., 2000; Razavi et al., 2002). Collateral flow via an ovarian artery may be a cause of uterine artery embolization treatment failure (Amato & Roberts, 2001). Collaterals may also be present through adhesions. In addition the rectal and vesicle branches of the internal iliac artery may simulate the uterine artery. The optimum occlusion of blood supply to the fibroid is achieved when uterine artery is embolised at the level of perforating branches. Proximal occlusion of larger arteries with coils or similar agents is not expected to provide clinical success and if the procedure needs to be repeated they will prevent re-entry of micro catheter (Spies et al., 2001). At present, distal embolization can best be accomplished with particulate agents suspended in contrast solution. Those in current use include polyvinyl alcohol (350 -500 μL), tris-acryl gelatin microspheres, and gelatin sponge particles and all three agents appear to be equally safe and effective and these particles have been used for embolization in many parts of the human body for more than 20 years without any significant reaction attributed to the agent (Castaneda-Zuniga et al., 1978). The main procedure involves catheter placement in femoral artery via single groin puncture. A 5-F angiographic catheter (3-French = 1mm diameter) is placed via the groin and advanced over the aortic bifurcation to the contralateral internal iliac artery, and digital angiography is done to identify the origin of the uterine artery. There is often a great deal of tortuosity at the origin, and catheter induced spasm is common. This can be avoided to some extent by coaxial placement of 3-F micro-catheter. After successful catheterization of uterine vessels, solution of polyvinyl alcohol particles mixed with sterile saline and iodinated contrast medium is injected into the vascular lumen. Because fibroids are very vascular, the particles flow to the fibroids first. The particles wedge in the vessels and cannot travel to any other parts of the body. Over several minutes the arteries are slowly blocked. The embolization is continued until there is nearly complete blockage of flow in the vessel. If necessary, after embolization of the artery with particles pledgets of an absorbable gelatin sponge may be placed via catheter to complete the embolization. The 5-French catheter is then formed into a loop, and the catheter is placed into the ipsilateral internal iliac artery; the embolization procedure is then repeated in the right uterine artery. Another postembolization angiogram is taken to confirm complete blockade and all catheters are then removed. The entire procedure takes approximately 60 to 100 minutes.

5.4 Postprocedural care

Of paramount importance is controlled and timely analgesia to treat pain during and after UAE. Periprocedural regimens should include administration of nonsteroidal antiinflammatory drugs (NSAIDs) such as diclofenac (i.m., p.o.), ibuprofene (p.o) or ketorolac (i.v.). Additional pain medication may include paracetamol (acetaminophen) which also has an antipyretic effect. Pain control, particularly in the first twelve hours, is important as some patients develop pelvic pain of severe intensity. Patient controlled analgesia with use of intravenous opioids morphine, meperidine, hydrocodone, or fentanyl has been used effectively in most centers (Ryan et al., 2002). Inadequate pain control is the most common reason for a patient's return or readmission to the emergency department after UAE and pain is the single most remembered side effect of the procedure. Women were given diclofenac, ibuprofene or ketorolac tablets to take home. Postprocedural pain cannot be predicted from baseline uterine or fibroid volume and the severity of pain experienced cannot be used to predict outcome. It varies significantly among patients and consists of an early ischemia-related component followed by pain that is modulated by the inflammatory response to tissue necrosis. Ischemic pain usually occurs by the end of the procedure. However, it may not become apparent until the patient is back in the ward. Pain levels peak within the first 6-8 hours and need to be addressed by a continuous and potent analgesia regimen. Pain may be constant, crampy or in waves, can be quite severe and is unrelated to the size, location or number of fibroids. Pain medication should be started after catheterization of the uterine artery and not after the procedure. Alternatives to intravenous opioids for pain control are spinal or epidural anesthesia. However, these analgesic regimens require the help of anesthesiologists, leading to a technically more complex scenario (Roth et al., 2002; Zhan et al., 2005).

Nausea is a common side effect of the embolization procedure and/or the medications used for pain control and hence there is a significant role for preoperatively administered antiemetic agent. During bedrest the patient should receive standard prophylaxis against deep vein thrombosis. Oral anti-inflammatory agents and narcotics are commonly used for several days after the procedure (usually 7-10 days). In the first postoperative week, approximately 10 to 15 percent of patients experience postembolization syndrome which is characterized by nausea, and/or vomiting, malaise, low grade fever, pain abdomen and elevated white blood count. The pain is due to ischemia induced by vascular occlusion and fever is probably because of the release of tissue breakdown products from degenerating uterine fibroids (Goodwin et al., 1997). Reported complication rates of UAE are low. Most complications were minor and occurred during the first 3 months after the procedure. A relatively common complication of UAE is vaginal expulsion of an infarcted fibroid, with a reported rate of up to 10% (Spies et al. 2002b; Walker & Pelage, 2002). This complication is more frequently seen in patients with submucosal fibroids or intramural fibroids with a submucosal component. Expulsion most often occurs within 6 months after the procedure, but there are reports of this event after a period of time as long as 4 years (Marret et al., 2004). In most cases, the infarcted fibroid is expelled spontaneously, and no additional treatment is necessary. Hysteroscopic resection or dilation and curettage is reserved for cases in which the fibroid is only partially infarcted and remains firmly attached to the uterine wall due to the increased risk of secondary infection (Marret et al., 2004; Spies et al. 2002b). When uncomplicated, fibroid expulsion can restore the uterine anatomy to nearer normal more rapidly than otherwise. In a minority of cases, however, retention of necrotic fibroid tissue may result in chronic vaginal discharge due to shedding of fibroid material into the endometrial cavity. This condition can be treated effectively by hysteroscopic resection of the necrotic fibroid material (Ogliari et al., 2005; Walker et al., 2004). The most serious, although rare, complication of UAE is the occurrence of intrauterine infection, which has been reported in less than 1% of procedures (Pron et al., 2003b; Walker & Pelage, 2002; Worthington-Kirsch et al., 2005).

If left untreated or refractory to antibiotics, uterine infection can lead to sepsis and the need for emergency hysterectomy. Sepsis is suspected when relatively high grade fever persists beyond the 24 to 48 hours typical of post embolization syndrome. Sepsis is more frequent when UAE is performed on a very large uterus; more than 20 cm in height, when a single fibroid is larger than 9 cm in diameter or when there is a large submucous fibroid (Aungst et al., 2004; Nikolic et al., 2004). Two deaths from uterine infection and overwhelming sepsis have also been reported after UAE (de Block et al., 2003; Vashist et al., 1999). Clinical experience and evidence from a case report (Vashist et al., 1999) suggest that infection may originate from the vagina and/or the urinary tract, which underlines the importance of pre-procedure screening for genitourinary infection. There is also evidence that certain pre-existing conditions, such as a coexistent adnexal pathology (Nikolic et al., 2004), and some minor post-procedure complications, in particular fibroid expulsion (Marret et al., 2004; Spies et al. 2002b), are associated with a higher risk of infection. In addition to two deaths from septic shock (de Block et al., 2003; Vashist et al., 1999), other three deaths following UAE have thus far been reported, one from pulmonary embolism and two from uncertain causes (Worthington-Kirsch et al., 2005), in more than 100 000 procedures performed worldwide. If we assume that all these deaths were related to the procedure, the mortality risk would be 0.05:1000, which compares favourably with the estimated mortality rate of 0.38:1000 following hysterectomy for non-obstetric benign disease (Maresh et al., 2002; Siskin et al., 2002; Vashist et al., 1999). An ischemic injury to the uterus of such severity necessitating hysterectomy is required in less than 1% of patients. Severe infection can occasionally require a hysterectomy (Pelage et al., 2000).

Temporary amenorrhea and post-procedure menopause are not uncommon after UAE. Because the blood supply to the ovaries is partially from the uterine arteries, the procedure of UAE invariably diminishes the blood supply to the ovaries and results in some reduced ovarian function. Postembolisation amenorrhea is usually limited to a few cycles and is not considered a major complication. Transient or permanent amenorrhea with other symptoms of ovarian failure has been reported in up to 5% of women after UAE. There have been anecdotal reports of ovarian failure in younger women (Pron et al., 2003b; Spies et al. 2002b; Walker & Pelage, 2002). Permanent loss of ovarian function after UAE resulting in menopause has been reported in several studies. This complication seems to occur mainly in women > 45 years of age (Rashid et al., 2010; Tulandi et al., 2002). Transient ovarian failure has also been described (Ahmad et al., 2002; Amato & Roberts, 2001) but other studies did not show any untoward effects on ovarian function from UAE (Ahmad et al., 2002; Tropeano et al., 2004). Ovarian damage is thought to occur after UAE because of passage of embolization particles through anastomotic vessels between uterine and ovarian arteries, causing hypoxic ovarian damage and tissue loss. Indeed, it has been confirmed that embolization particles can be found at histopathologic examination of ovarian tissue after UAE. Furthermore, loss of ovarian perfusion, as demonstrated by sonographic assessment, directly after treatment in a substantial number of patients has been observed (Tulandi et al., 2002).

Permanent ovarian failure can be demonstrated by increased FSH and LH levels, increased menopausal symptoms, decreased estradiol (E2) levels and ultrasound-based ovarian volume and antral follicle count. Ovarian reserve reduction can better be tested by measuring anti-Mullerian-hormone (AMH), a reliable marker of ovarian reserve, especially in relation to the quantity of remaining follicles in the ovaries (Hehenkamp, 2005, 2007; Tropeano et al., 2004). As a result of the abundant collateral arterial circulation, normal uterine tissue usually recovers from the reduction in uterine blood flow induced by bilateral UAE. Ultrasound and MRI follow-up examinations have documented rapid revascularization of the normal myometrium and an essentially normal appearance of the endometrium at 3-6 months after embolization (Pelage et al., 2000; Tropeano et al., 2003). In addition, there are some risks that are associated with any form of angiographic procedure, such as hematoma formation or infection at the catheter insertion site in the groin, contrast media reactions, and damage to blood vessels. There are few case reports of unintended embolization resulting in pelvic organ damage. Radiation exposure occurring during UAE is a significant concern because many women who are candidates for the procedure are of childbearing age. With operator experience and limiting fluoroscopy time, the use of magnified and oblique views, non-pulsed fluoroscopy and road-mapping, the absorbed ovarian dose may be minimized (Andrews & Brown 2000; Binkert et al., 2001).

Patients in the UAE cohort may have experienced severe complications such as death (de Block et al., 2003; Lanocita et al., 1999; Vashist et al., 1999), pulmonary embolus, myocardial infarction, and cerebrovascular accident (stroke) (Hascalik et al., 2004; Spies et al., 2002). These complications are very rare. Furthermore, major complications are thrombosis, septicaemia, and emergency myomectomy/hysterectomy (Spies, 2002, 2002b). In the EMMY Trial, Volkers et al. found that a larger fibroid volume (100 cm3) was associated with an increased risk of complications (Volkers et al., 2006). More often are minor complications like minor infections, haematoma requiring treatment, drug reaction, permanent amenorrhoea, retention of urine requiring catheterisation, and fibroid expulsion (Marret et al., 2004; Spies et al., 2002; Volkers et al., 2006).

5.5 Follow-up

Individual study variations in the definition of UAE failure: symptom persistence, or recurrence, or need for additional therapy. Large case series with less than 2 years of follow-up reported rates of treatment failure, defined as the need for subsequent interventions, ranging from 5.5 to 9.5% (Huang et al., 2006; Spies et al., 2005a; Walker & Pelage, 2002).

There are several possible reasons for UAE failure. First, since the procedure causes fibroid shrinkage but preserves normal uterine tissue, it is possible that new fibroids will develop and symptoms recur. The risk of fibroid recurrence after embolization has not yet been defined. A prospective study using transvaginal ultrasound reported appearance of new fibroids in 8.2% of patients at a median of 30 months after the procedure (Marret et al., 2003). On the other hand, results from MRI follow-up examinations up to 3 years after UAE indicated that many clinical recurrences were not caused by development of new fibroids but related to re-growth of incompletely infarcted fibroids (Pelage et al., 2004). Incomplete fibroid infarction is most often related to technical aspects of the procedure such as the presence of collateral blood supply to the fibroids (usually from the ovarian arteries) or difficulties in cannulating both uterine arteries as a result of anatomical variation or arterial spasm. Successful embolization of only one uterine artery is generally regarded as a technical UAE failure as, in most cases, both uterine arteries contribute to the fibroid blood supply (Spies, 2003).

After left hospital and coming home, an early phone interview allows to verify the expected gradual decrease in pain and physical weakness patients experience after UAE. Patients are reassured, minor problems such as minimally increased temperature, onset of minor vaginal bleeding etc. discussed, and adequate pain medication checked. Some centres with an outpatient interventional radiology clinic may also see the patient at 4 weeks for a regular check-up. Four week follow-up may also be performed by the patient's gynaecologist on condition that he or she is familiar with the typical clinical course after UAE (Pelage et al., 2000; Siskin et al., 2002). It is important to be aware that uterine or individual leiomyoma size reduction is not a good indicator of the clinical success of UAE. Symptom relief remains the single most important measure of clinical success. Improvement in clinical symptoms is generally seen three months after the procedure. At this time, only negligible size reduction of fibroids may be observed. Interventional radiologists should be aware of this discrepancy since patients might be irritated by imaging reports and may need reassurance regarding the course of symptomatic improvement and size reduction of the fibroids treated. While menorrhagia may improve as early as within the first cycle after UAE, bulk-related symptoms may take longer to recede (Hehenkamp et al., 2005; , Spies et al., 2005a). Transient amenorrhea for up to three cycles is common while permanent amenorrhea is uncommon. It is associated with patient age and rarely occurs in patients under the age of 45 years. Follow-up imaging can be done by transvaginal ultrasound in those women who improve. At least one follow-up imaging exam is recommended and should include size measurements to verify fibroid shrinkage. If patients do not report improvement of symptoms 4 months after UAE, the radiologist should investigate the causes of failure. A detailed history of signs and symptoms in the preceding months should be collected to differentiate true persistence of symptoms from symptoms that may be related to ongoing fibroid sloughing, intrauterine residual fibroid tissue or infectious complications. In collaboration with a skilled gynaecologist, the radiologist should initiate adequate measures such as evaluation for infection and hysteroscopy to assess the uterine cavity (including hysteroscopic removal of residual fibroid) (Pelage et al., 2000; Spies et al., 2005a). Patients with persistent symptoms and no decrease or even an increase in uterine fibroid size should undergo contrast-enhanced imaging to rule out incomplete fibroid infarction after UAE and the possibility of a leiomyosarcoma. MR imaging is particularly helpful in those patients who do not improve after 4 months following embolization. MR imaging depicts morphologic changes such as sloughing of fibroids in contact with the uterine cavity. The latter may be associated with vaginal discharge in patients having undergone UAE but do not require additional treatment in the majority of cases. MRI also identifies side effects and complications associated with UAE such as ongoing fibroid expulsion, endometritis, and uterine necrosis (Marret et al., 2004; Mehta et al., 2002; Walker et al., 2004). Endometritis is seen in 0.5% of cases after embolization, is associated with fibroid expulsion and usually responds well to antibiotics but may spread and result in septicaemia if left untreated (Spies, 2000, 2002b). Patient is asked to return for follow up 2 weeks after procedure for checking healing of the puncture site and screening for unusual symptoms or potential problems (Mehta et al., 2002). It is desirable to have follow-up imaging studies after 3, 6 and 12 months following the embolization. This is useful in determining whether all existing leiomyomata have been infarcted and begun to decrease in volume and will also help determine whether any uterine or adnexal complications have occurred. If a rapid increase in fibroid size is noted, one should try to rule out malignancy (mainly leiomyosarcoma) though this is a rare condition. Patients undergoing UAE should be available for long-term follow-up preferably under the same institution. This is important for monitoring the control of symptoms, but also for detecting complications that may occur (Hehenkamp et al., 2005; Spies et al., 2002a). Late infections, expulsion of portions of leiomyomata, chronic endometritis, chronic vaginal discharge, and cessation or irregularity of menses have all been described after UAE and may develop more than a year after the procedure (Marret et al., 2004; Mehta et al., 2002; Walker et al., 2004). If follow-up study indicates inadequate clinical improvement or volume reduction, a second arteriographic examination and repeat embolization may be necessary especially if there is evidence of continued perfusion of the leiomyomata (McLucas, 2009). However repeat embolization is unlikely to be of use if arteriogram demonstrates fibrotic change and absent perfusion. In indicated cases, it is important to counsel the patient regarding the risks of ovarian injury. This is important because ovarian collateral supply is a common cause for treatment failure, and more aggressive embolization during a second treatment may result in ovarian injury and cause accelerated ovarian failure (Ryu et al., 2001).

Successful embolization of bilateral uterine arteries is achievable in 96% of the cases (Freed & Spies, 2010; Spies & Sacks, 2004). Smaller baseline fibroid size and submucosal location are more likely to result in a positive outcome (Spies et al., 2002c). In the presence of a fibroid larger than 8.7cm the failure rate is higher than 15% and for every additional 1 cm increase in diameter there is an additional increase of 10% in the failure rate. Clinical results show that in approximately 80 to 90%, there is improvement in abnormal bleeding and bulk-related symptoms (Freed & Spies, 2010; Spies et al., 1999; Spies & Sacks, 2004). Of those presenting with menorrhagia 90% return to a normal cycle within three months following the procedure (Pron & Bennett, 2003). The volume shrinkage has been reported between 40 to 50% in most studies (Pron & Bennett, 2003; Spies et al., 2002c). Many fibroids under 5 cm in diameter may become undetectable after UAE. Patient satisfaction is very good in the vast majority, with 85-90% of patients indicating that they would again choose UAE as therapy, and would recommend it to others with symptomatic fibroids (Smith et al., 2004). An important element in the decision-making process is knowledge about possible outcomes, which can be gained only by appropriate follow-up of patients (Freed & Spies, 2010; Smith et al., 2004; Spies & Sacks, 2004). Initially UAE was a new and experimental procedure carried out under research conditions and information about possible side-effects and outcomes was not readily available to the first patients undergoing the treatment. Now that 16 years have elapsed, more information is readily available and patients are, in general, more carefully counselled prior to their treatment (Freed & Spies, 2010; Smith et al., 2004). Statistics show that 10 percent to 15 percent of women who have UAE will need a follow-up procedure, usually some years later, because of recurrent symptoms from fibroids that either did not fully succumb or from growth of new fibroids. UAE kills the majority of existing fibroids, but these women have already demonstrated that their uterus has a propensity to make fibroids (Hovsepian et al., 2004).

5.6 Effects on fertility

The reports from literature demonstrate that women can conceive and carry a pregnancy successfully to term after embolization (Berkane & Moutafoff-Borie, 2010; Carpenter & Walker, 2005; Ciraru-Vigneron & Ravina, 2001; Cook et al., 2010; D'Angelo et al., 2003; Forman et al., 1999; Homer & Saridogan, 2010; Kovacs et al., 2002; McLucas et al., 2001; Pinto Pabón et al., 2008; Pron et al., 2005; Ravina et al., 2000; Vashisht et al., 2001; Walker & McDowell, 2006). UAE appears to be viable in young women who still want to become pregnant. Potential effects of embolization on ovarian function are an important consideration if fertility preservation is desired. Reduction of ovarian reserve is of special importance when UAE is used in the treatment of women desiring future fertility, which is now still being discouraged (Tulandi et al., 2002; Hascalik et al., 2004). Few studies, however, have reported on gonadotropin levels. Clearly, the evidence is far too limited to make conclusive statements on premature menopause or ovarian failure after embolization (Ahmad et al., 2002; Spies et al., 2001; Tropeano et al., 2004; Tulandi et al., 2002).

Several pregnancy complications have been reported after UAE. In one survey involving 50 published articles on successful pregnancies following UAE, these complications were reported; malpresentations (17%), small for gestational age (7%), cesarean section (56%), preterm delivery (28%), and postpartum hemorrhage (13%) (Goldberg et al., 2002). The rates of abortions, preterm delivery, malpresentations and postpartum haemorrhage are significantly higher in patients treated with UAE compared to myomectomy group (Goldberg et al., 2004; Homer & Saridogan, 2010). Initially it was not known whether an embolized uterus could sustain a pregnancy, and it was thought that fetal losses could be high. Interpreting spontaneous abortion rates after embolization is difficult because of confounding factors such as advanced maternal age and the large leiomyoma burden present in most embolization study cohorts. Spontaneous abortions are known to increase with maternal age, ranging from 18% in the late 30s to 34% in the early 40s in the general population (Coronado et al., 2000). The study of the British embolization cohort reported 20% rate of spontaneous abortions (Walker & Pelage, 2002), but lower than the 35% and 29% reported in the French (Ravina et al., 2000; Ciraru-Vigneron & Ravina, 2001) and American (McLucas et al., 2001) studies. Because embolic techniques with respect to angiographic endpoints were similar in these studies, patient differences and variability due to small samples are likely to account for these discrepancies. The high rate in the French study could be accounted for to some extent by the use of smaller embolic particles (150 -300 μm) and the advanced maternal age of the women (all older than 40 years of age). Based on these initial reports, although the numbers of pregnancies are small, uterine embolization does not seem to confer an obvious increased risk of pregnancy wastage. Uterine embolization causes irreversible ischemia leading to leiomyoma degeneration. Because embolization cannot target exclusively the leiomyoma vascular supply, there is a concern for potential effects on the myometrium. Although the integrity of the myometrium after UAE is not known, results from histopathologic studies of failed embolization have concluded that the adjacent myometrium is generally spared (Colgan et al., 2003). Little is known about the optimal time to achieve pregnancy after embolization. Leiomyomata in most cases gradually shrink, and although most reductions are achieved within 6 months to a year (McLucas et al., 2001), the extent and timing of uterine healing associated with these changes are unknown. In general, patients intending to conceive after embolization were advised to wait several months, in keeping with the advice given women after myomectomy. The next complication is that UAE causes abnormal placentation. Placenta accreta, occurring when there is a focal or diffuse absence of the decidua basalis resulting in a poorly formed decidua that leads to deeper trophoblast invasion is also a rare complication (Miller et al., 1997). The incidence of placenta previa at delivery varies in published studies from 3 to 6 per 1,000 pregnancies (Ananth et al., 2003; Miller et al., 1997).

6. Our experience

6.1 Subjects and methods

The study cohort consisted of 347 premenopausal women with ultrasound documented symptomatic fibrods. All were consecutively selected from women presenting for evaluation for uterine artery embolisation at the Department of Obstetrics and Gynecology of the University Hospital Split, Croatia, between May 1999 and November 2009. According to our existing protocol, patients were considered suitable for UAE if they had single or multiple myomas causing symptoms (namely, heavy menstrual bleeding and bulk related symptoms, which included pelvic pain and pressure effects) sufficiently severe to warrant hysterectomy or myomectomy, and wished to avoid surgery. Eligibility was not restricted by age, fibroid size, location, or previous surgery. Although women desiring children were not excluded from the study, they were further informed of the uncertain effects of UAE on conception or carrying to full term. Exclusion criteria also included patients with pregnancy, active pelvic inflammatory disease, renal insufficiency, undiagnosed pelvic mass, or urogenital infection. A detailed gynecologic history was obtained from each patient, followed by a detailed description on the procedure including a discussion of its potential risks. This study was approved by the Hospital Ethic Committee, with written informed consent obtained from each participant at the time of enrollment.

During preprocedural testing each patient underwent venous blood sampling (complete blood count, blood urea nitrogen, creatinine, prothrombin time) and magnetic resonance imaging of the uterus. Measurements of the uterus and volume of the dominant fibroid were calculated. All the patients were admitted to department of gynecology the day before the procedure. They completed the questionnaire including information on demographics and medical and gynecologic history. All procedures were performed by the same interventional radiologist according to the same procedure protocol. Under local anesthesia vascular access was obtained with 5F catheter via the right femoral artery and aortic bifurcation to the contralateral internal iliac artery. Digital angiography was performed to identify the origin of the uterine artery, and thereafter, the left uterine artery was catheterized with coaxial 3F microcatheter. The tip of the microcatheter was placed in the distal third of the left uterine artery, and 350-500 μm sized polyvinyl alcohol particles (Ivalon, Nycomed, Paris) were injected until there was complete stasis of flow. After confirming the presence of a stagnant column of contrast in the left uterine artery, the right uterine artery was catheterized in similar fashion and embolized. The procedure is completed when there is no flow in either uterine artery. All catheters were removed and groin pressure was applied for 10 to 15 minutes, thus completing the procedure. The goal of the therapy was to occlude the uterine artery branches that supply only the fibroid tumors and spare normal myometrial vessels.The arteriograms obtained after embolization revealed complete occlusion of the branches supplying the fibroids. After the procedure, patients were kept in hospital for 24-48 hours for further observation hematoma formation at the arterial puncture site, and pain control. The patients had received intravenous medications for nausea, vomiting or pain control. The majority of the patients left the hospital next day after the procedure. They completed outcome questionnaires following their treatment. All patients with successful procedures were evaluated at 3, six and 12 months after embolization with gynecologic examination, magnetic resonance imaging, and questionnaire. They were asked whether their symptoms resolved completely, improved, remained unchanged or deteriorated. Furthermore, they were asked about their satisfaction with the procedure. Measurements of the uterus and volume of the dominant fibroid were calculated. The percent volume reduction was calculated for each patient. Symptom change and patient satisfaction was classified as markedly improved, moderately improved, slightly improved, unchanged and worse.

Descriptive statistics, including means and ranges were calculated for dominant fibroid and uterine volumes, demographic and clinical characteristics. Differences in dominant fibroid and uterine volumes before and after UAE were analyzed with Student's paired *t*-test. Statistical significance was set at a P value < 0.05.

6.2 Results

Baseline patient characteristics are summarized in Table 1. There were 347 patients included in the study, but bilateral UAE was successful in 336 (96.8%) cases. Eleven (3.2%) procedures were technically unsuccessful, four because of malformed vessels and one of them had allergic reaction to contrast medium. We excluded from statistical data processing unsuccessful procedures.

	Mean± SD	Range
Age (years)	42.9 ± 4.1	36 - 51
Weight (kg)	67.7 ± 4.7	55 - 87
Height (cm)	168.5 ± 3.2	157 - 181
Parity (number)	2.2 ± 0.4	1 - 4
Procedure time (min.)	37.0 ± 4.3	25 - 81
Duration of hospitalization (days)	1.4 ± 0.5	1 - 6

Table 1. Characteristics of patients with successful procedures (N=336)

	N	(%)
Moderate pain	47	(14)
Severe pain	17	(5)
Fever after procedure	30	(9)
Fibroid expulsion	3	(1)
Transient amenorrhea	17	(5)
Persisting amenorrhea	10	(3)

Table 2. Complications after uterine artery embolization (N=336)

Table 2. summarizes complications of the embolization. After the procedure, most patients experienced crampy pelvic pain, of variable intensity, which was well managed with the standard analgesia protocol (narcotics and non-steroidal anti-inflammatory drugs). Some of the participants had nausea, and only few of them had vomiting. The both symptoms were successfully cured with antiemetics. All patients had an uneventful recovery and were able to return to normal activity within two weeks of embolization. Ten (3%) of participants had persisting amenorrhea after procedure. All of them were older than 45 years. None reported any new gynecologic or medical problem during the follow-up period. There were no deaths and no major permanent injuries.

	FOLLOW – UP (months)				
	0	3	6	12	*P* – level*
Uterine volume (cm^3)	860	534 (-38%)	370 (-57%)	335 (-61%)	< 0.01
Dominant fibroid volume (cm^3)	385	214 (-46%)	155 (-61%)	134 (-66%)	< 0.01

*t-test

Table 3. Rate of regression of uterine and dominant fibroid volume determined by magnetic resonance scanning (N=336)

Rate of regression uterine and dominant fibroid volume determined by magnetic resonance scanning 3, 6 and 12 months after procedure shows Table 3. Median uterine volume decreased by 38%, 57%, and 61% after 3, 6 and 12 months after embolotherapy, respectively. Comparison of the regression of preprocedural and final uterine volume revealed statistical significance ($p < 0.01$). Median dominant fibroid volume decreased by 46%, 61%, and 66% after 3, 6 and 12 months from preprocedure values, respectively. The quantum regression of pretreatment to final dominant fibroid volume also revealed statistical significance ($p < 0.01$).

No patients were lost to follow-up.

	N	(%)
Markedly improved	239	(71)
Moderately improved	71	(21)
Slightly improved	20	(6)
Unchanged	7	(2)
Worse	0	

Table 4. Experience/satisfaction of the patients (N=336)

Patient satisfaction with UAE treatment paralleled symptomatic outcome, with moderate to great satisfaction expressed by 92 percent patients. All women reported resumption of regular menses except ten (3%) with persisting amenorrhea.

Therefore, during our research we tested 57 women younger than 40 years who were candidates for pregnancy. Our concern was to investigate ovarian function, vitality of the endometrium, existence of menstruation and menstrual cycle, and fertility. Ovarian reserve is best tested by a combination of serum hormones, Follicle Stimulating Hormone (FSH) and Anti-Mullerian hormone (AMH), and pelvic ultrasound (antral follicle count and ovarian volume). The combination of these tests is called the Egg Timer. However, the serum AMH is the most sensitive component of the Egg Timer, and this test alone can be used as an initial screening test for ovarian reserve. AMH levels are constant and the AMH test can be done on any day of a woman's cycle. AMH hormone levels be a fertility test. We serially measured FSH and AMH blood levels before and after UAE. To estimate the ovarian volume, each ovary was measured in three planes (anterior-posterior, longitudinal and transverse), and the volume was calculated with the prolate ellipsoid formula. To estimate the antral follicle number, all follicles up to 5 mm in diameter visible in each ovary were counted. Vitality of the endometrium has been tested on tissue biopsy of the endometrium. Endometrial tissue samples were immunohistochemically evaluated by monoclonal antibodies for protein Ki-67 and matrix metalloproteinases 1 and 2.

All of the patients were evaluated pre- end post-embolization. There was no statistical significance between all parameters studied before and post-embolization. These data are evidence that embolization does not affect the biology of the ovary and endometrium, or the fertility of women. Finally, our greatest successes were 22 pregnancies in 21 women among the tested women younger than 40 years (one woman had two pregnancies). Among them, ten women was duly born to live, full term and normal children. Unfortunately, the other had a miscarriage. However, our results are promising.

7. UAE compared to surgery

There are eight studies published that have compared the outcomes of UAE versus conventional surgical procedures for symptomatic fibroids. So far, three studies have been performed in which clinical outcomes of UAE were compared with those of abdominal myomectomy, two retrospective cohort studies (Broder et al., 2002; Razavi et al., 2003) and one prospective, but non-randomized, trial (Goodwin et al., 2006). Overall, these studies consistently reported that two procedures were equally safe and effective in relieving fibroid-related symptoms. The investigators also reported shorter hospital stays, faster recovery times and a lower overall morbidity rate for UAE than for myomectomy. Finally, they found no differences between the groups in the rate of subsequent interventions.

To date, there have been four studies, one multi-center prospective (Spies, 2004a, 2004b), one multi-center retrospective cohort (Dutton et al., 2007) and two randomized controlled trials (RCTs)(Pinto et al., 2003), and the EMMY trial published in four papers (Hehenkamp, 2005, 2006; Volkers, 2006, 2007) published that compared UAE with hysterectomy. In a third RCT, outcomes of UAE were compared with outcomes of a mixed group of hysterectomies and myomectomies (Edwards et al., 2007).

The investigators from all studies reported significant differences between the groups in the mean hospital stay and recovery time: both were significantly shorter in UAE cohorts. There were no differences between the groups in the degree of improvement in pressure symptoms, overall health assessment, and quality of life scores or the rate of patient satisfaction with outcomes. The investigators found no differences between the groups in the overall complication rate within the first 30 days of treatment, but hysterectomy women were more likely to experience major complications than UAE women. Women in the UAE group also reported significantly less pain during the first 24 h and first week postoperatively and returned to work sooner than hysterectomy patients. The investigators reported lower rates of overall morbidity in UAE group than in the hysterectomy cohort. The overall morbidity was higher in the hysterectomy than in the UAE group.

At the end, from all studies at 1 year of follow-up, 22 women in the UAE groups had required additional interventions (hysterectomy or repeated UAE) to treat persistent or recurrent symptoms. Of these re-interventions, two were due to bilaterally failed UAE procedures. Finally, based on these investigations, uterine artery embolization is equal to surgery in treating uterine fibroids.

8. Conclusion

Expanding non-surgical treatment options for fibroids are advancing care for women, who are now increasingly willing to be treated while keeping the constraints and sequelae of treatment to a minimum. At the same time, the new possibilities afforded by these minimally invasive options do raise challenging questions about changing indications for surgery in the management of uterine fibroids. So far, however, the availability of alternative treatments has failed to substantially change everyday clinical practice, and the majority of women with symptomatic fibroids are still managed surgically. It is more difficult to be sure of the reasons why UAE remains underused in spite of the accumulating good-quality evidence to support its safety and effectiveness. The major issues, however, seem to be about increasing the gynaecologists' awareness and acceptance of UAE as a viable treatment option for fibroids and improving the collaboration between gynaecologists and interventional radiologists to facilitate optimal care for patients.

Nevertheless, it is clear that UAE has good outcomes resulting in a similar complication-rate and similar health related quality of life scores and satisfaction-rates when compared to hysterectomy. In view of these findings, UAE deserves a place in the therapeutic arsenal for symptomatic uterine fibroids. In conclusion, after tens of thousands of successfully performed UAE worldwide, it is proved that this method is an effective alternative to surgery. UAE is a successful, minimal invasive treatment of myomas that preserves the uterus and requires shorter hospitalization and recovery times than surgery. The complication rate is low, and the results are rapid and impressive. In the near future, embolization might replace conventional medical and surgical treatments of uterine fibroids. The results of this study indicate that this procedure might be recommended as a primary treatment for young patients with fibroids who wish to preserve, or enhance, their fertility. In summary, UAE appears to be an excellent treatment option for most women with symptomatic fibroids, especially for those who no longer desire fertility but wish to avoid surgery or are poor surgical risks. Appropriate pre-procedure selection and careful follow-up of patients are necessary to optimize clinical outcomes from this therapy. For this reason, an interdisciplinary approach involving both gynaecologists and interventional radiologists, with gynaecologists taking a pivotal role in the selection, co-management and follow-up of patients undergoing UAE should be implemented into clinical practice.

9. References

ACOG Committee Opinion No. 444. (2009). Choosing the route of hysterectomy for benign disease. *Obstet Gynecol,* Vol. 114, No. 5, pp. 1156-1158, ISSN 0029-7844

Advincula AP, Song A, Burke W, et al.(2004). Preliminary experience with robot-assisted laparoscopic myomectomy. *J Am Assoc Gynecol Laparosc,* Vol. 11, No. 4, pp. 511–518, ISSN 0015-0282

Ahmad A, Qadan L, Hassan N, et al. (2002).Uterine artery embolization treatment of uterine fibroids: effect on ovarian function in younger women. *J Vasc Interv Radiol,* Vol. 13, No.10, pp. 1017–1020, ISSN 1051-0443

Altgassen C, Kuss S, Berger U, et al.(2006). Complications in laparoscopic myomectomy. *Surg Endosc,* Vol. 20, No. 4, pp. 614–618, ISSN 0930-2794

Amato P, Roberts AC.(2001). Transient ovarian failure: a complication of uterine artery embolization. *Fertil Steril,* Vol. 75, No. 2, pp. 438-439, ISSN 0015-0282

Ananth CV, Demissie K, Smulian JC, et al. (2003). The effect of placenta previa on neonatal mortality: a population based study in the United States, 1989 through 1997. *Am J Obstet Gynecol,* Vol. 188, No. 5, pp. 1299 –1304, ISSN 0002-9378

Andrews RT, Brown PH. (2000). Uterine arterial embolization: Factors influencing patient radiation exposure. *Radiology* , Vol. 217, No. 3, pp. 713-722, ISSN: 0033-8419 (printed), 1527-1315 (electronic)

Attilakos G, Fox R. (2005). Regression of tamoxifen-stimulated massive uterine fibroid after conversion to anastrozole. *J Obstet Gynaecol,* Vol. 25, No. 6, pp. 609–610, ISSN 0144-3615

Aungst M, Wilson M, Vournas K, et al. (2004). Necrotic leiomyoma and gram-negative sepsis eight weeks after uterine artery embolization. *Obstet Gynecol,* Vol. 104, No. 5, pp. 1161–1164, ISSN 0029-7844

Benassi L, Rossi T, Kaihura CT, et al. (2002). Abdominal or vaginal hysterectomy for enlarged uteri: a randomized clinical trial. *Am J Obstet Gynecol,* Vol. 187, No. 6, pp. 1561-1565, ISSN 0002-9378

Berkane N, Moutafoff-Borie C. (2010). Impact of previous uterine artery embolization on fertility. *Curr Opin Obstet Gynecol,* Vol. 22, No. 3, p. 242-247, ISSN 1040-872X

Binkert CA, Andrews RT, Kaufman JA.(2001). Utility of nonselective abdominal aortography in demonstrating ovarian artery collaterals in patients undergoing uterine artery embolization for fibroids. *J Vasc Interv Radiol,* Vol. 12, No. 7, pp. 841-845, ISSN 1051-0443

Broder MS, Goodwin S, Chen G, et al. (2002). Comparison of long-term outcomes of myomectomy and uterine artery embolization. *Obstet Gynecol,* Vol. 100, No. 5, pp. 864–868, ISSN 0029-7844

Carpenter TT, Walker WJ. (2005). Pregnancy following uterine artery embolisation for symptomatic fibroids: a series of 26 completed pregnancies. *BJOG,* Vol. 112, No. 3, pp. 321-325, ISSN 1471-0528

Castaneda-Zuniga WR, Sanchez R, Amplatz K.(1978). Experimental observations on short and long-term effects of arterial occlusion with Ivalon. *Radiology,* Vol. 126, No. 3, pp. 783-785, ISSN: 0033-8419 (printed), 1527- 1315 (electronic)

Chrisman HB, Saker MB, Ryu RK. (2000).The impact of uterine fibroid embolization on resumption of menses and ovarian function. *J Vasc Interv Radiol*, Vol. 11, No. 6, pp. 699–703, ISSN 1051-0443

Ciraru-Vigneron N, Ravina JH.(2001) Pregnancy subsequent to uterine artery embolization. *Fertil Steril*, Vol. 75, No. 6, pp. 1247-1248, ISSN 0015-0282

Colgan TJ, Pron G, Mocarski EJM, et al. (2003). Pathologic features of uteri and leiomyomas following uterine artery embolization for leiomyomas. *Am J Surg Pathol*, Vol. 27, No. 2, pp. 167–177, ISSN 0147-5185

Committee on Gynecologic Practice, American College of Obstetricians and Gynecologists. (2004). ACOG Committee Opinion: uterine artery embolization. *Obstet Gynecol*, Vol. 103, No. 2, pp. 403-404, ISSN 0029- 7844

Cook H, Ezzati M, Segars JH, et al. (2010).The impact of uterine leiomyomas on reproductive outcomes. *Minerva Ginecol*, Vol. 62, No. 3, pp. 225-236, ISSN 0026-4784

Coronado GD, Marshall LM, Schwartz SM. (2000). Complications in pregnancy, labor and delivery with uterine leiomyomas: a population-based study. *Obstet Gynecol*, Vol. 95, No. 5, pp. 764 –769, ISSN 0029-7844

D'Angelo AD, Amso NN, Wood A.(2003). Spontaneous multiple pregnancy after uterine artery embolization for uterine fibroid: a case report. *Eur J Obstet Gynecol Reprod Biol*, Vol. 110, No. 2, pp.245–246, ISSN 0301-2115

Day Baird D, Dunson DB, Hill MC, et al. (2003). High cumulative incidence of uterine leiomyoma in black and white women: ultrasound evidence. *Am J Obstet Gynecol*, Vol. 188, No. 1, pp. 100–107, ISSN 0002-9378

de Block S, de Vries C, Prinssen HM, et al.(2003). Fatal sepsis after uterine artery embolization with microspheres. *J Vasc Interv Radiol*, Vol. 14, No. 6, pp. 779–783, ISSN 1051-0443

Dodero D, Corticelli A, Pedretti L. (2005). Influence of a decisional tree on the route of hysterectomy for benign disease in Italy: personal experience. *Clin Exp Obstet Gynecol* , Vol. 32, No. 3, pp. 185-188, ISSN 0390-6663

Dutton S, Hirst A, McPherson K, et al.(2007). UK multicentre retrospective cohort study comparing hysterectomy and uterine artery embolisation for the treatment of symptomatic uterine fibroids (HOPEFUL study): main results on medium-term safety and efficacy. *BJOG*, Vol. 114, No. 11, pp. 1340–1351, ISSN 1471-0528

Edwards RD, Moss JG, Lumsden MA, et al. (2007). Uterine artery embolization versus surgery for symptomatic uterine fibroids. *N Engl J Med*, Vol. 356, No. 4, pp. 360–370, ISSN 0028-4793

Farquhar CM, Steiner CA.(2002). Hysterectomy rates in the United States 1990–1997. *Obstet Gynecol*, Vol. 99, No. 2, pp. 229–234, ISSN 0029-7844

Fennessy FM, Tempany CM, McDannold NJ, et al. (2007). Uterine leiomyomas: MR imaging-guided focused ultrasound surgery—results of different treatment protocols. *Radiology*, Vol. 243, No. 3, pp. 885–893, ISSN: 0033-8419 (printed), 1527-1315 (electronic)

Fiscella K, Eisinger SH, Meldrum S, et al. (2006). Effect of mifepristone for symptomatic leiomyomata on quality of life and uterine size: a randomized controlled trial. *Obstet Gynecol*, Vol. 108, No. 6, pp. 1381–1387, ISSN 0029-7844

Flake GP, Andersen J, Dixon D. (2003). Etiology and pathogenesis of uterine leiomyomas: a review. *Environ Health Perspect*, Vol. 111, No. 8, pp. 1037-1054, ISSN 0091-6765

Fogt F, Hinds N, Zimmerman RL. (2003). Histologic Features of Uterine Leiomyomata Treated With Microsphere Embolization. *Obstet Gynecol,* Vol. 102, No. 3, pp. 600-602, ISSN 0029-7844

Forman RG, Reidy J, Nott V, et al. (1999). Fibroids and fertility. *Min Invas Ther Allied Technol,* Vol. 8, No. 6, pp. 415-419, ISSN: 1364-5706 (printed), 1365-2931 (electronic), 1364-5706 (linking)

Fraser IS, Critchley HO, Munro MG, et al. (2007). A process designed to lead to international agreement on terminologies and definitions used to describe abnormalities of menstrual bleeding. Writing Group for this Menstrual Agreement Process. *Fertil Steril,* Vol. 87, No. 3, pp. 466–476, ISSN 0015-0282

Freed MM, Spies JB. (2010). Uterine artery embolization for fibroids: a review of current outcomes. *Semin Reprod Med,* Vol. 28, No. 3, pp. 235-241, ISSN 1526-8004

Friedman AJ, Daly M, Juneau-Norcross M, et al. (1992). Recurrence of myomas after myomectomy in women pretreated with leuprolide acetate depot or placebo. *Fertil Steril,* Vol. 58, No. 1, pp. 205–208, ISSN 0015- 0282

Gimbel H. (2007). Total or subtotal hysterectomy for benign uterine diseases? A metaanalysis. *Acta Obstet Gynecol Scand,* Vol. 86, No. 2, pp. 133-144, ISSN 0001-6349

Goldberg J, Pereira L, Berghella V.(2002). Pregnancy after uterine artery embolization. *Obstet Gynecol,* Vol. 100, No. 5, pp. 869-872, ISSN 0029-7844

Goldberg J, Pereira L, Berghella V. (2004). Pregnancy outcomes after treatment of uterine fibromyomata: UAE vs laparoscopic myomectomy. *Am J Obstet Gynecol,* Vol. 191, No. 1, pp. 18-21, ISSN 0002-9378

Goodwin SC, Vedantham S, McLucas B, et al. (1997). Preliminary experience with uterine artery embolization for uterine fibroids. *J Vasc Interv Radiol,* Vol. 8, No. 4, pp. 517-526, ISSN 1051-0443

Goodwin SC, Bradley LD, Lipman JC, et al. (2006). Uterine artery embolization versus myomectomy: a multicenter comparative study. *Fertil Steril,* Vol. 85, No. 1, pp. 14–21, ISSN 0015-0282

Guarnaccia MM, Rein MS. (2001).Traditional surgical approaches to uterine fibroids: abdominal myomectomy and hysterectomy. *Clin Obstet Gynecol,* Vol. 44, No. 2, pp. 385–400, ISSN 0028-4793

Harrison-Woolrych M, Robinson R. (1995). Fibroid growth in response to high-dose progestogen. *Fertil Steril,* Vol. 64, No. 1, p.p. 191–192, ISSN 0015-0282

Hascalik S, Celik O, Sarac K, et al. (2004). Transient ovarian failure: a rare complication of uterine fibroid embolization. *Acta Obstet Gynecol Scand,* Vol. 83, No. 7, pp. 682–685, ISSN 0001-6349

Heaston DK, Mineau DE, Brown BJ, et al. (1979). Transcatheter arterial embolization for the control of persistent massive puerperal hemorrhage after bilateral surgical hypogastric artery ligation. *Am J Roentgenol,* Vol. 133, No. 1, pp. 152–154, ISSN 0361-803X

Hehenkamp WJ, Volkers NA, Donderwinkel PF, et al. (2005). Uterine artery embolization versus hysterectomy in the treatment of symptomatic uterine fibroids (EMMY trial): peri- and postprocedural results from a randomized controlled trial. *Am J Obstet Gynecol,* Vol. 193, No. 5, pp. 1618–1629, ISSN 0002-9378

Hehenkamp WJ, Volkers NA, Brokemans FJ, et al. (2007). Loss of ovarian reserve after uterine artery embolization: a randomized comparison with hysterectomy. *Hum Reprod,* Vol. 22, No. 7, pp. 1996–2005, ISSN 0268-1161

Hehenkamp WJ, Volkers NA, Birnie E, et al. (2006). Pain and return to daily activities after uterine artery embolization and hysterectomy in the treatment of symptomatic uterine fibroids: results from the randomized EMMY trial. *Cardiovasc Interv Radiol*, Vol. 29, No. 2, pp. 179–187, ISSN 0174-1551

Holloway RW, Patel SD, Ahmad S. (2009). Robotic surgery in gynecology. *Scand J Surg*, Vol. 98, No. 2, pp. 96-109, ISSN 1457-4969

Homer H, Saridogan E. (2010). Uterine artery embolization for fibroids is associated with an increased risk of miscarriage. *Fertil Steril*, Vol. 94, No. 1, pp. 324-330, ISSN 0015-0282

Hovsepian DM, Siskin GP, Bonn J, et al. (2004). Quality improvement guidelines for uterine artery embolization for symptomatic leiomyomata. *J Vasc Interv Radiol*, Vol. 15, No. 6, pp. 535–541, ISSN 1051-0443

Huang JY, Kafy S, Dugas A, et al. (2006). Failure of uterine fibroid embolization. *Fertil Steril*, Vol. 85, No. 1, pp. 30–35, ISSN 0015-0282

Jacobson GF, Shaber RE, Armstrong MA, et al. (2006). Hysterectomy rates for benign indications. *Obstet Gynecol* Vol. 107, No. 6, pp. 1278-1283, ISSN 0029-7844

Johns A. (1997). Supracervical versus total hysterectomy. *Clin Obstet Gynecol*, Vol. 40, No. 4, pp. 903-913, 0009-9201

Kovacs P, Stangel JJ, Santoro NF, et al. (2002). Successful pregnancy after transient ovarian failure following treatment of symptomatic leiomyomata. *Fertil Steril*, Vol. 77, No. 6, pp. 1292–1295, ISSN 0015-0282

Kovac SR, Barhan S, Lister M, et al. (2002). Guidelines for the selection the route of hysterectomy: application in a resident clinic population. *Am J Obstet Gynecol*, Vol. 187, No. 6, pp. 1521-1527, ISSN 0002-9378

Manyonda I, Sinthamoney E, Belli AM. (2004). Controversies and challenges in the modern management of uterine fibroids. *BJOG*, Vol. 111, No. 2, pp. 95–102, ISSN 1471-0528

Maresh MJ, Metcalfe MA, McPherson K, et al. (2002). The VALUE national hysterectomy study: description of the patients and their surgery. *BJOG*, Vol. 109, No. 3, pp. 302–312, ISSN 1471-0528

Marret H, Alonso AM, Cottier JP, et al. (2003). Leiomyoma recurrence after uterine artery embolization. *J Vasc Interv Radiol*, Vol. 14, No. 11, pp. 1395–1400, ISSN 1051-0443

Marret H, Keris Yle B, Acker O, et al. (2004). Late leiomyoma expulsion after uterine artery embolization. *J Vasc Interv Radiol*, Vol. 15, No. 12, pp. 1483–1485, ISSN 1051-0443

McLucas B, Goodwin S, Adler L, et al. (2001). Pregnancy following uterine fibroid embolization. *Int J Gynaecol Obstet*, Vol. 74, No. 1, pp. 1–7, ISSN 0020-7292

McLucas B. (2009). Repeat uterine artery embolization following technical failure. *Minim Invasive Ther Allied Technol*, Vol. 18, No. 2, pp. 78-81, ISSN: 1364-5706 (print), 1365-2931 (electronic), 1364-5706 (linking)

Mehta H, Sandhu C, Matson M, et al. (2002). Review of readmissions due to complications from uterine fibroid embolization. *Clin Radiol*, Vol. 57, No. 12, pp. 1122-1124, ISSN 0009-9260

Mercorio F, De Simone R, Di Spiezio Sardo A, et al. (2003). The effect of a levonorgestrel-releasing intrauterine device in the treatment of myoma-related menorrhagia. *Contraception*, Vol. 67, No. 4, pp. 277–280, ISSN 0010-7824

Michael SB, Scott G, Gary C, et al. (2002). Comparison of Long-Term Outcomes of Myomectomy and Uterine Artery Embolization. *Obstet Gynecol*, Vol. 100, No. 5, pp. 864-868, ISSN 0029-7844

Miller DA, Chollet JA, Goodwin TM. (1997). Clinical risk factors for placenta previa–placenta accreta. *Am J Obstet Gynecol,* Vol. 177, No. 1, pp. 210–214, ISSN 0002-9378

Morita Y, Ito N, Ohashi H. (2007). Pregnancy following MR-guided focused ultrasound surgery for a uterine fibroid. *Int J Gynaecol Obstet,* Vol. 99, No. 1, pp. 56–57, ISSN 0020-7292

Myers ER, Barber MD, Gustilo-Ashby T, et al. (2002). Management of uterine leiomyomata: what do we really know? *Obstet Gynecol,* Vol. 100, No. 1, pp. 8–17, ISSN 0029-7844

Narayan A, Lee AS, Kuo GP, et al. (2010). Uterine artery embolization versus abdominal myomectomy: a long- term clinical outcome comparison. *J Vasc Interv Radiol,* Vol. 21, No. 7, pp. 1011-1017, ISSN 1051-0443

Nieboer TE, Johnson N, Lethaby E, et al. (2009). Surgical approach to hysterectomy for benign gynecological disease. *Cochrane Database Syst Rev,* (3): CD003677, ISSN 0020-7292

Nikolic B, Spies JB, Lundsten MJ, et al. (2000). Patient radiation dose association with uterine artery embolization. *Radiology,* Vol. 214, No. 1, pp. 121–125, ISSN: 0033-8419 (printed), 1527-1315 (electronic)

Nikolic B, Nguyen K, Martin LG, et al. (2004). Pyosalpinx developing from a preexisting hydrosalpinx after uterine artery embolization. *J Vasc Interv Radiol,* Vol. 15, No. 3, pp. 297–301, ISSN 1051-0443

Ogliari KS, Mohallem SV, Barrozo P, et al. (2005). A uterine cavity-myoma communication after uterine artery embolization: two case reports. *Fertil Steril,* Vol. 83, No. 1, pp. 220–222, ISSN 0015-0282

Olive DL, Lindheim SR, Pritts EA. (2004). Non-surgical management of leiomyoma: impact on fertility. *Curr Opin Obstet Gynecol,* Vol. 16, No. 3, pp. 239–243, ISSN 1040-872X

Oliver JA, Lance JS. (1979). Selective embolization to control massive hemorrhage following pelvic surgery. *Am J Obstet Gynecol,* Vol. 135, pp. 431-432, ISSN 0002-9378

Paxton BE, Lee JM, Kim HS. (2006). Treatment of Intrauterine and Large Pedunculated Subserosal Leiomyomata with Sequential Uterine Artery Embolization and Myomectomy. *JVIR,* Vol. 17, No. 12, pp. 1947-1950, ISSN 1051-0443

Pelage JP, Le Dref O, Jacob D. (2000). Uterine artery embolization: anatomical and technical considerations, indications results, and complications. *J Radiol,* Vol. 81, No. 12 Suppl., pp. 1863–1872, ISSN 0013-9580

Pelage JP, Le Dref O, Soyer P, et al. (2000). Fibroid related menorrhagia: treatment with superselective embolization of the uterine arteries and mid-term follow up. *Radiology,* Vol. 215, No. 2, pp. 428-431, ISSN: 0033-8419 (printed), 1527-1315 (electronic)

Pelage JP, Guaou NG, Jha RC, e al. (2004). Uterine fibroid tumors: long-term MR imaging outcome after embolization. *Radiology,* Vol. 230, No. 3, pp. 803–809, ISSN: 0033-8419 (printed), 1527-1315 (electronic)

Pinto I, Chimeno P, Romo A, et al. (2003). Uterine fibroids: Uterine artery embolization versus abdominal hysterectomy for treatment-a prospective, randomized, and controlled clinical trial. *Radiology* Vol. 226, No. 3, pp. 425–431, ISSN: 0033-8419 (printed), 1527-1315 (electronic)

Pinto Pabón I, Magret JP, Unzurrunzaga EA, et al. (2008). Pregnancy after uterine fibroid embolization: follow-up of 100 patients embolized using tris-acryl gelatin microspheres. *Fertil Steril,* Vol. 90, No. 6, pp. 2356-2360, ISSN 0015- 0282

Pron G, Bennett J. (2003a). The Ontario Uterine Fibroid Embolization Trial. Part 2: uterine fibroid reduction and symptom relief after uterine artery embolization for fibroids. *Fertil Steril*, Vol. 79, No. 1, pp. 120–127, ISSN 0015-0282

Pron G, Mocarski E, Bennet J, et al. (2003b). Tolerance, hospital stay, and recovery after uterine artery embolization for fibroids: the Ontario Uterine Fibroid Embolization Trial. *J Vasc Interv Radiol*, Vol. 14, No. 10, pp. 1243–1250, ISSN 1051-0443

Pron G, Mocarski E, Bennett J, et al. (2005). Pregnancy after uterine artery embolization for leiomyomata: the Ontario multicenter trial. *Obstet Gynecol*, Vol. 105, No. 1, pp. 67–76, ISSN 0029-7844

Rashid S, Khaund A, Murray LS, et al. (2010). The effects of uterine artery embolisation and surgical treatment on ovarian function in women with uterine fibroids. *BJOG*, Vol. 117, No. 8, pp. 985-989, ISSN 1471-0528

Ravina JH, Herbreteau D, Ciraru-Vigneron, et al. (1995). Arterial embolisation to treat uterine myomata. *Lancet*, Vol. 346, No. 8976, pp. 671-672, ISSN: 0140-6736 (print), 1474-547X (electronic)

Ravina JH, Ciraru-Vigneron N, Aymard A, et al. (1999). Uterine artery embolisation for fibroid disease: results of a 6 year study. *Minim Invas Ther Allied Technol*, Vol. 8, No. 6, pp. 441–447, ISSN: 1364-5706 (Print), 1365- 2931 (Electronic), 1364-5706 (Linking)

Ravina JH, Aymard A, Ciraru-Vigneron N. (2000). Arterial embolization of uterine myoma: results apropos of 286 cases. *J Gynecol Obstet Biol Reprod*, Vol. 29, No. 3, pp. 272-275, ISSN 0368-2315

Ravina JH, Vigneron NC, Aymard A, et al. (2000). Pregnancy after embolization of uterine myoma: report of 12 cases. *Fertil Steril*, Vol. 73, No. 6, pp. 1241–1243, ISSN 0015-0282

Razavi MK, Wolanske KA, Hwang GL, et al. (2002). Angiographic classification of ovarian artery-to-uterine artery anastomoses: initial observations in uterine fibroid embolization. *Radiology*,Vol. 224, No. 3, pp. 707-712, ISSN: 0033-8419 (printed), 1527-1315 (electronic)

Razavi MK, Hwang G, Jahed A, et al. (2003). Abdominal myomectomy versus uterine fibroid embolization in the treatment of symptomatic uterine leiomyomas. *Am J Roentgenol*, Vol. 180, No. 6, pp. 1571–1575, ISSN 0361-803X

Roth RA, Spies JB, Walsh SM, et al. (2000). Pain after uterine artery embolization for leiomyomata: Can its severity be predicted and does severity predict outcome? *J Vasc Interv Radiol*, Vol. 11, No. 8, pp. 1047-1052, ISSN 1051-0443

Ruuskanen A, Hippeläinen M, Sipola P, et al. (2010). Uterine artery embolisation versus hysterectomy for leiomyomas: primary- and 2-year follow-up results of a randomised prospective clinical trial. *European Radiology*, Vol. 20, No. 10, pp. 2524-2532, ISSN 0938-7994

Ryan JM, Gainey M, Glasson J, et al. (2002). Simplified pain-control protocol after uterine artery embolization. *Radiology*, Vol. 224, No. 2, pp. 610-611, ISSN (printed) 0033-8419, ISSN (electronic) 1527-1315

Ryu RK, Chrisman HB, Omary RA, et al. (2001). The vascular impact of uterine artery embolization: prospective sonographic assessment of ovarian arterial circulation. *J Vasc Interv Radiol*, Vol. 12, No. 9, pp. 1071-1074, ISSN 1051-0443

Shozu M, Murakami K, Segawa T, et al. (2003). Successful treatment of a symptomatic uterine leiomyoma in a perimenopausal woman with a nonsteroidal aromatase inhibitor. *Fertil Steril*, Vol. 79, No. 3, pp. 628–631, ISSN 0015-0282

Siskin GP, Stainken BF, Dowling K, et al. (2000). Outpatient uterine artery embolization for symptomatic uterine fibroids: experience in 49 patients. *J Vasc Interv Radiol*, Vol. 11, No. 3, pp. 305–311, ISSN 1051-0443

Sizzi O, Rossetti A, Malzoni M, et al. (2007). Italian multicenter study on complications of laparoscopic myomectomy. *J Minim Invasive Gynecol*, Vol. 14, No. 4, pp. 453–462, ISSN 1553-4650

Smith WJ, Upton E, Shuster EJ, et al. (2004). Patient satisfaction and disease specific quality of life after uterine artery embolization. *Am J Obstet Gynecol*, Vol. 190, No. 6, pp. 1697-1703, ISSN 0002-9378

Spies JB, Scialli AR, Jha RC, et al. (1999). Initial results from uterine fibroid embolization for symptomatic leiomyomata. *J Vasc Interv Radiol*, Vol. 10, No. 9, pp. 1149-1157, ISSN 1051-0443

Spies JB, Roth AR, Gonsalves SM, et al. (2001). Ovarian function after uterine artery embolization of leiomyomata: assessment with use of serum follicle stimulating hormone assay. *J Vasc Interv Radiol*, Vol. 12, No. 4, pp. 437–442, ISSN 1051-0443

Spies JB, Benenati JF, Worthington-Kirsch RL, et al. (2001). Initial experience with use of tris-acryl gelatin microspheres for uterine artery embolization for leiomyomata. *J Vasc Interv Radiol*, Vol. 12, No. 9, pp. 1059-1063, ISSN 1051-0443

Spies JB, Spector A, Roth AR, et al. (2002). Complications after uterine artery embolization for leiomyomas. *Obstet Gynecol*, Vol. 100, No. 5, pp. 873-880, ISSN 0029-7844

Spies JB, Roth AR, Jha RC, et al. (2002). Leiomyomata treated with uterine artery embolization: Factors associated with successful symptom and imaging outcome. *Radiology*, Vol. 222, No. 1, pp. 45-52, ISSN: 0033-8419 (printed), 1527-1315 (electronic)

Spies JB. (2003).Uterine artery embolization for fibroids: understanding the technical causes of failure. *J Vasc Interv Radiol*, Vol. 14, No. 1, pp. 11–14, ISSN 1051-0443

Spies JB, Allison S, Flick P, et al. (2004a). Polyvinyl alcohol particles and tris-acryl gelatin microspheres for uterine artery embolization for leiomyomas: results of a randomized comparative study. *J Vasc Interv Radiol*, Vol.15, No. 8, pp. 793–800, ISSN 1051-0443

Spies JB, Cooper JM, Worthington-Kirsch R, et al. (2004b). Outcome from uterine embolization and hysterectomy for leiomyomas: results of a multi-center study. *Am J Obstet Gynecol*, Vol. 191, No. 1, pp. 22–31, ISSN 0002-9378

Spies JB, Sacks D. (2004). Credentials for Uterine Artery Embolization. *J Vasc Interv Radiol*, Vol. 15, No. 2, pp. 111–113, ISSN 1051-0443

Spies JB, Myers ER, Worthington- Kirsch R, et al. (2005a). The FIBROID Registry: symptom and quality-of-life status 1 year after therapy. *Obstet Gynecol*, Vol. 106, No. 6, pp. 1309–1318, ISSN 0029-7844

Steinauer J, Pritts EA, Jackson R, et al. (2004). Systematic review of mifepristone for the treatment of uterine leiomyomata. *Obstet Gynecol*, Vol. 103, No. 6, pp. 1331–1336, ISSN 0029-7844

Stewart EA. (2001). Uterine fibroids. *Lancet*, Vol. 357, No. 9252, pp. 293-298, ISSN: 0140-6736 (print), 1474-547X (electronic)

Stewart EA, Rabinovici J, Tempany CM, et al. (2006). Clinical outcomes of focused ultrasound surgery for the treatment of uterine fibroids. *Fertil Steril*, Vol. 85, No. 1, pp. 22–29, ISSN 0015-0282

Tropeano G, Di Stasi C, Litwicka K, et al. (2004). Uterine artery embolization for fibroids does not have adverse effects on ovarian reserve in regularly cycling women younger than 40 years. *Fertil Steril*, Vol. 81, No. 4, pp. 1055– 1061, ISSN 0015-0282

Tulandi T, Sammour A, Valenti D, et al. (2002). Ovarian reserve after uterine artery embolization for leiomyomata. *Fertil Steril*, Vol. 78, No. 1, pp. 197-198, ISSN 0015-0282

Varelas FK, Papanicolaou AN, Vavatsi-Christaki N, et al. (2007). The effect of anastrazole on symptomatic uterine leiomyomata. *Obstet Gynecol*, Vol. 110, No. 3, pp. 643–649, ISSN 0029-7844

Vashist A, Studd J, Carey A, et al. (1999). Fatal septicaemia after fibroid embolization. *Lancet*, Vol. 354, No. 9175, pp. 307–308, ISSN: 0140-6736 (print), 1474-547X (electronic)

Vashisht A, Smith JR, Thorpe-Beeston G, et al. (2001). Pregnancy subsequent to uterine artery embolization. *Fertil Steril*, Vol. 75, No. 6, pp. 1246 –1247, ISSN 0015-0282

Venkatachalam S, Bagratee JS, Moodley J. (2004). Medical management of uterine fibroids with medroxyprogesterone acetate (Depo Provera): a pilot study. *J Obstet Gynaecol*, Vol. 24, No. 7, pp. 798–800, ISSN 0144-3615

Volkers NA, Hehenkamp WJ, Birnie E, et al. (2006). Uterine artery embolization in the treatment of symptomatic uterine fibroid tumors (EMMY trial): periprocedural results and complications. *J Vasc Interv Radiol*, Vol. 17, No. 3, pp. 471-480, ISSN 1051-0443

Volkers NA, Hehenkamp WJ, Birnie E, et al. (2007). Uterine artery embolization versus hysterectomy in the treatment of symptomatic uterine fibroids: 2 years' outcome from the randomized EMMY trial. *Am J Obstet Gynecol*, Vol. 196, No. 6, pp. 519.e1–519.e11, ISSN 0002-9378

Wallach EE, Vlahos NF. (2004). Uterine myomas: an overview of development, clinical features, and management. *Obstet Gynecol, Vol.* 104, No. 2, pp. 393–406, ISSN 0029-7844

Walker WJ, Pelage JP. (2002). Uterine artery embolisation for symptomatic fibroids: clinical results in 400 women with imaging follow-up. *Br J Obstet Gynecol*, Vol. 109, November, pp. 1263–1272, ISSN 1471-0528

Walker WJ, Carpenter TT, Kent AS. (2004). Persistent vaginal discharge after uterine artery embolization for fibroid tumors: cause of the condition, magnetic resonance imaging appearance, and surgical treatment. *Am J Obstet Gynecol, Vol.* 190, No. 5, pp. 1230–1233, ISSN 0002-9378

Walker WJ, McDowell SJ. (2006). Pregnancy after uterine artery embolization for leiomyomata: a series of 56 completed pregnancies. *Am J Obstet Gynecol*, Vol. 195, No. 5, pp. 1266-1271, ISSN 0002-9378

Weber AM, Lee JC. (1996). Use of alternative techniques of hysterectomy in Ohio, 1988–1994. *N Engl J Med*, Vol. 335, No. 7, pp. 483–489, ISSN 0028-4793

Worthington-Kirsch RL, Popky GL, Hutchins FL. (1998). Uterine arterial embolization for the management of leiomyomas: quality-of-life assessment and clinical response. *Radiology*, Vol. 208, No. 3, pp. 625-629, ISSN: 0033-8419 (print), 1527-1315 (electronic)

Worthington-Kirsch R, Spies JB, Myers ER, et al. (2005). The Fibroid Registry for Outcomes Data (FIBROID) for uterine embolization: short term outcomes. *Obstet Gynecol*, Vol. 106, No. 1, pp. 52–59, ISSN 0029-7844

Zhan S, Li Y, Wang G, Han H, et al. (2005). Effectiveness of intra-arterial anesthesia for uterine fibroid embolization using dilute lidocaine. *Eur Radiol*, Vol. 15, No. 8, pp. 1752-1756, ISSN 0028-4793

14

Pharmacotherapy of Massive Obstetric Bleedings as Alternative to Hysterectomy

Andrey Momot[1,2], Irina Molchanova[2],
Vitaly Tskhai[3] and Andrey Mamaev[1]
[1]*Russian Academy of Medical Sciences, Hematological Research Center, Altai department,*
[2]*Altai State Medical University,*
[3]*Krasnoyarsk State Medical University after V.F. Voino-Yasenetsky,*
Russia

1. Introduction

Modern society with its bad ecology, chronic stress and the prevalence of mental activities over physical no longer treats pregnancy as a physiological state with "natural" course of events but the state that requires intensive medical supervision, active, even invasive, intervention during pregnancy and delivery. In most cases such intervention is the only way to save life for a mother and her child. Therefore, modern obstetrics is primarily a surgical one. With the overall growth of obstetric operations a number of radical interventions to remove the reproductive organ is also increasing .The main cause of hysterectomy and sometimes death of a patient in obstetric practice is massive obstetric hemorrhage (post-partum haemorrhage - PPH). Life-threatening bleeding occurs in about 10% of deliveries worldwide (The Department of Health UK. Why mothers die. A report.., 2004). Obstetric hemorrhage is a major cause of maternal mortality, with 25 - 30% of overall death cases in prergnancy (Bonnar, 2000; Make Every Mather and Child count: the World Health Report.: WHO, 2005). The occurance of massive obstetric hemorrhage in developed and developing countries differs greatly (Ben Hamid et al., 2006; Sheiner et al., 2005). The risk to die from obstetric hemorrhage in developed countries is 1:100 000, while in developing countries the rate reaches 1: 1000 births (Mousa & Alfirevic, 2003). According to WHO bleeding is among the "big five" of causes of maternal mortality that leads to an on-going research to find various methods to stop bleeding, as well as blood transfusion (Baudo et al., 2001).

Cases with heavy bleeding, such as hysterorrhesis, premature detachment placenta increta and uterine atony require intensive resuscitation, and often result in hysterectomy. The problem of PPH treatment can be hardly overestimated in modern science and offers challenges to specialists in obstetrics, hematology and intensive care, in other words it requires inter-disciplinary approach to its solution.

It is known that only 62 - 65 % of vaginal deliveries are accompanied by physiological hemorrhage, and one third of patients lose from 500 ml to 1000 ml of blood and in 3 - 8 % hemorrhage exceeds 1.5 % of body weight and is to be massive and requires infusion of erythrocytes and hysterectomy. Definitions of PPH vary and relate to the patients with blood loss of 50 % of overall circulating blood within 3 hours, or hemorrhage > 150 ml/minute. WHO defines PPH as a loss of blood in volume of 500 ml or more during or after delivery, or any quantity of blood loss after the delivery which leads to instability of blood circulation (World Health Organization [WHO], 2009).

Most authors believe that uterine atony is the cause (75-90%) of early postpartum hemorrhage (Henrich et al., 2008; Ramanathan & Arulkumaran, 2006; Reynders et al., 2006). In this condition, uterus loses its ability to involution and does not react to medications and other types of stimulation (Roeal College of Obstetricians and Gynaecologists UK. Prevention .., 2009). Disorders of functional state of myometrium are possible due to prolonged labor, due to the of use of medication, reducing uterine tonus, due to greater amount of oxytocin in labor (Grotegut et al., 2011). Obstetric haemorrhage is characterized by suddenness and high temper of blood loss. Besides, reduced adaptive abilities of mother organism upon giving birth, her somatic diseases and pathology in pregnancy easily contribute to the rapid development of coagulopathy, to the shock phenomenon and multiple organ failure (Macphail & Talks, 2004). An increased number of caesarean section worldwide is one of the factors that cause the growth of postpartum haemorrhage (Deneux_Tharaux et al., 2006; Murkin, 2009). According to Ohkuchi et al. (2003), an average blood loss during vaginal delivery was 615 ml, whereas in cesarean section – 1530 ml.

Standard methods of treatment of massive PPH include therapeutic (hemotransfusion therapy and uterotonics) and surgical methods of hemorrhage control (Bouwmeester et al., 2005; Macphail & Talks, 2004; Mousa & Alfirevic, 2007). First aid in obstetric hemorrhage in most countries traditionally employs the use of uterotonics and prostaglandins, manual examination of uterus and birth canals and uterine massage (Abdel-Aleem et al., 2010; Henrich et al., 2008; Price & Lynch, 2005). If uterotonics and manual examination of the uterus prove to be ineffective, more complex surgical technics are traditionally employed - uterine artery ligation, internal iliac artery ligation and hysterectomy.

Many publications and reviews that relate to the problem of obstetric bleeding offer the opportunity and place to discuss new methods to stop postpartum bleeding. In recent years, a series of invasive manipulations is used as a rather effective measure to stop postpartum bleeding, for example - uterine balloon tamponade (Bakri et al., 2001; Dabelea et al., 2007; Penninx et al., 2010), uterine devascularization and compression sutures (Allam & B-Lynch, 2005; Sentilhes et al., 2008a; Sentilhes et al., 2008b), uterine artery embolization (Chauleur et al., 2008; Irion et al., 2008; Vedantham et al., 1997), internal iliac artery and uterine artery ligation (Api et al., 2005; O'Leary, 1995; Papp et al., 2006), that, to some extent, is an alternative to traditional hysterectomy (El-Hamamy & B-Lynch, 2005; Malibary, 2004; Smith & Baskett, 2003).

In the , in a majority of obstetric hospitals hysterectomy still plays a crucial role in the algorithm of surgical treatment of massive obstetric hemorrhage, and causes women to become infertile.

In accordance with nowadays approaches, to save a woman's life as well as her reproductive function in the course of solving the problem of bleedings upon pregnancy, delivery and early postpartum period is a priority. In this regard, research efforts for additional, effective methods of PPH management alternative to hysterectomy, is very important.

Recently advances for stopping PPH and decreasing the need in donor blood become crucial in the field of pharmacological correction of hemostasis as well. In particular, empirical use of recombinant factor VIIa (rFVIIa) is studied in the treatment of obstetric hemorrhage refractory to conventional conservative therapy.

2. Indications and clinical situations for rFVIIa administration

Originally rFVIIa (NovoSeven®; Novo Nordisk A/S, Bagsvaerd, Denmark) has been developed for treatment of spontaneous and/or surgical bleeding in patients, suffering from haemophilia A or B with formation of autoantibodies to FVIII or FIX as a result of compensation of their deficiency in the course of replacement therapy (Abshire & Kenet, 2004; Lusher et al., 1998; Negrier & Hay, 2000; Shapiro et al., 1998; Sobieszczyk & Breborowicz, 2006). Now rFVIIa is licensed for the use in a number of countries. In 1999 Food and Drug Administration (FDA), United States of America approved rFVIIa for treatment of hemophilia A or B in patients with inhibitors to FVIII or FIX. Further, in 2005, FDA also approved the use of rFVIIa in patients with congenital deficiency of factor VII (K.A. O'Connell et al., 2006). In Europe rFVIIa is also prescribed to stop bleeding in patients with acquired hemophilia and Glanzmann thrombasthenia (Franchini et al., 2005a; Hedner & Erhardtsen, 2002; Jurlander et al., 2001; Kessler, 2000).

Except above listed indications, any use of rFVIIa is reviewed «off-label» and responsibility for its decision remains for the attending physician. For the last decade, the use of rFVIIa, with more specified data about mechanisms of its action has been successfully approved «off-label» to stop other uncontrolled hemorrhages unassociated with haemophilia, to reduce the need for allogenic blood. They included intracranial hemorrhage, bleedings due to coumarin use, hepatic coagulopathy, major surgery and traumas (Aggarwal et al., 2004; Aldouri, 2002; Dutton al., 2004; Eikelboom et al., 2003; Franchini et al., 2007; Ghorashian & Hunt, 2004; Hedner, 2003; Mathew, 2004; Martinowitz et al., 2002; Martinowitz & Michaelson, 2005; Mayo et al., 2004; Mittal & Watson, 2006; O'Connell et al., 2003; Price et al., 2004; Roberts et al., 2004; Sobieszczyk & Breborowicz, 2004; Uhlmann & Eby, 2004; Vincent et al., 2006).

3. World experience of use of rFVIIa in treatment of PPH

The first experience of successful treatment of intractable obstetric bleeding in nonhaemophilic patients with rFVIIa was published by Moscardo et al. in 2001 (Moscardo et al., 2001), who reported that rFVIIa showed high hemostatic effect in life-threatening PPH after caesarean section in women with disseminated intravascular coagulation (DIC) syndrome, impaired liver and kidney failure. Later, Breborowicz et al. (2002) reported the results of the experience of PPH treatment when rFVIIa application helped to avoid hysterectomy in two of six cases.

Hossain et al. (2007) described the results of cohort retrospective study of 34 patients with blood loss more than 1500 ml, 18 of them received rFVIIa treatment. Ahonen et al. (2007) compared results of 26 women receiving rFVIIa with 22 women of control group, with PPH without rFVIIa. In both studies the causes of PPH were: uterine hypotension, abnormal placentation, premature placental detachment, as well as hysterorrhesis or vaginal laceration were. Before rFVIIa administration women received oxitocics, uterus massage, uterine artery ligation and, in some cases, hysterectomy.

Above-mentioned and other reports were very important, as treatment of life-threatening PPH still remains acute problem. Moreover it can demand hysterectomy with subsequent loss of reproductive function of woman, despite the fact that rendered aid was not included in the number of registered indications for this clinical situation (Franchini et al., 2007).

Presently there is a number of works available for successful empirical rFVIIa application in treatment of massive PPH, with introduced refractory to conservative methods of treatment. (Aggarwal et al., 2004; Ahonen & Jokela, 2005; Ahonen et al., 2007; Boehlen et al., 2004; Bomken et al., 2009; Bouwmeester et al., 2003; Boyer-Neumann et al., 2003; Breborowicz et al., 2002; Brueckner et. al., 2001; Dart et al., 2004; Dutton et al., 2004; Eikelboom et al., 2003; Franchini et al., 2007; Franchini et al., 2008; Hollnberger et al., 2005; Holub et al., 2005; Jansen et al., 2005; Jimenez-Yuste et al., 2000; Kale et al., 2004; Kretzschmar et al., 2003; Macphail et al., 2004; Martinowitz & Michaelson, 2005; Mayo et al., 2004; Merchant et al., 2004; Mittal & Watson, 2006; Moscardo et al., 2001; Mousa & Walkinshaw, 2001; Mousa & Alfirevic, 2003,2007; Nowacka et al., 2005; Palomino et al., 2006; Pepas et al., 2006; Price et al., 2004; Segal et al., 2004; Shamsi et al., 2005; Shander et al., 2005; Sobieszczyk et al., 2002, 2004, 2006; Sokolic et al., 2002; Tanchev et al., 2005; Verre et al., 2006; Vincent et al., 2006; Welsh et al., 2008; Zupancic et al., 2002).

There is also data about rFVIIa efficacy in hemorrhage prevention during delivery in pregnant women with acquired impaired coagulation. (Eskandari et al., 2002; O'Connell et al., 2006).

In Russia the first successful experience in this field took place in 2002 in Clinic of Professor Zinovij Barkagan (Russian Academy of Medical Sciences, Hematological Research Center, Altai department). The patient with severe postpartum hemorrhage and syndrome of massive hemotransfusions underwent a successful treatment and the followed long-term observations led to this publication.

Nevertheless, there is not enough evidence in favor of rFVIIa application in postpartum hemorrhage. According to the last recommendations of World Health Organization the use of rFVIIa should be limited to primary defect symptoms of hemostasis. (World Health Organization [WHO], 2009). The document also indicates that rFVIIa was given a priority interest to treat postpartum haemorrhage, mainly in industrialized developed countries due to its high cost. The broad use of rFVIIa is limited to the evidence in this area reporting that the use of rFVIIa is risky and even life-threatening . Despite the positive recommendations (Ahonen et al., 2007; Welsh et al., 2008) the practice of rFVIIa use in PPH is far from homogeneous (Haynes et al., 2007). Though it's available to be prescribed, experts need to determine its effectiveness, safety in obstetric hemorrhage and dosage recommendations. It is also clear that further accumulation and generalization of rFVIIa administration in obstetric practice may serve as the basis to register indications for its possible prescription in obstetrics.

4. Mechanism of hemostatic action of rFVIIa

FVII of natural origin, as well as a recombinant product, plays a key role in the haemostatic reactions in a human body. According to the cellular model of coagulation (Hoffman, 2003.)

after injury of vascular walls tissue factor (TF) gets into circulating blood to form a complex TF-FVII on the surface of cells containing TF. Complexes of TF-FVII activate factor X, which, in its turn, promotes the transformation of prothrombin to thrombin. A limited amount of formed thrombin activates cofactors V, VIII and XI, as well as platelets accumulated at the site of injury. Activated platelets secrete negatively charged phospholipids (phosphatidylserine) on membrane surface, and FIXa, FVIIIa and FXIa bound to their surface, which leads to further activation of FX and a massive thrombin formation (Monroe et al., 1997). The formation of large doses of thrombin leads to thrombin-activated fibrinolysis inhibitor (TAFI), which protects the fibrin clot from early dissolution (Bajzar et al., 1995). Direct activation of FX on the surface of activated platelets in the absence of TF, which leads to increased thrombin formation, may explain the mechanism of action of rFVIIa in the local cases of acquired coagulopathy due to trauma or surgery (Gabriel et al., 2004; Hedner, 2001; Hoffman et al., 1998; Lisman & De Groot, 2003; Monroe et al., 1997).

5. Original researches

Our research project offers a comparative assessment of rFVIIa effectiveness against (NovoSeven ®; Novo Nordisk A / S, Bagsvaerd, Denmark) PPH, due to the cause of bleeding, blood loss, dynamics of hemostatic disorders and period of drug administration from the start of bleeding. That is the main objective of the research.

In this study we obtained data on 75 patients with PPH in study conducted within the scope of prospective analysis, and 30 patients with PPH for the retrospective analysis. Recruitment campaign in patients was carried out randomly in accordance with internationally recognized protocol in major obstetric clinics in Russian cities - Barnaul, Krasnoyarsk, Bryansk, and Syktyvkar. The criterion for selection of patients for the research was the same pathology - a massive haemorrhage (PPH), which started during pregnancy, delivery and in the postpartum period. By "massive" we understand the blood loss that constitutes more than 1.5% of patient body weight or less, leading to hemodynamic disturbances.

The age range of women participating in this study varied: from 18 to 44, and average age was 28,6 ± 6,3 years. Gestational age at the time of bleeding was also different - from 24 to 43 weeks, average gestational age at delivery was 35,5 ± 5,5 weeks, that is, in the majority of patients (63.8%) bleeding occurred at full-term pregnancy.

Pregnancy which resulted in spontaneous vaginal birth is found only in 46 women (43.8%), the greater part of pregnant women (56.2%) required surgical delivery by cesarean section (93.2% women), or the use of obstetric forceps (6,8%). In more than half of the observations (56.2%) major bleeding occurred in the postpartum period, approximately in every fourth - during pregnancy (26.7%), almost in every sixth - during delivery (17.1%).

According to the study, all patients were divided into two groups – study group and control group (see pic. 1). The main principle of this division was the use of rFVIIa along with traditional therapy consisting of pharmacologic hemostasis in life-threatening obstetric hemorrhage in 75 patients (study group). rFVIIa was given intravenously at doses ranging from 13,6 to 146,5 mg / kg body weight, an average dose of rFVIIa was 65,4 ± 36,7 mg / kg.

Criteria for enrollment in the study group are: reproductive age 18 - 44 years, the presence of massive obstetric haemorrhage, rFVIIa administration to correct hemostasis. Negative factor for enrollment: physiological blood loss during delivery or in the postpartum period, the presence of massive obstetric haemorrhage without rFVIIa administration to correct hemostasis. The rFVIIa was used as a supplement to the traditional scheme against PPH.

The control group retrospectively consisted of 30 patients with PPH, and their treatment was delivered according to classical method, which includes the use of drugs that reduce uterus size, uterine massage, manual examination of the uterine cavity, infusion and transfusion therapy with fresh frozen plasma, blood cells - red blood cells and platelets, protease inhibitors, as well as surgical methods of hemostasis, which is consistent with the recommendations of several experts (Ahonen et al., 2010; Franchini et al., 2007; La Belle & Kitchens, 2007; Phillips et al., 2009; Shander et al., 2005; Sobieszczyk & Breborowicz, 2006a; Vincent et al., 2006; Welsh et al., 2008).

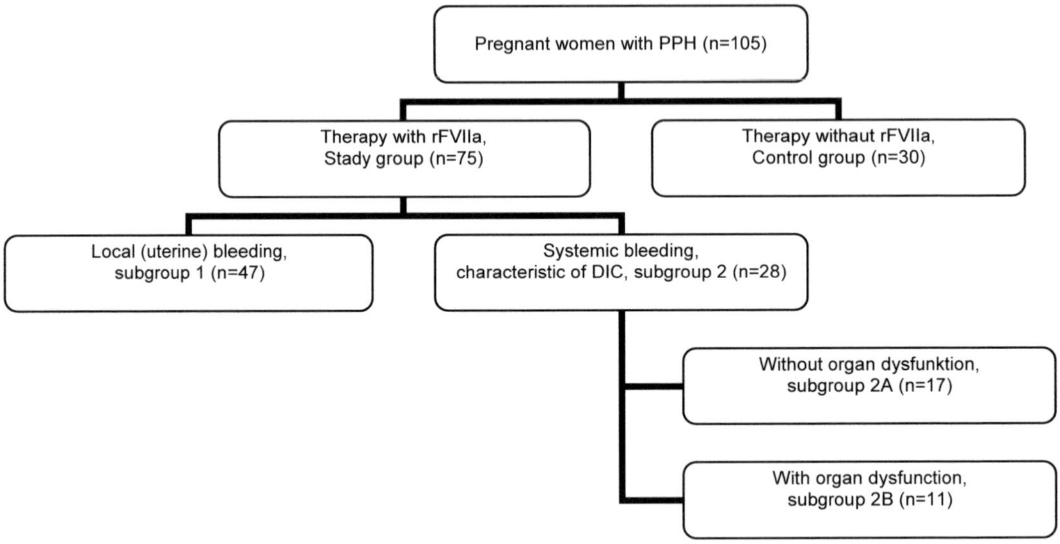

Pic. 1. The division of women with PPH into groups / subgroups in the study

The factors for the analysis in the study group: age of patients in the target group, gestational age at the time of massive bleeding, the methods of delivery, as well as obstetric data, reproductive and physical history, which in most patients characterized by the presence of several diseases in their reproductive system, abnormal cardiac and vascular system, presence of chronic infections, viral and toxic liver injury.

Analysis of the characteristics of hemorrhagic syndrome showed similar results in two groups compared to hemorrhage causes, the volume of blood loss, hemoglobin levels and bleeding tempo and other similar factors.

By the clinical manifestations of PPH we divided study group into two subgroups for further in-depth analysis. The first subgroup included 47 women with the classical picture of obstetric haemorrhage. rFVIIa was administered to stop PPH prior to the use of traumatic surgical methods of treatment. The purpose of rFVIIa administration in patients of this subgroup was to stop local uterine bleeding without a laparotomy and to preserve the uterus.

The second group which included 28 patients with obstetric DIC with massive blood loss, according to the criteria,offered by LaBelle & Kitchens (2007). Prior to the introduction of rFVIIa in this group, the classical scheme has been implemented in full, using the known methods of surgery, even a hysterectomy in 16 patients (57.1%). At the same time patients with DIC had systemic bleeding (hematoma under the skin, bleeding from the injection site, gastrointestinal bleeding, hematuria, and others in a variety of combinations), which threatened their lives. Thus, we introduced a special subgroup – 2B, which consisted of 11 patients in whom PPH was complicated with organ dysfunction.

To assess the effectiveness of rFVIIa in treatment PPH we indicated negative factors - early and late. Early negative factors are as follows:

- volume of blood loss ≥ 2.200 ml;
- rate of blood loss> 30 ml / min;
- hemoglobin level ≤ 60 g / l;
- period of time from the beginning of bleeding to rFVIIa administration > 120 min in the study group (the comparison group - the time from the beginning of bleeding to its termination);

Late negative factors -total hysterectomy and death of both mother and fetus.

In patients with PPH, with general clinical examination and measurement of parameters of blood loss, an analysis of core indicators of hemostasis was performed (Practical hemostasis and thrombosis, 2005). The number of platelets in blood, measurement of activated partial thromboplastin time (APTT), prothrombin time (PT) and fibrinogen concentrations according to Clauss were subject to the analysis.Moreover, the activity of antithrombin in plasma was evaluated by amidolytic method. Laboratory studies were conducted prior to bleeding, during (prior to use rFVIIa), and after 1-5 hours, 24 hours and 2-5 days after rFVII administration.

5.1 Statistical analysis

The results were statistically computed in Excel software by methods of calculations of indicators in descriptive statistics. Data analysis in small groups during the distribution was carried out by methods of nonparametric statistics, using Fisher angular transducer, criterion $\chi 2$ with Bonferroni correction, as well as T-score according to Wilcoxon (Wilcoxon F. et al., 1963). Assessment of the efficacy of rFVIIa for treatment of PPH was conducted according to the generally accepted criteria in evidence-based medicine, such as Absolute risk reduction (ARR), Relative risk (Rr), Relative Risk Reduction (RRR), Number needed to treat (NNT), Confidence interval (CI).

5.2 Study results

Upon the analysis of pregnancy complications in patients in the compared groups we obtained interesting results (Table 1). Complicated course of pregnancy due to the taken nosology was characteristic in patients with obstetrical DIC and organ dysfunction rather than in patients with uterine bleeding. Thus, systemic bleeding in the setting of massive obstetric blood loss (subgroup 2A) was more frequent than in patients with local hemorrhage (subgroup 1) and antenatal fetal death.

Pathology form	Study group (n=75)						P value
	Subgroup 1 (n=47)		Subgroup 2 (n=28)				
			Subgroup 2A(n=17)		Subgroup 2B(n=11)		
	abs.	%	abs.	%	abs.	%	
Pathologic placentation	7	14,89	4	23,53	1	9,09	≥0,05 ≥0,05 ≥0,05
Uterine scar	8	17,02	3	17,65	3	27,27	≥0,05 ≥0,05 ≥0,05
Premature detachment of physiological placenta	7	14,89	3	17,65	3	27,27	≥0,05 ≥0,05 ≥0,05
Preeclampsia	2	4,26	1	5,88	4	36,36	$P_{1\text{-}2B}$ = 0,001
Intrauterine growth retardation syndrome	5	10,64	1	5,88	3	27,27	P≥ 0,05
Fetus prenatal infection	14	29,79	8	47,06	8	72,73	$P_{1\text{-}2B}$ = 0,008
Antenatal fetal death	7	14,89	2	11,76	6	54,55	$P_{1\text{-}2B}$ = 0,004 $P_{2A\text{-}2B}$ = 0,01
Total number of women with pregnancy complications	30	63,83	15	88,24	11	100,00	$P_{1\text{-}2B}$ = 0,01

Table 1. Complications of pregnancy in women with pharmacological correction of hemostasis by rFVIIa

In a particularly severe clinical cases, namely in patients with severe DIC syndrome and the presence of multiple organ failure (subgroup 2B), the frequency of such pathological conditions like preeclampsia, intrauterine infection and antenatal fetal death as a consequence of placental dysfunction occurred more frequently than in the two other subgroups.

With regard to today's medical science and the latest scientific advances, it is likely that the high incidence of gestational complications such as preeclampsia, placental insufficiency with antenatal fetal death, are often caused by and associated with severe disorders of hemostasis, hereditary and acquired thrombophilia. High frequency of these complications in the subgroup of patients with massive blood loss, obstetrical DIC and organ dysfunction is consistent with the abovementioned.

Pregnancy pathologies partly determined the character of complications during delivery and the postpartum period, which caused the development of PPH (Table 2).

Pathology form	Study group (n=75)				
	Subgroup 1 (n=47)		Subgroup 2 (n=28)		
	abs.	%	abs.	%	P value
Uterine atony	17	36,17	6	21,43	0,08
Pathologic placentation	6	12,77	1	3,57	0,072
Premature detachment of physiological placenta	7	14,89	6	21,43	0,1
Coagulopathy caused by somatic diseases	3	6,38	2	7,14	0,1
Coagulopathy caused by pregnancy complications	7	14,89	1	3,57	0,045
Retained placenta	6	12,77	5	17,85	0,1
Obstetric trauma	1	2,13	4	14,30	0,022
Amniotic fluid embolism	0	0,00	2	7,14	-
Obstetric sepsis	0	0,00	1	3,57	-

Table 2. Causes of massive obstetric hemorrhage in women with pharmacological correction of hemostasis

Analysis of the characteristics of a hemorrhagic syndrome in the study group showed significant differences in subgroups (Table 3). Thus, the total volume of blood loss and blood loss before the drug administration in subgroup with local (uterine) bleeding were significantly lower than in subgroup 2 with the development of DIC.

Criteria of comparison	Study group (n=75)				P value
	Subgroup 1 (n=47)		Subgroup 2 (n=28)		
	X ± m		X ± m		
Volume of blood loss prior to rFVIIa administration, ml	1368,09 ± 77,14		2230,82 ± 198,20		0,01
Total volume of blood loss, ml	1740,21 ± 114,45		2605,16 ± 402,68		0,01
Blood loss rate, ml/min	30,89 ± 3,97		29,91 ± 7,81		0,1
Haemoglobin level at the moment of rFVIIa administration, g/L	71,48 ± 2,73		56,28 ± 4,07		0,05
Time from beginning of hemorrhage to rFVIIa administration, min	119,47 ± 22,82		318,02 ± 26,6		0,001
rFVIIa dose, mkg/kg	55,47 ± 4,24		70,37 ±-4,77		0,05
Repeated rFVIIa administration, number of cases	11	23,40%	8	28,55%	0,01
Volume of blood loss after rFVIIa administration, ml	340,21 ± 62,28		688,77 ± 88,80		0,001

Table 3. Indicators of blood loss and characteristics of the use of rFVIIa in patients with PPH in the study group

Time from the beginning of bleeding to rFVIIa administration was significantly higher among patients with obstetric DIC (subgroup 2). Obviously this is due to the fact that rFVIIa is considered by obstetricians and emergency physicians as a backup means to stop PPH after using known hemostatic technologies, including hysterectomy. However, one should pay attention to the fact that the dosage of rFVIIa in patients with DIC and pattern of administration were higher in patients with local (uterine) bleeding (subgroup 1). Despite this fact, PPH in subgroup 2 continued the use of rFVIIa, and estimated blood loss was higher compared to subgroup 1.

Effectiveness of rFVIIa in treatment PPH was assessed according to the prior given criteria of negative factors. The absolute number of early negative factors in the compared groups / subgroups is presented in Table 4.

Criteria of negative factors	Study group (n=75)				Control group (n=30)
	Subgroup 1 (n=47)	Subgroup 2(n=28)			
		Subgroup 2A (n=17)	Subgroup 2B (n=11)	Total	
	abs.	abs.	abs.	abs.	abs.
Volume of blood loss ≥2.200 ml	2	8	3	11	5
Blood loss rate >30 mL/min	15	5	1	6	4
Haemoglobin level in blood ≤ 60 g/L	13	8	8	16	15
Time from beginning of hemorrhage to rFVIIa administration > 120 min	10	6	7	13	19
Volume of blood loss after rFVIIa administration, >300 ml	14	10	7	17	2

Table 4. Early negative factors in women with PPH, depending on the use of rFVIIa in the therapy

Estimate of efficiency according to the blood loss criterion in patients of subgroup 1 (with local uterine bleeding) showed a relative risk reduction by 75%, according to the criterion of depth of anemia - by 45% and with the early administration of the preparation (less than 120 minutes since the beginning of bleeding) - by 66%, indicating a high clinical efficacy of rFVIIa in treatment of PPH not complicated by DIC (Table 5). To avoid adverse outcomes on all reflected criteria from 4, 5 to 7, 8 patients are needed to be treated in this group.

In contrast, in women with systemic bleeding due to underlying DIC (subgroup 2) absolute risk reduction was negative (Table 6). This suggests that the incidence of negative factors in the study group is higher than in the control group. The reduction of relative risk in patients of subgroup 2 accounted for 26%, suggesting that there is clinical effect from the use of rFVIIa, especially with the early introduction of preparation (≤ 120 min).

Factors	ARR	NNT	Rr	RRR	CI (95%)
Volume of blood loss ≥2.200 ml	0,128	7,8	0,25	75%	0,274; 0,018
Blood loss rate >30 mL/min	-0,189	-5,3	2,45	-1,45	-0,043; -0,335
Haemoglobin level in blood ≤ 60 g/L	0,224	4,5	0,55	45%	0,370; 0,078
Time from beginning of hemorrhage to rFVIIa administration >120 min	-0,418	-2,4	0,34	66%	0,272; 0,564

Table 5. The effectiveness of rFVIIa administration in patients with local uterine bleeding (subgroup 1)

Factors	ARR	NNT	Rr	RRR	CI (95%)
Volume of blood loss ≥2.200 ml	-0,222	-4,5	2,31	-1,31	-0,028; -0,416
Blood loss rate >30 mL/min	-0,084	-11,9	1,65	-65%	0,110; 0,278
Haemoglobin level in blood ≤ 60 g/L	-0,071	-14,1	1,14	-14%	0,123; 0,265
Time from beginning of hemorrhage to rFVIIa administration >120 min	-0,166	-6,0	0,74	26%	0,028; 0,360

Table 6. The effectiveness of rFVIIa administration in patients with PPH in the setting of DIC (subgroup 2)

This fact has motivated us to carry on more detailed analysis of the effectiveness of preparation in subgroups of women with DIC (Table 7).

The effectiveness of rFVIIa in systemic bleeding with simultaneous presence of organ dysfunction (in subgroup 2B) in prevention of large volume of blood loss was uncertain. According to the criterion of blood loss rate we obtained positive values of ARR, NNT, and RRR index was 31% in these patients, which corresponds to a positive clinical effect of rVIIa application in the "fast" bleeding. However, to prevent one negative factor in these cases 25 patients should be treated. At the same time, in systemic bleeding without development of organ dysfunction (subgroup 2A) with early introduction of rFVIIa clinical efficacy was even greater (RRR = 44%).

Thus, according to the results of this analysis we can conclude that the clinical efficacy of rFVIIa in treatment of PPH is the highest in patients with local (uterine) bleeding and only according to the selected criteria with the early rFVIIa administration in patients with the development of obstetrical DIC.

Factors	ARR (2A)	ARR (2B)	NNT (2A)	NNT (2 B)	Rr (2A)	Rr (2B)	RRR (2A)	RRR (2B)	CI (95%) (2A)	CI (95%) (2B)
Volume of blood loss ≥2.200 ml	-0,3	-0,1	-3,30	-10,0	2,76	1,59	-1,76	-59%	0,028; 0,416	-0,085; -0,285
Blood loss rate >30 mL/min	- 0,164	0,04	-6,1	25,0	2,26	0,69	- 126%	31%	0,032; -0,36	0,225; -0,145
Haemoglobin level in blood ≤ 60 g/L	0,03	-0,22	33,3	-4,5	0,94	1,44	6%	-44%	0,226; -0,166	-0,035; 0,405
Time from beginning of hemorrhage to rFVIIa administration >120 min	- 0,278	0,006	-3,6	166,7	0,56	1,01	44%	-1%	-0,082; -0,474	0,191; -0,179

Table 7. The effectiveness of rFVIIa administration in women with PPH, complicated by obstetrical DIC (subgroup 2A and 2B)

We also took into account the absolute number of late adverse outcomes in compared groups/subgroups that are shown in Table 8.

Criteria of negative factors	Groups / subgroups of patients				
	1 (n=47)	2A (n=17)	2B (n=11)	2 (n=28)	Control group (n=30)
	abs.	abs.	abs.	abs.	abs.
Maternal mortality	0	0	6	6	2
Perinatal mortality	4	7	3	10	3
Total hysterectomy	9	8	12	20	19

Table 8. Late adverse outcomes in the groups / subgroups of women with PPH

Below, we provide separate analysis for each criterion, except for the maternal mortality, as it was not registered in subgroup 1.

We did not obtain any data about the effect of rFVIIa administration in treatment of PPH on frequency of perinatal mortality in study groups (Table 9).

Absolute risk reduction for this criterion was indicated in women with DIC, but relative risk reduction was not indicated, so it is obvious that administration of rFVIIa has no significant effect on fetal loss. In contrast, we obtained positive clinical results for the total hysterectomy criterion, although somewhat different in the subgroups of study group (Table 10).

It is quite understandable that women with a local (uterine) bleeding according to the total hysterectomy criterion had negative rate of absolute risk reduction. This suggests that in

Values	Local (uterine) bleeding (subgroup 1)	Obstetric DIC, in general (subgroup 2)	Systemic bleeding without organ dysfunction (subgroup 2A)	Systemic bleeding with organ dysfunction (subgroup 2B)
ARR	-0,01	0,26	0,08	0,54
NNT	-67,1	3,9	13,1	1,9
Rr	0,85	3,57	1,76	6,36
RRR (%)	15	-2,57	-76	-5,36
CI 95% (+)	-0,030	0,514	0,153	1,073
CI 95% (-)	-0,104	0,131	-0,013	0,368

Table 9. The effectiveness of rFVIIa administration in women with PPH, according to the criterion of perinatal mortality

control group hysterectomy was performed much more frequently in order to stop bleeding than in the group with local (uterine) bleeding. Indicator for relative risk reduction in patients with massive local (uterine) bleeding recommended rFVIIa in their therapy was 70%, which was consistent with clinical effect to preserve healthy reproductive function. When we studied each case of hysterectomy in patients with local (uterine) bleeding (9 cases, or 19.1%) separately we found out that the use of rFVIIa was not effective in patients who had bleeding caused by pathologic placentation (placenta increta in 5 cases out of 9) and the development of Kuveler's uterus (4 cases out of 9) due to premature detachment of placenta.

Values	Local (uterine) bleeding (subgroup 1)	Obstetric DIC, in general (subgroup 2)	Systemic bleeding without organ dysfunction (subgroup 2A)	Systemic bleeding with organ dysfunction (subgroup 2B)
ARR	-0,44	0,08	0,09	0,07
NNT	-2,3	12,4	10,6	13,8
Rr	0,30	1,13	1,15	1,11
RRR (%)	70	-13	-15	-11
CI 95% (+)	-0,884	0,162	0,188	0,145
CI 95% (-)	-0,531	-0,045	-0,074	-0,017

Table 10. The effectiveness of rFVIIa administration in women with PPH, according to the total hysterectomy criterion

Further, we compared clinical manifestations of PPH to effects of rFVIIa in women under study who have abnormal changes in hemostatic system, and the research data gives the foundation for the formation of hemorrhagic syndrome, and to assess the effectiveness and safety of pharmacological correction of bleeding.

Based on coagulation results almost all patients (subgroups 1, 2) had the relative hypofibrinogenemia and hypocoagulation a few days prior to developing PPH (compared to the physiological norm for this gestational age) (Tables 11-13). We can assume that these changes can reduce the so-called physiological hypercoagulability in pregnancy and may serve as the pathological basis for the formation of severe hemorrhagic syndrome during delivery.

The manifestation of PPH was associated with thrombocytopenia, hypocoagulation on PT and dynamic lowering of fibrinogen concentrations. Later, the first hours after infusion of rFVIIa the termination or reduction of bleeding (see Table 11-13) was followed by depression of thrombocytopenia and hypofibrinogenemia which is to be the natural course, as the platelets and fibrinogen are the basis of a blood clot.

Haemostatic markers	The indicator for normal pregnancy in III trimester	In patients 1-7 days prior to administration of rFVIIa	During bleeding	After rFVIIa administration			
				In 30 min	In 1 - 5 hours	In 24 hours	In 2-5 days
Platelets, x10⁹/l	146-429	194,7±10,37	177,6± 8,2	109± 4,2	114± 7,9	146± 9,48	161± 5,8
PT, ratio	0,87	0,96	1,16	1,02	0,87	1,05	0,94
APPT, ratio	0,91	0,97	0,93	0,96	1,07	1,00	0,90
Fibrinogen, g/l	3,7-6,2	3,42± 0,16	2,15± 0,14	2,09± 0,13	2,02± 0,01	2,55± 0,12	3,09± 0,17
Antithrombin, %	82 - 116	93± 4,4	86± 3,5	87± 4,8	67,67± 1,8	91,38± 1,59	89,56± 2,9

Table 11. The dynamics of hemostasis in women of subgroup 1 (with local bleeding and uterine hypotension) before and after application of rFVIIa (X ± m); * - according to Abbassi-Ghanavati et al. (2009).

These shifts in patients of subgroup 1 were defined on the basis of shortening of PT and noticeable reduction of antithrombin activity. This indicates systemic, caused by rFVIIa interference increase of procoagulant properties of blood, along with moderate reduction of its anticoagulant potential, leading to clinically diagnosed hemostasis. Later, after 24 hours and more extended period of time , all abnormal changes appeared to be decreasing.

Haemostatic study of the second subgroup in women with obstetric DIC, showed direct (see the results for subgroup 1 given above), but more deep disorders of studied hemocoagulation markers in the period preceding and during PPH (Tables 12).

To determine the intensity, focus and accuracy of changes in hemostatic system in women after rFVIIa administration, we used a T-Wilcoxon test (Wilcoxon F, et al 1963). We analyzed changes in the pattern of bleeding, after 1-5 hours and 24 hours after the injection. The results were the following: the intensity of positive shift (in the direction of normal hemostasis) significantly prevails over the intensity of negative shift according to the following parameters: in patients with local uterine bleeding - protrombin time (P = 0.01), 24 hours after the administration, number of platelets (P = 0.05) 24 hours after the administration; level of fibrinogen (P = 0.05), 24 hours after the administration, in patients with DIC reliable shift only in number of platelets (P = 0.05) 24 hours after the administration . For all other parameters changes are not significant, and in patients with DIC there is no effect or negative shift in prothrombin time.

Haemostatic markers	The indicator for normal pregnancy in III trimester *	In patients 1-7 days prior to administration of rFVIIa	During bleeding	After rFVIIa administration			
				In 30 min	In 1-5 hours	In 24 hours	In 2-5 days
Platelets, $x10^9/l$	146-429	166,7±5,18	136,1± 8,8	65±5,9	62,67± 6,8	81,5± 9,2	104,7± 16,3
PT, ratio	0,87	1,31	1,04	1,2	1,3	1,6	1,1
APPT, ratio	0,91	1,9	1,0	0,81	0,89	1,0	1,5
Fibrinogen, g/l	3.7-6.2	3,07±0,32	2±0,09	-	1,27± 0,006	3,75± 0,55	2,94± 0,2
Antithrombin, %	82 - 116	108±0,75	59±6,2	55±0,2	42±0,15	82±0,09	91,86±2, 2

Table 12. Hemostasis markers in patients with obstetrical DIC (subgroup 2) before and after rFVIIa administration (X ± m)

Haemostatic markers	Subgroup 1			Subgroup 2		
	During bleeding	After rFVIIa administration		During bleeding	After rFVIIa administration	
		In 1-5 hours	In 24 hours		In 1-5 hours	In 24 hours
Platelets, $x10^9/l$	177,6±8,2	114±7,9	146±9,48	136,1±8,8	62,67±6,8	81,5±9,2
PT, ratio	1,16	0,87	1,05	1,04	1,3	1,6
Fibrinogen, g/l	2,15±0,14	2,02±0,01	2,55±0,12	2±0,09	1,27±0,006	3,75±0,55
Antithrombin, %	86±3,5	67,67±1,8	91,38±1,59	59±6,2	42±0,15	82±0,09

Table 13. The dynamics of main hemostatic markers in women with PPH after rFVIIa administration (X ± m)

With all the results shown, as well as the fact of the massive reduction of anticoagulant potential (antithrombin activity) in DIC-related PPH and rFVIIa administration , a higher risk of developing or enhancing organ dysfunction associated with blockade of microcirculation can be indicated in this subgroup, which is described and mentioned in a number of publications devoted to the study of aseptic and septic DIC (Eisele & Lamy, 1998; Macphail & Talks, 2004; Schouten et al., 2008; Vinazzer, 1995).

It is known that antithrombin acts as heparin cofactor and related to the most important inhibitors of blood clotting, it accounts approximately 80% of anticoagulant potential (LaBelle & Kitchens, 2007; Opal et al., 2002; Practical hemostasis and thrombosis, 2005; Rublee et al., 2002). When antithrombin activity in plasma falls below 70% the risk of pathological clotting progressively increases, and it is greater, the greater the anticoagulant deficiency. Decrease in antithrombin activity to the level of 30-50% of the physiological norm leads to a generalized, unrestrained thrombinemia and massive thrombosis in vessels of any size. In this case, antithrombin half-life shortens dramatically, and can be only a few hours (especially with therapeutic doses of heparin) (Vinazzer, 1995).

Decrease in antithrombin activity in patients below 70% in different types of pathology requires replacement therapy to recover the physiological norm (about 80-120%) (LaBelle & Kitchens, 2007; Schouten et al., 2008; Schwartz et al., 1989). To cover antithrombin small supply, commercial products of anticoagulants or fresh frozen plasma (FFP) can be used. Note, however, that the massive transfusion of FFP (20-25 ml/kg) may lead to hypervolemia and risk of interstitial pulmonary edema, if symptoms of renal failure and the termination of bleeding occur. In these cases, we believe, we can use combined application of antithrombin preparation and FFP (dose of 7-10 ml/kg).

We also believe that support of sustainable balance of pro- and anticoagulant systems of hemostasis in patients with systemic bleeding after rFVIIa administration will reduce the risk of thrombotic events, lessening or strengthening of potential multiple organ failure (Pic. 2).

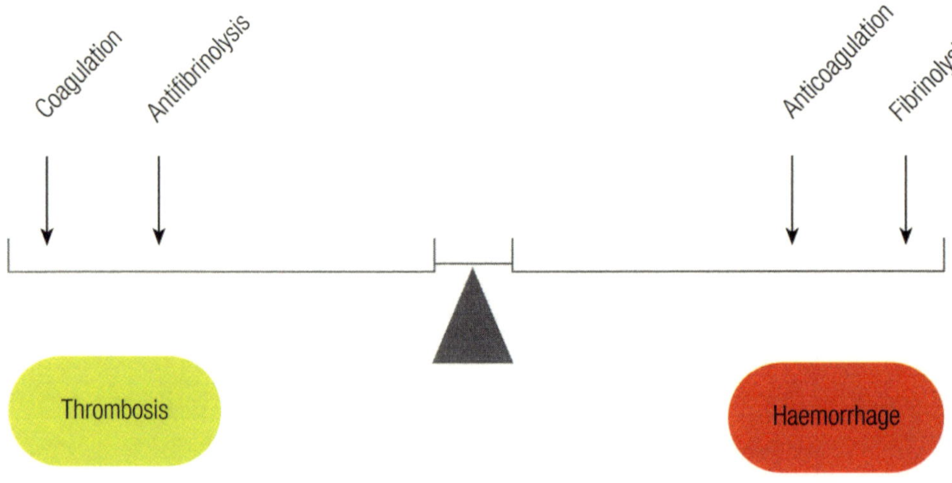

Pic. 2. Systematic hemostasis interaction in oder to balance coagulation / anticoagulation and fibrinolysis / antifibrinolysis, which when altered, results in haemorrage or thrombosis (after Buenso S.R., 2007)

If to look back at the reactions of hemostatic system to the introduction of rFVIIa in women with obstetric DIC and PPH, we conclude that PT, on average data, was not shortened, but in most cases, lengthened or remained normal at the time of registration of bleeding. In our view, the lack of shortening of PT in first two hours after rFVIIa administration may serve as a predictor of its low hemostatic activity, as well as the little impact of repeated injections of rFVIIa.

It was previously shown that the use of rFVIIa has the worst hemostatic effect in patients with severe coagulopathy, acidosis and hypothermia (Aggarwal et al., 2004; Bomken et al., 2009; Dutton, 2004; Eikelboom et al., 2003; Martinowitz & Michaelson, 2005; Mayo et al.,

2004; Mittal & Watson, 2006; O'Connell et al., 2003). It was shown in these studies that effective pharmacologic hemostasis with use of rFVIIa can be expected with the following parameters of blood:

- prothrombin time <1.5 hours upper limit of normal;
- Clauss fibrinogen> 1.0 g / L;
- platelet count > 50 × 10^9 / L;
- along with the above laboratory indices pH > 7.1 is also desirable for optimal effect;
- exclusion of hypothermia.

In the course of the research we have corrected the present parameters with the means of transfusion therapy, which was aimed at the recovery of hemostatic abilities in the blood, maintenance of the acid-base balance and the quantity of red blood cells to oxygenize tissues. It should be noted that in our research the volume and components of such a therapy were practically the same in the study and control groups. At the same time patients of the study group experiencing PPH and DIC (subgroup 2) received the bigger volume of the transfusion therapy as compared to subgroup 1 (table 14). The information we obtained about changes in hemostasis during haemostatic therapy allows us to estimate the importance of such studies in pregnant women and offer recommendations how to treat patients with PPH as evidenced by a number of experts (Ahonen et al., 2010; Bomken et al., 2009; Franchini et al., 2007; Sobieszczyk & Breborowicz, 2004).

Criteria of comparison	Study group (n=75)		P value
	Subgroup 1 (n=47)	Subgroup 2 (n=28)	
	X ± m	X ± m	
Total volume of transfusions, ml	2937,2 ± 630,1	5340,8 ± 1207,0	0,05
FFP, ml	1381,1 ± 314,9	2975,6 ± 702,7	0,01
Red blood cells, ml	1003,2 ± 213,7	1725,4 ± 770,1	P>0,05
Platelets concentrates, U	0	4,13 ± 1,1	-

Table 14. Transfusion therapy in women to study group

Among the questions raised above we were interested in the possibility of arterial and venous thrombosis development during treatment with rFVIIa. In the analysis of 75 cases of rFVIIa treatment of women with PPH, represented by Franchini et al. (2007) there were no evidence of venous thrombosis. The recent work of Bomken et al. (2009) also demonstrated the absence of thrombosis during treatment with rFVIIa, in spite of the increasing thrombogenicity inherent to physiological pregnancy. In addition, several reports indicated a low risk of venous thromboembolism in previously healthy patients, even with the development of DIC (Martinowitz & Michaelson, 2005; Moscardo et al., 2001.). In general, the majority of thrombotic events due to the application of rFVIIa, have arterial origin and are determined in patients with pre-existing thrombogenic risk factors (Biss & Hanley, 2006.). Nevertheless, as well as the number of authors, and according to materials of existing international recommendations (Franchini et al., 2007; Lim et al., 2004; Martinowitz & Michaelson, 2005; Ohkuchi et al., 2003; Vincent et al., 2006; Welsh et al., 2008; World Health

Organization [WHO], 2009), we recommend care in using this systemic haemostatic medicine in women with high risk of thromboembolism, such as cancer, including reproductive organs, air embolism, antiphospholipid syndrome, and thromboembolic syndrome present in history and in close blood relatives. In these cases it is vital to apply therapy or medication for thromboprophylaxis.

6. Discussion

In general the data that we obtained suggests that rFVIIa is a highly efficient hemostatic means to treat women with PPH, who are unable to respond to classical methods of haemostatic therapy. In accordance with the effectiveness criteria used in the present study women with massive local (uterine) bleeding, caused by uterine hypotony and atony in which the use of rFVIIa prescribed to avoid hysterectomy in most cases (80.9%) proved to have haemostatic effect, with no lethality among patients. Women with PPH due to the abruptio placentae combined with Kuveler's uterine and placenta increta had relatively lower hemostatic effectiveness. On the other hand patients with obstetrical DIC (without organ dysfunction) and PPH the use of rFVIIa can also be justified due to health reasons, though relatively less effective. In cases of obstetrical DIC, massive bleeding and developing of organ dysfunction haemostatic effect of rFVII is extremely doubtful.

Cases of failure of pharmacological correction of bleeding with rFVIIa can be attributed to resistance, for various reasons, of the blood coagulation system to activation of redundant quantity of factor VIIa (Franchini et al., 2007; Selo-Ojeme & Okonofua, 1997; Shander et al.,2005; Sobieszczyk & Breborowicz, 2004), as well as by the presence of organ dysfunction, which led to adverse outcome in 6 out of 11 women (54.5%) in our observations.

It is important to note that the use of rFVIIa in massive bleeding leads to further consumption of platelets and fibrinogen, which is consistent with the modern explanation of the mechanism of its hemostatic action, but to reduce the risk of development or strengthening of possible multiple organ failure in obstetrical DIC it is important to recover the deficit not only of platelets and clotting factors, but also of physiological anticoagulants. The optimal tactics in the period after rFVIIa administration is 3-7 days of corrective replacement therapy of fresh frozen plasma (at a dose of 7-10 ml / kg) in combination with antithrombin preparation, to restore the activity of the latter, tentatively, to 100-120% of normal levels. The role of efficient and high-quality laboratory diagnostics of dynamics and basic parameters of coagulation (platelet count, PT, fibrinogen concentration and antithrombin activity) goes without questioning.

Based on this data, we include rFVIIa in a scheme of therapy of obstetric hemorrhage, proposed by WHO, for the prevention of invasive and radical interventions in the treatment of PPH vital for haemostas management (World Health Organization [WHO], 2009) - See Pic. 3.

We also believe that the use of tranexamic acid in the therapeutic tactics proves to be effective in cases of PPH, due to local uterine bleeding. However, the threat of emerging or strengthening of organ dysfunction or venous thromboembolism based on fibrinolytic reaction suppression seems substantial and dangerous to mother's life.

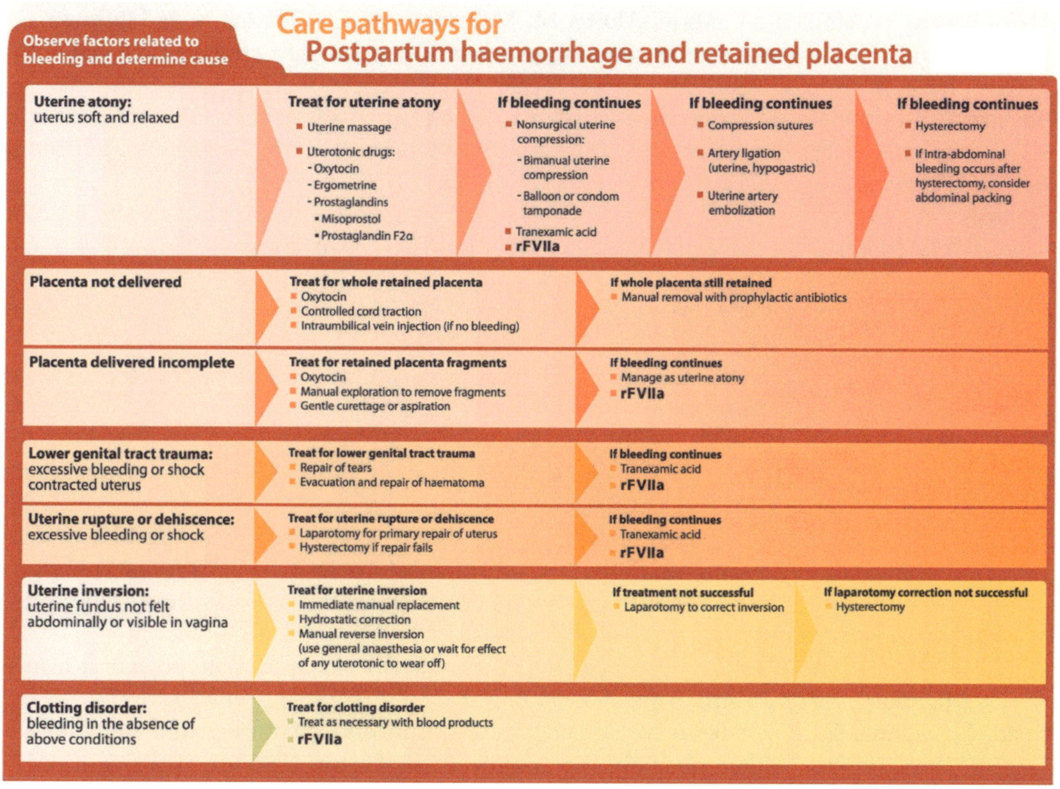

Pic. 3. Potential role of rFVIIa in treatment of PPH to reduce the number of radical operative interventions

7. Conclusion

We state that the resources of our own and those available publicly in regard to this issue received in non-controlled and nonrandomized studies, otherwise is impossible because of ethical reasons in obstetric practice of critical conditions (Bomken et al., 2009). Nevertheless, the accumulation and subsequent analysis of cases of rFVIIa administration in treating PPH will contribute to creating overall and clear recommendations for specialists in this field.

8. Acknowledgment

The authors thank Aleksandra Suvorova for critical reviewing of this manuscript and for her assistantship.

9. References

Abbassi-Ghanavati M, Greer LG. & Cunningham FG. (2009) Pregnancy and laboratory studies: a reference table for clinicians. Obstet Gynecol. Dec. 2009;114(6):1326-31.

Abdel-Aleem H, Singata M, Abdel-Aleem M, Mshweshwe N, Williams X. & Hofmeyr GJ (2010) Uterine massage to reduce postpartum hemorrhage after vaginal delivery. Int J Gynaecol Obstet. Oct. 2010;111(1):32-6.

Abshire T, Kenet G. (2004) Recombinant factor VIIa: review of efficacy, dosing regimens and safetyin patients with congenital and acquired factor VIII or IX inhibitors. J Thromb Haemost. Jun. 2004;2(6):899-909.

Aggarwal A., Malkovska V., Catlett J. P. & Alcorn K. (2004) Recombinant activated factor VII (rFVIIa) as salvage treatment for intractable hemorrhage. Thromb J. Nov. 2004;2(1):9.

Ahonen J, Jokela R. (2005) Recombinant factor VIIa for lifethreatening post-partum haemorrhage. Br J Anaesth. May. 2005;94(5):592-5.

Ahonen J, Jokela R. & Kortila K. (2007) An open non-randomized study of recombinant activated factor VII in major postpartum haemorrhage. Acta Anaesthesiol Scand. Aug. 2007;51(7):929-36.

Ahonen J, Stefanovic V. & Lassila R. (2010) Management of postpartum haemorrage. Acta Anaesthesiol Scand. Nov. 2010;54(10):1164-78.

Aldouri M. (2002) The use of recombinant factor VIIa in controlling surgical bleeding in nonhaemophiliac patients. Pathophysiol Haemost Thromb 2002;32(Suppl 1):41–6.

Allam MS, B-Lynch C. (2005) The B-Lync and other uterine compression suture techniques. Int J Gynaecol Obstet. Jun.2005;89(3):236-41.

Api M., Api O. & Yayla M. (2005) Fertility after B-Lynch suture and hypogastric artery ligation // Fertil Steril. Aug. 2005;84(2):509.

Bajzar L, Manuel R. & Nesheim ME. (1995) Purification and characterization of TAFI, a thrombin-activatable fibrinolysis inhibitor. J Biol Chem. 1995 Jun 16;270(24):14477-84.

Bakri Y.N., Amri A. & Abdul Jabbar F. (2001) Tamponade - balloon for obstetrical bleeding. Int J Gynaecol Obstet. Aug. 2001;74(2):139-42.

Baudo F, Caimi TM, Mostarda G, de Cataldo F. & Morra E. (2006) Critical bleeding in pregnancy: a novel therapeutic approach to bleeding. Minerva Anestesiol. Jun. 2006;72(6):389-93.

Ben Hmid R, El Houssaini S, Mahjoub S, Mourali M, Zeghal D, Zouari F, El Kamel M, Bouchnek M. & Maghrebi H. (2006) Haemorrhage delivery. About 65 case. Tunis Med. May. 2006;84(5):286-90.

Biss TT, Hanley JP. (2006) Recombinant activated factor VII (rFVIIa/NovoSeven) in intractable haemorrhage: use of a clinical scoring system to predict outcome Vox Sang. Jan. 2006;90(1):45-52.

Boehlen F, Morales MA, Fontana P, Ricou B, Irion O. & deMoerloose P. (2004) Prolonged treatment of massive postpartum haemorrhage with recombinant factor VIIa: case report and review of the literature. BJOG. Mar. 2004;111(3):284-7.

Bomken C, Mathai S, Biss T, Loughney A. & Hanley J. (2009) Recombinant activated factor VII (rFVIIa) in the management of major obstetric haemorrhage: a case series and a proposed guideline for use. Obstet Gynecol Int. 2009:364843.

Bonnar J. (2000) Massive obstetric haemorrhage. Baillieres Best Pract Res Clin Obstet Gynaecol. Feb. 2000;14(1):1-18.

Bouwmeester FW, Jonkhoff AR, Verheijen RHM & van Geijn HP. (2003) Successful treatment of life-threatening postpartum hemorrhage with recombinant activated factor VII. Obstet Gynecol. Jun. 2003;101(6):1174-6.

Bouwmeester FW, Bolte AC. & van Geijn HP. (2005) Pharmacological and surgical therapy for primary postpartum hemorrhage. Curr Pharm Des. 2005;11(6):759-73.

Boyer-Neumann C, Dreyfus M, Wolf M, Veyradier A. Meyer D. (2003) Multi-therapeutic approach to manage delivery in an alloimmunized patient with type 3 von Willebrand disease J Thromb Haemost. Jan. 2003 ;1(1):190-2.

Breborowicz GH, Sobieszczyk S, Szymankiewicz M. (2002) Efficacy of recombinant activated factor VII (rFVIIa, NovoSeven) in prenatal medicine. ArchPerinatMed2002; 8:21–7.

Brueckner S, Sedemund-Adib B, Malik E, Heringlake M, Schmucker P, Diedrich K. (2001) Treatment of a post partum bleeding complication with recombinant factor VIIa. Blood 2001; 98:80.

Bueno S.R. (2007) Atlas of haemostasis. 2007; II:1-126.

Chauleur C, Fanget C, Tourne G, Levy R, Larchez C. & Seffert P. (2008) Serious primary postpartum hemorrhage, arterial embolization and future fertility: a retrospective study of 46 cases. Hum Reprod. Jul. 2008;23(7):1553-9.

Dabelea V, Schultze P.M. & McDuffie R.S. (2007) Intrauterine balloon tamponade in the management of postpartum hemorrhage Am J Perinatol. Jun.2007;24(6):359-64.

Dart BW, Cockerham WT, Torres C, Kipikasa JH. & Maxwell RA. (2004) A novel use of recombinant factor VIIa in HELLP syndrome associated with spontaneous hepatic rupture and abdominal compartment syndrome. J Trauma. Jul.2004;57(1):171-4.

Deneux-Tharaux C, Carmona E, Bouvier-Colle M.H. & Breart G. (2006) Postpartum maternal mortality and cesarean delivery. Obstet Gynecol. Sep. 2006;108(3 Pt 1):541-8.

Dutton RP, McCunn M, Hyder M, D'Angelo M, O'Connor J, Hess JR. & Scalea TM. (2004) Factor VIIa for correction of traumatic coagulopathy. J Trauma. Oct. 2004;57(4):709-18.

Eikelboom JW, Bird R, Blythe D, Coyle L, Gan E, Harvey M, Isbister J, Leahy M, McIlroy D, Rahimpanah F, Ramanthan S, Strasser S, Ward C, Watts A, Towler S. & Yi Q. (2003) Recombinant activated factor VII for the treatment of life-threatening haemorrhage Blood Coagul Fibrinolysis. Dec. 2003;14(8):713-7.

Eisele B, Lamy M. (1998) Clinical experience with antithrombin III concentrates in critically ill patients with sepsis and multiple organ failure. Semin Thromb Hemost. 1998;24(1):71-80.

El-Hamamy E, B-Lynch C. (2005) A worldwide review of the uses of the uterine compression suture techniques as alternative to hysterectomy in the management of severe postpartum hemorrhage. J Obstet Gynaecol. Feb.2005;25(2):143-149.

Eskandari N, Feldman N. & Greenspoon JS. (2002) Factor VII deficiency in pregnancy treated with recombinant factor VIIa. Obstet Gynecol. May.2002;99(5 Pt 2):935-7.

Franchini M, Zaffanello M. & Veneri D. (2005) Recombinant factor VIIa. An update on its clinical use. Thromb Haemost. Jun.2005;93(6):1027-35.

Franchini M, Lippi G. & Franchi M. (2007) The use of recombinant activated factor VII in obstetric and gynaecological haemorrhage. BJOG. Jan.2007;114(1):8-15.

Franchini M, Franchi M, Bergamini V, Salvagno GL, Montagnana M. & Lippi G. (2008) A critical review on the use of recombinant factor VIIa in life-threatening obstetric postpartum hemorrhage. Semin Thromb Hemost. Feb.2008;34(1):104-12.

Gabriel DA, Li X, Monroe DM 3rd & Roberts HR. (2004) Recombinant human factor VIIa (rFVIIa) can activate factor FIX on activated platelets. J Thromb Haemost. 2004 Oct;2(10):1816-22.

Ghorashian S, Hunt BJ. (2004) "Off-license" use of recombinant activated factor VII. Blood Rev. 2004 Dec;18(4):245-59.Transfusion. Sep.2004;44(9):1325-31.

Grotegut CA, Paglia MJ, Johnson LNC, Thames B. & James AH. (2011) Oxytocin exposure during labor among women with postpartum hemorrhage secondary to uterine atony. Am J Obstet Gynecol. Jan.2011;204(1):56.

Haynes J, Laffan M, & Plaat F. (2007) Use of recombinant activated factor VII in massive obstetric haemorrhage. Int J Obstet Anesth. Jan.2007;16(1):40-9.

Hedner U. (2001) Recombinant factor VIIa (Novoseven) as a hemostatic agent. Semin Hematol. Oct.2001;38(4 Suppl 12):43-7.

Hedner U, Erhardtsen E. (2002) Potential role for rFVIIa in transfusion medicine. Transfusion. Jan.2002;42(1):114-24.

Hedner U. (2003) Recombinant factor VIIa (NovoSeven) as a hemostatic agent. Dis Mon. Jan.2003;49(1):39-48.

Henrich W., Surbek D., Kainer F., Grottke O, Hopp H, Kiesewetter H, Koscielny J, Maul H, Schlembach D, von Tempelhoff GF. & Rath W. (2008) Diagnosis and treatment of peripartum bleeding. // J Perinat. Med. - 2008; 36(6):467-78.

Hoffman M, Monroe DM. & Roberts HR. (1998) Activated Factor VII activates Factor IX and X on surface of activated platelets: thoughts on the mechanism of action of high-dose activated Factor VII. Blood Coagul Fibrinolysis. Mar.1998;9 Suppl 1:S61-5.

Hoffman M. (2003) A cell-based model of haemostasis. Blood Rev. Sep.2003;17 Suppl 1:S1-5.

Hollnberger H, Gruber E. & Seelbach GB. (2005) Major post-partum hemorrhage and treatment with recombinant factor VIIa. Anesth Analg. Dec.2005;101(6):1886-7.

Holub Z, Feyereisl J, Kabelik L. & Rittstein T. (2005) Successful treatment of severe post-partum bleeding after caesarean section using recombinant activated factor VII. Ceska Gynekol. Mar.2005;70(2):144, 146-8.

Hossain N, Shamsi T, Haider S, Soomro N, Khan NH, Memon GU, Farzana T, Ansari S, Triche EW, Kuczynski E, Lockwood CJ. & Paidas MJ. (2007) Use of recombinant activated factor VII for massive postpartum haemorrhage. Acta Obstet Gynecol Scand. Aug. 2007; 29:1-7.

Irion O, Terraz S, Boulvain M, Boehlen F. & Becker CD. (2008) Postpartum hemmorhage: prevention and treatment by arterial embolization and activated recombinant factor VII. Rev Med Suisse. Oct.2008; 22;4(176):2269-2270.

Jansen A, van Rhenen D, Steegers E. & Duvekot J. (2005) Postpartum hemorrhage and transfusion of blood components. Obstet Gynekol Surv. Okt.2005;60(10):663-71.

Jimenez-Yuste V, Villar A, Morado M, Canales M, Hernandez MC, Sanjurjo MJ, Quintana M. & Hernбndez-Navarro F. (2000) Continuous infusion of recombinant activated factor VII during caesarean section delivery in a patient with congenital factor VII deficiency. Haemophilia. Sep.2000;6(5):588-90.

Jurlander B, Thim L, Klausen NK, Persson E, Kjalke M, Rexen P, Jшrgensen TB, Шstergaard PB, Erhardtsen E. & Bjшrn SE. (2001) Recombinant activated factor VII (rFVIIa): characterization, manufacturing and clinical development. Semin Thromb Hemost. Aug.2001;27(4):373-84.

Kale A, Bayhan G, Yalinkaya A. & Yayla M. (2004) The use of recombinant factor VIIa in a primigravida with Glanzmann's thrombasthenia during delivery. J Perinat Med. 2004;32(5):456-8.

Kessler CM. (2000) New products for managing inhibitors to coagulation factors: a focus on recombinant factor VIIa concentrate. Curr Opin Hematol. Nov.2000;7(6):408-13.

Kretzschmar M, Zahm DM, Remmler K, Pfeiffer L, Victor L. & Schirmeister W. (2003) Pathophysiological and therapeutic aspects of amniotic fluid embolism (anaphylactoid syndrome of pregnancy): case report with lethal outcome and overview. Anaesthesist. May.2003;52(5):419-26.

LaBelle C, Kitchens CS. (2007) Disseminated Intravascular Coagulation, Chapter 12, in Kitchens CS, Alving BM, Kessler CM, eds, in Consultative Hemostasis and Thrombosis, ed 2, Elsevier, Philadelphia, 2007:183-209.

Lim Y, Loo CC, Chia V. & Fun W. (2004) Recombinant factor VIIa after amniotic fluid embolism and disseminated intravascular coagulopathy. Int J Gynaecol Obstet. Nov. 2004;87(2):178-9.

Lisman T, De Groot PG. (2003) Mechanism of action of recombinant factor VIIa. J Thromb Haemost. Jun. 2003;1(6):1138-9.

Lusher JM, Roberts HR, Davignon G, Joist JH, Smith H, Shapiro A, Laurian Y, Kasper CK. & Mannucci PM. (1998) A randomized, double-blind comparison of two doses of recombinant factor VIIa in the treatment of joint, muscle and mucocutaneous haemorrhages in persons with haemophilia A and B, with and without inhibitors. rFVIIa Study Group. Haemophilia. Nov. 1998;4(6):790-8.

Macphail S, Talks K. (2004) Massive post-partum haemorrhage and management of disseminated intravascular coagulation Curr Obstet Gynaecol 2004; 14 (2) : 123–131.

Make Every Mother and Child count: the World Health Report. - Geneva: WHO, 2005:219.

Mittal S, Watson H. G. (2006) A critical appraisal of the use of recombinant factor VIIa in acquired bleeding conditions. Br J Haematol. May. 2006;133(4):355-63.

Monroe DM, Hoffman M, Oliver JA. & Roberts HR. (1997) Platelet activity of high-dose factor VIIa is independent of tissue factor. Br J Haematol. Dec.1997;99(3):542-7.

Moscardo F, Perez F, de la Rubia J, Balerdi B, Lorenzo JI, Senent ML, Aznar I, Carceller S. & Sanz MA. (2001) Successful treatment of severe intra-abdominal bleeding associated with disseminated intravascular coagulation using recombinant activated factor VII. Br J Haematol. Jul.2001;114(1):174-6.

Mousa H.A, Walkinshaw S. (2001) Major postpartum haemorrhage // Curr Opin Obstet Gynecol. Dec.2001;13(6):595-603.

Mousa HA, Alfirevic Z. (2003) Treatment of primary postpartum haemorrhage. Cochrane Rev 2003:CD003249.

Mousa HA, Alfirevic Z. (2007) Treatment for primary postpartum haemorrhage. Cochrane Rev 2007, 1:CD 003249.

Murkin JM. (2009) Efficacy of recombinant activated Factor VII in patients with massive uncontrolled bleeding: a retrospective observational analysis. Transfusion. Mar.2009;49(3):570-7.

Negrier C, Hay CR (2000) The treatment of bleeding in hemophilic patients with inhibitors with recombinant factor VIIa. Semin Thromb Hemost. 2000;26(4):407-12.

Nowacka E, Krawczynska-Wichrzycka R, Teliga-Czajkowska J, Czajkowski K, Mayzner-Zawadzka E, Schubert W, et al. (2005) Recombinant factor VIIa for severe bleeding during cesarean section for quadruplet pregnancy. Anest Intens Ter 2005; 37:259–62.

O'Leary, J. A. (1995) Uterine artery ligation in the control of postcesarean hemorrhage. J Reprod Med. Mar.1995;40(3):189-93.

O'Connell NM., Perry DJ, Hodgson AJ, O'Shaughnessy DF, Laffan M. A. & Smith OP. (2003) Recombinant FVIIa in the management of uncontrolled hemorrhage. Transfusion. Dec.2003;43(12):1711-6.

O'Connell KA, Wood JJ, Wise RP, Lozier JN. & Braun MM. (2006) Thromboembolic adverse events after use of recombinant human coagulation factor VIIa. JAMA. 2006 Jan.18;295(3):293-8.

Ohkuchi A, Onagawa T, Usui R, Koike T, Hiratsuka M, Izumi A, Ohkusa T, Matsubara S, Sato I, Suzuki M. & Minakami H. (2003) Effect of maternal age on blood loss during parturition: a retrospective multivariate analysis of 10,053 cases. J Perinat Med.2003;31(3):209-15.

Opal SM, Kessler CM, Roemisch J. & Knaub S. (2002) Antithrombin, heparin, and heparan sulfate. Crit Care Med. May.2002;30(5 Suppl):S325-31.

Palomino MA, Chaparro MJ, de Elvira MJ. & Curiel EB. (2006) Recombinant activated factor VII in the management of massive obstetric bleeding. Blood Coagul Fibrinolysis. Apr.2006;17(3):226-7.

Papp Z, Tyth-P6l E, Papp C, Sziller I, G6vai M. & Silhavy M, Hupuczi P. (206) Hypogastric artery ligation for intractable pelvic hemorrhage. Int J Gynaecol Obstet. Jan.2006;92(1):27-31

Penninx JPM., Pasmans HLM. & Oei SG. (2010) Arterial balloon occlusion of the internal iliac arteries for treatment of life-threatening massive postpartum haemorrhage: a series of 15 consecutive cases. Eur J Obstet Gynecol Reprod Biol. Feb.2010;148(2):131-4.

Pepas LP, Arif-Adib M, & Kadir RA. (2006) Factor VIIa in puerperal hemorrhage with disseminated intravascular coagulation. Obstet Gynecol. Sep.2006;108(4, Part 2):757-761.

Phillips LE, McLintock C, Pollock W, Gatt S, Popham P, Jankelowitz G, Ogle R. & Cameron PA. (2009) Recombinant activated factor VII in obstetric hemorrhage: experiences from the Australian and New Zealand haemostasis registry. Anesth Analg. Dec.2009;109(6):1908-15.

Practical hemostasis and thrombosis. / Ed. by O'Shaughnessy D, Makris M, Lillicrap D. // Blackwell Publishing Ltd, 2005.- 224 p.

Price G, Kaplan J. & Skowronski G. (2004) Use of recombinant factor VIIa to treat life-threatening non-surgical bleeding in a post-partum patient. Br J Anaesth. Aug.2004;93(2):298-300.

Price N., B-Lynch C. (2005) Technical description of the B-Lynch brace suture for treatment of massive postpartum hemorrhage and review of published cases. Int J Fertil Womens Med. Jul-Aug.2005;50(4):148-63.

Ramanathan G., Arulkumaran S. (2006) Postpartum hemorrhage. // J Obstet Gynaecol Can Nov.2006;28(11):967-73.

Reynders FC, Senten L, Tjaima W. & Jacquemyn Y. (2006) Postpartum hemorrhage: practical approach to a life-threatening complication. Clin Exp Obstet Gynecol. 2006;33:81–84.

Roberts HR, Monroe DM. & White GC. (2004) The use of recombinant factor VIIa in the treatment of bleeding disorders. Blood. 2004 Dec 15;104(13):3858-64.

Royal College of Obstetricians and Gynaecologists UK (2009). Prevention and management of postpartum haemorrhage (Green-top Guideline) No. 52; May 2009:1-24.

Rublee D, Opal SM, Schramm W, Keinecke HO. & Knaub S. (2002) Quality of life effects of antithrombin III in sepsis survivors: results from the KyberSept trial. Crit Care. Aug.2002;6(4):349-56.

Schouten M, Wiersinga WJ, Levi M, Poll T (2008) Inflammation, endotelium, and coagulation in sepsis. J Leukoc Biol 2008, 83:536-545.

Segal S, Shemesh IY, Blumental R, Yoffe B, Laufer N, Mankuta D, Mazor M, Zohar S, Schiff E. & Martinovitz U. (2004) The use of recombinant factor VIIa in severe postpartum hemorrhage. Acta Obstet Gynecol Scand. Aug.2004;83(8):771-2.

Selo-Ojeme DO, Okonofua FE. (1997) Risk factors for primary postpartum haemorrhage. A case control study. Arch Gynecol Obstet. 1997;259(4):179-87.

Sentilhes L, Gromez A, Razzouk K. Resch B, Verrspyck E. & Marpeau L. (2008) B-Lynch suture for massive persistent postpartum hemorrhage following stepwise uterine devascularization Acta Obstet Gynecol Scand. Oct.2008;87(10):1020-6.

Schwartz RS, Bauer KA, Rosenberg RD, Kavanaugh EJ, Davies DC, Bogdanoff DA. (1989) Clinical experience with antithrombin III concentrate in treatment of congenital and aquired deficiency of antithrombin. Am J Med. 1989 Sep 11;87(3B):53-60.

Sentilhes L., Gomez A., Tricot C. et al. (2009) Fertility after B-Lynch suture and stepwise uterine devascularization. Fertil Steril. Mar.2009;91(3):934.

Shamsi TS, Hossain N, Soomro N, Hasan JA, Noorani M, Kazi S, Quraishy MS, Jameel B, Sultan ST. & Haider S. (2005) Use of recombinant factor VIIa for massive postpartum haemorrhage: case series and review of literature. J Pak Med Assoc. 2005 Nov;55(11):512-5.

Shander A, Goodnough LT, Ratko T et al. (2005) Consensus recommendations for the off-label use of recombinant human factor VIIa (NovoSeven) therapy. Pharma Ther 2005; 30: 644.

Shapiro AD, Gilchrist GS, Hoots WK, Cooper HA. & Gastineau DA. (1998) Prospective, randomised trial of two doses of rFVIIa (NovoSeven) in haemophilia patients with inhibitors undergoing surgery. Thromb Haemost. Nov.1998;80(5):773-8.

Sheiner E, Sarid L, Levy A, Seidman DS. & Hallak M. (2005) Obstetric risk factors and outcome of pregnancies complicated with early postpartum hemorrhage: a population-based study. J Matern Fetal Neonatal Med. 2005 Sep;18(3):149-54.

Smith K.L., Baskett T.F. (2003) Uterine compression sutures as an alternative to hysterectomy for severe postpartum hemorrhage. J Obstet Gynaecol Can. Mar.2003;25(3):197-200.

Sobieszczyk S, Breborowicz GH, Markwitz W, Mallinger S, Adamski D. & Kruszycski Z. (2002) Effect of recombinant activated factor VII (RFVIIA; NovoSeven) in a patient in haemorrhagic shock after obstetrical hysterectomy. Ginekol Pol. Mar.2002;73(3):230-3.

Sobieszczyk S, Breborowicz GH. (2004) Management recommendations for postpartum hemorrhage. Arch Perinat Med 2004; 10:1–4.

Sobieszczyk S, Breborowicz GH, Platicanov V, Tanchev S. & Kessler CM. (2006) Recombinant factor VIIa in the management of postpartum bleeds: an audit of clinical use. Acta Obstet Gynecol Scand. 2006;85(10):1239-47.

Sobieszczyk S, Breborowicz GH. The use of recombinant factor VIIa in A Textbook of Post Partum Hemorrhage (ed C. B-Lynch et al.). Sapiens Publishing 2006:250.

Sokolic V, Bukovic D, Fures R, Zadro M, Scuric I, Colak F, Celovec K. & Вожан A. (2002) Recombinant factor VIIa (rFVIIa) is effective at massive bleeding after cesarean section—a case report. Coll Antropol. Dec.2002;26 Suppl:155-7.

Tanchev S, Platikanov V. & Karadimov D. (2005) Administration of recombinant factor VIIa for the management of massive bleeding due to uterine atonia in the post-placental period. Acta Obstet Gynecol Scand. Apr.2005;84(4):402-3.

The Department of Health. Why mothers die. A report on confidential enquiries into maternal deaths in the UK 2000–2002. (2004) Confidential Enquiry into maternal and child health. - London: RCOG Press; 2004.

Uhlmann EJ, Eby CS. (2004) Recombinant activated factor VIII for non-hemophiliac bleeding patients. Curr Opin Hematol. May.2004;11(3):198-204.

Vedantham S, Goodwin SC, McLucas B. & Mohr G. (1997) Uterine artery embolization: an underused method of controlling pelvic hemorrhage. Am J Obstet Gynecol. Apr.1997;176(4):938-48.

Verre M, Bossio F, Mammone A, Piccirillo M, Tancioni F. & Varano M. (2006) Use of recombinant activated factor VII in a case of severe postpartum haemorrhage. Minerva Ginecol. Feb.2006;58(1):81-4.

Vinazzer H.A. Antitrombin III in shock and disseminated intravascular coagulation. Clin. Appl. Thromb. Haemost. 1995;1:62-65.

Vincent JL, Rossaint R, Riou B, Ozier Y, Zideman D, Spahn DR. (2006) Recommendations on the use of recombinant activated factor VII as an adjunctive treatment for massive bleeding—a European perspective. Crit Care. 2006;10(4):R120.

Welsh A, McLintock C, Gatt S, Somerset D, Popham P, Ogle R. (2008) Guidelines for the use of recombinant activated factor VII in massive obstetric haemorrhage. Aust N Z J Obstet Gynaecol. Feb.2008;48(1):12-6.

WHO Guidelines for the Management of Postpartum Haemorrhage and Retained Placenta. World Health Organization. - Geneva: WHO, 2009

Zupancic SS, Sokolic V, Viskovic T, Sanjug J, Simic M, Kastelan M. (2002) Successful use of recombinant factor VIIa for massive bleeding after cesarean section due to HELLP syndrome. Acta Haematol. 2002;108(3):162-3.

Part 3

Hysterectomy Pre-Operative Considerations

15

Hysterectomy: Advances in Perioperative Care

Kenneth Jensen and Jens Børglum
Copenhagen University Hospital: Bispebjerg, Denmark

1. Introduction

1.1 Perioperative medicine

Perioperative medicine is an ever growing field of interest that encompasses the care of the patient preparing for, undergoing and recuperating from surgery. Medical professionals, interest groups and societies each year convene at congresses dedicated to the field of evidence-based perioperative medicine (e.g., www.ebpom.org). Since many interventions during the hospital stay have ramifications extending into the first six months after discharge, many choose to define "perioperative" broadly to include this extended period as well. Our topics of interest are equally broadly defined and include psychological, physiological, anaesthesiological and surgical issues. We have chosen this overview to increase our understanding of the interplay of factors that in all make up the experience of the hysterectomy patients, hopefully to explain and justify the value of treatment regimens.

1.2 Purpose and methods

Much has happened within the past 10 years. In spite of an ever-growing and unwieldy amount of scientific information appearing every month, unmet needs may still be readily identified in many fields of endeavor. To highlight the current evidence, we have performed a Medline search on "hysterectomy" limited to randomized studies published in the past decade. This should expand the evidence-based website www.postoppain.org, which provides an analysis of all randomized studies on abdominal hysterectomy since 1966 (and until 2004). Our aim is to provide the anaesthesia-unqualified reader with an extensive and easily accessible presentation of the psychology, physiology, pharmacology and operative logistics that we find relevant to the subject of hysterectomy; characteristics of the patients, the importance of anaesthetic and surgical techniques, the prevention and treatment of postoperative complaints, and why established treatments may not work. While not striving to be completely exhaustive, our review nevertheless includes a thorough reference list that may inspire the reader to further in-depth study.

2. Psychology

2.1 Preoperative psychology and coping skills

Understandably, undergoing surgery is often the cause of great concern for patients. We know that as many as 60% of patients are anxious (Hashimato, 1993), with females, depressed and patients in pain being particularly prone (Caumo, 2002; Karanci, 2003). This anxiety is caused by uncertainty/lack of information about what is going to happen and an existential component (Caumo, 2002; Sjölin, 2003). While uncertainties about oncoming events may be reduced by relevant information and proper expectations, existential anxieties are often resistant to intervention (Kain, 2001). Studies have shown that most patients are scared of thoughts of the unknown, severe pain, nausea and vomiting, or imminent death (Kindler, 2000). Previous experiences and personality usually dictate the style and ability of coping and dealing with serious life events such as surgery. Studies using the Spielberger State and Trait Anxiety Index (Johnson, 1968) or the Amsterdam Preoperative Anxiety and Information Scale (Moerman, 1996) have documented that particular personality structures and coping skills of the patient are in part responsible for the intensity and duration of postoperative pain, with subsequent self-imposed limitations to mobilization and restoration of normal activities (Riddle, 2010). Such psychological traits may in fact be so strong that they overshadow effective pain treatment (Maranets, 1999; Caumo, 2002; Kalkman, 2003). Neurologically, the interaction between the amygdala (fear-avoidance centre), the frontal cortex (centre of experience and value-setting), and the nucleus accumbens (reward centre) are pivotal, all of which are influenced by personality, obesity, alcoholism, depressive disorders and more (Di Chiara, 2002). The personality structure that is most reliably used is the five factor model (Big Five Inventory) which uses five independent personality measures (openness to change, conscientiousness, extroversion, agreeableness, and neuroticism) (Digman, 1990). The variability of these measures is dynamic, and at least three measures rapidly change following surgery: patients become less open to changes, more introvert, and more negative in thought. These changes lead to distorted and inefficient coping skills, depressive or defeatist mood swings, and catastrophizing (imagining unlikely and potentially catastrophic events from simple and harmless signs and symptoms). These emotions are strong and overwhelming and must be addressed in order to secure a return to postoperative well-being.

2.2 The impact on postoperative well-being

Preoperative pain or depression may be seen in as many as 50% (Davies, 2002). In a study on chronic pain following hysterectomy, most patients having pain at four months after surgery had pain that resembled the preoperative pain; preoperative "pain problems elsewhere" and strong acute postoperative pain were associated with the development of chronic pain, again emphasizing the psychological dimension (Brandsborg, 2009). Women with preoperative depression and pain had 3 to 5 times the odds of continued impaired quality of life for both physical function, mental health, social function and dyspareunia, compared to those who did not have depression or pain (Hartmann, 2004). The extent (subtotal vs total hysterectomy) or method (laparoscopic vs abdominal) of surgery does not seem to influence these long-term effects (Thakar, 2004; Flory, 2006). Most studies support a general increase in psychosocial well-being at 6 months following surgery (Davies, 2002; Persson, 2010), and it is worth noting that this long-term well-being does not seem to be associated with perioperative complications or hormone disturbances (Persson, 2010).

2.3 Long-term psychological effects following hysterectomy

Women undergoing hysterectomy are in a particularly difficult position, since surgery may alter both their perception of body image and sexuality, and impose hormonal changes after oophorectomy with surgical menopause. As a case in point, quality-of-life estimates are clearly rated as worse by a surgical menopause than by a natural menopause (Bhattacharya, 2010). Surgical menopause also adversely affects perceptions of body image and sleep quality at six months compared to ovarian conservation surgery (Teplin, 2007). Women who undergo prophylactic oophorectomy in addition to hysterectomy are found to have higher anxiety-related scores, lower sexuality scores and poorer emotional partner relationships (Aziz, 2005). In terms of sexual function, extent of surgery (subtotal vs total hysterectomy) does not seem to affect overall sexual activity, but total hysterectomy does reduce the perception of body image at one year (Gorlero, 2008). Recently, however, some have found that women who had subtotal hysterectomy report significantly greater positive change in the frequency of orgasm and sexual pleasure than women who have had total hysterectomy (Ellström, 2010). Method of surgery (laparoscopic vs vaginal vs abdominal) yields conflicting results on the influence on sexual activity (Ellström, 2003; Roovers, 2003). Women having abdominal hysterectomy may be dissatisfied with their body image because of the abdominal scar (Gütl, 2002). Quality of life following hysterectomy for malignant reasons seems to be affected even stronger: sexual function worsens considerably, regardless of surgical technique (Serati, 2009). Anxiety and depression following surgery for cervical cancer is commonly associated with financial difficulty, poor body image, sexual inactivity, and low existential well-being. Low support and insomnia are related to anxiety, with older age and decrement role function related to depression (Kim, 2010). These substantial effects seem to cling to an inherent personality profile rather than disease-related clinical factors.

2.4 Prevention and treatment of anxiety and its effects

Trait and existential anxiety seem to be resistant to preventive informational or cognitive interventions. Procedure-specific concerns, however, lend themselves to several psychological og medical approaches (Caumo, 2002). A preoperative 24-minute videotape of a nurse showing breathing and movement skills with four postoperative mobility activities (The Foster Pain Intervention) reduces pain, increases mobility, preoperative self-efficacy and speeds up home readiness more than a control group receiving standard information (Heye, 2002). Cognitive interventions using distraction and reappraisal combined with information are associated with lower postoperative anxiety, less pain and higher levels of satisfaction (Cheung, 2003). Therapeutic touch may be equally effective (Vitale, 2006). Intraoperative music is associated with increased levels of sedation and satisfaction (Zhang, 2005). Patient-carer interactions using negative words on the surgical wards has significant influence on pain in the early postoperative period by increasing pain, opioid consumption and stress hormone levels, whereas positive words or no words at all has little influence (Wang, 2008). These studies again underline the importance of optimal information-handling, pragmatic instructions, simple psychological interventions and decent patient-carer interactions as the basic premise for the prevention of postoperative complaints following hysterectomy. It makes perfect sense to identify beforehand the psychological traits that predispose to inappropriate coping abilities, exaggerated pain processing and distorted body image perceptions, since they seem to share similar psychological profiles (Persson, 2008).

3. Pharmacology

3.1 Opioid-free analgesia

Opioid-free analgesia has long been considered the holy grail of pain treatment. Opioids reduce nociceptive signal processing in the spinal cord and central nervous system by acting on, among others, the μ receptor. The analgesic potential for blockade of this receptor is limitless, and the mode of administration of an opioid is largely independent of its efficacy. No other type of drug has a similar potential, and for this reason, opioids are of immense value. Opioids are widely distributed and are subsequently found in most compartments of the body by any route of administration. In terms of analgesic effect, no strong opioid is superior to any other; their only differences rest in mode of administration, dosage and duration of action (Macintyre, 2010). Surgical stress and analgesic efficacy during and after abdominal hysterectomy proceeds regardless of the opioid used (Rodriguez, 2007); one report argues that morphine in combination with the weak opioid tramadol may confer better postoperative pain scores than morphine alone (Kocabas, 2005), but the result should be replicated before firm conclusions can be made. Spinal morphine seems to attenuate several measures of the surgical stress response, in particular serum values of catecholamines and glucose (Karaman, 2006). However, preoperative intravenous morphine fails to attenuate the stress response measured by serum cortisol, glucose and leukocytes (Kilickan, 2001); the socalled "preemptive effect" has been largely abandoned in clinical life because many studies fail to document better pain relief when opioids are administered preoperatively than postoperatively, even though studies appear from time to time arguing the case of preemptive analgesia from the viewpoint of minor effects on immune function, parameters which may be clinically redundant (Akural, 2002; Akural, 2004).

3.2 Opioid side effects and preventive strategies

In terms of side effects, however, opioids do have differences, primarily due to pharmacokinetics (administration, distribution, metabolism, excretion), where the most basic opioid, morphine, may accumulate metabolites that are neurotoxic under certain conditions such as renal insufficiency, advanced age or immense doses (Murphy, 2005). The quest for opioid-free analgesia, however, stems from the autonomic side effects of the drugs: impaired cognitive function, dizziness, sedation bordering on coma; respiratory depression and apnoe; nausea, vomiting and increased gastrointestinal sphincter contraction causing obstipation; urinary bladder paralysis, pruritus and excessive sweating. Many of these side effects occur at random and with different intensities, but they all counteract the primary content of recuperation: eating, drinking, passing urine, defecating and ambulating. All opioids act similarly in this respect, and although side effects usually occur at higher doses than analgesic effects, they still remain a major clinical problem which render many patients helpless, unable to get out of bed, with the subsequent risk of more severe complications such as hypoxia, pneumonia, deep venous thrombosis, pulmonary embolism, ileus and decubitus. The apparent discord between the obvious need for opioids and the abhorred side effects have led clinicians to try various methods of alleviating opioid-related side effects: 1) the combination of intravenous morphine with a μ-receptor antagonist such as naloxone by patient-controlled analgesia (PCA) has been largely disappointing (Sartain, 2003; Zhao, 2005); 2) a similar combination using a μ-receptor antagonist, alvimopan, with limited oral bioavailibility (thus only acting in the GI tract) has fared better and has been shown to improve tolerance to solid foods, time to first bowel movement and passage of stool, although the magnitude of improvements were moderate (Herzog, 2006; Tan, 2007); 3) the use of simple osmotic laxatives have been shown to reduce time to first defecation from 69 to 45 hours with subsequent early hospital discharge (Hansen, 2007); 4) early postoperative oral intake seems to be superior to delayed intake by reducing time to first solid diet, presence of bowel sounds, and shorter hospital stay, at the expense of slightly increased nausea (Charoenkwan, 2007); 5) the combination of intravenous morphine with butorphanol reduces opioid requirements and some opioid-related side effects, but causes sedation, sweating and dry mouth (Wang, 2009); 6) the combination with nalbuphine, a mixed opioid agonist-antagonist, also seems to attenuate opioid-related nausea, but other opioid-related side effects remain unchanged (Yeh, 2009); 7) the omission of a background rate of infusion of morphine for intravenous patient-controlled analgesia (PCA) seems to reduce overall morphine consumption, reduce nausea, vomiting and dizziness but, again, other opioid-related side effects remain unchanged (Chen, 2011); 8) intravenous oxycodone seems to cause less opioid-related sedation than intravenous morphine, but other side effects are similar, suggesting a difference caused by stochastic variation (Lenz, 2009).

3.3 Gender-specific pharmacogenetics

Variations between opioids aside, even more pronounced differences may be found between individuals in terms of pharmacokinetics and, in particular, pharmacodynamics. In the past decade, research has given us a great amount of knowledge on the genetic disposition that explains these differences, and to what extent people react differently to pain. The opioid receptor and its determining gene (OPRM1) has been shown to have 17 variations (socalled polymorhism) that are unequally distributed between the sexes (Samer, 2010; Kolesnikov, 2011). Women are found to have μ receptor variations that predispose to longer clinical effects of an opioid, and twice as many side effects as men (Sarton, 2003; Niesters, 2010). In a study on A118G polymorphisms, patients homozygous for G118 required more morphine doses to achieve adequate pain relief compared with patients homozygous for A118 (Chou, 2006). Furthermore, the experience of pain may be unevenly distributed. Women experience more pain than men, and even among women major differences in the tolerance to each pain modality exist. Studies that address these variations suggest that at least six modalities may be identified (Lariviere, 2002; Hastie, 2005). The clinical relevance is enormous because several modalities of pain are at work following hysterectomy: nociceptive, ischaemic, pressure, temporal, neurogenic, chemical/irritative. The individual contribution of each pain modality may be difficult to assess in a particular patient, but each patient will react to certain pain sensations according to her particular sensitivity. Investigations into other postoperative complaints are also emerging and seem to share similar gender differences. These gender differences may include the actions of commonly used drugs for intraoperative sedation and pain relief, causing prolonged sedative effects and ill health in the post-anaesthesia care unit (Jensen, 2009).

4. Physiology

4.1 Physiological changes during surgery

Acute physiological changes during surgery are determined by the disposition and preoperative state of the patient, the type and depth of anaesthesia, and the surgical technique. Important preoperative patient factors include heart and lung function, body mass index, metabolic disorders, concurrent medications or alcohol, and level of hydration; such factors determine the mechanistic vascular responses to surgery and the sensitivity to drugs, fluids and body positioning. Serious complications include hypotension, bradycardia, atelectasis, hypoxia and awareness, all of which may be adequately prevented and treated. Particular interest should be paid to surgical techniques involving laparoscopy. Pneumoperitoneum increases intraabdominal pressure and, either alone or with Trendelenburg positioning, may increase/decrease cardiac preload, increase cardiac afterload, reduce pulmonary volumes, decrease functional residual capacity and increase closing volume. This may lead to circulatory instability, atelectases and hypoxia (Strang, 2009; Hedenstierna, 2010). Oxygenation may be considerably improved by alveolar recruitment maneuvres and positive end-expiratory pressure, and these measures are considered mandatory for pulmonary protection (Park, 2009). The immune system seems resistant to most types of anaesthesia. Metabolic changes such as cortisol rise is more pronounced in vaginal than laparoscopic surgery, although stress response with catecholamine levels are high in both types of surgery (Lattermann, 2001). Laparotomy is associated with increased levels of C-reactive protein, creatine phosphokinase and lactic dehydrogenase compared to laparoscopic-assisted vaginal technique, corresponding to the greater amount of tissue damage inflicted; these immunological differences are in turn reflected in clinically useful measures such as length of stay (Atabekoglu, 2004). Although the clinical value remains controversial, preoperative epidural blockade may in fact attenuate interleukin levels associated with the inflammatory response after abdominal hysterectomy (Beilin, 2003).

4.2 Anaesthetic technique

The type of anaesthesia is highly variable between surgical centres and is in a limited way dictated by type of surgery. General anaesthesia is the preferred method, with supplemental epidural analgesia, perineural or infiltrative analgesia when major postoperative pain is anticipated. Spinal anaesthesia may be an alternative for abdominal or vaginal hysterectomy allowing for less postoperative morphine demands, but the use of intrathecal morphine also includes more postoperative itching (Sprung, 2006; Massicotte, 2009; Wodlin, 2011). Fast-track programmes using spinal anaesthesia with intrathecal morphine may even be associated with improved quality of life measures several weeks after surgery compared to general anaesthesia, because even minor complications adversely affect the mental component of quality of life and duration of sick leave (Ottesen, 2002; Penketh, 2007; Wodlin, 2011). General anaesthesia counteracts the cardiovascular effects of the physiological stress response by dilating peripheral vasculature, reducing cardiac output, blood pressure and heart rate in a dose-dependent fashion. Metabolic responses to surgery are, however, largely unaffected by sedative agents alone, and in order to suppress these responses as well, opioids or neuraxial anaesthesia should be used (Demirbilek, 2004; Hong, 2008; Ihn, 2009). Sedation is almost always combined with an efficient intraoperative opioid, and all opioids may in principle be adequate; controllability of dosage and effect is the primary concern for the clinician. Level of sleep may be estimated by bispectral index monitoring, although some controversy exists regarding the applicability and usefulness of its largely unknown algorithm for interpreting depth of anaesthesia (Meyhoff, 2009). Autonomic signs such as hypertension, tachycardia, pupil dilation, sweating and reflex movement are useless for identifying patients that may be partially awake and at risk of awareness. A particular side effect of inhalational anaesthesia is the increased risk of postoperative nausea and vomiting (PONV), suggesting that intravenous drugs may be preferable. Propofol may in itself be antiemetic. The decision between inhalational anaesthesia and TIVA does, however, remain difficult. Studies comparing the two anaesthetic methods are equivocal, with a tendency towards superiority in the TIVA groups in terms of less nausea and earlier start of oral fluid intake (Fassoulaki, 2008; Kroon, 2010). A recent study suggests that deep levels of intraoperative sedation (as measured by auditory evoked potentials) may reduce postoperative morphine demands (Henneberg, 2005). It was conducted using TIVA, but it remains unknown if a similar relationship may be seen with inhalational agents. This would justify a more widespread use of monitoring devices for depth of sedation.

4.3 Epidural blockade as an adjuvant technique

The use of an adjuvant epidural has had strong support for many years. It reduces surgical stress response, reduces sedative requirements (Morley, 2002), shortens length of stay in the post-anaesthesia care unit (Jensen, 2009) and may serve as route of administration for other adjuvant drugs beside local anaesthetics and opioids. Duration or quality of analgesia has been shown to be increased by the addition of butorphanol (Bharti, 2009), magnesium (Farouk, 2008) or clonidine (Topcu, 2005). The combination of epidural local anaesthetics with opioids does however remain a basic requirement (Niiyama, 2005), and epidural opioids carry with them an increased risk of gastric paresis, obstipation, nausea and bladder paresis. Furthermore, while the use of an epidural may reduce pain and opioid demands, it seems to have only limited effects on gastrointestinal function and patient recovery (Jørgensen, 2001). In conclusion, the epidural technique has several shortcomings as an adjuvant technique and does not convincingly seem to solve the basic clinical problems in the immediate postoperative period.

4.4 Surgical technique

The type of surgery probably has the greatest impact on the physiological changes during surgery. Many of these are expected from a mechanistic point of view in relation to Trendelenburg positioning, increased abdominal pressure, variations in cardiac preload and afterload, positive pressure ventilation, fluid therapy and depth of anaesthesia, but some are also infrequent. They include hypothermia, deep vein thrombosis, cardiac arhythmias, circulatory collapse from sympathetic trunk block and metabolic changes during surgical stress response. The choice between surgical techniques is often made by the surgeon in conference with the patient, but the reasons are often unclear. From the view of an anaesthesiologist, only in the past few years do we have strong scientific support for the effect of surgical technique on postoperative complaints. It seems evident that a minimally invasive technique using laparoscopy and/or vaginal approach is superior to laparotomy, in terms of less postoperative pain, less morphine demand, shorter duration of bladder catheterisation, better immune function, length of stay in hospital, and measures of postoperative vitality (Ribeiro, 2003; Garry, 2004; Ghezzi, 2010; Naik, 2010). Minilaparotomy has similar advantages to ordinary laparotomy (Sharma, 2004). Laparoscopic technique seems superior to vaginal approach in terms of reduced postoperative pain and length of stay in hospital (Candiani, 2009). Recent advances such as single-port-access laparoscopy techniques may reduce pain scores even further (Kim, 2010). The extent of surgery (subtotal vs total hysterectomy) does not seem to affect short-term or long-term recovery (Lethaby, 2006; Persson, 2010).

5. Pain and discomfort

5.1 Management of postoperative pain

A complete list of randomized trials investigating the analgesic value of pharmacological and psychological interventions in abdominal hysterectomy is available at the website by the Prospect Research Group (www.postoppain.org). The site covers the entire period 1966-2004, with additions into 2006 for some drugs, and a complete reference list is available. An extracted summary of the available procedure-specific evidence has been derived in Table 1, but caution should be observed in taking information at face value. With the advent of new, minimally invasive surgical techniques, thoughts about laparotomy procedures may be posthoc. It may only represent our abilities to attenuate problems caused by the most traumatic surgical technique possible, and it may not be up-to-date in regard to the spectrum of currently available analgesic techniques. This chapter therefore warrants some notes on developments in pain management that have taken place within the last few years.

Intervention	Preoperative	Intraoperative	Postoperative
Intravenous/oral opioids	0	2	2
Intravenous/oral NSAIDS or coxibs	0-1	2	2
Oral gapabentin or pregabalin	2	?	2
Oral/rectal/intravenous paracetamol	1	?	1
Intravenous tramadol	?	?	1
Intravenous ketamine	0	0-1	1
Epidural local anaesthetics	0-1	2	1-2
Epidural ketamine	0	1	?
Epidural opioids	2	0-2	2
Epidural clonidine	2	0-2	1-2
Spinal local anaesthetics	2	?	2
Spinal opioids	1-2	?	?
Wound infiltration with local anaesthetics	0-1	0-1	0-1
Intraperitoneal local anaesthetics	-	0	-
Cognitive treatment	2	0-1	?
Music	?	1	0
Acupuncture	1	0	1

Table 1. Summary effects of selected interventions on postoperative pain after abdominal hysterectomy according to the timing of administration. *Notes:* 0, no analgesic effect; 1, some analgesic effect; 2, considerable analgesic effect; ?, data not available; -, data irrelevant.

5.2 Extent of tissue trauma

The anatomical basis of pain following hysterectomy is complex. In chapter 2, we have outlined some psychological and neurophysiological aspects of importance, and highlighted the importance of tissue trauma as the cornerstone of surgical stress response and subsequent activation of prostaglandins, cytokines, and nociceptive impulses for central nervous system modulation. These reactions are best known in the skin, in which a variety of vasoactive and irritative substances are released by tissue damage, causing a primary area of hypersensitivity, and a secondary activation of metabolites and nerve impulses in the spinal cord and central nervous system, in turn causing an additional hypersensitivity around the initial skin damage (Dirks, 2002). Brain centres value-set these painful impulses, affecting cognition, emotions, motor cortex and the autonomous nervous system. In the abdomen, the most pronounced effect during hysterectomy is activation of the vagus part of the autonomous nervous system, arising from stimulation of the neural tissue surrounding the uterus, leading to bradycardia, hypotension and nausea. Since the extent of cutaneous tissue damage during surgery determines the frame of postoperative pain complaints, the potential methods of prevention and treatment should mirror the desired clinical effect and the acceptability of side effects. In this respect, clinicians may judge inconsistently because priorities may vary according to specific demands afforded by the patient or the specific situation.

5.3 Weak analgesics

Tramadol is a weak opioid that has failed to convincingly show benefits (Wang, 2009). Intravenous paracetamol, a weak cyclooxygenase-inhibitor in the CNS, has gained interest in a recent study that implies an additional opioid-sparing effect when given preoperatively in abdominal hysterectomy (Arici, 2009). Rectal paracetamol, on the other hand, has almost no effect (Kvalsvik, 2003). As for NSAIDs and cox-2 inhibitors (which only differ in their side effect profiles and duration of action), many studies continue to be done by the pharmaceutical companies. New intravenous formulations given during surgery clearly confirm the almost ubiquitous opioid-sparing quality of these drugs, but they add nothing new to our spectrum of useful drugs, other than handy iv formulations. A much more interesting study using intrathecal ketorolac as adjuvant in patients with chronic or postoperative pain following vaginal hysterectomy showed that, while contributions of prostaglandins from the spinal cord must be evident in the development of pain, it is clearly only of value to block prostaglandin production (by ketorolac) if levels of prostaglandin E2 are high in the cerebrospinal fluid, an event which only occurs in a subset of patients. In addition, intrathecal ketorolac does not alter time to first morphine demand after surgery (Eisenach, 2010).

5.4 New drugs

Dexamethasone has been the focus of several studies, and when used alone in laparoscopic hysterectomy, it has clinically relevant opioid-sparing properties, as well as reducing the risk of dizziness (Jokela, 2009; Thangaswamy, 2010). When used in combination with pregabalin for abdominal hysterectomy, however, one study did not replicate these properties (Mathiesen, 2009), suggesting a potentially weak analgesic effect. It should also be noted that dexamethasone at 8 mg dose given before surgery causes significant hyperglycaemia within the first six postoperative hours (Eberhart, 2011). The value of gabapentin and pregabalin are confirmed in studies published after the Prospect review and may in fact also lead to faster recovery of bowel function (Turan, 2006; Durmus, 2007). The combination of gabapentin and a cox-2 inhibitor seems to be superior to either single agent for postoperative pain, as well as improvements in mood and sleep quality (Gilron, 2005). For gabapentin, 1200 mg/day is the appropriate dosage, whereas for pregabalin it is 300 mg/day (Ittichaikulthol, 2009). When compared to ketamine (low dose infusion), gabapentin seems to improve pain scores, but either drug seems equally efficacious as opioid-sparing agents (Sen, 2009; Pirim, 2006). For gabapentin, side effects include dizziness and sedation, and for ketamine, side effects include sleep disorders, hallucinations and a condition known as "dissociative anaesthesia" (to feel present, yet distant; to feel pain, yet not to care). When used within proposed dose limits, these side effects are exceedingly rare. The alpha-2 antagonist dexmedetomidine may be used as a continuous infusion during surgery or as an effective adjuvant to iv PCA morphine after abdominal hysterectomy, decreasing pain levels without increasing the incidence of side effects such as sedation or hemodynamic instability (Gurbet, 2006; Lin, 2009). Intraoperative dexmedetomidine may also reduce the risk of postoperative shivering (Elvan, 2008). Other CNS-active drugs such as droperidol, cyclizine and promethazine reduce postoperative morphine consumption and the frequency of nausea and vomiting compared to placebo (Chia, 2004; Lo, 2005). The biologically active drug melatonin, which is used for circadian rhythms and sleep, has recently been highlighted in two interesting studies. When given as an oral dose of 5 mg the night before and one hour before surgery, it has reduced opioid requirements and postoperative anxiety, and patients regain their circadian rhythm more quickly after surgery (Caumo, 2007). Given the demonstration that melatonin has both analgesic, anti-inflammatory, and anxiolytic properties, and that higher anxiety makes the control of postoperative pain more difficult, one can hypothesize that melatonin is a promising agent to improve the control of postoperative pain. The efficacy of melatonin equals that of clonidine after abdominal hysterectomy (Caumo, 2009). Finally, intravenous lidocaine has both analgesic and antiinflammatory properties, which decrease the upregulation of proinflammatory cytokines, but clinical results have been disappointing (Yardeni, 2009; Bryson, 2010).

5.5 Acupuncture

Intraoperative use of acupuncture has been investigated and has been found to have no value in abdominal hysterectomy (Table 1). However, when applying classical needle acupuncture, electroacupuncture or capsicum plaster at certain acupoints (Zusanli, ST-36) preoperatively or postoperatively after abdominal hysterectomy, requests for morphine and antiemetics are significantly reduced (Lin, 2002; Kim, 2006; Grube, 2009). Other studies using electroacupuncture at 10 Hz have failed to confirm these findings, suggesting that acupuncture points need to be clearly defined and that the procedure itself requires special knowledge to perform (El-Rakshy, 2009).

5.6 Local anaesthetic techniques

The paradigm of blocking nerve conduction at the site of injury without the need for additional systemic analgesics is an enduring and very enticing proposition. While the need for such techniques are decidedly relevant in scenarios with considerable tissue damage such as conventional laparotomy, it seems appropriate to consider their use in laparoscopic surgery as well. The overall efficacy of local anaesthetic infiltration around the surgical wound is not entirely convincing. The main problem is duration of action, which is usually only a few hours. Due to the enhanced blood flow caused by inflammation, instilled drugs are washed out very quickly. For this reason, continuous catheter solutions seem promising (Gomez Rios, 2009). The placement of the catheter, however, is important and must be situated above the fascia to have any effect (Hafizoglu, 2008; Perniola, 2009). The physiological reason is perfectly straightforward, since most pain-conducting nerves are located in this area.

5.7 Transverse Abdominis Plane (TAP) block

The administration of various forms of TAP blocks has attracted a substantial interest during the last decade. The emergence of anaesthetic ultrasound, the simplicity of the block and the rapid effect on postoperative pain following many abdominal procedures are among the primary movers for the widespread use of the TAP block (Petersen, 2010; Børglum, 2011, Koscielniak-Nielsen, 2011). The block has evolved from an abdominal wall block administered blindly and based on anatomical landmarks to an ultrasound guided block, where the spread of the injectate can be seen to be deposited in the right compartment; i.e. in the neurovascular plane between the internal oblique and the transversus abdominis muscles (Rafi, 2001; McDonnell, 2007; Petersen, 2010). Recently, the block has been refined and described in more detail when the aim of various studies was to expand and ensure the analgesic efficacy of the block to cover the entire abdominal wall (Th6-Th12(L1)) (Hebbard, 2010; Børglum, 2011). Most interestingly, the TAP block administered blindly prior to surgical incision for total abdominal hysterectomy using the double loss-of-resistance technique together with the traditional landmark assistance has been proven to provide superior analgesia when compared to a placebo group (Carney, 2008). Patients in the active group had reduced 48-h morphine requirements, and a longer time to first PCA morphine request. Postoperative VAS pain scores at rest and on movement were reduced after TAP block at most time points assessed (over 48 hours) (Carney, 2008). It would seem that promising results in this area could merit further studies. An internet search provided proof to this matter, since novel studies registered on ClinicalTrials.com exhibited research projects concerning laparoscopic vaginal hysterectomy and the efficacy of pre-operative TAP block on postoperative pain management. In addition, it would seem plausible that other types of truncal blocks such as ultrasound-guided thoracic paravertebral (TPV) blocks and rectus sheath blocks could well provide benefits in postoperative pain management following either abdominal or laparoscopic hysterectomy. Recently, TPV and rectus sheath blocks were given grade B and A recommendations for ultrasound guidance (United States Agency for health Care Policy and Research), respectively (Abrahams, 2010). An anatomically more caudal, but equally effective block option is bilateral ilioinguinal nerve block (Oriola, 2007). Thus, it seems straightforward to include any of these blocks in a multimodal analgesic regime.

5.8 Postoperative Nausea And Vomiting (PONV)

Nausea and vomiting rank high among feared postoperative complaints. Even to this day, they are also among the most common after any kind of hysterectomy. PONV may be caused by a variety of factors (Table 2). Commonly used algorithms for prevention should be taken as guidelines rather than statements of fact, because new techniques have changed the foundation for the specific frequencies of PONV cited in the algorithms (Eberhart, 2000; Gan, 2007). Another methodological problem is frequency of PONV, which often differs considerably (0-80%) in comparable studies. The good part of the story is that PONV usually abates within 24 hours, but because of its frequency and enormous impact on well-being, clinicians must hold a strong focus on its prevention. While studies on PONV are heterogeneous, randomized data suggest that combinations of at least two antiemetics are effective for prophylaxis, reducing the risk of PONV to less than 20% (Piper, 2003; Chu, 2008). Antiemetics may also with advantage be added to patient-controlled analgesia infusions (Boonmak, 2007). The specific type of antiemetic is less important and should be guided by the desired effect and potential side effects (Bilgin, 2010). For instance, when PONV may be aggravated by anxiety, a benzodiazepine or sedative antiemetic is preferable (Elhakim, 2009; Fujii 2010; Huh, 2010). Antiemetics used for prophylaxis may also be used for treatment. Again, the use of acupuncture has reliably been shown to prevent PONV. Of special importance is the P6 point at the wrist (Frey, 2009; Kim, 2011). The Korean K-D2 or auricular points are equally useful (Ki, 2002; Kim, 2003).

DEFINITE risk factors for PONV	
Females	Non-smokers
Previous PONV	Motion sickness
Opioids	Inhalational anaesthetics and N2O
Neostigmine	General anaesthesia
Prolonged surgery	
PRESUMED risk factors for PONV	
Hormonal imbalance	Obesity
Pain	Anxiety
Early mobilization and transport	Laparoscopy

Table 2. Definite or presumed risk factors for PONV in females undergoing hysterectomy.

Benzodiazepines	Propofol	Chlorpromazine
Antihistamines	Droperidol, haloperidol	Metoclopramide
Dexamethasone	Serotonine antagonists	Ephedrine
Effective pain management	P6 acupressure	

Table 3. Modalities in prevention and treatment of PONV.

5.9 Development of chronic pain

Chronic pain is frequently observed several months after laparotomy (7 to 37%, depending on incision) (Perkins, 2000); the most apparent cause is direct nerve damage by severance or compression, leading to a host of nerve changes including peripheral receptor and spinal neuron changes, hyperalgesia/allodynia, ectopic activity and wind-up phenomena. Prevention is of key importance, since major breakthroughs in treatment have not yet emerged. In spite of an enormous amount of literature dealing with the prevention, pathophysiology and treatment of chronic pain, we are still at the very beginning of our understanding. Every effort should therefore be directed at minimally invasive surgical techniques. Persistent nerve damage resulting from epidural, spinal or regional anaesthesia is exceedingly rare and occurs in the order of 1:5000. Transient nerve damage (neuropraxia) lasting weeks to months is more common following regional anaesthesia, but the incidence is largely unknown. Its pathophysiology also remains murky but may include compression or stretching effects of nerve fibres, toxic effects of local anaesthetic drugs, and an inherent increased susceptibility to compression effects (known as HNPP, hereditary liability to neuropathic pressure palsies). Patients having HNPP often complain of prolonged dys-aesthesias, wrist pain, and strange sensory sensations after even banal experiences. Nerve damage resulting from inadequate positioning during surgery in the lithotomy position, for instance, may be prevented by soft padding, frequent movement during surgery, and continuous monitoring of vascular supply by pulse oximetry. Brachial plexus damage may occur if arms are hyperextended from the axis of the body in steep Trendelenburg positioning (Ben-David, 1997).

6. Administrative logistics

6.1 Fast-track protocols

The concept of a fast-track surgical protocol for hysterectomy was introduced by Kehlet and associates a decade ago (Møller, 2001). The protocol included optimized information, well-defined anaesthesia and fluid therapy, early mobilization, early food intake and the concept of multimodal pain treatment. The idea was to combine several modalities of analgesic techniques, systemic to neuraxial, in order to harvest tbe benefits of synergistic effects. Using these concepts, the authors were even then able to optimize length of stay in abdominal hysterectomy to approximate that of laparoscopically-assisted vaginal hysterectomy, which strongly suggests that 1) the concept works, and that 2) benefits from randomized trials were until then not adequately transformed and utilized in clinical practice. Patients were simply not asked to get out of bed and take care of themselves, in spite of several well-meaning treatments and preventive measures that should facilitate ambulation and self-sufficiency. While the concept of fast-track protocols have continued to expand in recent years, there are however limits to the number of complaints that can be prevented by this paradigm. In a comprehensive cohort study looking at the immediate recovery profile after abdominal hysterectomy, several important points emerge (Jensen, 2009): 25% experience severe pain in spite of preoperatively placed epidurals, but only 8% experience PONV (patients were pretreated with three antiemetics). However, a complicated recovery, defined as the presence of severe complaints (pain or PONV), with more than five treatment interventions in the postanaesthesia care unit or a length of stay more than two hours, was observed in half the patients. The patency of the epidural was a key issue, and failed epidurals or patients not wishing/having epidurals were at particularly high risk of complaints. Inadequate pain treatment was the principal factor responsible for prolonged stay in the postanaesthesia care unit, causing increased opioid demands, nausea, dependency on oxygen supply, and sedation. Recent studies rightfully discuss the optimal surgical and anaesthetic techniques, but there are no clear answers (Sarmini, 2005; Abdelmonem, 2006; Wodlin, 2011). Spinal anaesthesia has some advantages to general anaesthesia by reducing immediate postoperative discomfort, opioid demands and duration of sick leave, but spinal opioids increase the risk of itching, with no differences in PONV (Wodlin, 2011a; Wodlin, 2011b). A similar fast-track study seems to imply that total intravenous anaesthesia may be superior to inhalational anaesthesia by reducing nausea, length of hospital stay, and duration of an indwelling urinary catheter (Kroon,

2010). The case for early urinary catheter removal, however, is offset by an increased risk of urinary retention episodes requiring re-catheterisation (Chai, 2011).

6.2 The economics of hysterectomy

Hot on the heels of the fast-track protocols, hospital administrators have become aware of the potential to reap the benefits of this new paradigm. Optimal logistics in the surgical suite, short durations of surgery, few necessary interventions or short length of stay in the postanaesthesia care unit are pivotal issues for increasing the number of surgeries that can be performed in a day. In the surgical ward, severity of activity-limiting and treatment-necessary complaints determine, besides surgical complications, the degree of observation and the level of competency that needs to be present, and ultimately the length of hospital stay. This length of stay in turn determines which days elective patients can be scheduled for surgery (typically monday through wednesday), so that only residual problems persist in the weekend and a clean slate of patients can be admitted the following monday (Roumm, 2005). Day surgery may be placed in the extreme end of the spectrum, facilitating quick patient flow, fewer overnight beds and lower costs (Levy, 2005), while complicated (acute, laparotomic) surgery may be placed in the other end. From the administrative point, the balance between the two extremes is as delicate as a double-edged sword: day surgery may reduce costs per patient, but increasing number of patients puts considerable pressure on optimized flow, well-functioning protocols, teamwork, the implementation of lean principles, patient profiles (ASA health status 1-2), and staff enthusiasm. Complicated cases puts pressure on staff competency, individual solutions and across-department collaborations. It is for these very reasons that medical technology assessments are important in determining the true logistical value of new anaesthetic or surgical techniques, because each new intervention affects the entire system of people and work descriptions in the surgical food chain. Studies investigating financial costs, e.g. the introduction of robotic surgery, should not uncritically be taken at face value: they often fail to take these issues into account and merely represent fictive scenarios that may or may not be applicable (Barnett, 2010; Oehler, 2011). In a wider perspective, the cost for the society may not be reflected in the immediate hospital costs. A recent study suggests that the majority of women extend their sick leave beyond the recommended period on their own initiative, despite the ward's long recommended period of sick leave (Johansen, 2008).

7. Conclusions

From the topics discussed above, several unmet patient needs and clear avenues of research still need to be pursued; even though multimodal, evidence-based treatment regimens are conducted efficiently and in detail, many patients still suffer from unacceptable postoperative complaints. The reasons are complex and include definite limitations in the current potentials of anaesthesia and surgery, stress response, variability among patients in psychological or genetic disposition, and downright treatment failures or withdrawals because of unacceptable side effects. Certain surgical techniques are related to more complaints. Pharmacologically, new drugs have not lived up to their potential to facilitate opioid-free analgesia. Recent advances in local anaesthetic techniques such as the transverse abdominis plane block may help solve this problem, but we are still in want of a magic bullet to alleviate nausea, dizziness, exhaustion and failed ambulation. From a patient perspective, there is a need for adequate information to properly balance expectations and coping strategies, and a need for focused postoperative follow-up, since people are nowadays discharged early with health complaints and limitations in activities of daily living persisting for weeks or even months after surgery. A useful method for transferring procedure-specific evidence from controlled studies into the very real and heterogeneous world of uncontrolled patients and health care professionals is also highly welcomed. Can we succeed in this? Only the future will tell.

8. References

Abdelmonem A, Wilson H, Pasic R. Observational comparison of abdominal, vaginal and laparoscopic hysterectomy as performed at a university teaching hospital. *J Reprod Med* 2006; 51: 945-54

Abrahams MS, Horn J-L, Noles LM, Aziz MF. Evidence-based medicine. Ultrasound guidance for truncal blocks. *Res Anesth Pain Med* 2010; 35:36-42

Akural EI, Salomäki TE, Bloigu AH, Ryhänen P, Tekay AH, Alahuhta SM, Surcel HM. The effects of pre-emptive epidural sufentanil on human immune function. *Acta Anaesth Scand* 2004; 48: 750-5

Akural EI, Salomäki TE, Tekay AH, Bloigu AH, Alahuhta SM. Pre-emptive effect of epidural sufentanil in abdominal hysterectomy. *Br J Anaesth* 2002; 88: 803-8

Arici S, Gurbet A, Türker G, Yavascaoglu B, Sahin S. Preemptive analgesic effects of intravenous paracetamol in total abdominal hysterectomy. *Agri* 2009; 21: 54-61

Aziz A, bergquist C, Brännström M, Nordholm L, Silfverstolpe G. Differences in aspects of personality and sexuality between perimenopausal women making different choices regarding prophylactic oophorectomy at elective hysterectomy. *Acta Obstet Gynecol Scand* 2005; 84: 854-9

Barnett JC, Judd JP, Wu JM, Scales CD, Myers ER, Havrilesky LJ. Cost comparison among robotic, laparoscopic, and open hysterectomy for endometrial cancer. *Obstet Gynecol* 2010; 116: 685-93

Beilin B, Bessler H, Mayburd E, Smirnov G et al. Effects of preemptive analgesia on pain and cytokine production in the postoperative period. *Anesthesiology* 2003; 98: 151-5

Ben-David B, Stahl S. Prognosis of intraoperaive brachial plexus injury: a review of 22 cases. *Br J Anaesthesia* 1997; 79: 440-5

Bharti N, Chari P. Epidural butorphanol-bupivacaine analgesia for postoperative pain relief after abdominal hysterectomy. *J Clin Anesth* 2009; 21: 19-22

Bhattacharya SM, Jha A. A comparison of health-related quality of life (HRQOL) after natural and surgical menopause. *Maturitas* 2010; 66: 431-4

Bilgin TE, Birbicer H, Ozer Z, Doruk N, Tok E, Oral U. A comparative study of the antiemetic efficacy of dexamethasone, ondansetron, and metoclopramide in patients undergoing gynecological surgery. *Med Sci Monit* 2010; 16: CR336-41

Boonmak P, Boonmak S, Bunsaengjaroen P et al. Antiemetic effect of ondansetron 0.2 mg mL-1 in PCA morphine solution. *Eur J Anaesthesiol* 2007; 24: 664-7

Brandsborg B, Dueholm M, Nikolajsen L, Kehlet H, Jensen TS. A prospective study of risk factors for pain persisting 4 months after hysterectomy. *Clin J Pain* 2009; 25: 263-8

Bryson GL, Charapov I, Krolczyk G, Taljaard M, Reid D. Intravenous lidocaine does not reduce length of hospital stay following abdominal hysterectomy. *Can J Anaesth* 2010; 57: 759-66

Børglum J, Maschmann C, Belhage B, Jensen K. Ultrasound-guided bilateral dual transversus abdominis plane block: a new four-point approach. *Acta Anaesth Scand* 2011; 55: 658-663

Candiani M, Izzo S, Bulfoni A, Riparini J, Ronzoni S, Marconi A. Laparoscopic vs vaginal hysterectomy for benign pathology. *Am J Obstet Gynecol* 2009; 200: 368.e1-7

Carney J, McDonnell, JG, Ochna A, Bhinder R, Laffey JG. The transversus abdominis plane block provides effective postoperative analgesia in patients undergoing total abdominal hysterectomy. *Anesth Analg* 2008; 107: 2056-2060

Caumo W, Hidalgo MP, Schmidt AP, Iwamoto CW, Adamatti LC, Bergmann J, Ferreira MB. Effect of pre-operative anxiolysis on postoperative pain response in patients undergoing total abdominal hysterectomy. *Anaesthesia* 2002; 57: 740-6

Caumo W, Levandovski R, Hidalgo MP. Preoperative anxiolytic effect of melatonin and clonidine on postoperative pain and morphine in patients undergoing abdominal hysterectomy. *J Pain* 2009; 10: 100-8

Caumo W, Schmidt AP, Schneider CN, Bergmann J, Iwamoto CW, Bandeira D, Ferreira MB. Preoperative predictors of moderate to intense acute postoperative pain in patients undergoing abdominal surgery. *Acta Anaesth Scand* 2002; 46: 1265-71

Caumo W, Torres F, Moreira NL, Auzani JA, Monteiro CA, Londero G, Ribeiro DF, Hidalgo MP. The clinical impact of preoperative melatonin on postoperative outcomes in patients undergoing abdominal hysterectomy. *Anesth Analg* 2007; 105: 1263-71

Chai J, Pun TC. A prospective randomized trial to compare immediate and 24-hour delayed catheter removal following total abdominal hysterectomy. *Acta Obstet Gynecol Scand* 2011; 90: 478-82

Charoenkwan K, Phillipson G, Vutyavanich T. Early versus delayed (traditional) oral fluids and food for reducing complications after major abdominal gynaecologic surgery. *Cochrane Database Syst Rev* 2007; 17: CD004508

Chen WH, Liu K, Tan PH, Chia YY. Effects of postoperative background PCA morphine infusion on pain management and related side effects in patients undergoing abdominal hysterectomy. *J Clin Anesth* 2011; 23: 124-9

Cheung LH, Callaghan P, Chang AM. A controlled trial of psycho-educational interventions in preparing Chinese women for elective hysterectomy. *Int J Nurs Stud* 2003; 40: 207-16

Chia YY, Lo Y, Liu K, Tan PH, Chung NC, Ko NH. The effect of promethazine on postoperative pain: a comparison of preoperative, postoperative, and placebo administration in patients following total abdominal hysterectomy. *Acta Anaesth Scand* 2004; 48: 625-30

Chou WY, Wang CH, Liu PH, Liu CC, Tseng CC, Jawan B. Human opioid receptor A118G polymorphism affects intravenous patient-controlled analgesia morphine consumption after total abdominal hysterectomy. *Anesthesiology* 2006; 105: 334-7

Chu CC, Shieh JP, Tzeng JI, Chen JY, Lee Y, Wang JJ. The prophylactic effect of haloperidol plus dexamethasone on postoperative nausea and vomiting in patients undergoing laparoscopically assisted vaginal hysterectomy. *Anesth Analg* 2008; 106: 1402-6

Davies JE, Doyle PM. Quality of life studies in unselected gynaecological outpatients and inpatients before and after hysterectomy. *J Obstet Gynaecol* 2002; 22: 523-6

Demirbilek S, Ganidagli S, Aksoy N, Becerik C, Baysal Z. The effects of remifentanil and alfentanil-based total intravenous anesthesia (TIVA) on the endocrine response to abdominal hysterectomy. *J Clin Anesth* 2004; 16: 358-63

Di Chiara G. Nucleus accumbens shell and core dopamine: differential role in behavior and addiction. *Behav Brain Res* 2002; 137: 75-114

Digman JM. Personality structure: emergence of the five-factor model. *Ann Rev Psychology* 1990; 41: 417-40

Dirks J, Møiniche S, Hilsted KL, Dahl JB. Mechanisms of postoperative pain: clinical indications for a contribution of central neuronal sensitization. *Anesthesiology* 2002; 97: 1591-6

Durmus M, Kadir But A, Saricicek V, Ilksen Toprak H. The post-operative analgesic effects of a combination of gabapentin and paracetamol in patients undergoing abdominal hysterectomy: a randomized clinical trial. *Acta Anaesth Scand* 2007; 51: 299-304

Eberhart LH, Graf J, Morin AM, Stief T, Kalder M, Lattermann R, Schricker T. Randomised controlled trial of the effect of oral premedication with dexamethasone on hyperglycaemic response to abdominal hysterectomy. *Eur J Anaesthesiol* 2011; 28: 195-201

Eberhart LH, Högel J, Seeling W, Staack AM, Geldner G. Evaluation of three risk scores to predict postoperative nausea and vomiting. *Acta Anaesth Scand* 2000; 44: 480-8

Eisenach JC, Curry R, Rauck R, Pan P, Yaksh TL. Role of spinal cyclooxygenase in human postoperative and chronic pain. *Anesthesiology* 2010; 112: 1225-33

El-Rakshy M, Clark SC, Thompson J, Thant M. Effect of intraoperative electroacupuncture on postoperative pain, analgesic requirements, nausea and sedation: a randomised controlled trial. *Acupunct Med* 2009; 27: 9-12

Elhakim M, Abd-elfattah H, El-Din DN et al. Midazolam as an antiemetic in patients receiving epidural morphine for postoperative pain relief. *J Opioid Manag* 2009; 5: 189-95

Ellström MA, Aström M, Möller A, Olsson JH, Hahlin M. A randomized trial comparing changes in psychological well-being and sexuality after laparoscopic and abdominal hysterectomy. *Acta Obstet Gynecol Scand* 2003; 82: 871-5

Ellström MA, Jerhamre K, Junskog K. A randomized trial comparing changes in sexual health and psychological well-being after subtotal and total hysterectomies. *Acta Obstet Gynecol Scand* 2010; 89: 65-70

Elvan EG, Oc B, Uzun S, Karabulut E, Coskun F, Aypar U. Dexmedetomidine and postoperative shivering in patients undergoing elective abdominal hysterectomy. *Eur J Anaesthesiol* 2008; 25: 357-64

Farouk S. Pre-incisional epidural magnesium provides pre-emptive and preventive analgesia in patients undergoing abdominal hysterectomy. *Br J Anaesth* 2008; 101: 694-9.

Fassoulaki A, Melemeni A, Paraskeva A, Siafaka I, Sarantopoulos C. Postoperative pain and analgesic requirements after anesthesia with sevoflurane, desflurane or propofol. *Anesth Analg* 2008; 107: 1715-9

Flory N, Bissonnette F, Amsel RT, Binik YM. The psychosocial outcomes of total and subtotal hysterectomy: a randomized controlled trial. *J Sex Med* 2006; 3: 483-91

Frey UH, Scharmann P, Löhlein C, Peters J. P6 acustimulation effectively decreases postoperative nausea and vomiting in high-risk patients. *Br J Anaesth* 2009; 102: 620-5

Fujii Y, Itakura M. A prospective, randomized, double-blind, placebo-controlled study to assess the antiemetic effects of midazolam on postoperative nausea and vomiting in women undergoing laparoscopic gynecologic surgery. *Clin Ther* 2010; 32: 1633-7

Gan TJ, Meyer TA, Apfel CC, Chung F, Davis PJ, Habib AS et al. Society for Ambulatory Anesthesia guidelines for the management of postoperative nausea and vomiting. *Anesth Analg* 2007; 105: 1615-28

Garry R, Fountain J, Brown J, Manca A, Mason S, Sculpher M, Napp V, Bridgman S, Gray J, Lilford R. EVALUATE hysterectomy trial: a multicentre randomised trial comparing abdominal, vaginal and laparoscopic methods of hysterectomy. *Health Technol Assess* 2004; 8: 1-154

Ghezzi F, Uccella S, Cromi A, Siesto G, Serati M, Bogani G, Bolis P. Postoperative pain after laparoscopic and vaginal hysterectomy for benign gynecologic disease: a randomized trial. *Am J Obstet Gynecol* 2010; 203: 118.e1-8

Gilron I, Orr E, Tu D, O'Neill JP, Zamora JE, Bell AC. A placebo-controlled randomized clinical trial of perioperative administration of gabapentin, rofecoxib and their combination for spontaneous and movement-evoked pain after abdominal hysterectomy. *Pain* 2005; 113: 191-200

Gomez Rios MA, Vázquez Barreiro L, Nieto Serradilla L, Diz Gomez JC, Lopez Alvarez S. Efficacy of a continuous infusion of local anesthetic into the surgical wound for pain relief after abdominal hysterectomy. *Rev Esp Anestesiol Reanim* 2009; 56: 417-24

Gorlero F, Lijoi D, Biamonti M, Lorenzi P, Pullé A, Ragni N. Hysterectomy and women satisfaction: total versus subtotal technique. *Arch Gynecol Obstet* 2008; 278: 405-10

Grube T, Uhlemann C, Weiss T, Meissner W. Influence of acupuncture on postoperative pain, nausea and vomiting after visceral surgery: a prospective, randomized comparative study of metamizole and standard treatment. *Schmerz* 2009; 23: 370-6

Gurbet A, Basagan-Mogol E, Turker G, Ugun F, Kaya FN, Ozcan B. Intraoperative infusion of dexmedetomidine reduces perioperative analgesic requirements. *Can J Anaesth* 2006; 53: 646-52

Gütl P, Greimel ER, Roth R, Winter R. Women's sexual behavior, body image and satisfaction with surgical outcomes after hysterectomy: a comparison of vaginal and abdominal surgery. *J Psychosom Obstet Gynaecol* 2002; 23: 51-9

Hafizoglu MC, Katircioglu K, Ozkalkanli MY, Savaci S. Bupivacaine infusion above or below the fascia for postoperative pain treatment after abdominal hysterectomy. *Anesth Analg* 2008; 107: 2068-72

Hansen CT, Sørensen M, Møller C, Ottesen B, Kehlet H. Effect of laxatives on gastrointestinal functional recovery in fast-track hysterectomy: a double-blind, placebo-controlled randomized study. *Am J Obstet Gynecol* 2007; 196: 311.e1-7

Hartmann KE, Ma C, Lamvu GM, Langenberg PW, Steege JF, Kjerulff KH. Quality of life and sexual function after hysterectomy in women with preoperative pain and depression. *Obstet Gynecol* 2004; 104: 701-9

Hashimoto Y, Baba S, Koh H, Takagi H, Ishihara H. Anxiolytic effect of preoperative showing of anesthesia video for surgical patients. *Anesth Analg* 1993; 42: 611-6

Hastie BA, Riley JL, Robinson ME, Glover T, Campbell CM, Staud R, Fillingim RB. Cluster analysis of multiple experimental pain modalities. *Pain* 2005; 116: 227-37

Hebbard PD, Barrington MJ, Vasey C. Ultrasound-guided continuous oblique subcostal transversus abdominis plane blockade: description of anatomy and clinical technique. *Reg Anesth Pain Med* 2010; 35: 436-441

Hedenstierna G, Edmark L. Mechanisms of atelectasis in the perioperative period. *Best Pract Res Clin Anaesthesiol* 2010; 24: 157-69

Henneberg SW, Rosenborg D, Weber Jensen E, Ahn P, Burgdorff B, Thomsen LL. Peroperative depth of anaesthesia may influence postoperative opioid requirements. *Acta Anaesth Scand* 2005; 49: 293-6

Herzog TJ, Coleman RL, Guerrieri JP, Gabriel K, Du W, Techner L, Fort JG, Wallin B. A double-blind, randomized, placebo-controlled phase III study of the safety of alvimopan in patients who undergo simple total abdominal hysterectomy. *Am J Obstet Gynecol* 2006; 195: 445-53

Heye ML, Foster L, Bartlett MK, Adkins S. A preoperative intervention for pain reduction, improved mobility, and self-efficacy. *Appl Nurs Res* 2002; 15: 174-83

Hong JY, Lim KT. Effect of preemptive epidural analgesia on cytokine response and postoperative pain in laparoscopic radical hysterectomy for cervical cancer. *Reg Anesth Pain Med* 2008; 33: 44-51

Huh BK, Jung S, White W, Jeon Y. Anti-emetic effect of midazolam added to morphine patient-controlled analgesia after total abdominal hysterectomy. *Anaesth Intensive Care* 2010; 38: 481-5

Ihn CH, Joo JD, Choi JW, Kim DW, Jeon YS et al. Comparison of stress hormone response, interleukin-6 and anaesthetic characteristics of two anaesthetic techniques: volatile induction and maintenance of anaesthesia using sevoflurane versus total intravenous anaesthesia using propofol and remifentanil. *J Int Med Res* 2009; 37: 1760-71

Ittichaikulthol W, Virankabutra T, Kunopart M, Khamhom W, Putarawuthichai P, Rungphet S. Effects of pregabalin on post operative morphine consumption and pain after abdominal hysterectomy with/without salpingo-oophorectomy: a randomized, double-blind trial. *J Med Assoc Thai* 2009; 92: 1318-23

Jensen K, Kehlet H, Lund CM. Postoperative recovery profile after elective abdominal hysterectomy: a prospective, observational study of a multimodal anaesthetic regime. *Eur J Anaesthesiol* 2009; 26: 382-8

Johansen P, Al-Khafagi SK, Thøstesen LM, Lauszus FF, Rasmussen KL. Analysis of need for sick leave after hysterectomy. *Ugeskr Læger* 2008; 170: 1465-8

Johnson DT, Spielberger CD. The effects of relaxation training and the passage of time on measures of state- and trait-anxiety. *J Clin Psychol* 1968; 24: 20-3

Jokela RM, Ahonen JV, Tallgren MK, Marjakangas PC et al. The effective analgesic dose of dexamethasone after laparoscopic hysterectomy. *Anesth Analg* 2009; 109: 607-15

Jørgensen H, Fomsgaard JS, Dirks J, Wetterslev J, Andreasson B, Dahl JB. Effect of peri- and postoperative epidural anaesthesia on pain and gastrointestinal function after abdominal hysterectomy. *Br J Anaesth* 2001; 87: 577-83

Kain ZN, Sevarino FB, Rinder C, Pincus S, Alexander GM, Ivy M, Heninger G. Preoperative anxiolysis and postoperative recovery in women undergoing abdominal hysterectomy. *Anesthesiology* 2001; 94: 415-22

Kalkman CJ, Visser K, Moen J, Bonsel GJ, Grobbee DE, Moons KG. Preoperative prediction of severe postoperative pain. *Pain* 2003; 105: 415-23

Karaman S, Kocabas S, Uyar M, Zincircioglu C, Firat V. Intrathecal morphine: effects on perioperative hemodynamics, postoperative analgesia, and stress response for total abdominal hysterectomy. *Adv Ther* 2006; 23: 295-306

Karanci AN, Dirik G. Predictors of pre- and postoperative anxiety in emergency surgery patients. *J Psychosom Res* 203; 55: 363-9

Kilickan L, Toker K. The effect of preemptive intravenous morphine on postoperative analgesia and surgical stress response. *Panminerva Med* 2001; 43: 171-5

Kim KS, Koo MS, Jeon JW, Park Hs, Seung IS. Capsicum plaster at the korean hand acupuncture point reduces postoperative nausea and vomiting after abdominal hysterectomy. *Anesth Analg* 2002; 95: 1103-7

Kim KS, Nam YM. The analgesic effects of capsicum plaster at the Zusanli point after abdominal hysterectomy. *Anesth Analg* 2006; 103: 709-13

Kim SH, Kang S, Kim YM, Kim BG, Seong SJ, Cha SD, Park CY, Yun YH. Prevalence and predictors of anxiety and depression among cervical cancer survivors in Korea. *Int J Gynecol Cancer* 2010; 20: 1017-24

Kim TJ, Lee YY, Cha HH, Kim CJ, Choi CH, Lee JW, Bae DS, Lee JH, Kim BG. Single-port-access laparoscopic-assisted vaginal hysterectomy versus conventional laparoscopic-assisted vaginal hysterectomy: a comparison of perioperative outcomes. *Surg Endosc* 2010; 24: 2248-52

Kim YH, Kim CW, Kim KS. Clinical observations on postoperative vomiting treated by auricular acupuncture. *Am J Chin Med* 2003; 31: 475-80

Kim YH, Kim KS, Lee HJ, Shim JC, Yoon SW. The efficacy of several neuromuscular monitoring modes at the P6 acupuncture point in preventing postoperative nausea and vomiting. *Anesth Analg* 2011; 112: 819-23

Kindler CH, Harms C, Amsler F, Ihde-Scholl T, Scheidegger D. The visual analog scale allows effective measurement of preoperative anxiety and detection of patients' anesthetic concerns. *Anesth Analg* 2000; 90: 706-12

Kocabas S, Karaman S, Uysallar E, Firat V. The use of tramadol and morphine for pain relief after abdominal hysterectomy. *Clin Exp Obstet Gynecol* 2005; 32: 45-8

Kolesnikov Y, Gabovits B, Levin A, Voiko E, Veske A. Combined catechol-O-methyltransferase and mu-opioid receptor gene polymorphisms affect morphine postoperative analgesia and central side effects. *Anesth Analg* 2011; 112: 448-53

Koscielniak-Nielsen ZJ. Transversus abdominis plane blocks for rescue analgesia after major abdominal surgery. *Acta Anaesthesiol Scand* 2011; 55: 635-637

Kroon UB, Rådström M, Hjelthe C, Dahlin C, Kroon L. Fast-track hysterectomy: a randomised, controlled study. *Eur J Obstet Gynecol Reprod Biol* 2010; 151: 203-7

Kvalsvik O, Borchgrevink PC, Hagen L, Dale O. Randomized, double-blind, placebo-controlled study of the effect of rectal paracetamol on morphine consumption after abdominal hysterectomy. *Acta Anaesthesiol Scand* 2003; 47: 451-6

Lariviere WR, Wilson SG, Laughlin TM, Kokayeff A, West EE, Adhikari SM, Wan Y, Mogil JS. Heritability of nociception. III. genetic relationships among commonly used assays of nociception and hypersensitivity. *Pain* 2002; 97: 75-86

Lattermann R, Schricker T, Wachter U, Georgieff M, Schreiber M. Laparoscopic-assisted vaginal hysterectomy and the hyperglycemic response to surgery: an observational study. *Can J Anaesth* 2001; 48: 871-5

Lenz H, Sandvik L, Qvigstad E, Bjerkelund CE, Ræder J. A comparison of intravenous oxycodone and intravenous morphine in patient-controlled postoperative analgesia after laparoscopic hysterectomy. *Anesth Analg* 2009; 109: 1279-83

Lethaby A, Ivanova V, Johnson NP. Total versus subtotal hysterectomy for benign gynaecological conditions. *Cochrane Database Syst Rev* 2006; 2: CD004993

Levy BS, Luciano DE, Emery LL. Outpatient vaginal hysterectomy is safe for patients and reduces institutional cost. *J Minim Invasive Gynecol* 2005; 12: 494-501

Lin JG, Lo MW, Wen YR, Hsieh CL, Tsai SK, Sun WZ. The effect of high an low frequency electrpoacupuncture in pain after lower abdominal surgery. *Pain* 2002; 99: 509-14

Lin TF, Yeh YC, Lin FS, Wang YP, Lin CJ, Sun WZ, Fan SZ. Effect of combining dexmedetomidine and morphine for intravenous patient-controlled analgesia. *Br J Anaesth* 2009; 102: 117-22

Lo Y, Chia YY, Liu K, Ko NH. Morphine sparing with droperidol in patient-controlled analgesia. *J Clin Anesth* 2005; 17: 271-5

Macintyre PE, Scott DA, Schug SA, Visser EJ, Walker SM. Acute pain management: scientific evidence (3rd edition), Melbourne 2010

Maranets I, Kain ZN. Preoperative anxiety and intraoperative anesthetic requirements. *Anesth Analg* 1999; 89: 1346-51

Massicotte L, Chalaoui KD, Beaulieu D, Roy JD, Bissonnette F. Comparison of spinal anesthesia with general anesthesia on morphine requirement after abdominal hysterectomy. *Acta Anaesth Scand* 2009; 53: 641-7

Mathiesen O, Rasmussen ML, Dierking G, Lech K, Hilsted KL, Fomsgaard JS, Lose G, Dahl JB. Pregabalin and dexamethasone in combination with paracetamol for postoperative pain control after abdominal hysterectomy. *Acta Anaesth Scand* 2009; 53: 227-35

McDonnell J, Laffey J. Transversus abdominis plane block. *Anesth Analg* 2007; 105: 883

Meyhoff CS, Henneberg SW, Jørgensen BG, Gätke MR, Rasmussen LS. Depth of anaesthesia monitoring in obese patients: a randomized study of propofol-remifentanil. *Acta Anaesth Scand* 2009; 53: 369-75

Moerman N, van Dam FS, Muller MJ, Oosting H. The Amsterdam preoperative anxiety and information scale (APAIS). *Anesth Analg* 1996; 82: 445-51

Morley AP, Derrick J, Seed PT, Tan PE, Chung DC, Short TG. Isoflurane dosage for equivalent intraoperative electroencephalographic suppression in patients with and without epidural blockade. *Anesth Analg* 2002; 95: 1412-8

Murphy EJ. Acute pain management pharmacology for the patient with concurrent renal or hepatic disease. *Anaesth Intensive Care* 2005; 33: 311-22

Møller C, Kehlet H, Friland SG, Schouenborg LO, Lund C, Ottesen B. Fast track hysterectomy. *Eur J Obstet Gynecol Reprod Biol* 2001; 98: 18-22

Naik R, Jackson KS, Lopes A, Cross P, Henry JA. Laparoscopic assisted radical vaginal hysterectomy versus radical abdominal hysterectomy - a randomised phase II trial. *BJOG* 2010; 117: 746-51

Niesters M, Dahan A, Kest B, Zacny J, Stijnen T, Aarts L, Sarton E. Do sex differences exist in opioid analgeisa? A systematic review and meta-analysis of human experimental and clinical studies. *Pain* 2010; 151: 61-8

Niiyama Y, Kawamata T, Shimizu H, Omote K, Namiki A. The addition of epidural morphine to ropivacaine improves epidural analgesia after lower abdominal surgery. *Can J Anaesth* 2005; 52: 181-5

Oehler MK. Robotic surgery in gynaecology and gynaecologic oncology: program initiation and operative outcomes at the Royal Adelaide Hospital. *Aust N Z J Obstet Gynaecol* 2011; 51: 119-24

Oriola F, Toque Y, Mary A, Gagneur O, Beloucif S, Dupont H. Bilateral ilioinguinal nerve block decreases morphine consumption in female patients undergoing nonlaparoscopic gynecologic surgery. *Anesth Analg* 2007; 104: 731-4

Ottesen M, Sørensen M, Rasmussen Y, Smidt-Jensen S, Kehlet H, Ottesen B. Fast track vaginal surgery. *Acta Obstet Gynecol Scand* 2002; 81: 138-46

Park HP, Hwang JW, Kim YB, Jeon YT, Park SH, Yun MJ, Do SH. Effect of pre-emptive alveolar recruitment strategy before pneumoperitoneum on arterial oxygenation during laparoscopic hysterectomy. *Anaesth Intensive Care* 2009; 37: 593-7

Penketh R, Griffiths A, Chawathe S. A prospective observational study of the safety and acceptability of vaginal hysterectomy performed in a 24-hour day case surgery setting. *BJOG* 2007; 114: 430-6

Perkins FM, Kehlet H. Chronic pain as an outcome of surgery. A review of predictive factors. *Anesthesiology* 2000; 93: 1123-33

Perniola A, Gupta A, Crafoord K, Darvish B, Magnuson A, Axelsson K. Intraabdominal local anesthetics for postoperative pain relief following abdominal hysterectomy: a randomized, double-blind, dose-finding study. *Eur J Anaesthesiol* 2009; 26: 421-9

Persson P, Brynhildsen J, Kjølhede P. Short-term recovery after subtotal and total abdominal hysterectomy – a randomised clinical trial. *BJOG* 2010; 117: 469-78

Persson P, Kjølhede P. Factors associated with postoperative recovery after laparoscopic and abdominal hysterectomy. *Eur J Obstet Gynecol Reprod Biol* 2008; 140: 108-13

Petersen PL, Mathiesen O, Thorup H, Dahl JB. The transversus abdominis plane block: a valuable option for post-operative analgesia? A topical review. *Acta Anaesthesiol Scand* 2010; 54: 529-539

Piper SN, Triem JG, Röhm KD, Kranke P, Maleck WH, Boldt J. Prevention of post-operative nausea and vomiting. Randomised comparison of dolasetron versus dolasetron plus dexamethasone. *Anaesthesist* 2003; 52: 120-6

Pirim A, Karaman S, Uyar M. Addition of ketamine infusion to patient controlled analgesia with intravenous morphine after abdominal hysterectomy. *Agri* 2006; 18: 52-8

Rafi A. Abdominal field block: a new approach via the lumbar triangle. *Anesthesia* 2001; 56: 1024-26

Ribeiro SC, Ribeiro RM, Santos NC, Pinotti JA. A randomized study of total abdominal, vaginal and laparoscopic hysterectomy. *Int J Gynaecol Obstet* 2003; 83: 37-43

Riddle DL, Wade JB, Jiranek WA, Kong X. Preoperative pain catastrophizing predicts pain outcome after knee arthroplasty. *Clin Orthop Relat Res* 2010; 468: 798-806

Rodriguez R, Martinez E, Santana M, Rodriguez Huertas E. Stress response under continuous infusion of remifentanil compared to bolus doses of fentanyl assessed by levels of cytokines, C-reactive protein, and cortisol during and after abdominal hysterectomy. *Rev Esp Anestesiol Reanim* 2007; 54: 221-6

Roovers JP, van der Bom JG, van der Vaart CH, Heintz AP. Hysterectomy and sexual wellbeing: prospective observational study of vaginal hysterectomy, subtotal abdominal hysterectomy, and total abdominal hysterectomy. *BMJ* 2003; 327: 774-8

Roumm AR, Pizzi L, Goldfarb NI, Cohn H. Minimally invasive: minimally reimbursed? An examination of six laparoscopic surgical procedures. *Surg Innov* 2005; 12: 261-87

Samer CF, Daali Y, Wagner M, Hopfgartner G, Eap CB et al. Genetic polymorphisms and drug interactions modulating CYP2D6 and CYP3A activities have a major effect on oxycodone analgesic efficacy and safety. *Br J Pharmacol* 2010; 160: 919-30

Sarmini OR, Lefholz K, Froeschke HP. A comparison of laparoscopic supracervical hysterectomy and total abdominal hysterectomy outcomes. *J Minim Invasive Gynecol* 2005; 12: 121-4

Sartain JB, Barry JJ, Richardson CA, Branagan HC. Effect of combining naloxone and morphine for intravenous patient-controlled analgesia. *Anesthesiology* 2003; 99: 148-51

Sarton E, Romberg R, Dahan A. Gender differences in morphine pharmacokinetics and dynamics. *Adv Exp Med Biol* 2003; 523: 71-80

Sen H, Sizlan A, Yanarates O, Emirkadi H, Ozkan S, Dagli G, Turan A. A comparison of gabapentin and ketamine in acute and chronic pain after hysterectomy. *Anesth Analg* 2009; 109: 1645-50

Serati M, Salvatore S, Uccella S, Laterza RM, Cromi A, Ghezzi F, Bolis P. Sexual function after radical hysterectomy for early-stage cervical cancer: is there a difference between laparoscopy and laparotomy? *J Sex Med* 2009; 6: 2516-22

Sharma JB, Wadhwa L, Malhotra M, Arora R. Mini laparotomy versus conventional laparotomy for abdominal hysterectomy: a comparative study. *Indian J Med Sci* 2004; 58: 196-202

Sjöling M, Nordahl G, Olofsson N, Asplund K. The impact of preoperative information on state anxiety, postoperative pain and satisfaction with pain management. *Patient Educ Couns* 2003; 51: 169-76

Sprung J, Sanders Ms, Warner ME, Gebhart JB, Stanhope CR, Jankowski CJ et al. Pain relief and functional status after vaginal hysterectomy: intrathecal versus general anesthesia. *Can J Anaesth* 2006; 53: 690-700

Strang CM, Hachenberg T, Fredén F, Hedenstierna G. Development of atelectasis and arterial to end-tidal PCO2-difference in a porcine model of pneumoperitoneum. *Br J Anaesth* 2009; 103: 298-303

Tan EK, Cornish J, Darzi AW, Tekkis PP. Meta-analysis: alvimopan vs placebo in the treatment of post-operative ileus. *Aliment Pharmacol Ther* 2007; 25: 47-57

Teplin V, Vittinghoff E, Lin F, Learman LA, Richter HE, Kuppermann M. Oophorectomy in premenopausal women: health-related quality of life and sexual functioning. *Obstet Gynecol* 2007; 109: 347-54

Thangaswamy CR, Rewari V, Trikha A, Dehran M, Chandralekha. Dexamethasone before total laparoscopic hyerectomy: a randomized controlled dose-response study. *J Anesth* 2010; 24: 24-30

Topcu I, Luleci N, Tekin S, Kefi A, Erincler T. Effectiveness of clonidine and fentanyl addition to bupivacaine in postoperative patient controlled epidural analgesia. *Anasthesiol Intensivmed Notfallmed Schmerzther* 2005; 40: 521-5

Turan A, White PF, Karamanlioglu B, Memis D, Tasdogan M, Pamukcu Z, Yavuz E. Gabapentin: an alternative to the cyclooxygenase-2 inhibitors for perioperative pain management. *Anesth Analg* 2006; 102: 175-81

Vitale AT, O'Connor PC. The effect of Reiki on pain and anxiety in women with abdominal hysterectomies: a quasi-experimental pilot study. *Holist Nurs Pract* 2006; 263-72

Wang F, Shen X, Liu Y, Xu S, Guo X. Continuous infusion of butorphanol combined with intravenous morphine patient-controlled analgesia after total abdominal hysterectomy a randomized, double-blind controlled trial. *Eur J Anaesth* 2009; 26: 28-34

Wang F, Shen X, Xu S, Liu Y, Ma L, Zhao Q, Fu D, Feng S, Li X. Negative words on surgical wards result in therapeutic failure of patient-controlled analgesia and further release of cortisol after abdominal surgeries. *Minerva Anestesiol* 2008; 74: 353-65

Wang F, Shen X, Xu S, Liu Y. Preoperative tramadol combined with postoperative small-dose tramadol infusion after total abdominal hysterectomy: a double-blind, randomized, controlled trial. *Pharmacol Rep* 2009; 61: 1198-205

Wodlin NB, Nilsson L, Arestedt K, Kjølhede P. Mode of anesthesia and postoperative symptoms following abdominal hysterectomy in a fast-track setting. *Acta Obstet Gynecol Scand* 2011; 90: 369-79

Wodlin NB, Nilsson L, Kjølhede P. Health-related quality of life and postoperative recovery in fast-track hysterectomy. *Acta Obstet Gynecol Scand* 2011; 90: 362-8

Wodlin NB, Nilsson L, Kjølhede P. The impact of mode of anaesthesia on postoperative recovery from fast-track abdominal hysterectomy: a randomised clinical trial. *BJOG* 2011; 118: 299-308

Yardeni IZ, Beilin B, Mayburd E, Levinson Y, Bessler H. The effect of perioperative intravenous lidocaine on postoperative pain and immune function. *Anesth Analg* 2009; 109: 1464-9

Yeh YC, Lin TF, Chang HC, Chan WS, Wang YP, Lin CJ, Sun WZ. Combination of low-dose nalbuphine and morphine in patient-controlled analgesia decreases incidence of opioid-related side effects. *J Formos Med Assoc* 2009; 108: 548-53

Zhang XW, Fan Y, Manyande A, Tian YK, Yin P. Effects of music on target-controlled infusion of propofol requirements during combined spinal-epidural anaesthesia. *Anaesthesia* 2005; 60: 990-4

Zhao LY, Ye TH,Zhang YZ, Zhao H. Combination of morphine with low-dose naloxone for intravenous patient-controlled analgesia. *Zhongguo Yi Xue Ke Xue Yuan Xue Bao* 2005; 27: 228-31

Part 4

Hysterectomy Post-Operative Care

16

Innovations in the Care of Postoperative Hysterectomy Patients

Sepeedeh Saleh and Amitabha Majumdar
East Lancashire NHS Trust, Lancashire, United Kingdom

1. Introduction

Hysterectomy, removal of the uterus, has traditionally been regarded as the definitive surgical treatment for heavy menstrual bleeding. And is one of the most commonly performed operations in the UK. (Marjoribanks, 2006) Whilst menstrual disorders are the most frequent reasons for performing hysterectomy other common indications include chronic pelvic pain, fibroids, malignancy of the uterus, cervix or ovaries and genital prolapse. Hysterectomy is a major surgical procedure with potential for significant physical and emotional complications. It also carries additional social and economic costs. (Lethaby, 1999)

Hysterectomy rates have been decreasing in recent years, but there remain large variations in population-based rates of hysterectomy across primary care organisations in England, from fewer than 10 per 100,000 to 100 per 100,000 in female populations. (Information for hospital episode statistics) Although hysterectomies were originally all performed via the abdominal route, alternative types of hysterectomy (for example vaginal and laparoscopic hysterectomies) are increasingly popular, particularly when carried out for benign disease. Vaginal hysterectomy is the procedure of choice for uterovaginal prolapse amongst practitioners in the UK. (Jha, 2007) This move away from abdominal surgery is in part due to the less invasive nature of the vaginal and laparoscopic procedures which, as a result, produce arguably better outcomes: an effect most marked when considering post-operative recovery. Current evidence on the safety and efficacy of laparoscopic techniques for hysterectomy (including laparoscopic-assisted vaginal hysterectomy, laparoscopic hysterectomy, laparoscopic supracervical hysterectomy and total laparoscopic hysterectomy) appears adequate to support their use, provided arrangements are in place for consent, audit and clinical governance.

Although hysterectomy is generally considered safe several possible complications are associated with the procedure. These complications can result in mild to severe morbidity and even (in rare cases) mortality. Although their incidence is low, it is important to be aware of the immediate and longer-term complications that may arise from hysterectomy. Immediate complications include haemorrhage, bladder and ureteric injury, bowel injury, infection and venous thromboembolism. Long-term complications include the psychological and emotional aspects of such surgery in addition to complications arising from the surgical menopause and the use of hormone replacement therapies.

In recent years there has been increasing pressure on the health service for faster return to normal activity following major surgical procedures including hysterectomy, irrespective of the route of surgery. Demand for these changes has been driven not only by economic considerations but also by the healthcare needs of working population. There is also greater awareness among women undergoing major surgery, presumably due to increased health education, about the need for faster recovery. In order to ensure a safe and quick recovery after surgery effective preoperative preparation and intraoperative planning are essential and it is important that the patient play an active role in this pathway. It is against this background that enhanced recovery after surgery (ERAS) has been discussed in this chapter, with special emphasis on hysterectomy.

2. ERAS overview

In recent years the concept of 'Enhanced Recovery After Surgery' (ERAS), initially pioneered in colonic surgery by Kehlet et al. (2008) has led to great improvements in postoperative recovery.

Enhanced Recovery after Surgery (or 'Fast-track' surgery) is an evidence-based, multidisciplinary approach to perioperative care. It aims to empower the patient to take an active role in their own care and integrates preoperative, intraoperative and postoperative techniques to reduce the stress response to surgery. These interventions help to lessen the degree of organ dysfunction postoperatively. This can lead to reduced complication rates and better overall recovery from surgery which in turn allows earlier hospital discharge without an increase in perioperative morbidity. As well as being an indicator of quicker postoperative recovery, and therefore earlier return to normal activity, reduced hospital stay also increases NHS productivity and reduces the risk of hospital acquired infection. (NHS Better Care, 2011 & Delgado- Rodriguez, 1990)

2.1 The stress response

It is thought that one of the primary causes of postoperative morbidity in an otherwise uncomplicated surgical procedure is the system of reactive changes to injury or trauma known as the surgical stress response. (Kehlet M, 1997) This is a complex neuroendocrine response mediated by the sympathetic autonomic nervous system and hypothalamic-pituitary axis and involving activation of several biological cascade systems (See below). The stress response is commenced within minutes of hysterectomy, first with adrenocorticotrophic hormone (ACTH) stimulating increased cortisol production, and within the next few hours with increased interleukin levels in the circulation. The magnitude of the reaction is dependent on the degree of trauma meaning that significant differences in the response are seen between vaginal or laparoscopic hysterectomies and open procedures. We will now discuss in more detail the various constituents of the stress response resulting from hysterectomy procedures.

2.2 Constituents of the stress response

2.2.1 Initiation

Somatic and autonomic afferents from the area of trauma (or surgery) activate both the sympathetic nervous system and the hypothalamic-pituitary axis initiating both systems of response.

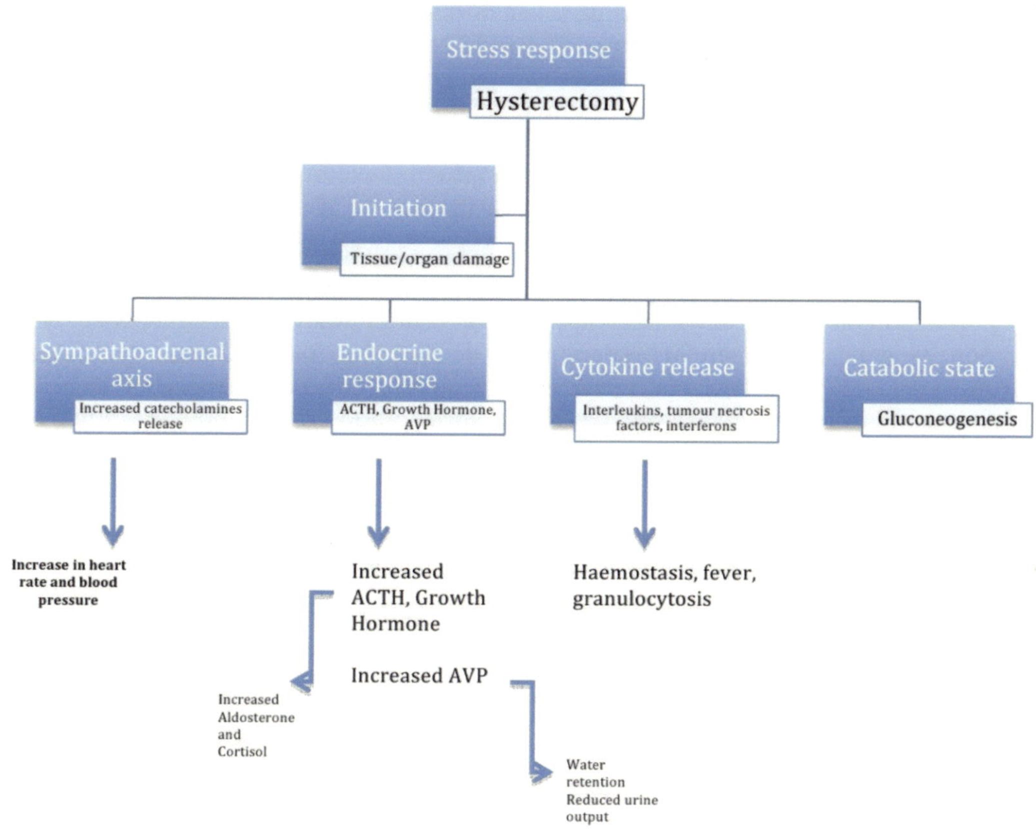

Fig. 1. The Stress Response in Hysterectomy

2.2.2 Sympathoadrenal response

Hypothalamic activation of the sympathetic nervous system leads to increased catecholamine secretion from the adrenal medulla. There is also spillover of norepinephrine into the circulation from the presynaptic nerve terminals. This results in cardiovascular effects such as tachycardia and hypertension as well as modifications in end organs, namely the liver, pancreas and kidneys.

2.2.3 Endocrine response

There is increased secretion of ACTH and growth hormone from the anterior pituitary gland and arginine vasopressin (AVP) from the posterior pituitary. These hormones have effects on target organs including increased cortisol and aldosterone secretion from the adrenal cortex. Furthermore, the usual negative feedback mechanism between ACTH and cortisol fails postoperatively and there is a persistent rise in the concentrations of both hormones. A catabolic state results in which substrates are mobilised to release energy sources and salt and water are retained to increase the intravascular fluid volume. Specifically, cortisol promotes protein catabolism and gluconeogenesis and reduces glucose use by cells thus creating an increase in blood glucose levels. These actions are augmented by an inhibition of insulin secretion from the β cells of the pancreas during surgery and a postoperative state of insulin resistance in the cells. A reduction in the effects of insulin means reduced uptake of glucose into adipose tissue and muscle and reduced glucose storage in the form of glycogen and triglycerides as well as additional catabolic effects on protein and lipids. Glucagon release from the pancreas results in further breakdown of glycogen and muscle. Growth hormone, mainly mediated through insulin-like growth factors (IGFs) such as IGF-1, also has anti-insulin effects and promotes lipolysis, furthering the general catabolic state during and after surgery.

Increased secretion of AVP by the posterior pituitary gland in response to trauma promotes water retention in the kidneys resulting in more concentrated urine. Increased renin secretion by the juxtaglomerular apparatus of the kidneys (partly due to sympathetic activation) adds to this effect by converting angiotensin I to angiotensin II which then stimulates aldosterone secretion from the adrenal cortex. Aldosterone amplifies sodium and water reabsorption by the kidneys.

This osmotic diuresis combined with the hypoinsulinaemia and relative insulin resistance occurring intra- and postoperatively is particularly problematic in diabetic patients who can suffer perioperatively from ketoacidosis or hyperosmolar syndrome.

Changes in the thyroid hormones, gonadotrophins, prolactin and β-endorphin also take place in response to surgery but these are not central to the present discussion.

Cytokines are a group of low molecular weight proteins including the interleukins (IL), interferons and tumour necrosis factor (TNF). They play a major role in immunity and inflammation, acting on target cell receptors both locally and systemically. Initially, IL-1 and TNF-α are released from activated macrophages and monocytes in damaged tissues. This triggers further cytokine release, particularly IL-6, the main cytokine causing the systemic changes comprising the acute phase response. Production of IL-6 increases within 30 to 60 minutes of the start of surgery and its serum concentration is in direct proportion to the degree of tissue damage occurring. Cytokines also mediate other effects such as fever, granulocytosis and haemostasis.

2.2.4 Summary

The stress response is characterised by catabolism, fluid retention, pain, immunosupression and coagulatory system changes favouring coagulation and thrombosis. In addition, there is increased cardiac work due to autonomic activation, impaired pulmonary function and gastrointestinal dysfunction including nausea and ileus.

In terms of development the changes described above were likely to have evolved to help survival of an injured animal, mobilising stored body fuels and activating repair processes. In modern medicine, however, it is argued that these systems are more likely to have negative effects, catabolising cell mass and disrupting physiological reserve. These factors could greatly impede the recovery process after hysterectomy. In recent years research has been done into perioperative interventions to modify the response in an attempt to reduce postoperative morbidity. Addressing the stress response to surgery constitutes a major part of the ERAS system. We go on to discuss these in more detail in the next section.

2.3 Components of the ERAS system

Enhanced recovery after surgery is a comprehensive programme combining many facets, each of which has been individually explored and validated. (Enhanced Recovery Partnership Programme, 2010) The system relies on full cooperation of the multidisciplinary team throughout. This allows a smooth operative journey from patient preparation (starting prior to hospital referral) to a proactive approach to analgesia, nutrition and mobilization on the hospital ward postoperatively.

2.3.1 Preoperative factors

2.3.1.1 Preoperative assessment/optimization

As shown by the American Society of Anesthesiologists' (ASA) grading system, a patients' preoperative physical status plays a key role in predicting their overall perioperative outcome. A normal healthy patient (ASA I) has an absolute surgical mortality risk of 0.1%. This risk increases to 1.8% for patients with severe systemic diseases such as chronic obstructive pulmonary disease (COPD), who would be graded ASA III. (ASA Task Force publication, 2002) It is therefore vital to optimise women's physical (as well as psychological) condition prior to undertaking the hysterectomy procedure. The first step in doing this is to quantify each individual woman's risk from the surgical procedure planned: an assessment which may involve further investigations depending on the patient's comorbidities. Women with asthma or COPD, for example, may need specialist tests of pulmonary function; women with known heart murmurs or a degree of cardiac failure may need cardiac investigations. Optimising comorbidities is a key step in hysterectomy planning. Patients undergoing hysterectomy due to menorrhagia or malignancy may require correction of anaemia with iron therapy, blood transfusion or other measures. Similarly, optimisation of diabetic control and nutritional status preoperatively can yield benefits in operative outcome.

In all cases complete risk assessment must be carried out for venous thromboembolism (VTE) and appropriate measures must be in place for thromboprophylaxis prior to commencing surgery, in accordance with national guidance. (NICE Guidance CG92, 2011)

Lastly, as part of the preoperative evaluation process, the type and route of surgery planned must be carefully considered, along with the indications for surgery and any alternatives to surgery in each case. This involves full discussion with the patient, ensuring their understanding and consent at each stage. Patient education, including information regarding the anticipated postoperative course (in particular, analgesia mobilisation and discharge) is central to improving postoperative recovery and reducing length of stay. Studies have shown that preoperative patient education programmes can work to improve patient outcomes after surgery, including significant reductions in the length of hospital stay, and increase patient satisfaction with the surgical experience. (Kruzik, 2009 & Jones, 2011)

2.3.1.2 Preoperative hydration status

Patients for elective surgery under general anaesthetic are traditionally fasted overnight with a view to reducing the volume and acidity of the gastric contents and minimising the risk of aspiration. However, it is important that patients are adequately hydrated before surgery and research on the subject has found that fasting from midnight is not only potentially unnecessary for most patients but may also have negative effects on postoperative recovery. (Nygren, 2007) Guidance from anaesthetic associations agrees that, in general, clear fluids should be allowed up to two hours before administration of general anaesthesia, and light meals up to six hours before and recent ASA guidelines made no changes to this recommendation. (ASA Guideline, 2011 & Powell-Tuck, 2008). A Cochrane review supports this advice stating that there was no evidence to suggest that shortened fasting times for fluids results in increased risks of aspiration, regurgitation or related morbidity compared with the standard 'nil by mouth from midnight' policy, and encourages clinicians to evaluate the evidence for themselves, adjusting existing fasting policies where necessary. (Brady, 2003)

A traditional overnight fasting regime, apart from producing dehydration, also heightens the insulin resistance which, as discussed above, constitutes a key element of the surgical stress response. It has been found in many settings that an oral carbohydrate load administered prior to surgery reduces postoperative insulin resistance and is associated with improved postoperative wellbeing. This has, in addition, translated to reduced hospital stays postoperatively. (Ljungqvist, 2002 & 2009, Noblett, 2006)

2.3.1.3 Premedication

In the enhanced recovery setting, consideration is given to premedication with a view to further reducing the surgical stress response. Research initially focused on β-blockers, which aim to reduce the catecholamine response to surgery and therefore improve cardiovascular function. However the POISE trial demonstrated an increased death rate with perioperative commencement of high-dose β-blockers (Devereaux, 2008) so the use of β-blockers as premedication has largely been discontinued. Work is now focusing on α_2-agonists such as clonidine which mainly have opioid-sparing effects, but have also been found to have positive effects on blood loss, nausea and vomiting. (Goyagi, 1999, Wu, 2004, Mohseni, 2011 & Oddby-Muhrbeck, 2002)

2.3.2 Intraoperative factors

2.3.2.1 Surgical technique

It is known that minimally invasive surgery leads to less of a systemic immune response than open access surgery and that it is generally associated with shorter hospital stays and reduced pain postoperatively. (Fuchs, 2002)

Looking specifically at hysterectomy procedures for benign indications, a Cochrane review reported improved recovery from vaginal hysterectomy compared with abdominal and laparoscopically assisted procedures. Laparoscopic procedures were found to be similarly advantageous compared with abdominal hysterectomy. With comparison of overall, particularly longer-term, outcome measures, however, there is not necessarily a clear advantage to minimal access surgery (Nieboer, 2009 & Kehlet, 2006) over open surgery when considered apart from other aspects of a fast-track programme.

Consideration must be given to the type of incision employed: transverse incisions tend to reduce postoperative pain and should be used preferentially where all other factors are equal. Lastly, surgeons must bear in mind that wound drains can hinder pain control and slow recovery. Their use must therefore be judicious and any drains or urinary catheters which are used must be removed at the earliest possible stage postoperatively to minimise the potential for negative effects.

In general, it is important to evaluate each case individually when making decisions regarding surgical technique and to integrate components of a multimodal enhanced recovery programme to yield significant benefits.

2.3.2.2 Anaesthetic technique

Detailed discussion of anaesthetic techniques is outside the remit of this chapter, however, enhanced recovery programmes aim, in general, to achieve good pain control with minimal opioid 'hang-over' effects postoperatively. For this reason short acting anaesthetics and analgesics are preferred. Regional blocks can be useful, reducing the dose of opioids required and minimising the stress response to surgery as well as providing postoperative analgesia and expediting recovery of bowel function thereby reducing the occurrence of postoperative ileus, as shown by a recent study. (Wodlin, 2011) Other benefits from epidural use include a reduction in the rates of respiratory failure and venous thromboembolism, as shown by the MASTER trial. (Rigg, 2002) Research does not, however, draw any definite conclusions regarding superiority of one anaesthetic technique over another and the optimal approach remains to evaluate anaesthetic choices on a case-by-case basis.

2.3.2.3 Fluid management

A good balance must be stuck when managing patients' hydration status perioperatively. Adequate hydration is effective in minimising postoperative nausea and vomiting and drowsiness. The effects of good hydration have been found to include reductions in postoperative complication rates and in length of hospital stay. (Walsh, 2008) Overhydration could, however, be harmful carrying risks of pulmonary and cardiac dysfunction and potentially impeding wound healing. These effects could potentially be inflated by the effects of the surgical stress response leading to increased salt and water retention. Perioperative fluid balance is dependent on many factors including nature and magnitude of the surgery. A radical open hysterectomy would create more opportunity for evaporative fluid loss than a vaginal or laparoscopic procedure and if bowel became involved further oedema and third-spacing of fluids would be more likely. The ideal approach, therefore, is that of tailored, goal-directed fluid therapy. Consensus guidance on operative fluid therapy suggests intravenous fluid administration to achieve optimal values of stroke volume in certain types of orthopaedic and abdominal surgery. (Powell-Tuck, 2008) This is achieved using either central venous pressure monitoring or the less invasive oesophageal Doppler ultrasound intraoperatively to guide fluid management. Evidence for such 'goal-directed' fluid therapy evidence shows benefits including reduction of complications and shortening of hospital stay where it is used in more major surgery. (Giglio, 2009 & Wakeling, 2005) It is not, however, currently suggested for use during routine hysterectomy procedures, although it could be useful in more extensive hysterectomy surgery (for example in cancer surgery) or in cases requiring more precise fluid management.

2.3.2.4 Temperature control

Hypothermia, even if mild, can exacerbate the stress response to surgery by sympathetic activation and there is evidence that it can impair coagulation and wound healing and predispose to infection. (Frank, 2001) These effects become more pertinent as the operative time increases as thermoregulatory heat-preserving mechanisms are impaired by anaesthetic and patients' behaviour responses to cold are lost. NICE guidelines on perioperative temperature regulation are extensive, recommending, amongst other measures, close monitoring of patient temperatures intraoperatively, warming of intravenous fluids if more than 500ml are given intraoperatively and use of a forced air warming device if patients are under anaesthetic for more than half 30 minutes. (NICE Guideline 29, 2011)

2.3.2.5 Avoidance of postoperative nausea and vomiting (PONV)

Nausea and vomiting following surgery is a common complication and can be highly distressing for patients. Furthermore, it can interfere with oral intake and analgesia creating further problems with postoperative recovery. It is recommended that patients are risk-assessed for postoperative nausea and vomiting and given prophylactic antiemetic therapy if they are found to be at moderate or high risk. (Lassen, 2009) Risk stratification is commonly carried out using the 'Apfel' scoring system which awards a point for each of the following four risk factors: female sex, history of motion sickness or postoperative nausea and vomiting, non-smoker status and planned opioid use. (Apfel, 1999) This demonstrates that most hysterectomy patients are at moderate if not high risk of PONV due to their female gender and the frequent use of opioid analgesia in the immediate postoperative period.

2.3.3 Postoperative factors

2.3.3.1 Balanced analgesia

Effective pain relief postoperatively is vital in minimising the surgical stress response as well as easing return to normal activity (mobilisation, oral intake, etc) thus further improving recovery. The central aim of balanced (or multimodal) analgesia as a constituent of the enhanced recovery system is to maximise analgesic efficacy and minimise side effects by combining various modes of analgesia. The use of paracetamol and non-steroidals can help to reduce the doses of opioids and therefore minimise opioid side effects such as sedation, ileus and respiratory complications. Other opioid-sparing adjuncts which can be helpful include gabapentin and pregabalin. For major surgical procedures techniques such as transversus abdominis plane (TAP) blocks and epidural analgesia may also be used. (Petersen, 2010 & Kehlet, 1997)

2.3.3.2 Early enteral nutrition

The catabolic response to surgery is known to reduce muscle mass, compromise immune function and delay the healing process as well as increasing patient fatigue which itself further impedes recovery. (Wilmore, 2000) It has been traditional to delay oral intake after major abdominal surgery, mainly due to concerns over ileus and nausea and vomiting, however, recent work has demonstrated the safety of early feeding, even after major bowel surgery. (Andersen, 2006) A Cochrane review comparing early and delayed feeding after major gynaecological surgery also illustrated benefits of early oral intake in terms of shorter times to the presence of bowel sounds; shorter times to first solid diet and, ultimately, shorter hospital stays. Early feeding was defined as having oral intake of fluids or food within the first 24 hours after surgery regardless of the presence or absence of the signs that indicate the return of bowel function and delayed feeding was defined after first 24 hours following surgery and only after clinical signs of resolution of postoperative ileus. There was an increased risk of nausea noted with early feeding and it was recommended that the decision regarding commencement of oral intake should be individualised. (Charoenkwan, 2007)

There is some evidence that routine provision of laxatives postoperatively also improves gastrointestinal function after procedures such as hysterectomy. (Hansen, 2007) This is not yet an established element of the fast-track programme, however, and in most cases laxatives are reserved for use on an 'as required' basis.

2.3.3.3 Early mobilisation

Mobilisation helps to reduce the catabolic effects of surgery on skeletal muscle, improves pulmonary function and stimulates the circulation, thus improving oxygen delivery to tissues and reducing chances of venous thromboembolism. In terms of the gastrointestinal system ambulation promotes the return of gut function and can help to prevent postoperative ileus. Early postoperative mobilisation is a key part of the fast-track system. It should be discussed preoperatively to allow the patient to create positive goals in recovery and adequate analgesia should be maintained to allow the patient to mobilise comfortably. Multidisciplinary teams are important with physiotherapy staff playing major roles in aiding early mobilisation. This facilitates a smooth postoperative journey towards a planned, criteria-based discharge in which the patient is a partner throughout their rehabilitation.

3. Enhanced recovery after surgery with reference to hysterectomy

Enhanced recovery is a relatively new concept in gynaecological surgery although it has been in vogue in colorectal and other surgeries for a few years. The authors reviewed the current literature and present the existing evidence regarding the use of enhanced recovery techniques with hysterectomy. The authors will discuss the findings of nine papers published after 1990, with clear endpoints addressing aspects of enhanced recovery programmes in use for hysterectomy. It is felt that enhanced recovery programmes applied to other aspects of obstetrics and gynaecological surgery, i.e. caesarean sections and prolapse surgery, are beyond the scope of this chapter.

We looked first at the study by Borendal Wodlin et al. for the 'GASPI' study group. This was a multicentre randomised controlled trial initially involving 180 women scheduled for benign hysterectomy, although only 162 of these patients completed the study. The patients were randomised and allocated to either spinal (82 women) or general anaesthetic (80 women) for the procedure. A range of outcome measures were assessed using the 'Swedish Postoperative Symptoms Questionnaire'. These outcomes were reported separately as discussed above. The first paper we examined was entitled 'The impact of mode of anaesthesia on postoperative recovery from fast-track abdominal hysterectomy: a randomised clinical trial' (Wodlin, 2011a). This compared the duration of stay postoperatively between the two groups as well as postoperative morphine requirements. It was found that duration of hospital stay after any fast-track abdominal hysterectomy was less than 50 hours, regardless of the mode of anaesthetic used. No significant difference was detected between the two groups with regard to this endpoint. It was noted, however, that there was a reduced need for postoperative morphine with hysterectomy performed under spinal anaesthesia compared with general anaesthesia.

The next paper we considered was 'Mode of anaesthesia and postoperative symptoms following abdominal hysterectomy in a fast-track setting' (Wodlin, 2011b) which reported the differences in postoperative symptoms within the first 5 weeks post-hysterectomy found between the two groups in the 'GASPI' study described above. The main findings here were that, in general, spinal had advantages over general anaesthetic in terms of postoperative symptoms and recovery. It was found that abdominal pain, drowsiness and fatigue occurred significantly less often and with lower intensity with spinal anaesthesia but that there were more episodes of vomiting after spinal anaesthetics.

A later paper in the same journal issue entitled 'Health-related quality of life and postoperative recovery in fast-track hysterectomy'(Wodlin, 2011c) reported differences in health-related quality of life and duration of sick leave between the two study groups in the 'GASPI' study. Faster postoperative improvements in health-related quality of life and shorter sick leave were seen after surgery under spinal anaesthetic than with general anaesthetic although it was noted that these outcomes were influenced by complications in both groups. Finally the 'GASPI' study group published an article entitled 'Cost-effectiveness of general anesthesia versus spinal anesthesia in fast track abdominal benign hysterectomy'. (Wodlin, 2011d) This compared total healthcare costs between the two groups as described previously and concluded that the surgery was more cost effective under spinal than under general anaesthesia.

The next study examined at was 'The effect of accelerated rehabilitation on recovery after surgery for ovarian malignancy' by Marx et al. (Marx, 2006) This was a case control study looking at surgery for ovarian malignancy (undertaken according to guidelines from the International Federation of Gynecology and Obstetrics). A total of 141 women were included: 72 patients receiving conventional perioperative care were compared with 69 patients receiving multimodal, fast-track rehabilitation. The main outcome measures were postoperative hospital stay and morbidity during the first postoperative month. In this study the fast-track programme was found to reduce the median postoperative hospital stay as well as the rate of severe medical complications and the readmission rate. There was, however, no significant difference in overall complication rates between the two groups.

An article by Møller et al. entitled 'Fast track hysterectomy' (Moller, 2001) was found very interesting in this context. It was a prospective descriptive study involving 32 women and aimed to identify factors limiting early discharge after Laparoscopically Assisted Vaginal Hysterectomy (LAVH) and abdominal hysterectomy in a fast track setting. Outcome measures analysed included length of postoperative hospital stay and resumption of work. This study found no significant benefits to either surgical route in terms of convalescence or hospitalisation and concluded that further studies involving active rehabilitation would be required to demonstrate any such differences.

A later paper on the topic by Kroon et al. was entitled 'Fast-track hysterectomy: a randomised, controlled study'. (Kroon, 2010) This was a randomised controlled trial in which 53 women undergoing hysterectomy were randomised to receive either patient-controlled analgesia (PCA) combined with anaesthesia based on volatile anaesthetics or intrathecally administered morphine combined with a low-dose mode of total intravenous anaesthesia (TIVA). A few outcomes were considered, all related to accelerated recovery: the primary endpoints being length of stay on the postoperative ward and total length of hospital stay. Other outcomes included time to commencement of oral fluids, time to removal of catheter, postoperative nausea and complication rates. Significant advantages were demonstrated with TIVA in all outcomes except complication rates which were not significantly different between the two groups.

The next study was 'Effect of laxatives on gastrointestinal functional recovery in fast-track hysterectomy: a double-blind, placebo-controlled randomized study' by Hansen et al. (Hansen, 2007) This double-blind, placebo-controlled study involved the allocation of 53 women undergoing fast-track radical hysterectomy to postoperative osmotic laxative or placebo. Amongst the various endpoints those considered primary outcomes were postoperative pain and time to first defaecation postoperatively (considered a marker for recovery of gastrointestinal function). The main conclusion drawn by this study was that postoperative laxative administration improves recovery of gastrointestinal function after fast-track hysterectomy (demonstrated by a significant reduction in the median time to first defaecation in the laxative group compared with the placebo group). No differences were seen, however, in postoperative pain or nausea and vomiting between the two groups.

The final article considered was 'Perioperative care of patients with stage IIIC ovarian cancer' by Jakobsen et al. (Jakobsen, 2010) This was a retrospective audit involving 90 patients across 6 centres undergoing surgery for stage IIIC ovarian cancer. Its stated aim was to assess multimodal evidence-based perioperative care within the fast track programme and to determine whether it enhanced postoperative recovery and reduced morbidity. Outcomes included mobilization, nutrition, nausea and pain. The paper had no clear conclusions but stated that optimised perioperative care was required, including a procedure-specific, evidence-based clinical guideline for patients receiving extensive surgery.

4. Discussion

Enhanced Recovery after Surgery (or "Fast-track" surgery) is an evidence-based, multidisciplinary approach to perioperative care in which patient empowerment is central, encouraging active involvement of patients in their care. It is multimodal in nature integrating preoperative, intraoperative and postoperative techniques to reduce complication rates and improve overall recovery from surgery. The studies that have been discussed in this chapter addressed various components of the enhanced recovery programme, either individually or in combinations. These components have been discussed in detail above but are outlined in box 1 for reference.

We continue the discussion with an analysis of the studies with reference to aspects of the programme addressed by each.

No studies were found to specifically evaluate the effects of preoperative fast-track interventions. One study compared different routes of hysterectomy (abdominal vs. laparoscopically assisted vaginal hysterectomy) in a fast-track setting. (Moller, 2001) This was a relatively small study comprising 16 women in each group. The selection of patients for each group was not randomised and was done by a gynaecologist, almost certainly in view of factors leading to suitability for open or laparoscopic surgery in each case. Apart from route of hysterectomy the two groups experienced the same fast-track approach to perioperative care, specifically in terms of preoperative information-giving, postoperative mobilisation and oral food intake and pain management throughout. With reference to routes of hysterectomy the study does not create a medium for fair comparison of the two, indeed, no advantages were reported in either route above the other. This maintains the

Preoperative factors
Preoperative assessment/optimisation
Preoperative hydration status
Premedication
Intraoperative factors
Surgical technique
Anaesthetic techniques
Fluid management
Temperature control
Avoidance of postoperative nausea and vomiting
Postoperative factors
Balanced analgesia
Early enteral nutrition
Laxative use
Early mobilisation

Box 1. Components of the ERAS system

principle, as discussed earlier, that route of surgery is a factor best decided on an individual basis by the surgeon in discussion with the patient and multidisciplinary team. The report did, however, quote the benefits in terms of postoperative recovery from employing the fast-track programme in both groups.

Two studies addressed mode of anaesthesia for hysterectomy. (Wodlin, 2011a, 2011b, 2011c, Kroon, 2010) The work by the 'GASPI' study group was a multicentre randomised controlled trial involving a total of 162 women undergoing total or subtotal hysterectomy for benign indications. The patients were relatively fit: contraindications to participation in the trial included an ASA score of ≥3, gynaecological malignancy and physical or psychiatric disability. They were randomised to two groups for the different modes of anaesthesia as described above but all patients received identical fast-track care. The main components taken up in this study included, preoperatively, patient information, paracetamol premedication and a two-hour fluid fast and postoperatively, approaches to feeding, mobilisation and analgesia in keeping with enhanced recovery principles. It was concluded that the duration of hospital stay, the stated primary aim of the study, was reduced in both groups as a result of the fast-track techniques with no significant difference in this measure between the two groups. Other findings reported from this work suggested benefits with spinal over general anaesthesia for some endpoints, for example, the opioid-sparing effects of regional anaesthesia and resultant faster recovery of gastrointestinal function in the patients receiving spinal anaesthetic. Side effects of spinal anaesthetic were, however also clearly demonstrated with increases in vomiting and pruritis after spinal anaesthetic. (Wodlin, 2011b, 2011c, 2011d)

The second trial looking at mode of anaesthesia, by Kroon et al. (2010), compared different anaesthetic methods (PCA and volatile anaesthesia vs. intrathecally administered morphine and TIVA) in 53 randomised patients undergoing abdominal hysterectomy for benign indications. It was noted that most of the uteri in the study were oversized as normal practice in the unit in question was to opt for vaginal hysterectomy for normal-sized uteri. As a result 11 of the 26 or 27 women in each group required midline incisions. Preoperatively the patients in both groups experienced fast-track interventions including information-giving and premedication. Patients in the TIVA group were encouraged to drink clear fluids two hours preoperatively. Postoperatively, outcomes related to accelerated recovery were focal findings of the study. The outcome of hospital discharge after two days in the TIVA group compared with three days in the volatile anaesthesia group constituted a significant improvement. Other fast-track-related outcomes which were superior in the TIVA group included length of stay on postoperative ward, time to commencement of oral fluids, time to removal of catheter and postoperative nausea. (Kroon, 2010) Detailed discussion of these anaesthetic techniques falls outside the remit of this chapter, however, this paper appears to support the use of intrathecal morphine and TIVA in the fast-track approach to hysterectomy.

Perhaps surprisingly given the important role of postoperative care in the enhanced recovery system, the only postoperative intervention addressed was that of laxative administration. The article in question was a study by Hansen et al. (Hansen, 2007) This was a double blind, placebo-controlled study that looked at the effects of postoperative administration of magnesium oxide and disodium phosphate on gastrointestinal function and postoperative symptoms after fast-track abdominal hysterectomy. A total of 53 women were involved in the completed study, which was the only one of its kind in terms of the intervention assessed. The results were encouraging in that the median time to first defecation was significantly reduced in the group given laxatives evidencing a quicker normalisation of gastrointestinal function. Postoperative hospitalization showed a trend towards reduction in the laxative group but this did not reach significance. Other endpoints again failed to demonstrate significant benefits in laxative administration with similar pain scores and incidences of nausea and vomiting in the two groups.

The two last papers both discussed hysterectomy for ovarian malignancy and both considered the fast-track programme as a whole. (Marx, 2006 & Jakobsen, 2010) The first of these, published in Acta Obstetricia et Gynecologica in 2006, was a case control study involving a total of 141 women. One group (comprising 72 women) received conventional care and were analysed retrospectively whilst the second group (69 women) received multimodal rehabilitation and were studied prospectively. Surgery in all cases was carried out by the same the surgeons and according to international (Federation Internationale Gynecologie et Obstetrique) guidelines. Patients in the accelerated recovery group received a complete bundle of care in keeping with enhanced recovery principles and outlined in detail in the paper. This included preoperative information, a well defined programme of nursing care postoperatively and a criteria-driven plan for discharge on the fourth postoperative day (although patients were actually discharged on the fifth postoperative day). This trial showed significant advantages to the fast-track system with reductions in postoperative stay, severe medical complication rates and readmission rates in the fast-track group. In addition it was noted that none of the readmissions of the fast-track patients were connected with acute life-threatening conditions whereas the reasons for readmission in the conventional care group were potentially life threatening in six out of the seven cases.

Finally, a further paper examining fast-track perioperative care in patients undergoing surgery for ovarian cancer was found in the Danish journal, Ugeskr Laeger. (Jakobsen, 2010. This was a fairly large study, involving a total of 90 consecutive patients across six Danish centres, but was a retrospective audit which obtained data from patient files to assess the fast-track principles of perioperative care employed in these cases. The patients were divided into two groups according to the extent of surgery carried out and endpoints measured included hospital stay, postoperative mobilisation and recommencement of oral intake postoperatively. The nature of the work (a retrospective audit) made it difficult to draw any firm conclusions, as there was no control group for comparison to assess the effects of the interventions. This was compounded by the fact that, due to language restrictions, it was not possible to access the full article so information could only be gained from the article abstract. The results mainly addressed the differences between outcomes in the patients with and without extensive surgery. These included, predictably, longer hospital stays and slower return to mobilisation postoperatively in the extensive surgery group). No conclusions relating to the effects of the fast-track interventions could be drawn. The authors concluded that procedure-specific; evidence-based clinical guidelines should be produced for patients undergoing extensive surgery to optimise perioperative care.

Three further articles were studied which showed some relevance to the subject in question. The first of these was a prospective study entitled 'fast-track vaginal surgery'. (Ottesen, 2002) This initially appeared pertinent to the literature search but, on closer analysis, was found to discuss vaginal surgery for uterovaginal prolapse: only 46% of the procedures carried out (19 of the total of 41) involved hysterectomy. This paper did, however, explore fast-track surgery with generally favourable results.

The next paper, though descriptive in nature, took an interesting look into the introduction of the enhanced recovery system to a gynaecology ward and the impact on ward nursing practices. (Sjetne, 2009) Positive outcomes were reported including reductions in mean length of hospital stay and in time spent on nursing activities per patient stay. This demonstrated that the expected gains of implementing an enhanced recovery system may be achieved without compromising the workload or work environment of ward nursing staff.

The last article was an examination of patient and staff experiences of fast-track hysterectomy. (Wagner, 2004) This, again, was exploratory and descriptive in nature with no objective outcome measures. Conclusions from the authors included recommendations that, in the future, staff must be fully informed regarding the system and that a new unit be set up dedicated to the recovery programme.

Two reviews from the Cochrane database of Systematic Reviews displayed some relevance to our discussion and their contents will be discussed forthwith. (Charoenkwan, 2007 & Nieboer, 2009)

The first of these reviews was regarding early versus delayed oral fluids and food for reducing complications after major abdominal gynaecologic surgery. (Charoenkwan, 2007) The review looked into the presence of multiple postoperative parameters in patients recommencing oral food and fluid intake within the first 24 hours after surgery and those in whom it was delayed beyond 24 hours. No significant differences were found between the two in most parameters including postoperative ileus, vomiting and first passage of flatus and stool postoperatively, although there was an associated increase in postoperative nausea associated with early feeding. A possibility of shorter hospital stay in patients with early oral intake was raised in the review although this would require further research. It was concluded that early feeding after major abdominal gynaecologic surgery is safe but that the approach must be individualised.

The other Cochrane review examined the subject of surgical approach to hysterectomy for benign gynaecological disease. (Nieboer, 2009) Studies comparing vaginal, abdominal and laparopscopic hysterectomy were included and, again, various outcome measures were taken into account. It was found, predictably, that the different routes of hysterectomy each carried their own benefits and risks. In conclusion it was stated that vaginal hysterectomy would be preferable to abdominal hysterectomy where possible, and that laparoscopic hysterectomy may have advantages in cases where vaginal hysterectomy was not possible. The route of hysterectomy must, however, be decided on an individual basis after discussion between the patient and surgeon.

5. Conclusion

The Enhanced Recovery after Surgery programme was first introduced and is now commonly used in colorectal surgery. It is increasingly becoming a part of the surgical system in many hospitals in disciplines including gynaecology, urology and orthopaedics. In gynaecology some of the elements of the programme already constitute established practice in many hospitals, but the complete system requires a smooth flowing process from preoperative patient preparation to postoperative measures, including engagement of patients and staff throughout. In the UK the aim is for this programme of care to be delivered in all surgical specialties over the next 18 months. This, however, requires more widespread evidence of the type considered in this review to demonstrate the potential benefits of the enhanced recovery programme to patients and staff across the country.

6. References

American Society of Anesthesiologists Task Force on Preoperative Fasting. (2011). Practice Guidelines for Preoperative Fasting and the Use of Pharmacologic Agents to Reduce the Risk of Pulmonary Aspiration: Application to Healthy Patients Undergoing Elective Procedures: An Updated Report by the American Society of Anesthesiologists Committee on Standards and Practice Parameters. *Anesthesiology* 114(3): pp 495-511.

Andersen, HK. Lewis, SJ. Thomas, S. (2006) Early enteral nutrition within 24h of colorectal surgery versus later commencement of feeding for postoperative complications. *Cochrane Database Syst Rev*. CD004080

Apfel, CC. Laara, E. Koivuranta, M. Greim, CA. Roewer, N. (1999) A simplified risk score for predicting postoperative nausea and vomiting: conclusions from crossvalidations between two centers. *Anesthesiology*. pp 91:693–700

Brady, M. Kinn, S. Stuart, P. Preoperative fasting for adults to prevent perioperative complications. (2003) *Cochrane Database Syst Rev* CD004423.

Charoenkwan, K. Phillipson, G. Vutyavanich, T. (2007) Early versus delayed oral fluids and food for reducing complications after major abdominal gynaecologic surgery. *Cochrane Database Syst Rev*. CD004508.

Delgado-Rodriguez, M. Bueno-Cavanillas, A. Lopez-Gigosos, R. et al. (1990) Hospital stay length as an effect modifier of other risk factors for nosocomial infections. *Eur Journal of Epidemiol* pp 6: 34-9

Devereaux, PJ. Yang, H. Yusuf, S. et al.(2008) Effects of extended-release metoprolol succinate in patients undergoing non-cardiac surgery (POISE trial): a randomised controlled trial. *Lancet*. pp 371:1839–47.

Enhanced Recovery Partnership Programme (2010), Delivering enhanced recovery- Helping patients to get better sooner after surgery, viewed 21 March 2011, *www.dh.gov.uk/publications*.

Fuchs, KH. Minimally invasive surgery. (2002) *Endoscopy*. pp 34(2):154-9

Frank, SM. (2001) Consequences of hypothermia. Current *Anaesthesia & Critical Care* pp 12, 79-86

Giglio, MT. Marucci, M. Testini, M. Brienza, N. (2009) Goal-directed haemodynamic therapy and gastrointestinal complications in major surgery: a meta-analysis of randomized controlled trials. *Br.J.Anaesth*. pp 103 (5): 637-646.

Goyagi, T. Tanaka, M. Nishikawa, T. (1999) Oral clonidine premedication enhances postoperative analgesia by epidural morphine. *Anesth Analg*. pp 89(6):1487-91.

Hansen, CT. Sørensen, M. Møller, C. et al.(2007) Effect of laxatives on gastrointestinal functional recovery in fast-track hysterectomy: a double-blind, placebo-controlled randomized study. *Am J Obstet Gynaecol*. pp 196: 311.e1-7.

Information from hospital episode statistics. The Information Centre for Health and Social Care (2007).

Institute for Innovation and Improvement (2010), NHS Better Care, Better Value Indicates, viewed 21 March 2011,
www.productivity.nhs.uk

Jakobsen, DH. Høgdall, C. Kehlet, H. (2010) Perioperative care of patients with stage IIIC ovarian cancer. *Ugeskr Laeger*. pp 27;172(39):2688-91

Jha, S. Moran, PA. (2007) National survey on the management of prolapse in the UK. *Neurouorlogy and Urdynamics*. Pp 26(3):325-31.

Jones, S. Alnaib, M. Kokkinakis, M. Wilkinson, M. et al. (2011) Pre-operative patient education reduces length of stay after knee joint arthroplasty. *Ann R Coll Surg Engl*. pp 93(1):71-5.

Kehlet, H. (1997) Multimodal approach to control postoperative pathophysiology and rehabilitation.*Br J Anaesth* pp 78:606–617

Kehlet, H. Kennedy, RH. (2006) Laparoscopic colonic surgery--mission accomplished or work in progress? *Colorectal Dis*. pp 8(6):514-7

Kehlet, H. (2008) Fast-track colorectal surgery. *Lancet*. Pp 371:791-3

Kroon, UB. Rådström, M. Hjelthe, C., Dahlin, C. Kroon, L. (2010) Fast-track hysterectomy: a randomised, controlled study. *Eur J Obstet Gynecol Reprod Biol.* pp 151(2):203-7

Kruzik, N. (2009) Benefits of preoperative education for adult elective surgery patients. *AORN J.* pp 90(3):381-7.

Lassen, K. Soop, M. Nygren, J. et al. (2009) Consensus review of optimal perioperative care in colorectal surgery. Enhanced Recovery After Surgery (ERAS) Group Recommendations. *Arch Surg.* pp 144:961-969

Lethaby, A. Shepperd, S. Cook, I. et al. (1999) Endometrial resection and ablation versus hysterectomy for heavy menstrual bleeding. *Cochrane Database of Systematic Reviews.* Issue 2.

Ljungqvist, O. Nygren, J. Thorell, A. (2002) Modulation of post-operative insulin resistance by pre-operative carbohydrate loading. *Proc Nutr* pp 61(3):329-36.

Ljungqvist, O. (2009) Modulating postoperative insulin resistance by preoperative carbohydrate loading. *Best Pract Res Clin Anaesthesiol.* pp 23(4):401-9.

Marjoribanks, J. Lethaby, A. Farquhar, C. (2006) Surgery versus medical therapy for heavy menstrual bleeding. *Cochrane Database of Systematic Reviews.* Issue 2

Marx, C. Rasmussen, T. Jakobsen, DH. Ottosen, C. Lundvall, L. Ottesen, B. Callesen, T. Kehlet, H. (2006) The effect of accelerated rehabilitation on recovery after surgery for ovarian malignancy. *Acta Obstet Gynecol Scand.* pp 85(4):488-92

Mohseni, M. Ebneshahidi, A. (2011) The effect of oral clonidine premedication on blood loss and the quality of the surgical field during endoscopic sinus surgery: a placebo-controlled clinical trial. *J Anesth.* [Epub ahead of print]

Møller, C. Kehlet, H. Groth Friland, S. Schouenborg, LO. Lund, C. Ottesen, B. (2001)Fast track hysterectomy. *Eur J Obstet Gynecol Reprod Biol* pp 98:18-22

No authors listed. (2002) Practice advisory for preanesthesia evaluation: a report by the American Society of Anesthesiologists Task Force on Preanesthesia Evaluation. *Anesthesiology.* pp Feb; 96(2):485-96.

NICE Clinical Guideline 29. London. (2008). *National Institute for Health and Clinical Excellence;* Perioperative hypothermia (inadvertent): the management of inadvertent perioperative hypothermia in adults.

NICE Clinical Guideline 92. (2011) Reducing the risk of venous thromboembolism (deep vein thrombosis and pulmonary embolism) in patients admitted to hospital *guidance.nice.org.uk/CG92.*

Nieboer, TE. Johnson, N. Lethaby, A. Tavender, E. Curr, E. Garry, R. van Voorst, S. Mol, BW. Kluivers, KB. (2009) Surgical approach to hysterectomy for benign gynaecological disease. *Cochrane Database Syst Rev.*CD003677

Nieboer, TE. Johnson, N. Lethaby, A. Tavender, E. Curr, E. Garry, R. van Voorst, S. Mol, BWJ. Kluivers, KB. (2009) Surgical approach to hysterectomy for benign gynaecological disease. *Cochrane Database of Systematic Reviews.* Issue 3. Art. No.: CD003677. DOI: 10.1002/14651858.CD003677.pub4

Noblett, SE. Watson, DS. Huong, H. Davison, B. Hainsworth, PJ. Horgan, AF. (2006) Pre-operative oral carbohydrate loading in colorectal surgery: a randomized controlled trial. *Colorectal Dis.* pp 8(7):563-9.

Nygren, .J, Thorell, A. Ljungqvist, O. (2007) Are there any benefits from minimizing fasting and optimization of nutrition and fluid management for patients undergoing day surgery? *Curr Opin Anaesthesiol.* pp 20(6):540-4.

Oddby-Muhrbeck, E. Eksborg, S. Bergendahl, HT. Muhrbeck, O. Lönnqvist, PA. (2002) Effects of clonidine on postoperative nausea and vomiting in breast cancer surgery. *Anesthesiology*. pp 96(5):1109-14.

Ottesen, M. Sørensen, M. Rasmussen, Y. Smidt-Jensen, S. Kehlet, H. Ottesen, B. (2002)Fast track vaginal surgery. *Acta Obstet Gynecol Scand*. pp 281(2):138-46

Pre-operative Assessment: The Role of the Anaesthetist. London: (2001) *The Association of Anaesthetists of Great Britain and Ireland.*

Petersen, PL. Mathiesen, O. Torup, H. Dahl, JB. (2010) The transversus abdominis plane block: a valuable option for postoperative analgesia? A topical review. *Acta Anaesthesiol Scand*. pp 54(5):529-35.

Powell-Tuck, J. Gosling, P. Lobo, DN. Allison, SP. et al. (2008) *British consensus guidelines on intravenous fluid therapy for adult surgical patients – GIFTASUP.* <www.bapen.org.uk/pdfs/bapen_pubs/giftasup.pdf>

Rigg, JR. Jamrozik, K. Myles, PS. et al. MASTER Anaesthesia Trial Study Group. (2002) Epidural Wodlin, BN. Nilsson, L. Kjølhede, P. for the GASPI study group. (2011) The impact of mode of anaesthesia on postoperative recovery from fast-track abdominal hysterectomy: a randomised clinical trial. *BJOG*. pp 118:299–308.

Sjetne, IS. Krogstad, U. Ødegård, S. Engh, ME. (2009) Improving quality by introducing enhanced recovery after surgery in a gynaecological department: consequences for ward nursing practice. *Qual Saf Health Care*. pp 18(3):236-40

Wagner, L. Carlslund, AM. Møller, C. Ottesen, B. (2004) Patient and staff (doctors and nurses) experiences of abdominal hysterectomy in accelerated recovery programme. A qualitative study. *Dan Med Bull*. pp 51(4):418-21

Walsh, SR. Tang, T. Bass, S. Gaunt, ME. (2008) Doppler-guided intra-operative fluid management during major abdominal surgery: systematic review and meta-analysis. *Int J Clin Pract* pp 62:466-470

Wakeling, HG. McFall, MR. Jenkins, CS. Woods, WGA. Miles, WFA. Barclay, GR. Fleming, SC. (2005) Intraoperative oesophageal Doppler guided fluid management shortens postoperative hospital stay after major bowel surgery. *Br.J.Anaesth*. pp 95 (5): 634-642

Wilmore, DW. (2000) Metabolic response to severe surgical illness: overview. *World J Surg* pp24:705

Wodlin, NB. Nilsson, L. Kjølhede, P. for the GASPI study group. (2011a) The impact of mode of anaesthesia on postoperative recovery from fast-track abdominal hysterectomy: a randomised clinical trial. *BJOG*. pp 118:299-308

Wodlin, NB. Nilsson, L. Arestedt, K. Kjølhede, P. (2011b) Mode of anesthesia and postoperative symptoms following abdominal hysterectomy in a fast-track setting. *Acta Obstet Gynecol Scand* pp 90(4): 369-379

Wodlin, NB, Nilsson L, Kjølhede P. (2011c) Health-related quality of life and postoperative recovery in fast-track hysterectomy. *Acta Obstet Gynecol Scand*. pp 90(4):362-8

Wodlin, NB. Nilsson, L. Carlsson, P. Kjølhede, P. for the GASPI study group. (2011d) Cost-effectiveness of general anesthesia versus spinal anesthesia in fast track abdominal benign hysterectomy. *AJOG*doi:10.1016/j.ajog.2011.05.043

Wu, CT. Jao, SW. Borel, CO. et al. (2004) The effect of epidural clonidine on perioperative cytokine response, postoperative pain and bowel function in patients undergoing colorectal surgery. *Anesth Anal* pp 99:502–9

17

Postoperative Pain Management After Hysterectomy – A Simple Approach

Mariana Calderon, Guillermo Castorena and Emina Pasic
Hospital Medica Sur,
Universidad Nacional Autonoma de Mexico UNAM,
Mexico

1. Introduction

Surgery is often physically and psychologically stressful and in the postoperative period, many patients experience significant amounts of pain and discomfort. The International Association for the Study of Pain defines pain as "an unpleasant sensory and emotional experience associated with actual or potential damage, or described in terms of such damage".

Although acute pain and associated responses can be unpleasant and often debilitating, they serve important adaptive purposes. They identify and localize noxious stimuli, initiate withdrawal responses that limit tissue injury, inhibit mobility thereby enhancing wound healing[1]. Nevertheless, intense and prolonged pain transmission[2], as well as analgesic undermedication, can increase surgical postsurgical / traumatic morbidity, delay recovery, and lead to development of chronic pain. Despite the obviously simple nature of surgical incision, however, perioperative and specifically postoperative pain remain underevaluated and poorly treated. Recent surveys suggest that 80% of patients experience pain after surgery[3], 11% having severe pain, and that pain delays recovery in 24% of patients undergoing ambulatory surgery[4].

2. Pathophisiology of acute pain

A number of theories have been formulated to explain noxious perception: The specificity theory by Descartes, the intensity theory by Sydenham, and recently the gate control theory by Melzack and Wall where they suggested that sensory fibers of differing specificity stimulate second-order spinal neurons fire at a different intensity.[5] Pain perception is dependent on the degree of noxious stimulation, local descending inhibition from CNS centers, and responses of second order transmissions cells. Woolf and coworkers have proposed a new theory to explain pain-processing, suggesting that primary and secondary hyperalgesia as well as qualitative differences among physiologic, inflammatory, and neuropathic pain reflect sensitization of both peripheral nociceptors and spinal neurons. Noxious perception is the result of several distinct processes that begin in the periphery, extended up the neuraxis, and terminate at supraspinal regions responsible for interpretation and reaction. [6]

Pain can only be experienced when nociceptive afference reaches the cortex. Most brain imaging studies report an activation of the sensory and affective brain structures following a nociceptive stimulus, demonstrating that pain perception is a complex experience with emotion, cognitive factors, and previous experience playing an important role in perceived pain. It can therefore be understood why the clinician should address pain from both the physical as well the emotional aspect.

Injured tissues will release various substances, such as potassium, prostaglandins, histamine, of bradykinins that are pronociceptive, and will also evoke an immune response. [7]These inflammatory and immune factors will sensitize the nociceptive receptors directly within the lesion and in the surrounding neurons. Primary hyperalgesia, which follows the release of these factors, may be measured as a lowered pain threshold in and around the lesion.

The most important fibers in the transmission of nociceptive stimulus are the Aδ and C fibers. The first ones will rapidly transmit a brief and acute pinprick-like sensation, perceived to be precisely located at the point of stimulation. Following this activity, C fibers will transmit their information with a relatively long delay (100 millisenconds to a second, depending on the stimulus location). This second sensory input results in a more diffuse deep pain sensation. [8]

Secondary hyperalgesia is a phenomenon that refers to sensitization that occurs within the central nervous system[9]. Repeated recruitment of C-fibers following an injury will produce central sensitization by changing the respose properties of the membranes of secondary neurons. This will result in an increase of the firing rate, a phenomenon known as windup[10]. The high frequency recruitment of C fibers, either by increased repetitive stimuli or by a tonic stimulation[11], will induce an increase of the perceived pain, even if the intensity of the stimulation remains constant. The spinal sensitization can persist for minutes, but can also be present for hours and even days[12]. The prolonged activation of the NMDA receptors will induce the transcription of rapidly expressed genes (c-fos, c-jun), resulting in sensitization of nociceptors. This neuronal plasticity of the secondary neuron will result in a reduced threshold in the spinal cord, producing hyperalgesic and allodynic responses that may persist even after the healing of the injury. Considering the impact of sensitization, an aggressive and early treatment plan to reduce pain will help in preventing ongoing chronic pain[6].

After reviewing some of the above mentioned theories, we can conclude that pain is a dynamic phenomenon; all the nociceptive signals will be modulated at all levels from the periphery to the brain but we still have to take into account genetic and environmental factors that will influence the acute perception and the development of persistent pain. Understanding the neurophysiologic mechanisms involved in the development and maintenance of pain will help the clinician to devise a more effective treatment plan.

3. Risk factors for developing chronic pain

Three factors have been proposed to play a role in the chronicity of pain: personal predisposition, environmental factors, and psychologic factors.

It is also well known that chronic pain syndromes more frequently affect women than men; the reason for this predisposition is probably multifactorial, with sex hormones likely playing an important role. The age is also a factor in this sort of patients; literature suggests that in the 50s it begins a reduction in endogenous pain control which contributes to the higher prevalence of chronic pain in the older population. Expectations of pain, which has not previously been experienced, may confound pain memory, especially when anxiety levels are high. Hysterectomy procedure is a high-risk surgery in terms of psychological and environmental ambience for most of the patients where the surgical team must be aware of these factors.

4. Physiology and anatomy of pain in hysterectomy

Uterine innervation stems from a variety of sources. Parasympathetic nerves stemming from S2 to S4 conglomerate into the cervical ganglion of Frankenhauser. Sympathetic nerves, the predominant influence in uterine innervation, descend from T7-T8 to the internal iliac plexi bilaterally to meet their parasympathetic counterparts. Together these nerves innervate not only the uterus, but also the bladder and upper vagina. Within the uterus nerves terminate both within muscle fibers and the endometrium itself. The perineum is innervated by the pudendal nerve, which also enters the spinal cord at the S2-S4 levels.

Although these systems are primarily responsible for the function of the uterus, the perception of pain stems from different sites. Visceral afferent fibers from the uterine corpus transmit pain signals to the brain by entering the spinal cord at the T11-T12 levels, whereas spinal cord levels S2-S4 receive signals from the cervis, vagina, and perineum. Recognition of this divergence is the key[13], because of the pain fibers' high entry point in the spinal cord the block of lower stems will be insufficient for relieving pain independently of the type of surgery (laparoscopic vs open procedure).

Recent advances in minimally invasive surgery have made procedures to be less traumatic however abdominal pain must be avoided because it can restrict ventilation and prevent ambulation; this statement is particularly important in the obese population.[14]

5. Mechanistic approach to pain treatment

The different types of pain may be divided into two categories: nociceptive and neurogenic. Acute postoperative pain relies in the nociceptive category where there is a transitory response to nociceptive stimuli that could be mechanical, thermal or chemical. Nociceptive pain plays an important protective role and is normally present for as long as the protection of the organism in necessary; however if not treated well it will persist even after healing of the initial injury.

Postoperative pain management is based on a number of principles. Pain prevention is preferable to, and more efficacious than, treatment of established pain[15]. Multimodal analgesia is a rational approach to pain management and is more effective. The aim of multimodal analgesia combinations is to reduce postoperative pain. Theoretically, multimodal analgesia is achieved by a combination of opioids, and regional blocks, which attenuate the pain-related signals in the central nervous system, and nonsteroidal anti-inflammatory drugs, which act mainly in the periphery to inhibit the initiation of pain signals.

Abdominal hysterectomy is refered among the most frequently procedures associated to pain in the gynecologic population.[16]

Whether is an open or laparoscopic procedure, abdominal or vaginal approach, the clinician has many options for providing multimodal analgesia: patient control analgesia, epidural analgesia, intratecal opioids, wound infiltration, nonsteroidal anti-inflammatory drugs and adjuvant drugs.

5.1 Nonselective nonsteroidal anti-inflammatory drugs, COX-2 inhibitors, and acetaminophen

Nonsteroidal anti-inflammatory drugs (NSAIDs) form a heterogeneous group of organic acids that have analgesic, antipyretic, anti-inflammatory, and platelet inhibitory actions.

NSAIDs have long been used in the treatment of nonoperative pain syndromes; their mechanism of action is through the nonspecific inhibition of COX, which therefore blocks both the constitutive COX-1 isoform, responsible for gastric protection and platelet function, and the inducible proinflamatory isoform, COX-2. Thus, the actions of the NSAIDs result in both the desired analgesic effects and the unwanted adverse effects of the COX isoforms.

Some systematic reviews have concluded that there are no significant differences in the analgesic efficacy between different NSAIDs, but they do have different levels of toxicities, especially at high or increased doses[17]. The use of the NSAIDs in preemptive analgesic therapy has been debated and is still controversial with non measurable long-term advantage when compared with its postoperative use[18]

The postoperative use of NSAIDs has been evaluated in several types of surgical procedures and in several dosages forms either as a single therapy compared with other analgesics or placebo or in a multimodal approach in combination with different kinds of analgesics to determine their efficacy, opiate-sparing effects and safety. One example is the postoperative use of ketorolac in combination with tramadol in patients who underwent abdominal surgery; the use of this combination was found to be safe and effective with similar pain relief when compared to a higher dose of tramadol used as monotherapy[19]

In another study a group of patients with open gynecologic surgery, received a loading dose of parecoxib on day one and continued their analgesic regimen with morphine through a PCA. After day one they were separated in two groups: placebo vs parecoxib 20mg twice daily on days 2-5. The results were that in the parecoxib treatment group, 24-hour summed pain intensity scores were significantly lower than in the placebo treatment group on days 2 and 3 and consumed less rescue medication compared with the placebo-treated patients[20]

In an effort to minimize the risk of bleeding and the risk of gastrointestinal complications that have traditionally been associated with the use of the nonselective NSAIDs, the use of COX-2 inhibitors as non opioid adjuvants has become increasingly popular to reduce pain during the perioperative period[21]. They haven't shown increased analgesic potency in the treatment of postoperative pain; even more valdecoxib was not approved by the US FDA for the management of acute pain. Actually valdecoxib and rofecoxib were voluntarily withdrawn from the market because of concerns of increasing the risk of cardiovascular events.

Unless there is a major contraindication for the use of the NSAIDs, they are generally accepted for the management of mild to moderate postoperative pain and as adjuncts for use with other analgesics in moderate to severe postoperative pain (table 1). The concomitant inhibition of physiological COX-1 leads to renal toxicity, platelet dysfunction, and gastrointestinal toxicity.

	COX Selectivity	COX-2:COX-1 ratio	Vd (I)	$T_{1/2\beta}$ (h)	Clearance (I h^{-1})
Ibuprofen	None	1:1	10	2.4	4.4
Diclofenac	None	1:1	30	2	15.6
Ketorolac	None	1:1	14	5.4	2.3
Meloxicam	Moderate	10-13:1	10-15	20-22	0.5
Celecoxib	High	375:1	400	11	30
Rofecoxib	High	>800:1	86	17	7.2

Table 1. Preparing for the primary FRCA, Non-steroidal anti-inflammatory drugs, Sharpe P. and Thompson J.
Bulletin 6. The Royal College of Anaesthetists, March 2001

The group of patients who are at higher risk of adverse reactions when treated with NSAIDs are well known; they include the elderly, pregnant women (and their fetuses), neonates, patients with liver, kidney, or cardiac disorders, and those with hypertension, multiple myeloma, peptic disorders, or active rheumatoid arthritis.

The dosage of any NSAIDs must be according to specific recommendations and prescribing practices. It is well known that many of the medication errors in the hospital setting are due to analgesic overdose and misused[16].

5.2 Acetaminophen (paracetamol)

Acetaminophen was first used in 1883 but gained widespread acceptance only after 1948. It possesses a wide safety profile. The WHO has recommended it to be used as the first line medication for mild, moderate, or severe pain and to add opioids and other analgesics as the pain remains persistent or increases. This multimodal approach has been adopted in the European Union and has effectively resulted in a 33% decrease in opioids use and their adverse effects.

Although paracetamol is acceptably safe in usual dosages, there have been some reports that in patients with significant hepatic dysfunction or those taking substances that induce hepatic enzymes even common doses may aggravate liver dysfunction, sometimes to the point of causing hepatic failure. Stable mild chronic liver disease does not seem to be a contraindication.[22]

Paracetamol is one of the most commonly ingested medications in deliberate self-poisoning and accidental ingestion by children. The problem of overdosage is substantial. Fulminant hepatic failure occurs in 1-5% of cases of paracetamol overdosage 3-6 days after ingestion[23] with frequent deaths in people who take 20-25g. There is noly a narrow margin betwwn the normal maxium 24-hour dosage and that which can cause liver damage and acute hepatic failure.

Available in oral, rectal and intravenous administration (most of the countries)

5.3 Opioids

Opioids represent a class of analgesics that provide powerful dose-dependent pain relief for patients suffering moderate to severe pain. This class of drug includes a large number of compounds with variable pharmacokinetics and pharmacodynamics and a dosing versatility for its administration.

Opioids interact with specific transmembrane G-protein coupled binding sites termed opiate or opioid receptors. These receptors are located primarily in the spinal dorsal horn, central gray, medial thalamus, amygdala, limbic cortex, and other regions of the central nervous system that process affective and suffering aspects of pain perception[24]. Opioid receptors serve as binding sites for endogenous ligands, including endorphins and the enkephalins, which naturally modulate pain transmission and perception. Opiates ad synthetic opioids have structural/chemical similarities that enable them to bind and activate opioid receptors resulting in powerful, dose-dependent analgesia[25]

Three principal opioid receptor subtypes, designated as μ, κ and δ have been isolated and characterized. μ receptor (also known as OPR1) is the main responsible for the analgesic and side effects of opiates; its primary agonist includes β-endorphin and morphine.[26]

According to their binging affinities and intrinsic activity at receptor subtypes, opioids are classified as agonists, partial agonists, mixed agonist-antagonists, and complete antagonists[17,18]. (tables 2 and 3)

Opiates			
Agonists	Partial Agonist	Agonist/Antagonist	Antagonist
Morphine and derivates Codeine Fentanyl Sulfentanil Alfentanil Remifentanil Meperidine	Buprenorphine	Nalbuphine Butorphanol Pentazocine	Naloxone Naltrexone

Table 2.

In acute pain scenarios, most opioid-related adverse events are transient and tend to resolve with ongoing treatment. The common adverse events are nausea, vomiting, sedation, pruritus, and constipation. Patients recovery from abdominal and gynecological surgery are generally at risk for opioid-induced bowel dysfunction and ileus with recommendation that such therapy may be supplemented with stool softeners, bulk laxatives, and occasional enemas[27].

When using opioids for acute pain management it is recommended to have safety rules that must be applied mainly in high risk patients. Neonates, infants, and children are at risk of adverse effects of opioids, owing to pharmacokinetic and pharmacodynamic changes. Routine use of pulse oximetry is recommended in all children receiving opioids[28].

Elderly patients are particularly at risk, as a number of other susceptibility factors can co-exist. Renal insufficiency can result in clinically significant accumulation of

Opiates	
Morphine	Standard of comparison of all opioid analgesics Moderate analgesic potency Slow onset to peak effect Intermediate duration of activity Dose dependent adverse effects Release of histamine which may precipitate hypotension and bronchospasm Increases smooth muscle tone which exacerbate biliary, tubular, and ureteral colic
Oxycodone	Semisynthetic mu receptor agonist High oral bioavailability Less sedation than equivalent doses of morphine
Hydromorphone	Semysinthetic mu selective opioid agonist Analgesic potency 5-6 times greater than morphine with a greater ability to penetrate the blood brain barrier Less histamine release
Fentanyl	Mu-specific opioid agonist related to meperidine Analgesic potency 35-60 times greater than morphine Rapid onset and variable dose-dependent duration of effect Rapidly penetrate blood brain barrier and bind opioid receptors in central nervous system Provide hemodynamic stability Major adverse effects include rapid and profound respiratory depression and chest wall rigidity
Methadone	Opioid agonist Analgesic potency 1.5-2 times greater than morphine Oral bioavailability greater than 80% Accumulates in tissues so analgesic duration and risk of overdosing may increase with doses Prolongation of QTc interval and may initiate or exacerbate torsades de pointes and Wolff-Parkinson-White syndrome Good choice for patients with highly opioid dependent disorders
Meperidine	Opioid agonist Analgesic potency one tenth that of morphine Produces smooth muscle relaxing effect
Codeine	Opiate-derived analgesic Analgesic potency one-third to one-fourth as potent as morphine High incidence of nausea and vomiting
Tramadol	Weak mu-receptor opioid agonist Also inhibits re-uptake of both 5-HT and noradrenaline and stimulates the presynaptic release of 5-HT Analgesic potency similar to codeine Not recommended for severe acute pain
Sufentanil	Synthetic mu-specific opioid agonist related to fentanyl Analgesic potency 500-700 times greater than morphine Rapid onset and dose dependent duration of effect
Buprenorphine	Partial agonist-type opioid Available in a sublingual formulation

Table 3.

pharmacologically active opioid metabolites and prolonged narcosis; such patients must be monitored for signs of toxicity. To date, this effect has only been reported with codeine, morphine, and pethidine. Dextropropoxyphene is not recommended in renal insufficiency.[29]

The use of oxygen supply, highly trained nurses, monitoring to avoid respiratory and cardiovascular adverse events is highly recommended.

5.4 Patient control analgesia

Patient control analgesia (PCA) is the standard technique for the management of moderate or severe postoperative pain. The concept of intravenous PCA is described as a technique that allows patients to self-administer intravenous opioids as required and dates back to the mid-1960s. Nowadays the drugs used in this kind of devices vary according to hospital facilities and clinician preferences. Opioids are the first line drugs used in PCA, however in many hospitals a combination of opioids and NSAIDs for background infusions with a extra shot at patient request are now used. Regular paracetamol and NSAIDs can be used simultaneously. Supplementary oxygen should be considered, particularly on the first and second postoperative nights.

Over the years, further improvements were made to the design of PCA devices. These have resulted in increases in security and data output capacity, introduction of error reduction programs, and a choice of mains in battery power. In addition, a variety of disposable delivery systems are now available. Before PCA can be used safely and effectively it is mandatory to educate the patients, all medical and nursing staff involved in its utilization.

5.5 Intravenous PCA

Most authors use morphine as the opioid of choice beginning with a small dose (1mg of morphine) at patient request, with a lockout period (5 minutes) to prevent overdosing. However there are many side effects of morphine that has lead a vary of studies searching for the optimal opioid for PCA analgesia. Lenz et al. showed in their study that oxycodone was more potent than morphine for visceral pain relief but not for sedation in patients after laparoscopic hysterectomy[30].

For abdominal hysterectomies in a teaching hospital in Mexico City a combination of fentanyl (1mg) plus ketorolac (90-120mg of ketorolac) in a mix of 100cc of total volume is given to the patients at a rate of 0.4mcg/kg/hr of fentanyl with the same dose for patient request with a lockout of 30minutes[16].

5.6 Epidural analgesia

Epidural analgesia provides excellent pain management after major surgery. It is only safe to use on wards with trained staff under pain service supervision. Usually, a combined local anesthetic and opiate infusion is used. These drugs act synergistically, but can be given separately. The level and density of block must be regularly assessed. Ideally, the local anesthetic will provide blockade of small nerve fibers (pain and temperature) but maintain fine sensation and motor power. The opiates augment the analgesic effect at spinal level.

The sympathetic blockade associated with local anesthetics can result in vasodilation and subsequent hypotension. The location of the epidural catheter placement affects the efficacy of epidural analgesia and influences patient outcomes. Epidural catheters should be inserted in a location congruent to the incisional dermatome. Discrepancy between epidural catheter insertion level and incision site may lead to an increased rate of side effects secondary to an increased infusion rate and increased volumes of local anesthetics used. Inadequate pain relief can lead to early termination of epidural analgesia and masking the potential beneficial effects of epidural analgesia[31]

Side effects of epidural opiates include pruritus, nausea and vomiting, urinary retention, and respiratory depression. Continuous supplementary oxygen should be used.

The choice of analgesic agents administered in the epidural space play a significant role in the achievement of optimal analgesia. The most common agents used are opioids and local anesthetics. Other agents include clonidine, neostigmine, adenosine, ketamine.

Removal of epidural catheters may need to be timed to match a therapeutic trough after prophylactic heparin or low molecular weight heparin is given.

5.7 Epidural PCA

Two meta-analysis have concluded that IV PCA is less effective than continuous epidural and PCA-epidural analgesia.[32, 33]

Local anesthetics are not widely used as the sole agent in postoperative epidural analgesia. To achieve effective analgesia using local anesthetics alone, patients will require higher concentrations of the drugs that could result in hypotension and motor block. Nevertheless, epidural of local anesthetics alone may be warranted in situations in which the side effects of opioids are troublesome to the patient.

The most commonly used local anesthetics in epidural analgesic preparations are bupivacaine, ropivacaine and levobupivacaine. Nowadays for many clinicians ropivacaine is the local anesthetic of choice for background infusions because of their unique property of minimum motor blockade. Most authors recommend an infusion with a 1-2% concentration of ropivacaine at a 4-6ml/hr. An additional opioid could be used in the same mixture.

5.8 Other pain management techniques

This includes the use of non-opiate drugs such as clonidine or tramadol, continuous nerve blocks, and novel drugs used epidurally. The management of a surgical patient with coexisting substance abuse issues or chronic pain problems of any cause is complex and requires the early involvement of a pain specialist.

5.9 Glucocorticoids for pain management

Glucocorticoids have a number of beneficial properties in a surgical setting. In addition to being antiemetic, they are antiinflammatory, analgesic, antipyretic, and antiallergic[34]. Glucocorticoids exert their effects by binding to a glucocorticoid receptor (GR) localized in the cytoplasm of target cells. There is a single class of GR that binds glucocorticoids, with no evidence for subtypes of differing affinity in different tissues[35].

Glucocorticoids may control inflammation by inhibiting many aspects of the inflammatory process through increasing the transcription of anti-inflammatory genes and decreasing the transcription of inflammatory genes.

Glucocorticoids inhibit the transcription of several cytokines that are relevant in inflammatory diseases, including IL-1b, IL-2, IL-3, IL-6, IL-11, TNF-a, GM-CSF and chemokines that attract inflammatory cells to the site of inflammation, including IL8, RANTES, MCP-1, MCP-3, MCP-4, MIP-1a and eotaxin.

The analgesic effect of glucocorticoids was first shown with betamethasone in patients undergoing third molar extraction[36]. A group of doctors from the Helsinki University Hospital chose to investigate the analgesic potency of different doses of dexamethasone for postoperative pain management of patients who underwent laparoscopic hysterectomy[37]. IV dexamethasone 15 mg before induction of anesthesia decreases the oxycodone consumption during the first 24 h after laparoscopic hysterectomy. During first 2 h after surgery, dexamethasone 10 mg reduces the oxycodone consumption as effectively as the 15 mg dose. The opioid-sparing potency of dexamethasone is dose dependent. The effect of the 5 mg dose on postoperative oxycodone consumption was negligible, whereas the 10 and 15 mg doses reduced oxycodone consumption during the first 2 h after surgery.

There is also some studies that presumed the prolonged analgesic effect of non steroidal anti-inflammatory drugs with dexamethasone; a group of experts from Scandinavia, have demonstrated that the association of 16 mg of dexamethasone with rofecoxib has prolonged its analgesic effect[38]. It is also worth mentioning a cost related benefit of the use of dexamethasone. Compared to costs of multiple doses of non-steroidal antiinflammatory drugs used during and after this procedure sounds reasonable to use a single dose of dexamethasone in order to reduce consumption of analgesics.

5.10 Adjuvants in anesthesia and postoperative pain

A number of adjuvants have been added to the intrathecal local anaesthetics for supplementation of intraoperative anaesthesia and postoperative analgesia. They have advantages as they reduce the dose of local anaesthetic; provide long lasting postoperative analgesia with reduced incidence of central nervous system depression, motor effects or hypotension.

Ketamine is an intravenous (IV) anesthetic with analgesic properties in subanesthetic doses, secondary to its action on the NMDA receptor. Several trials are investigating the use of low-dose ketamine for managing postoperative pain. The effect of adding ketamine to morphine for postoperative patient-controlled analgesia (PCA), compared with using morphine alone was investigated in six trials involving 330 patients. Only one trial in patients undergoing lumbar microdiscectomy[39] showed a beneficial effect of adding ketamine. There were no analgesic effects of ketamine in the other five studies in patients undergoing abdominal surgery [41]. Adverse effects including vivid dreams, hallucinations, dysphoria, and disorientation were increased in ketamine-treated patients in two studies.

Dextromethorphan is a weak, noncompetitive NMDA antagonist that has been used as an antitussive agent. It has been shown to inhibit development of cutaneous secondary hyperalgesia in people after peripheral burn injury and to reduce temporal summation of pain[40]. Several studies investigated the effect of the perioperative administration of dextromethorphan on acute postoperative pain. Opiate-related adverse effects were similar between patients who received dextromethorphan and control patients. Postoperative administration of IM dextromethorphan at a dose of 40 mg and oral dextromethorphan (200 mg every 8 hours) also were associated with a significant reduction in postoperative opioid consumption[41].

Analgesic effect of intrathecal neostigmine is secondary to acetylcholine release in the spinal cord tissue[42]. During surgical stimuli, a pre-existent spinal cholinergic tonus is activated. Neostigmine, an anticholinsterase drug increases the concentration of acetylcholine in the cerebrospinal fluid and acetylcholine bioavailability at the cholinergic nerves within the spinal cord. The existence of a cholinergic system in the spinal dorsal horn involved in sensory transmission and modulation is supported by anatomical, pharmacological and electrophysiological studies. Electrophysiological studies have demonstrated that cholinergic receptor agonists produce inhibitory effects on spinal dorsal horn neurons, including spinothalamic tract neurons[43]. This suggests that a spinal cholinergic system plays an important inhibitory role in the modulation of nociceptive transmission.

Nitric oxide (NO) was shown to be a central neurotransmitter and to act as a second messenger in the central nervous system. There are several reports of the relationship between NO and pain processing in the brain and the spinal cord. Acetylcholine and morphine induce analgesia via activation of the arginine-NO-cGMP pathway. Guanylate cyclase activity in the brain is markedly stimulated by NO, generated from L-arginine or provided through an exogenous source. The transdermal nitroglycerine patch has been related to NO formation during degradation of organic nitrates.

There is a significant increase in postoperative analgesia when neostigmine is added to intrathecal bupivacaine in patients undergoing total abdominal hysterectomy. A combination of 5 mg/day transdermal nitroglycerine patch and intrathecal low dose neostigmine (5 mcg) resulted in an average of 10 hours of postoperative analgesia after total abdominal hysterectomy during bupivacaine spinal block, compared to 3.5 hours in the control group. Also the use of intrathecal neostigmine and transdermal nitroglycerine delays the first requirement of rescue analgesia by 6.5 hours. Transdermal nitroglycerine has been shown to increase the postoperative analgesia of intrathecal opioids[44].

6. Conclusions

Recent developments in our understanding of incisional pain have highlighted the complexity of perioperative pain and the need for optimal management not only to provide rapid recovery but also to prevent long-term consequences.

More than 100 NSAIDs are marketed or at an advance stage of development worldwide. There is no a single compound with proven efficacy better than other in the treatment of postoperative pain. The search for more efficacious and better-tolerated compounds is still being persued.

Principles of safe IV treatment:

- Acetaminophen or pure NSAIDs alone
- Acetaminophen + NSAIDs
- Weak opioid + acetaminophen or
- Weak opioid + NSAIDs

7. References

[1] Vadivelu N, Whitney C, Sinatra R: Pain Pathways and Acute Pain Processing in: Sinatra R, De Leon Casadola O, Ginsberg B, VIscusi E: Acute Pain Management. 2009

[2] Woolf CJ, Salter MW. Neuronal Pasticity: Increasing the Gain in Pain. Science, 2000: 1765- 1769

[3] Apfelbaum JL, Chen C, Mehta SS, gan TJ. Postoperative pain experience: results from a national survey suggest postoperative pain continues to be undermanaged. Anesth Analg 2003; 97: 534-540

[4] Pavlin DJ, Chen C, Penaloza DA, et al. Pain as a factor complicating recovery and discharge after ambulatory surgery. Anesth Analg 2002; 95: 627-634

[5] Melzack R, Wall PD. Pain Mechanisms: a new theory. New York, NY. Science. 1965; 150 (699): 971-979.

[6] Ji RR, Woolf CJ. Neuronal plasticity and signal transduction in nociceptive neurons: implications for the initiation and maintenance of pathological pain. Neurobiol. Dis. 2001;8 (1): 1-10

[7] Byers MR, Bonica JJ. Periperral pain mechanisms and nociceptor plasticity. In: Loeser JD, editor. Management of pain. New York: Lippincott Williams & Wilkins; 2001. P 26-72

[8] Marchand S: The Physiology of Pain Mechanisms: From the periphery to the brain. Rheum Dis Clin N Am, 2008: 285-309

[9] Byers MR, Bonica JJ. Periperral pain mechanisms and nociceptor plasticity. In: Loeser JD, editor. Management of pain. New York: Lippincott Williams & Wilkins; 2001. P 73-152

[10] Mendel LM. Physiological properties of unmyelinated fiber prohections to the spinal cord. Exp Neurol 1966; 16 (3): 316 - 32

[11] Granot M, Granovsky Y, Sprecher E, et al. Contact heat-evoked temporal summation: tonic versus repetitive-phasic stimulation. Pain 2006; 122 (3)295-305

[12] Woolf CJ. Windup and central sensitization are not equivalent. Pain 1996;66(2-3):105-8.

[13] Althaus J, Wax J: Analgesia and Anestehsia in Labor. Obst Gynecol Clin N Am, 2005: 231-244

[14] Lamvu G, Zolnoun D, Boggess J, Steege J. Obesity: Phsiologic changes and challenges during laparoscopy. Am J Obs & Gyn 2004; 669-74

[15] Kerridge R. Perioperative patient management. Best Practice and Research Clinical Obstetrics and Gunaecology. 2006: 23-40

[16] Calderón VM, Zamora MR, Zavaleta BM, Santa Rita EM, y col. Analgesia posoperatoria en ginecoobstetricia. Ginecol Obstet Mex 2009;77(2):82-88

[17] Gotche PC. Extracts from clinical evidence: non-steroidal anti-inflammatory drugs. Br Med J.2000;320:1058-1061

[18] Rosaeg OP, Krepski B, Cicutti N, et al. Effect of preemptive multimodal analgesia for arthroscopic knee ligament repair. Reg Anesth Pain Med. 2001;26:125-130

[19] Lepri A, Sia S, Catinelli S, et al. Patient controlled analgesia with tramadol versus tramadolplus ketorolac. Minerva Anestesiol.2006;72:59-67

[20] Snabes M, Jakimiuk A, Kotarski J, et al. Parecoxib sodium administered over several days reduces pain after gynecologic surgery via laparotomy. Journal of Clin Anesth, 2007;19:448-455

[21] Gajraj NM, Joshi GP. Role of cycloosygenase-2 inhibitors in postoperative pain management. Anesthesiology Clin N Am. 2005;23:49-72

[22] Benson GD. Acetaminophen in chronic liver disease. Clin Pharmacol Ther 1983;33:95-101

[23] Brotodihardjo AE, Batey RG, Farrel GC, Byth K. Hepatotoxicity from paracetamol self-poisoning in western Sydney: a continuing challenge. Med J Aus 1992;157:382-5

[24] Gutstein HB, Akil H. Opioid analgesics. In Hardman JG, Limbird LE, Gilman AG, eds. Goodman & Gilman's The Pharmacological Basis of Therapeutics. 10th ed. New York, NY: Mc Graw Hill; 2002:569-619

[25] Reisine T, Pasternak G. Opioid analgesics and antagonists. In Goodman LS, Gilman A, eds. The Pharmacological Basis of Therapeutics. 9th ed. New York, NY: Mcmillan;1997.

[26] Bonica JJ. Biochemistry and modulation of nociception and pain. In Bonica, JJ ed. The Management of Pain. 2nd Ed. Philadelphia, PA: Lea & Febiger; 1990: 94-121

[27] Sinatra R: Oral and Parenteral Opioid analgesics for Acute Pain Management. In Sinatra R, de Leon O, Ginsberg B, BIscusi E. Acute Pain Management, Cambrige University Press; 2009.181-203

[28] Wright IV C, Kramer D, Zalman M, Smith MY, Haddox JD. Risk identification, risk assessment, and risk management of abusable drugs formulation. Drug Alcohol Depend 2006;83S:S68-S76

[29] Littlejohn C, Baldacchino A, Bannister J. Comorbid chronic non-cancer pain and opioid use disorders. Hospt Med 2004;65:206-9

[30] Lenz H, Sandvik L, Qvigstad E, Bjerkelund C, Raeder J. A comparison of intravenous oxydocone and intravenous morphine in patient-controlled postoperative analgesia after laparoscopic hysterectomy. Anesth Analg 2009;109:1279 –83

[31] Ready LB. Acte pain: lessons learned from 25,000 patients. Reg Anesth Pain Med. 1999;24:499-505

[32] Werawatganon T, Charuluxanun S. Patient controlled intravenous opioid analgesia versus continuous epidural analgesia for pain after intra-abdominal surgery. Cochrane Database Syst Rev. 2005;CD004088

[33] Wu CL, Cohen SR, Richman JM et al. Efficacy of postoperative patient-controlled and continuous infusion epidural analgesia versus intravenous patient-controlled analgesia with opioids: a meta-analysis. Anesthesiology.2005;103:1079-1088

[34] Lieberman BA, Nordeen SK. (1997) DNA intersegment transfer, how steroid receptors search for a target site. J Biol Chem **272:** 1061-8

[35] Drouin J, Sun YL, Chamberland M, et al. (1993) Novel glucocorticoid receptor complex with DNA element of the hormone-repressed POMC gene. EMBO J **12:** 145-56.

[36] Skjelbred P, Løkken P. Post-operative pain and inflammatory reaction reduced by injection of corticosteroid. Eur J Clin Pharmacol 1982;21:391–6

[37] Bisgaard T, Klarskov B, Kehlet H, Rosenberg J. Preoperative dexamethasone improves surgical outcome after laparoscopic cholecystectomy. A randomized double-blind placebo-controlled trial. Ann Surg 2003;238:651–60

[38] Hval K, Thagaard KS, Schlichting E, Raeder J. The prolonged postoperative analgesic effect when dexamethasone is added to a nonsteroidal anti-inflammatory drug (rofecoxib) before breast surgery. Anesth Analg 2007;105:481–6

[39] Javery KB, Ussery TW, Steger HG, et al. Comparison of morphine and morphine with ketamine for postoperative analgesia. Can J Anaesth 1996;43:212- 5.
[40] Price DD, Mao J, Frenk H, Mayer DJ. The N-methyl-D-aspartate receptor antagonist dextromethorphan selectively reduces temporal summation of second pain in man. Pain 1994; 59:165- 74.
[41] Habib A, Gan T. Role of Analgesic Adjuncts in Postoperative Pain Management. Anesthesiology Clin N Am;23:85-107
[42] Shibuki K, Okada D. Endogenous nitric oxide release required for long-term synaptic depression in the cerebellum. Nature 1991;349:326-8.
[43] Kitto KF, Haley JE, Wilcox GL. Involvement of nitric oxide in spinally-mediated hyperalgesia in the mouse. Neurosci Lett 1992;148:1-5.
[44] Kaur G, Osahan N, Afzal L. Effect of transdermal nitroglycerine patch on analgesia of low dose intrathecal neostigmine: An evaluation. J Anesth Clin Pharmacol 2007;23:159-62.

Part 5

Hysterectomy Complications

18

Ureter: How to Avoid Injuries in Various Hysterectomy Techniques

Manoel Afonso Guimarães Gonçalves, Fernando Anschau,
Daniela Martins Gonçalves and Chrystiane da Silva Marc
Pontifical Catholic University of Rio Grande do Sul
Brazil

1. Introduction

Hysterectomy is one of the most common surgical procedures in the practice of gynecology. The various surgical techniques for hysterectomy, including those by the abdominal approach as well as those by the vaginal route, deserve special attention with regard to possible transoperative urological injuries. These complications raise questions about the anatomic knowledge for all gynecologists. The ureters are vulnerable to injuries during gynecological surgeries and even obstetric ones due to the anatomic proximity to the organs of the female reproductive system. [1] The general incidence of ureteral injuries is estimated to be 0.03% to 2.0% for abdominal hysterectomy, 0.02% to 0.5% for vaginal hysterectomy, and 0.2% to 6.0% for laparoscopy-assisted vaginal hysterectomy. [2, 3, 4, 5, 6] There are four critical points of potential ureteral injury during a hysterectomy. The first critical point is situated at the entrance of the ureter in the pelvic bone, when the ovarian vessels cross over it. The second critical point is identified next to the uterosacral ligament, where the ureter is situated lateral to this ligament. The third critical point is at the level of the uterine artery, where the ureter crosses below the uterine artery through the cardinal ligament at the level of the ischial spine. The fourth critical points occurs in the bladder, where the ureter turns medially, crossing the anterior portion of the vaginal dome and entering the bladder wall. [7] Certainly, the ability to recognize the anatomy, as well the ability of the surgeon in recognizing the points of greater risk of ureter injury, will help in lowering these percentages.

2. Anatomy

The ureter is a tube that is part of the urinary tract and that connects the renal pelvis to the bladder. Its function is to transport the urine from the kidney to the bladder, which involves peristaltic or wave-like movements by contraction of its smooth muscle layer. The ureters have three layers, like other tubular organs: (i) the **outermost** layer consists of connective tissue, partially covered by the serosa in the regions where the ureter is in contact with the peritoneum; (ii) in the **intermediate** portion, there is a middle layer consisting of smooth muscle tissue of three types, circular, longitudinal and oblique; (iii) the **inner** layer is composed of mucosa – with transition epithelium - and submucosa – with connective tissue.

The ureters each have a length of 25 to 30 cm and a diameter of 3 mm. They originate from the confluence of the various renal calyces, coming together in the renal pelvis. The ureters exit the kidney at the level of the superior abdomen, going down to the pelvis bone behind the organs of the gastrointestinal tract, in the retroperitoneum, medial to the greater psoas muscle. On penetrating the pelvic cavity, crossing over the bifurcation of the common iliac vessels, we also observe the crossing of the ovarian vessels (first critical point of injury). The ureters form the posterior border of the ovarian fossa; they continue caudal to the lateral edge of the uterosacral ligaments (second critical point of injury) up to the cardinal ligament. The uterine artery accompanies the ureter along the lateral part of the cervix and the upper part of the vagina. At the base of the cardinal ligament, the ureter passes below the uterine artery (third critical point of injury), at the level of the ischial spine. At this point it goes initially forward and then medially, under the wide extensive ligament, between the uterine and vaginal arteries, toward the bottom of the lateral sac of the vagina - lying approximately 2 cm lateral to the cervix. Here, the ureter ascends anterior to the vagina for a short distance finally reaching the base of the bladder, where it opens at a lateral angle of the vesical trigone, obliquely perforating the wall of the bladder (fourth critical point of injury).

In relation to the blood supply of the ureter, it is well established that it is variable and that it is provided from various sources. The abdominal part of the ureter is irrigated regularly by a branch from the abdominal aorta or by a branch of the renal or ovarian artery. At the level of the arched line (the transition point from the abdominal portion to the pelvic portion), the middle portion in general is irrigated by branches of the common or internal iliac arteries. The pelvic portion is irrigated by the superior and inferior vesical arteries, as well as branches from the uterine, mid-rectal and internal pudendal arteries. At its upper and middle portions, blood supply to the ureter comes from the medial side. In contrast, the pelvic ureter receives its vascular supply mainly from the lateral part. Therefore, medial dissection in this distal pelvic portion produces the least vascular damage. Periureteral tissues are also irrigated by the subperitoneal arteries, which allows us to conclude that dissection of the ureters should be minimal in separating them from the peritoneum.

Despite good anatomic knowledge and an experienced surgeon, ureteral injuries can occur due to anatomic distortions. The risk of ureteral injury increases in cases of endometriosis, pelvic adherences or pelvic tumors, which distort the normal course of the ureter. [8] Abnormalities of the urinary tract, which occur in 17 to 20% of the population, could be documented by preoperative excretory urography; meanwhile, the majority of ureteral injuries occur when there is no indication for excretory urography. [9] The use of this diagnostic technology , like other examinations, for example, cystoscopy, are not indicated in routine preoperative assessment in patients who are going to have a hysterectomy, due to morbidities that, although small, are present in these procedures. The preoperative introduction of ureteral catheters, another method for the identification of ureteral abnormalities and even identification of normal ureteral anatomy, is undesirable because of the cost and associated morbidity. In patients with large pelvic masses that distort anatomy, small uterine segment, cervical myomas or cervical cancer, preoperative imaging studies such as endovenous pyelogram, ultrasound, retrograde pyelography and other studies can be particularly useful. [8]

The direct visualization of the ureter should constitute an initial necessary in all pelvic dissections, particularly hysterectomies. The surgeon should feel at ease with the ureteral trajectory and well familiarized with the locations of frequent injuries during an abdominal surgery. It is important to recall that routine dissection and repair of the ureters, a procedure to prevent injuries cited by some authors, increases the risks of injury of the ureter and should not be routinely done. [10]

3. Injuries and their repair

The adage "just happens to those who make" holds true when we discuss ureteral injuries. Even experienced surgeons, with a substantial volume of pelvic surgeries, at some moment will end up injuring the ureter. Despite being less common than injuries of the bladder and rectum, ureteral injury is one of the most serious complications in gynecological surgery, with high morbidity. The major concern in this case is not always the injury itself, but rather not knowing of its occurrence. The inability to recognize and repair this injury constitutes a great risk for the patient. [11] Transoperative identification of a ureteral injury occurs in only 11% to 12% of cases. [12, 13]

Unexpected pain in the flank region in the postoperative period, fever or vaginal discharge can suggest ureteral injury. Sometimes, the ureteral injuries can go unnoticed because the signs and symptoms are not specific. The 1.7% incidence of ureteral injuries in hysterectomies concerns some authors when referring to the question of their early identification. Persistent peristalsis was identified in 5 of 6 injured ureters, demonstrating that this sign is a poor marker for determining the integrity of the ureter. [12]

The ureter can be injured in numerous ways: fulgurated, ligated, pinched, jostled and sectioned partially or completely. Besides these injuries, trauma to the sheath of the ureter and to its longitudinal blood supply can occur (devascularization), despite a technique of meticulous dissection.

Injuries due to ligature, pinching or jostling of the ureter occur more often in the locations where the ovarian and uterine vessels are ligated or clamped. [14] If they are soon noticed, the simple removal of a wrongly placed suture can be sufficient for repair. However, injuries caused by clamping produce significant damage of the crush type. After removal of the hemostat, the tissues should be examined with respect to their viability, and if there is still vitality, it is likely that the placement of ureteral catheters will be sufficient. If any segment appears to be nonviable, it should be excised.

The ureteral sections can be partial or complete. The partially sectioned ureters should also be evaluated with respect to their vitality. Vascularized tissue can be reapproximated by an absorbable suture on a ureteral catheter. Repair of complete sections can vary with localization and extent of vascular damage. If the injury occurs distant from the bladder, it can be repaired on a ureteral catheter. The proximal and distal ends should be mobilized and resutured without any tension.

The location of the injury constitutes an important element in the choice of the repair technique. Approximately 80 to 90% of the injuries occur in the terminal ureter. In this situation, a form of ureteral reimplantation can be indicated. For the injuries less than 5 cm of the ureterovesical junction, a simple reimplantation can be complicated by urinary reflux, and therefore, some authors, recommend the creation of a submucosal tunnel of the vesical wall. In this technique, the dome of the bladder is opened to choose the most inclined part of the vesical base, where a tunnel is made, creating a submucosal passage of approximately 1.5 cm. The ureter should be drawn through the tunnel with delicate traction. A mucosa-mucosa anastomosis over a catheter is made utilizing a fine absorbable suture. A second set of sutures supports the anastomosis, uniting the ureteral adventitia and the vesical muscle. The closing of the bladder should be done with double plane suturing with a fine absorbable suture.

For higher injuries - above 5 cm from the ureterovesical junction- and in those in which it is not possible to unblock the ureter or where a complete sectioning has occurred or the ureter crushed, some procedure will be necessary to mobilize the ureter and/or bladder so that the reimplantation site is not under tension. This method can consist of the dissection of the healthy portion of the ureter and its sectioning above the location of the injury. [15] The injured end of the ureter should be ligated to avoid extravasation of urine from the bladder, proceeding then to the choice of a site for reimplantation of the ureter in the posterior portion of the vesical fundus. The bladder is opened and its wall is transfixed from inside to outside with curved forceps, pulling the ureter through this orifice. The ureteral orifice is sutured to the muscle and mucosa layers of the bladder with a fine 4-0 absorbable suture. The ureter can also be tunnelized in the vesical submucosa before performing the anastomosis. A double J ureteral catheter is introduced, where it is removed after about 6 weeks. The vesical wall is sutured in planes with a 3-0 absorbable suture, and the bladder examined for 7 to 10 days by the supra-pubic and urethral route with two No. 20 Foley probes. One of these probes can be removed as soon as the patient no longer shows macroscopic hematuria, where excretory urography is performed after the removal of the double J catheter for anatomic evaluation of the urinary tract. The success of ureteral reimplantation surgery (ureteroneocystostomy) described here depends on the realization of an anastomosis between the ureter and bladder absolutely free of tension. To achieve this, it is often necessary to fix the bladder on the major psoas muscle of the compromised side. [16]

Various conditions contribute in determining the incidence of ureteral injuries in gynecological practice. The relations of contiguity between the pelvic ureter and the genital tract, on the one hand, and the possible direct or indirect participation of the ureter in genital pathology, on the other hand, represent the presumptions about the ureteral pathology of gynecological interest. The intimate relation that the pelvic ureter has with the genital tract explains how many inflammatory or tumor processes can compromise it directly or cause its topographic modification.

In the classification of ureteral injuries, a very useful difference for clinical purposes is separately considering the ureteral injuries diagnosed at the moment of the surgical act and others in which clinical manifestations emerged after some time. In injuries found during the surgical intervention, its repair requires only technical knowledge of its resolution, generally with low morbidity. However, for injuries diagnosed later, the problems will be of various natures, showing variable symptomatology and complex diagnostic and therapeutic possibilities.

When there is ureteral injury, the therapy is in general subordinated to the type and site of the ureteral injury, to the type of intervention during which the injury was caused, and to the nature and extent of the disease which determined the surgical intervention.

We describe below the ureteral injuries during abdominal interventions for benign problems.

4. Abdominal hysterectomy

It is in this intervention that a large number of ureteral injuries are found. For a clear description of the various possibilities of the ureteral injuries in relation to various techniques, we will consider separately the various times of this intervention in which the injury can be produced. Certainly, we should make an essential observation in the approach of the abdominal hysterectomy and ureteral injuries: some authors believe that there is increased risk of injury for the laparoscopic route that, although small - with 1.1% prevalence, representing 7.2 times the risk demonstrated in laparotomy procedures. [17] However, based on meta-analysis that considered all the complications of major severity, including ureteral injuries, there would be no difference in the incidence of these major complications between laparotomic and laparoscopic techniques. [18]

4.1 At the level of the ovarian pedicle

The injury that can occur during the clamping and sectioning of the ovarian vessels is a relatively rare incident under normal conditions. However, some congenital or acquired situations can favor the injury, such as congenitally short ovarian pedicle, presence of an adnexial inflammatory process or the growth of a tumor with intra-ligamentary development. Besides, it should be pointed out that an injury can occur during the ligature of the ovarian vessels with an insufficient clipping of the vessels and their consequent retraction, with the approximation of the ureter. The attempt at successive hemostasis in these situations can lead to a ureteral injury. A better prophylaxis of ureteral injuries at this level would be a careful and precise preparation of the ovarian pedicle and freeing it from pathological adherences before the ligature of the ovarian vessels. [19]

4.2 At the level of the uterosacral ligament

In the sectioning of the uterosacral ligament, the possibility of a ureteral injury often becomes real due to the retractions caused by pelvic peritonitis or especially in not very rare cases of endometriosis next to this ligament. As we know, the ureter passes below and lateral to the uterosacral ligament, and therefore, when sectioning this ligament, the ureter can be injured.

This accident can be avoided with the sectioning of the peritoneum at the bottom of Douglas' sac and with traction of the uterus upward toward the pubic symphysis. With this maneuver, the ureter is separated and we can observe the rectal columns better, which can also be retracted. These ligaments can be sectioned by electrosurgery or clamped and sectioned horizontally and separate from the cardinal or Mackenrodt ligament, through which the ureter passes.

4.3 At the level of mackenrodt's ligament

At this point, we have the crossing of the ureter with the uterine artery. The most frequent injuries in total hysterectomy occur at the moment of the sectioning of Mackenrodt's ligament. Various determinants can be responsible for this, but those that deserve special attention are the inflammatory abnormalities that favor the retraction of the parametrium and allow the most frequent occurrence of this accident. Prophylaxis of this injury is done respecting the surgical technique in which the bladder is first mobilized, especially in the middle zone, individualizing the vesical columns, which should be distended laterally, allowing the ureters to be separated. [15] The ureters, in this way, remain laterally, which allows the secure ligatura of the uterine vessels followed by Mackenrodt's ligament. Inflammatory reactions or neoplasms that cause a blockage in this region can result in difficulties in executing this technique.

In these cases, the ureter should be first individualized and dissected up to its entrance into the parametrium. In many situations, this is the moment for making a tunnel between the ureter and the parametrium, identifying clearly the artery and the uterine vein, which are above the ureter. On sectioning the roof of the tunel, after its clamping, hemostasis of the uterine vascular bundle is also performed. In this way, this surgical time, even in adverse situations, can be done with little chance of accidents.

4.4 At level of the bladder

Ureteral injuries at level of the bladder are of concern when there is large dissection of the tissues in this related anatomic region, for example, in extrafascial total hysterectomy and radical hysterectomy. Even so, after the surgical time of the sectioning of Mackenrodt's ligament, taking the usual technical precautions, these injuries are infrequent. Surgical precautions include dissection with caudal separation of the bladder after ligature of the uterine vessels, associated with contralateral traction of the uterus, and moving the ureter away from the surgical field, increasing the distance between the ureter and the cervix. This maneuver positions the ureter more inferior and lateral to Mackenrodt's ligament (already sectioned). In this way, the sectioning of the vaginal wall for the extraction of the uterus will be free of risks of ureteral injury at the level of its entrance in the bladder.

4.5 In the presence of myoma

Injury of the ureter during a surgical intervention with myomatous uterus remains subordinate to the location and volume of the myoma and to the degree of topographic dislocation of the ureter that the myoma may have caused. Myomas located in the cervical or intra-ligamentary regions can make the surgery more difficult, providing a greater chance of ureteral injuries.

Generally, the ureter remains compromised, in these cases below the myoma, but can sometimes be over the myoma. This situation occurs when the myoma develops in the lower part of the isthmus. A better prophylaxis of this accident is to individualize the ureter by dissection of the retroperitoneum.

4.6 Adnexectomy

Adnexectomy when performed alone or together with hysterectomy can favor surgical injuries of the ureter. We can have infectious clinical situations, pictures of endometriosis, ectopic pregnancies with involvement of all tube, malignant or benign neoplastic problems such as intra-ligamentary cysts, which favor an injury of the ureter.

Operative maneuvers should adapt to each circumstance where there is always the possibility of the injury of the ureter, which with the growth of a cystic formation can undergo modifications in its topography.

5. Vaginal hysterectomy

Even if ureteral injuries can happen in the course of this intervention, we should point that this accident can be avoided simply by carrying out the surgical technique in a correct manner. The rate of ureteral injuries is low, around 0.88%, and remain less than that of vesical injury, around 1.76%, in vaginal hysterectomy without prolapse. [20]

The possibility of injury of the ureter can occur soon after sectioning Mackenrodt's ligament, when we proceed with the ligature of the uterine artery, when there can be the need for of successive attempts at hemostasis. To avoid the injury, it is sufficient to mobilize the bladder in the direction of the vesico-uterine peritoneal fold and even to pull the cervix down and in the direction opposite to the side of the parametrium to be sectioned.

5.1 In adnexectomy

Another moment in which an injury of the ureter can occur in vaginal hysterectomy is when there is the need for an adnexectomy. On the occasion of ligature of the ovarian pedicle, by slipping the loop of the suture over the vessels, these can withdraw, causing bleeding and in the attempt of successive hemostasis, with new hemostats, the ureter can be included, leading to its injury. The care that should taken when this happens is to isolate the bleeding vessel, and to clamp it individually, never blindly or en masse. If during the surgery, it is decided to close the peritoneum, there is the risk of the angulation of the ureter at the level of the ovarian pedicle.

6. Radical hysterectomy (Wertheim-Meigs)

Even though it may appear paradoxical, direct ureteral injuries in these interventions are less frequent than in the execution of total hysterectomy due to benign injuries. The description of ureteral injuries in radical hysterectomy is on the order of 0.77% to 1.32%. [21, 22] In performing a radical hysterectomy, injuries can occur by contusion of the ureter which can translate into later fistulas. Eventual accidents can occur in unfavorable situations such as in deeper planes, with an imperfect exposure of the surgical field or with difficult hemostatic control, leading to failure in a routine surgical technique.

7. References

[1] Jung SK, Huh CY. Ureteral injuries during classic intrafascial supracervical hysterectomy: an 11-years experience in 1163 patients. J Minim Invasive Gynecol. 2008;15(4):440-445.

[2] Goodno JA Jr, Powers TW, Harris VD. Ureteral injury in gynecologic surgery: a ten year review in a community hospital. Am J Obstet Gynecol. 1995; 172:1817-1820.

[3] Harkki-Siren P, Sjoberg J, Tiitinen A. Urinary tract injuries after hysterectomy. Obstet Gynecol. 1998; 92:113-118.

[4] Stanhope CR, Wilson TO, Utz WJ, Smith LH, O'Brien PC. Suture entrapment and secondary ureteral obstruction. Am J Obstet Gynecol. 1991; 164:1513-1517.

[5] Wu HH, Yang PY, Yeh GP, Chou PH, Hsu JC, Lin KC. The detection of ureteral injuries after hysterectomy. J Minim Invasive Gynecol. 2006; 13:403-408.

[6] Gilmour DT, of the S, Flowerdew G. Rates of urinary tract injury from gynecologic surgery and the role of intraoperative cystoscopy. Obstet Gynecol. 2006; 107(6):1366-1372.
[7] Berek J. Berek and Novak's Gynecology. 14th ed. Philadelphia, PA: Lippincott Williams and Wilkins; 2006. p.123-124.
[8] Ferro A, Byck D, Gallup D. Am J Obstet Gynecol. 2003;189(2):354-357.
[9] Piscitelli JT, Simel DL, Addison WA : Who should have intravenous pyelograms before hysterectomy for benign disease. Obstet Gynecol. 1987;69:541-544
[10] Buller JL,Thompson JR, Cundiff GW, et al. Uterosacral ligament: description of anatomic relatioships to optimize surgical safety. Obstet Gynecol. 2001;97:873-879.
[11] Higgins CC: Ureteral injuries during surgery: a review of 87 cases. JAMA. 1967;199:82-86.
[12] Vakili B, Chesson RR, Kyle BL, et al. The incidence of urinary tract injury during hysterectomy: a prospective analysis based on universal cystoscopy. Am J Obstet Gynecol. 2005; 192:1599-1604.
[13] Gilmour DT, Dwyer PL, Carey MP. Lower urinary tract injury during gynecologic surgery and its detection by intraoperative cystoscopy. Obstet Gynecol. 1999; 94:883-889.
[14] Daly, JW, Higgins KA: Injury to the ureter during gynecologic surgical procedures. Surg Gynecol Obstet. 1988;167:19-22.
[15] Utrie JW. Bladder and ureteral injury: prevention and management. Clin Obstet Gynecol. 1998; 41:755-763.
[16] Ehrlich RM, Melman A, Skinner DG. The use of the vesico-psoas hitch in urologic surgery. J Urol. 1978; 119:322-326.
[17] Mäkinen J, Johansson J, Tomás C, et al. Morbidity of 10110 hysterectomies by type approach. Human Reprod. 2001; 16(7):1473-1478.
[18] Walsh CA, Walsh SR, Tang TY, Slack M. Total abdominal hysterectomy versus total laparoscopic hysterectomy for benign disease: a meta-analysis. Eur J Obstet Gynecol Reprod Biol. 2009; 144:3-7.
[19] Messaoudi F, Ben Jemaa S, Yazidi M, et al. Lower urinary trauma complication gyneacologic and obstetrical surgery. Tunis Med. 2008; 86(8):740-744.
[20] Ibeanu AO, Chesson RR, Echols KT, et al. Urinary tract injury during hysterectomy based on universal cystoscopy. Obstet Gynecol. 2009; 113:6-10.
[21] Frankman EA, Wang L, Bunker CH, Lowder JL. Lower urinary tract injury in women in the United States, 1976-2006. Am J Obstet Gynecol. 2010; 202(5):495.e1-5.
[22] Likic IS, Kadija S, Ladjevic NG, et al. Analysis of urologic complications after radical hysterectomy. Am J Obstet Gynecol. 2008; 199(6):644.e1-3.

19

Sacrocolpopexy for Post Hysterectomy Vault Prolapse

Serge P. Marinkovic, Lisa M. Gillin and Christina M. Marinkovic
Department of Surgery/Division of Urology,
Female Pelvic Medicine and Reconstructive Surgery Specialist
St Joseph Hospital, Fort Wayne, Indiana,
USA

1. Introduction

Pelvic organ prolapse is most likely the result of one or more clinical entities that gradually assist in weakening the pelvic floor [Connell KA, 2011]. Direct childbirth trauma to the levator ani and surrounding pelvic floor tissue will decrease strength over the course of recurrent childbirth and time. These injuries compromise support of the pelvic floor and may deviate its apical S_3 horizontal orientation, while constant collagen and elastin remodelling may lead to further pelvic floor demise and upstage pelvic organ prolapse [Connell KA, 2011]. Over two hundred thousand women undergo the repair of pelvic organ prolapse in the United States every year. In fact, the cost for diagnosis and treatment exceeds two billion dollars annually [Subak LL, 2001]. A Kaiser Permanente retrospective, observational study surveyed 149,554 female patients over the age of twenty and estimated that the lifetime risk of undergoing a single surgery for pelvic organ prolapse or urinary incontinence by age eighty was eleven percent [Olsen 1997].

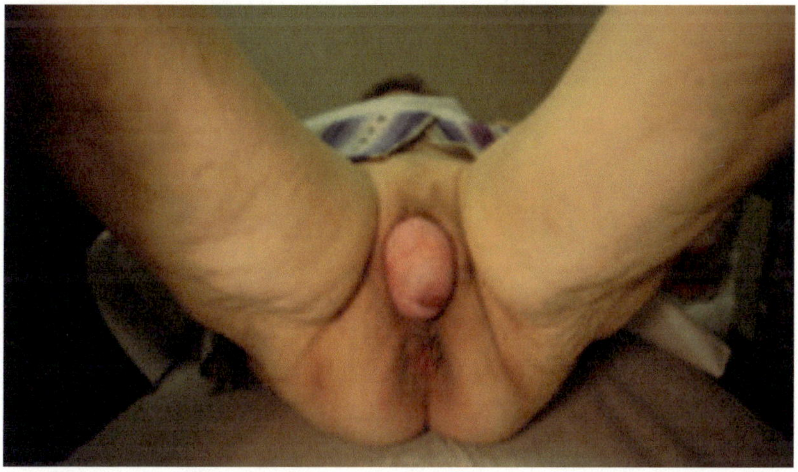

Fig. 1. Stage 4 Complete Procidentia. The cervix is the dimple in the middle of the photograph. Patient underwent a total hysterectomy and a double mesh, anterior and posterior polypropylene mesh [Scali Method, 1974] sacrocolpopexy.

The need for recurrent pelvic organ prolapse surgery [within four years of prolapse surgery] has been estimated to be twenty-nine percent. Post-hysterectomy vault prolapse ranges from ten to forty percent and appears to have an equal occurrence regardless of whether the abdominal or vaginal approach is utilized [Maher C, 2010].

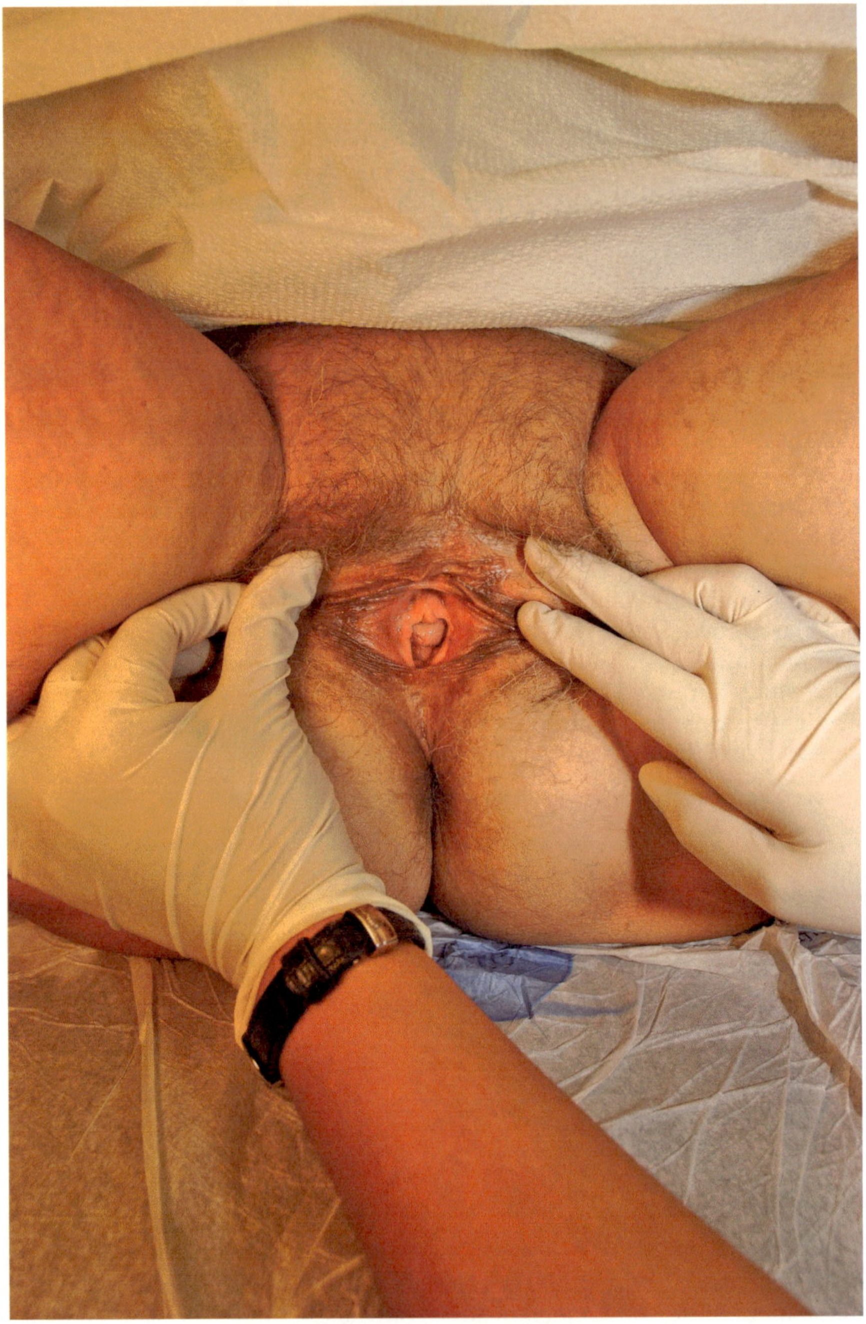

Fig. 2. Figure 1 patient five years after her sacrocolpopexy with no recurrent prolapse.

The high rates of failed pelvic organ prolapse surgeries have led to a long history of new surgical procedural development. The Frenchman, Dr. Ameline [Ameline, 1957] first published abdominal sacrocolpopexy in 1957 while in the United States, Dr. Lane [Lane, 1962] published a series of four patients undergoing abdominal sacrocolpopexy in the Journal of Obstetrics and Gynecology. Abdominal Sacrocolpopexy entails an extensive abdominal procedure that has potential complications of mesh exposure, hemorrhage, dyspareunia, injury to bladder or ureter and prolapse recurrence. Newer approaches such as laparoscopic and robotic-assisted sacrocolpopexy have proven short-term benefits of expedited convalescence and reduced morbidity; disadvantages, however, are that the procedure is less accessible, higher in cost, and still with no results approaching ten years. [Gilleran JP, 2010].

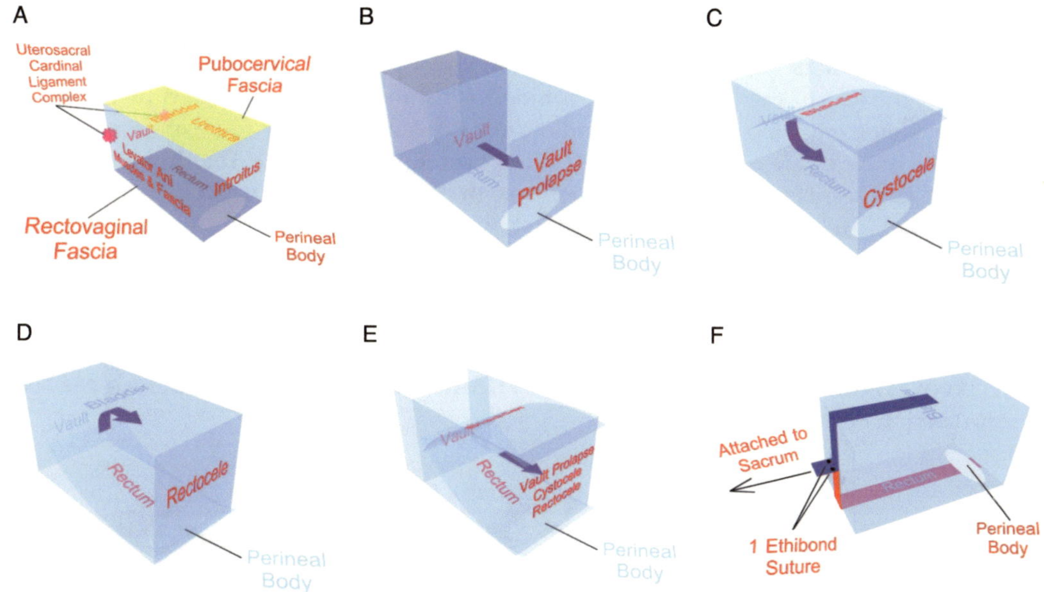

Fig. 1. A. Normal support anatomy of the vagina. B. Vault Prolapse. C. Cystocele D. Rectocele. E. Triple compartment prolapse. F. Anterior and posterior mesh extensions to sacral anterior longitudinal ligament.

2. Pertinent procedural anatomy

To perform a sacrocolpopexy, the uterus and cervix need to be excised concomitant with sacrocolpopexy or separately; similar support can be obtained with an intact uterus and cervix by performing a sacrohysteropexy [Lewis, 2011]. Once the uterus is excised, the main supporting structures of the vault, anterior and posterior vaginal walls are three-fold: Uterosacral-cardinal ligament complex [Level One support], Pubocervical/Rectovaginal fascia, and their attachments to the arcus tendineus fascia pelvic and levator ani fascia provide mid-vaginal compartment reinforcement [Level Two support], Levator ani and perineal body [Level Three support] [**Figure 1a,** Marinkovic & Stanton 2004]. These three fascial ligament components comprise John Delancey's three autonomous layers of pelvic organ support [Delancey JO, 1992]. The presacral space [Shiozawa, 2010] is the pelvic floor nerve center and has the following anatomic landmark boundaries. Superiorly, we have the lumbosacral intervertebral disc, while with the right pelvic lateral side, we have the right common iliac artery/vein and right ureter. On the contralateral pelvic side we have the left common iliac artery/vein and left ureter. The middle presacral area's hallmarks include the middle sacral artery [final branch off the posterior abdominal aorta] and the pelvic plexus, which lie on the medial aspect of the sacrum and can often be seen and venturously prodded. Tread carefully while in this venue because the middle sacral vein develops below the left common iliac vein while draining superiorly into the inferior vena cava and can easily be injured potentiating severe pelvic bleeding. The pelvic venous plexus can in some patients be widely divergent and easily friable to the application of DeBakey or Russian forceps, the gloved-hand, scissors or cautery device and the ensuing brisk, low pressure bleeding is often very difficult to control. When brisk, heavy pelvic plexus bleeding occurs, immediately apply direct digital pressure or a sponge stick to the bleeding vessels. Obtain three units of packed red blood cells into the operating room with visual confirmation of the packed red blood units' physical presence in your room prior to attempting vessel ligature. Once ready, the loss of the least amount of blood and time may be improved by excising a rectangular shape piece of rectus fascia and muscle measuring two by four centimeters, then applying the muscle side directly to the bleeding vessel [Remzi, 2002]. The thrombin within the muscle bed assists in thrombosis along with the applied graft occlusion pressure. Suturing the rectus muscle/fascial graft first with four, interrupted side applied (3-0) polypropylene sutures is recommended. An alternative method is to apply absorbable [Figure 3a, left] copolymer or non-absorbable titanium tacks [Protack, Covidien, Mansfield, MA, USA]. Another prompt and useful method is to directly apply sterile metal thumbtacks with its corequisite applicator [Figure 3b, Hemorrhage Occluder Pin, Tools for Surgery, Stoneybrook, **Figure 3b**, New York, 11790-2201, USA]. Unfortunately this approach has been less studied [Nivatvongs, 1986].

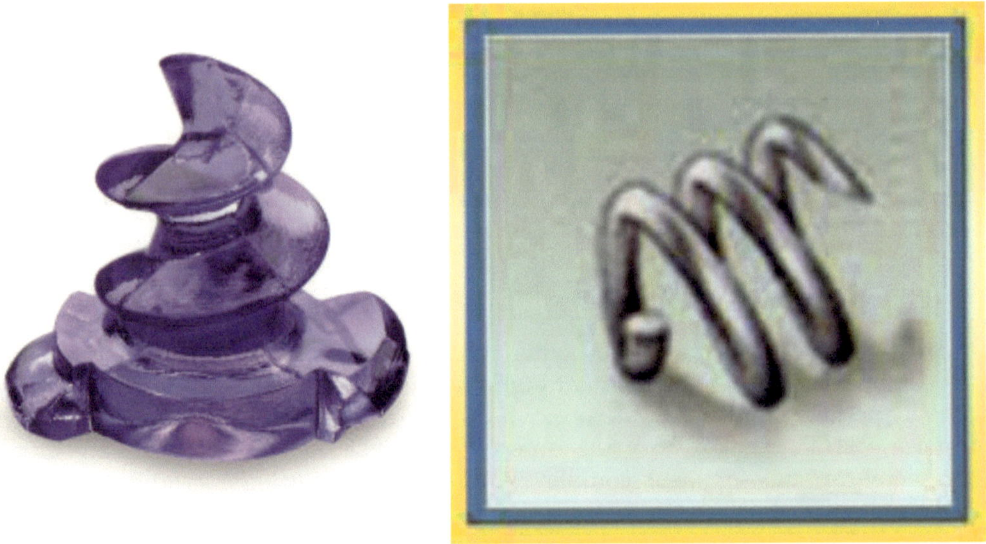

Fig. 3a. [Left] A copolymer delayed absorbable tack [Absorbatack, Covidien, Mansfield, USA] for fixation of polypropylene mesh to the anterior and posterior vaginal walls. [Right] A 5-millimeter titanium tack [Protack, Covidien, Mansfield, USA] for sacral fixation of the polypropylene mesh to the anterior and posterior vaginal walls and/or for the application of a rectus fascia/muscle graft for brisk sacral pelvic plexus venous bleeding.

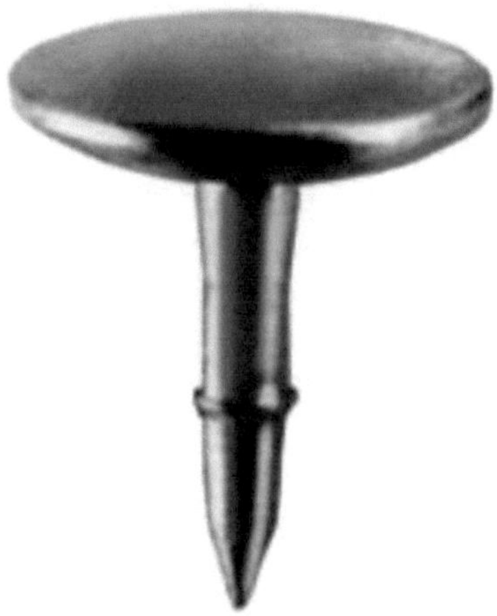

Fig. 3b. A Sterile thumbtack for presacral vascular occlusion

These methods are successful with achieving containment of blood loss in addition to direct closure of the plexus vessel injury. Another important aspect of this procedure is the securing of the double or single Y mesh to the sacrum. The author prefers to perform a suturing or tack fixation of both or singular Y meshes by loosely fixating each mesh to the sacral anterior longitudinal ligament at the S_2 -S_3 level [Marinkovic, 2008]. There is an increased injury risk to pelvic plexus blood vessels but attaining a normal vaginal axis is important to prevent the pelvic floor hyperextension which occurs with sacral promontory fixation and potentially increasing the occurrence of iatrogenic enteroceles and/or rectoceles post-operatively. Surgeon comfort level operating in the presacral space is most important and occurs only through mentorship and experience. Additional manners of fixation have been well described including permanent, delayed absorbable suture, bone anchors or similar absorbable and non-absorbable tacks.

The author recommends a bowel preparation with each patient. This should be initiated the day before and continued with a clear liquid diet and nothing by mouth after midnight the night before surgery. This may enhance landmark anatomical details by debulking the stool content of the sigmoid colon while allowing the surgery to carry on with less circumventing effort. Should an enterotomy occur, mesh must not be utilized at this time [whether or not a bowel preparation has been performed or not] and a reoperation considered in three to six months time. In this short-term, there should be prophylactic antibiotic utilized and a methodical bowel rest with a return to oral intake with the initiation of bowel sounds and the development of flatus.

3. Preoperative assessment and indications for surgery

A detailed Pelvic Floor Distress Inventory questionnaire [Teleman 2011] can be utilized to accurately assess patient preoperative and postoperative symptom improvement or worsening over time. Clinical assessment should be multidimensional and performed with observation by the responsible surgeon and staff. The consultation initiates with a detailed history and physical examination. Assessment of prolapse can be performed in the left recumbent or lithotomy position although the former may provide a overall assessment for prolapse. The patient should be asked to serially and incrementally cough [or strain] with pronounced inspiration to its maximum capacity, and then hold for three seconds to better gauge the prolapse breadth and width. The author recommends the utilization of the International Continence Society Pelvic Organ Prolapse score [Persu, 2011] for all three compartments and ancillary points of pelvic floor interest. Using a graduated Q-tip with one-centimeter increments on its shaft assists in determining the pelvic organ prolapse score and can be performed ergonomically and in a comfortable setting for both the patient and physician. With indeterminate cases, the patient may be asked to stand and repeat serial, graduated coughs or Valsalva maneuvers while holding for three seconds at their deepest ebb to see the full prominence of the prolapse or stress incontinence episodes. Whether or not the bladder is prefilled, many times patients do not leak with their prolapse reduced in the lithotomy or left lateral recumbent position. Once standing, the patient's stress incontinence may be facilitated. With digitation, the idea is to reduce the prolapse without compressing the bladder neck to avoid closing the bladder neck and iatrogenically causing the recording of a false negative stress test evaluation. Your digit should carefully proceed to the apex of the vault without concomitant applied pressure to either the anterior or posterior vaginal walls. The latter can lead to a false negative enterocele determination. If there is still doubt, you can access with a physiological study to give a dynamic impression of the severity of prolapse and rectal symptoms by utilizing defecography [Steensma, 2007] with corequisite defecation pressure assessment [rectal manometry]. If the dynamic quality of the patient's symptoms is not apparent, we can also utilize Magnetic Resonance Imaging of the Abdomen and Pelvis with intravenous and rectal gadolinium contrast [Groenendijk 2009]. This study can also determine whether hydronephrosis is apparent in which case a pessary should be placed and renal function assessed. Additionally, to better determine preoperative bladder characteristics, multichannel urodynamics [Mueller, 2007] may also be performed with and without their prolapse reduced [with prolapse unreduced -to assess current condition and perhaps bladder urgency while with the prolapse reduced to assess the bladder's post-operative function] to accurately determine the urethral pressure profile and videourodynamics which may become useful with Stage Three or more prolapse of any one compartment.

The bladder has an associated potential for urethral kinking and/or urethral obstruction from urethral hypermobility, cystocele, rectocele/enterocele or prolapsed uterus. In the latter, contrast can be placed into the apex of the vault or into the rectum simultaneously to access the pelvic floor rectal dynamics and with the fluoroscopy arm positioned laterally or in the anterior/posterior position.

Indications for surgery are controversial and are not clearly defined and keen individual patient assessment is important. A useful guide is symptomatic Stage Two or more prolapse patients and potentially all asymptomatic Stage Three or more prolapsed compartments may be successfully managed with the sacrocolpopexy approach. Patients always need to be reminded that pelvic organ prolapse is a systemic disease with a multitude of causative factors including pelvic floor collagen and elastin processing inequities and with several analogous determinant causes, so no surgery can ever be expected to be a one hundred percent symptom remedy.

- **Classification of Synthetic Meshes (Amid, 1997)**
- **Type 1: Totally macroporous**
  - **Pore size > 75μ**
    - **PROLENE**
    - **GYNEMESH PS**
    - **GYNECARE TVT**
    - **SPARC**
- **Type 2: Totally microporous**
  - **Pore size < 10μ**
    - **GORETEX**
- **Type 3: Macroporous with multifilaments or microporous component**
    - **IVS**
    - **URATAPE**
    - **SURGIPRO**
    - **MERSILENE**
    - **PARIETEX**
- **Type 4: Submicronic pore size**
  - **Pore size < 1μ**

Table 1. Types of Synthetic materials

4. Types of synthetic materials for prolapse support and potential infections

There are four types of material utilized for pelvic organ prolapse surgery, each varying in their potential contributions to pelvic floor reconstructive surgery. Dr. Amid [Amid, 1997] initiated the classification of synthetic materials for inguinal and abdominal herniorrhaphys in 1997 and system is still in use to better understand macroporous and microporous operative mesh characteristics.

Type 1 macroporous synthetic materials [Ostergard, 2010] have a pore size greater than 75 microns allowing white blood cells [diameter of 7-20 microns] to penetrate through and fight infection and their leukotriene by-products. They also allow for substantial collagen and elastin ingrowth allowing the material to act as supportive platform. Type 2 (microporous mesh) materials have a much smaller pore size diameter of less than 10 microns making it improbable for larger white blood cells to penetrate the material's interstices to combat an infection and its harmful by-products. Collagen and elastin ingrowth may also be impeded. Type 3 mesh materials demonstrate a combination of both Type 1 and Type 2 material properties and because of the type 2 microporous elements the host defenses against infection can be compromised making treatment more difficult and likely less successful with mesh infections. Type 2, 3 and 4 with their submicroporous may make their molecular properties a concern by potentially impairing the host defense mechanisms. Understanding these basic principles is important because mesh infections with Types 2, 3, and 4 materials may necessitate a shorter tolerance with signs and symptoms of mesh infections in lieu of surgery to remove the entire mesh system. Although all four types of mesh have been utilized in sacrocolpopexy, it appears that Type 1 Polypropylene in particular has a manageable incidence of infection. Once the decision to remove an infected piece of mesh has been made the entire material contents. [**Finding the original operative report or speaking to the original surgeon is paramount to practicing**

meticulous surgical care]. If a Type 1 mesh infection is suspected, treatment with antibiotics can be pursued and the patient's improvement monitored. Once the mesh has been removed we should wait at least three to six months prior to placement of another synthetic material. The most common bacteria [Falagas, 2004] encountered in both my literature search and Female Reconstructive Surgery practice have been Staphylococcus, Streptococcus subtypes, and Pseudomonas. Treatment should be initiated with a third generation cephalosporin and aminoglycoside. Consideration for not using a third generation penicillin or cephalosporin because of a penicillin allergy may be successfully treated by the substitution of Vancomycin with the continuation of an aminoglycoside. It is equally pertinent to closely monitor aminoglycode peaks and trough levels unless a single aminoglycoside QD dosing regimen is implemented, serial white counts with differential analysis, while blood and infection site cultures with sensitivities are necessary. If the infection is not improving, remember to consider performing a flexible cystoscopy and/or anoscopy to establish whether mesh organ erosion into the bladder or rectum has occurred. If the latter is evident, a consultation with a general or colorectal surgeon is recommended.

5. Description of the open surgical approach and complications

To decrease the intrusion of the sigmoid colon contents into the operative field, a bowel preparation with polyethylene glycol-electrolyte solution [Golytely, Braintree laboratories, Braintree, MA 02185, USA] one gallon administered with a clear liquid diet the day before surgery with nothing by mouth after midnight the night before surgery. Bowel preparations with antibiotics have been utilized including a Nichols bowel preparation [Nichols, 1973] with oral neomycin and erythromycin, but these are not encouraged, recommended or, necessary. Intravenous antibiotics are administered in preoperative holding one hour prior to the incision continued for a minimum of twenty-four hours postoperatively. Afterwards the patient is switched to an oral quinolone like Ciprofloxin 500 mg po twice daily, then sent home on the same for an additional ten days. The patient is placed in modified lithotomy position in Allen stirrups. Ample space is created between the patient's legs because an assistant is soon needed once the peritoneum is opened to place within the vagina a large bore disposable number 25 EEA sizer [Autosuture, Covidien, Mansfield, MA, USA]. The EEA sizer helps to define the edges of the vaginal vault, bladder and perineal body facilitating future suture or absorbable tack placement. A Bookwalter retractor will be needed for abdominal compartmentalization of the small and large bowels. The abdominal incision is approached with either a eight to ten-centimeter Phannenstiel incision or a subumbilical vertical incision. The rectus fascia is incised and the superior and inferior rectus fascial flaps are created so their closure is easily performed with one-two centimeters rectal fascial bites. The midline is found with the Metzenbaum scissors by gently opening the Metzenbaum and placing your dominant finger through the incision until the opening in the peritoneum is palpated and subsequently extended both superiorly and inferiorly. Care needs to be taken and this point in time to minimize the opportunity for the creation of an enterotomy or more likely, a cystotomy. An enterotomy should be closed with running 3-0 monofilament suture then Lembertized over the top of the closure with the same type suture this approach is also repeated for cystotomies. The Bookwalter retractor [Codman, Johnson and Johnson, Raynham, MA 02767] is placed for retraction of the sigmoid colon to the patient's left side [closest to the lead surgeon] and with a Kelly retractor blade (two inch by six inch) attached to the Bookwalter with a bowel facing wet lap. The midline abdominal contents are held with a Balfour retractor blade. Each Bookwalter blade should be set to use with a bowel facing wet lap to protect the bowel and surrounding blood vessels from iatrogenic injury. A bladder blade is placed on the circular ring (an oval ring for the Bookwalter is utilized for patients with Body Mass Index greater than thirty-five while a two-part circular ring is used for patients with a Body Mass Index less than thirty-four) to retract the bladder caudally and away from the vault and bladder clearly exposing the commonly atretic and weak anterior vaginal wall **[Figure 4].** We first approach the placement of the large disposable EEA sizer one inch into the vagina to clearly demarcate the perineal body and distal posterior vaginal wall. We carefully use a Finochetti needle driver with 0 Delayed absorbable [PDS, polydioxanone, Ethicon, Somerset, New Jersey, USA] suture or 0 monofilament permanent suture Polypropylene [Ethicon, Somerville, New Jersey, USA]. The suture is placed once through the right and another suture through the left sides of the perineal body without removing the suture's needle. A hemostat is placed over the needle and the hemostat placed on the outer edge of the Bookwalter retractor. Next, we place the same on the right and left sides up the posterior vaginal every two or three centimeters towards the vault usually for a total of six to eight sutures [two columns of three or four sutures]. Then the posterior mesh consisting of a two inch by twelve inch narrow strip of pre-fabricated and pre-cut Polypropylene mesh [Ethicon, Somerset, New Jersey, USA] has the eight sutures carefully threaded through the top of the mesh and tied on the meshes undersurface [the side facing the bowel]. The authors' concerns for placing the Polyprophylene mesh against the posterior vaginal wall from the onset include that our bite of the posterior vaginal wall may become too compromised and may be too superficial or conversely too deep into the vaginal wall and epithelium. Be mindful that the mesh is

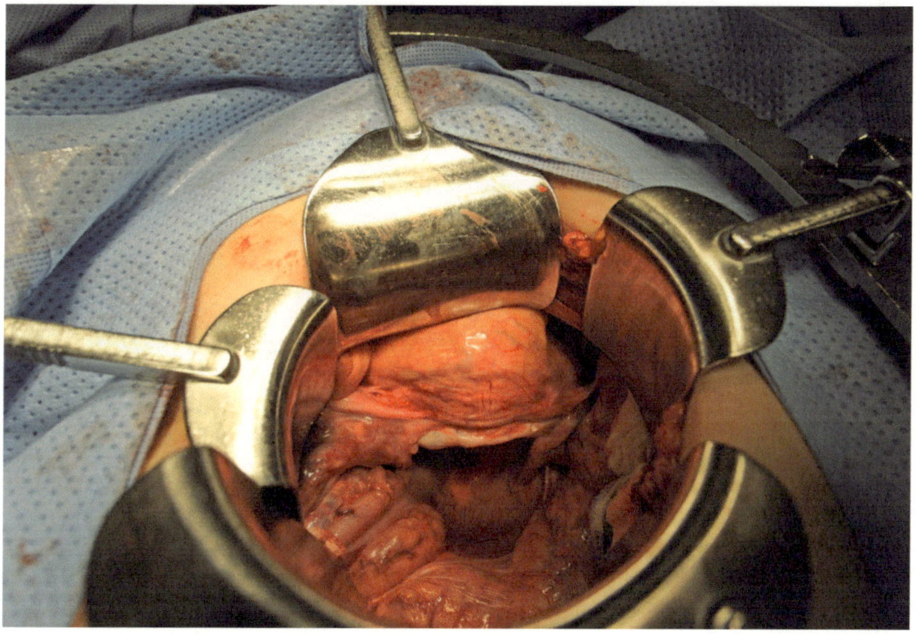

Fig. 4. The Bookwalter retractor has been placed giving us a clear view of the bladder, vault, anterior and posterior vaginal walls.

also difficult to place a suture through with good control of its depth. This may lead to poor suture fixation and potentially the patient may develop attenuated mesh fixated areas that later succumb to detachment from either vaginal wall and sacral anterior longitudinal ligament. To optimize your suture placement, attempt to get a full bite through the bulk of the vaginal wall first, while not including the epithelium of the vagina. Remember the anterior vaginal wall more commonly attenuated than the posterior vaginal wall and likely more readily pierced through to the vaginal epithelium and may become only apparent with a careful well lit examination during surgery or with colposcopy. Mentally attempt to proceed within two or three millimeters of the vaginal epithelium to prevent a potential suture and/or mesh exposure and accompanying dyspareunia. When starting these cases, performing a concomitant colposcopy with a digital video tower will allow you to see and palpate each individual suture placement to avoid piercing the vaginal epithelium. With gained experience, colposcopy can wait until both meshes have been placed vaginally. Once each suture throw is placed through the mesh, remember that for the posterior mesh, the knots of the suture will be tied onto the bowel facing side of the mesh [side directly facing and juxtaposed to the bowel) as in **[Figure 5].**

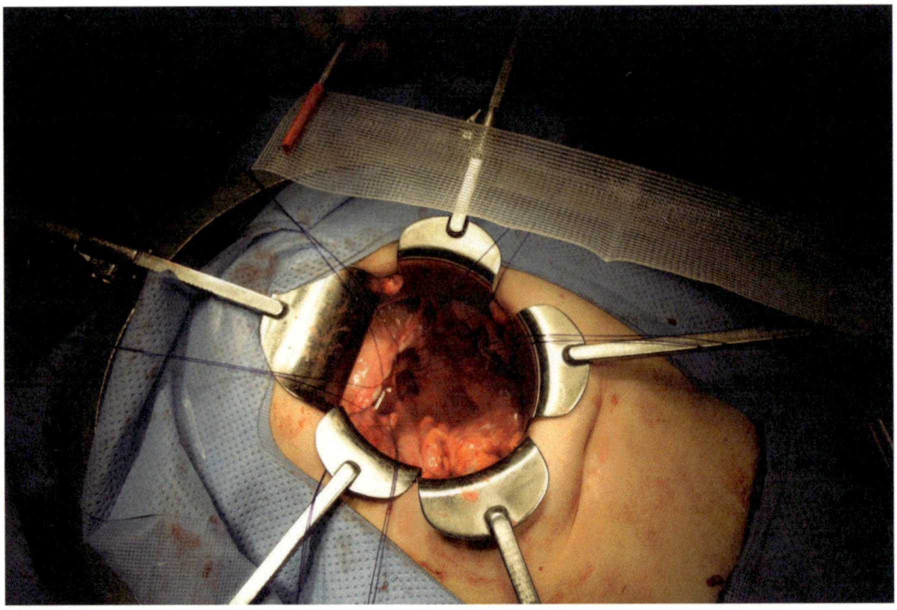

Fig. 5. Represents when the sutures are placed through the posterior vaginal wall and now the sutures are passed from the top of the mesh so the knots are tied on its underside.

Once the sutures have been placed through the mesh in right and left columns, they can be tied from the bottom to the top. If tied from top to bottom, the sutures at the bottom will be more difficult to tie and the mesh will move from one side to the other from the midline. The resulting mesh may not be placed straight but angled to the right or left side instead of straight towards the sacrum.

Starting with the perineal body [**Figure 6**] towards the vault is the most ergonomic approach still allowing the surgeon the opportunity to adjust the mesh from side to side as they proceed to maximize a straight and horizontal plane. This same principle can be applied to the anterior mesh.

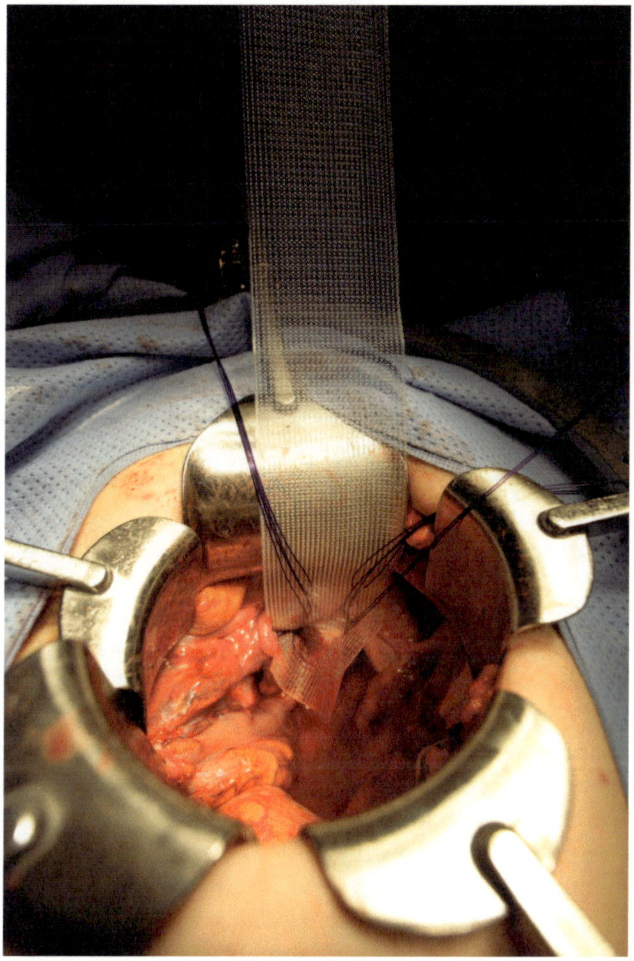

Fig. 6. The perineal body has its two sutures [one right and left sided] and are strung through the mesh and tied. Usually this is not done until all sutures are placed through the posterior vaginal wall then strung through the mesh and tied on the bowel facing side of the Polypropylene mesh.

The anterior mesh is placed on the apical anterior vaginal wall. To better gauge the cephalic aspect of the bladder and prevent cystotomy, the bladder can be filled with two hundred milliliters of indigo carmine. If a cystotomy is made, the dye will venture out and delineate the area in need of closure. Once the surgeon is experienced with mobilization of the bladder off the anterior vaginal wall, the author still recommends that the bladder be filled and carefully checked for cystotomies after mobilization is completed. The best time to correct cystotomies is during the case and not post-operatively. We recommend for closure of a cystotomy 2-0 Polyglactin 910 or similar monofilament absorbable suture with the deep layer being a continuous running closure then the more superficial layer with the same Polyglactin 910 suture in a Lembert interrupted fashion. With a cystotomy, the patient should have a 16 F Foley catheter left in place for ten days and a voiding cystourethrogram performed. If there is no leakage, the Foley can be discontinued. If there is still some leakage, leave the Foley in for an additional ten days and repeat the voiding cystourethrogram. Once the case is almost completed and closure initiated, it is recommended to perform a colposcopy with video guidance to ascertain whether there is any vaginal enterotomy or suture/tack penetrating through the vaginal epithelium. If penetration occurs-the suture or tack should be removed and carefully replaced.

Once both meshes have been sutured to both the anterior and posterior vaginal walls, we need to open the sacral peritoneum from the sacral promontory (palpable by hand and three centimeters below the aortic bifurcation) with the electrocautery set at fifteen watts. Cut and coagulate [blend] to minimize potential radiating heat injury to the underlying blood vessels and ureters. The right ureter is also important to visualize and/or palpate to ascertain its pelvic course. [The right or left ureter is most commonly injured with suture when closing both sacral peritoneal flaps during the retroperitonealizing of both meshes to prevent bowel adherence and obstruction. This is ascertained when there is no flow out the right ureter with a cystoscopic examination. Usually untying and removing the multiple interrupted retroperitonealizing sutures will safely restore flow to the affected ureter]. Once we are oriented, we carefully incise the peritoneum from the sacral promontory down to S_5. Then carefully and methodically cauterize the underlying tissue toward the right side of the sacrum. The normal vaginal axis for vault orientation is towards S_3. We must always be prepared for rapid venous bleeding when creating the right and left flaps for future retroperitonealizing of both meshes. If rapid bleeding occurs, take long-ring forceps with a sponge tip and apply pressure to the area while asking for three units of packed red blood cells to be held for potential infusion. Long DeBakey forceps are used to hold the bleeding vessel and the electrocautery should be increased to thirty watts. Apply significant electrocautery at least twice before abandoning cautery. The next means can be suture ligation with 4-0 double-edged polypropylene or the author's two favorite alternatives, which may also be quicker and more secure from the beginning. First, a sterile ten-millimeter wide and seven millimeter deep thumbtack can be applied directly into the bleeder or a two inch by three inch rectus fascial graft [preferably not a flap although either can be utilized] is taken from the abdominal incision with its accompanying rectal muscle. Apply the muscle side onto the bleeder first and apply pressure and suture the rectus fascia to the underlying tissue. Any of these four methods should successfully manage rapid bleeding. Another useful alternative is to apply packing with a later return to the operating room and/or to request a radiology vessel embolization.

Alternative methods for mesh attachments to the sacral anterior longitudinal ligament include titanium tacks [**Figure 10**][Tan-Kim, 2011]. With either method, the mesh needs to be secured loosely to the longitudinal ligament to prevent detachment, since the mesh may contract ten to twenty percent along its longitudinal length over time. After both meshes

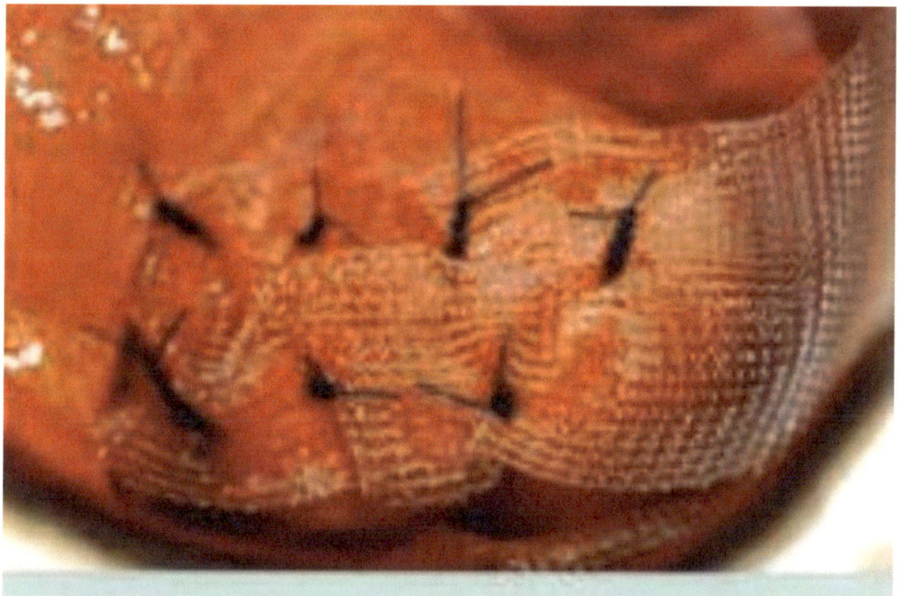

Fig. 7. The bladder has been mobilized two centimeters off the apical vault and the same size polypropylene mesh applied to the anterior vaginal wall with only two columns [right and left] of four sutures for a total of eight sutures on the anterior mesh. In this figure the eighth left top suture has not been placed.

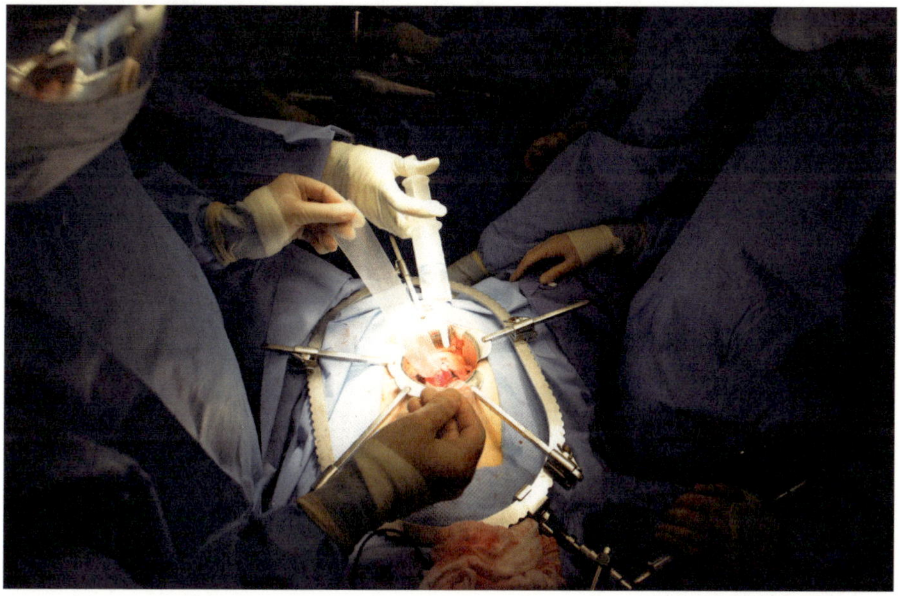

Fig. 8. Both the anterior and posterior meshes have been applied with suture and the sacral peritoneum overlying the sacrum needs to be incised with cautery to allow access to the sacral anterior longitudinal ligament for the anchoring of both meshes.

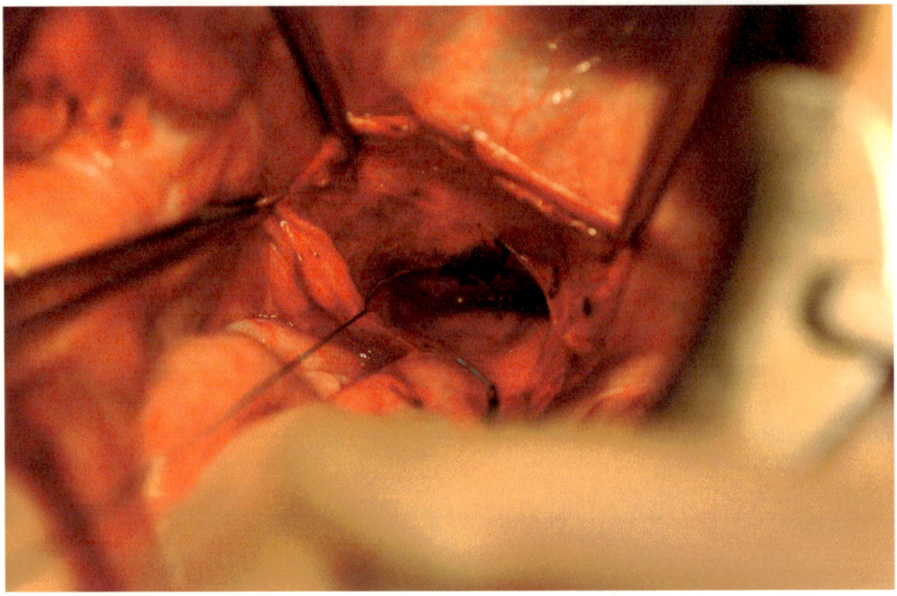

Fig. 9. Both meshes can be anchored to the sacral anterior longitudinal ligament with 0 permanent suture.

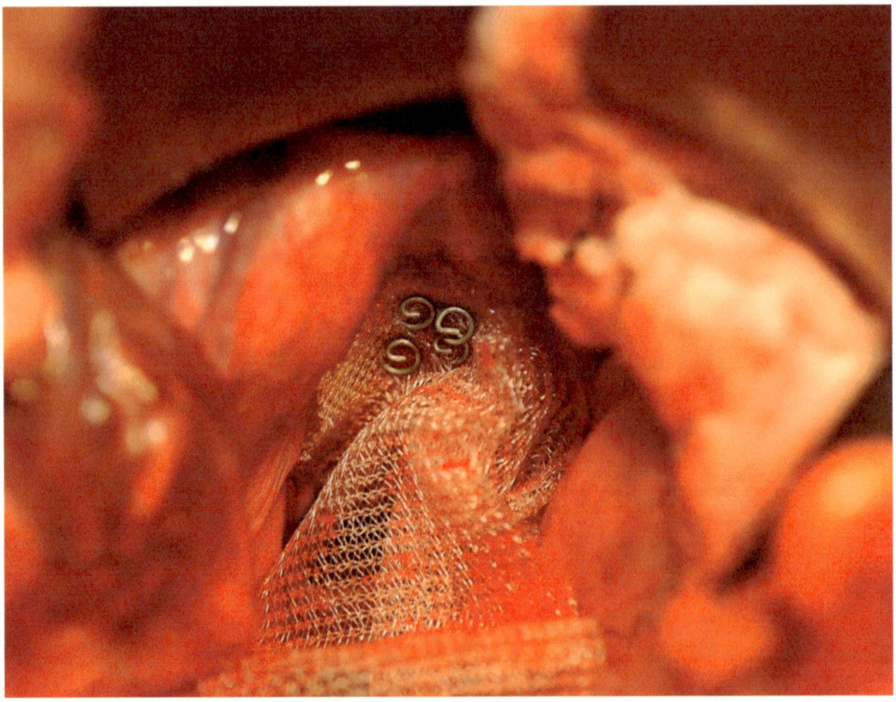

Fig. 10. One alternative sacral fixation method is the use of titanium tacks. Both polypropylene meshes here have been anchored by a series of rectangular oriented titanium tacks [**Figure 3a**].

have been successfully anchored to the sacrum, we must digitally feel some looseness or bend in the middle to prevent detachment or severing of the polypropylene monofilament mesh.

To complete the sacrocolpopexy, close the sacrum peritoneum while retroperitonealizing both meshes [Figure 11 & 12]. Take the serosa and muscularis of the bladder's most cephalad aspect and attach it to the beginning of your sacral peritoneal incision or directly to the most cephalic aspect of either mesh so the entire length of the either mesh is not exposed to the surrounding small or large bowel for potential obstructive bowel complications. Once closed, the rectus muscle is re-approximated in the midline with running polyglactin 910 suture and the rectus fascia with 0 loop Polydioxanone suture. The subcutaneous area is irrigated to prevent a seroma and both sides are re-approximated with interrupted polyglactin 910. The skin may be closed with interrupted subcuticular 4-0 chromic sutures followed by a Tegaderm transparent 8″x 2″ dressing. Staples may be used in obese patients

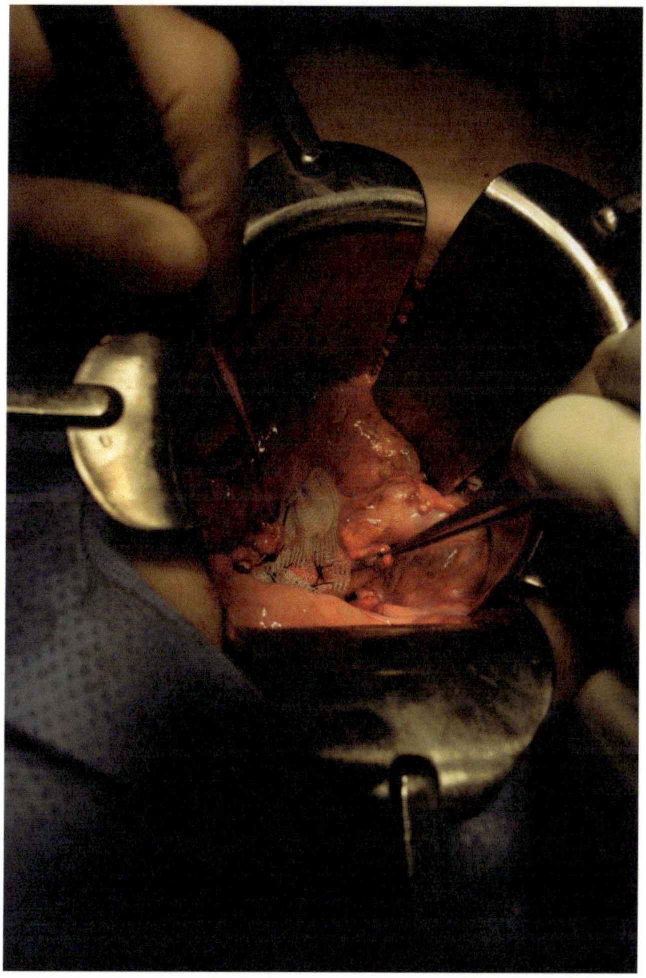

Fig. 11. Both meshes have been secured to the sacral anterior ligament and now the sacral peritoneum flaps are re-approximated.

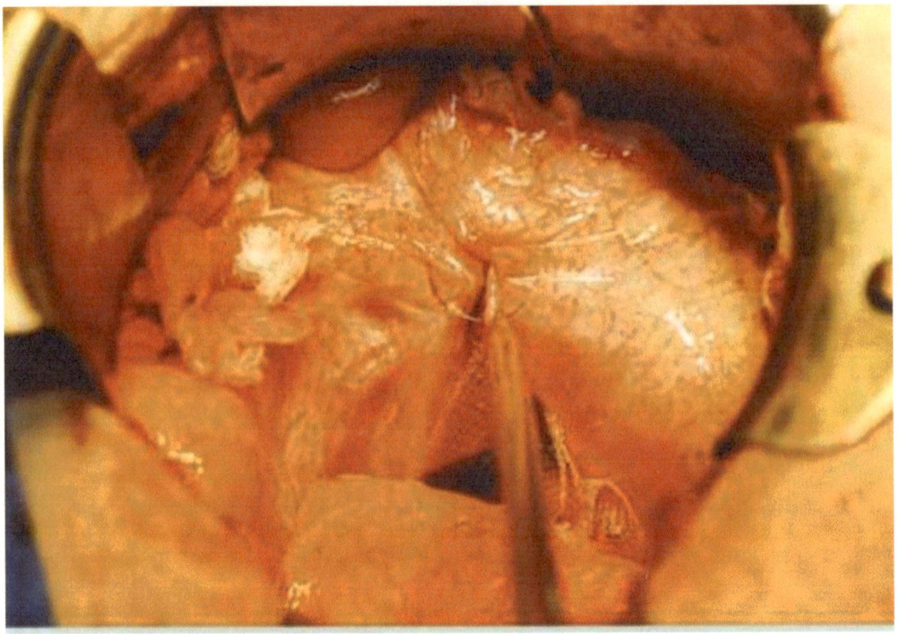

Fig. 12. Both meshes have been closed over their top by the sacral peritoneum. If there is not enough peritoneum to cover both meshes you can use the serosa of the cephalic part of the bladder and suture directly to the sacral peritoneum or to the most cephalic section of visible mesh.

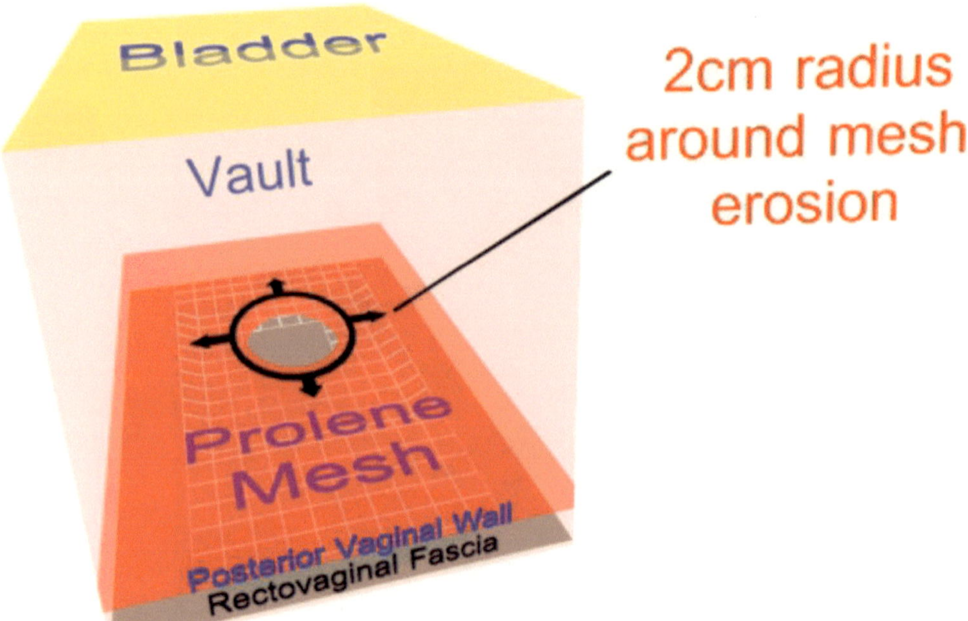

Fig. 13. An illustration of a macroporous mesh exposure through the posterior vaginal wall.

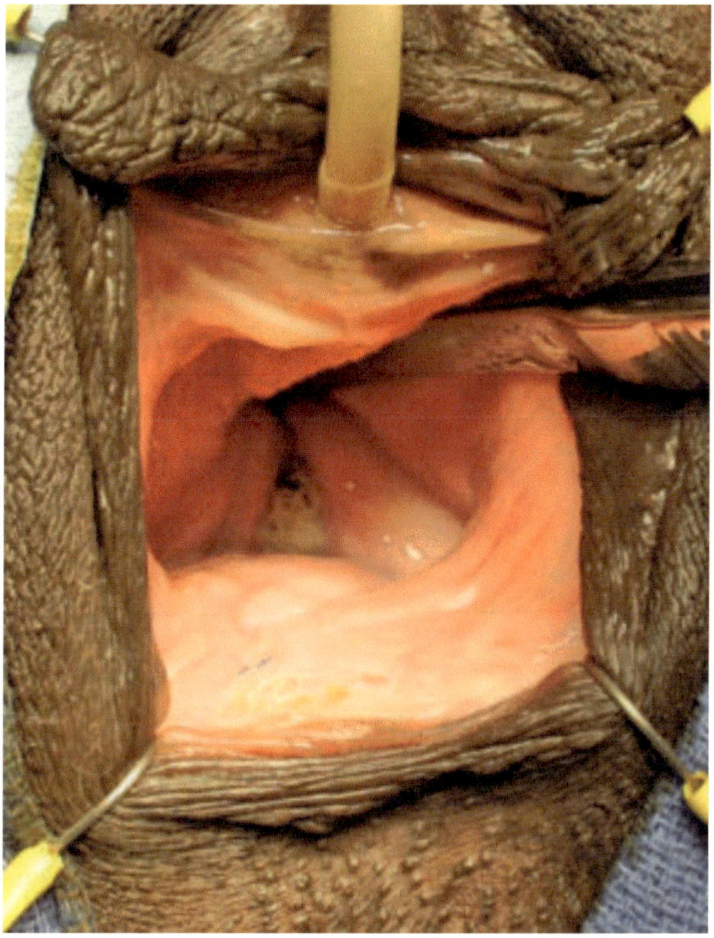

Fig. 14. A Mersilene mesh exposure through the posterior vaginal wall at the perineal body and posteriorly at the vaginal vault.

or those with frail skin. Retention sutures for those at risk by history for fascial dehiscence can also be considered. The usefulness of transparent dressing is the ability and ease of checking the incision by all heath care professionals at all times without having to consistently traumatize the patients with the reapplication and removal of bandages.

6. Mesh exposure management

Mesh exposure is an important complication. Rates may range from zero to twenty percent [Skala, 2011] in the first two post-operative years. It can occur with the patient complaining of a rough and painful vaginal area, a draining sinus, or without any symptoms. This is why when mesh is utilized, we need to periodically follow up with the patient. My recommended conservative follow-up course is 6 weeks, 3 months, 6 months, 12 months, 24 months, and 36 months, then as needed thereafter. When examining the patient, the lithotomy position is the standard by which all other examination position's are compared. But always entertain utilizing the left recumbent position which is also very helpful to examine the vaginal walls. If

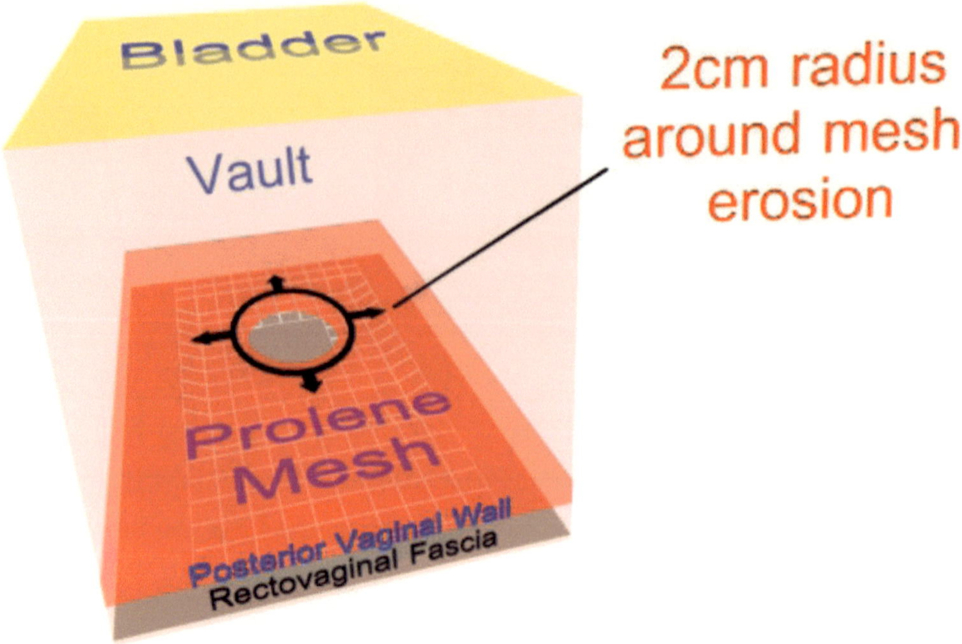

Fig. 15. The first step in this repair is to grasp the mesh with an Alice clamp and circumscribe a two-centimeter perimeter around the mesh exposure. Then excise the protruding mesh with the Metsenbaum scissors. The right and left edges should be undermined with scissors for an additional one to two centimeter's circumferentially then closed with a tension free approach utilizing a deep running layer with 3-0 Polyglactin 910. Followed by a superficial Lembertizing layer with interrupted monofilament.

readily available, colposcopy is also a useful office procedure to ascertain early supple and pre-exposure development or signs of mesh infection that may be missed on a standard physical examination. I recommend that all post sacrocolpopexy patients have a colposcopy at least once post-operatively and as needed thereafter. When an exposure has surfaced during your examination some aspects are important to note and guide your treatment. If the exposure size when measured with a malleable ruler or a graduated Q-tip is less than one centimeter or involves two or less areas of this size, it may be amenable to apply estrogen cream for six weeks and then schedule a follow-up re-examination. If it has not been re-epithelized, consideration for outpatient surgery should be entertained. If exposures are more than one centimeter and/or are located in two or more analogous locations this correction should be performed in the operating room. Two or more areas of concern may foreshadow a seriously thin operative flap problem, erosion, or infection.

Repairs need to be performed with a two centimeter, circumferential, mesh mobilization and excision followed by in a deep continuous closure followed by a superficial interrupted Lembertizing layer closure with 3-0 polyglactin 910. A Lembert closure approach embodies an incisional closure initiating with a deep continuous closure followed by a superficial interrupted closure of the same incision. For the latter, the surgeon starts at the beginning of the incision and goes through the area five millimeters lateral to the right and left sides of the incision and buries the original incision within this superficial interrupted suture line. This approach affords the closure with a good-healing tissue process.

The important point is to make the closure tension free and if the incision is close to the introitus to cut your sutures long to prevent the patient feeling a sticking sensation from the tips of the short suture when they are sitting. New monofilament antibacterial-coated [poliglecaprone 25 plus] suture is available that may add infection assistance with these closures.

7. Conclusion

Sacrocolpopexy is an effective option for the correction of advanced pelvic organ prolapse and can be performed in either one of three manners including open, laparoscopy and robot-assisted approaches. Its major advantage is that it has a greater than ten-year success rate and a fifty year history of experience in the control of pelvic organ prolapse. Sacrocolpopexy may be more enduring than a vaginal approach and for the sexually active patient provides the longest possible vaginal length. Currently many of the common complications are amenable to medical or surgical therapy usually as an outpatient visit or same-day surgery.

8. References

Ameline A, Huguier J. La suspension posterieure aux disques lombo-sacres: technique de remplacement des ligaments utero-sacres par voie abdominale. J Gynecol Obstet Biol Reprod 1957; 56:94-99.

Amid, PK. Classification of biomaterials and their related complications in abdominal wall hernia surgery. Hernia 1997 1:15-21.

Connell, KA. Elastogenesis in the vaginal wall and pelvic organ prolapse. N Engl J Med 2011 Jun16; 364(24): 2356-2358.

Delancey JO. Anatomic aspects of vaginal eversion after hysterectomy. Am J. Obstet Gynecol 1992 Jun; 166:1717-1724.

Falagas ME, Kasiakou SK. Mesh-related infections after hernia repair surgery. Clin Microbiol Infect 2005; 11:3-8.

Gilleran JP, Johnson M, Hundley A. Robotic-assisted laparoscopic mesh sacrocolpopexy. Ther Adv Urol 2010; 2(5): 195-208.

Groenendijk AG, Birnie E, de Blok S, Adriaanse AH, Ankum WM, Roovers JP, Bonsel GJ. Clinical decision taking in primary pelvic organ prolapse; the effects of diagnostic tests on treatment selection in comparison with a consensus meeting. Int Urogynecol J Pelvic Floor Dysfunct 2009 Jun; 20(6): 711-719.

Lane, F.E. Repair of post hysterectomy vaginal vault prolapse. *Obstet Gynecol*(1962) 20: 72–77.

Lewis CM, Culligan P. Sacrohysteropexy followed by successful pregnancy and eventual reoperation for prolapse. Int Urogynecol J 2011; PMID 22179338.

Maher C, Feiner B, Baessler K, Adams EJ, Hagen S, Glazener CM. Surgical management of pelvic organ prolapse in women. Cochrane Database Syst Rev 2010 Apr 14;(4): CD004014.

Marinkovic SP. Will hysterectomy at the time of sacrocolpopexy increase the rate of polypropylene mesh erosion? Int Urogynecol J Pelvic Floor Dysfunction 2008 Feb; 19(2): 199-203.

Mainkovic SP, Stanton SL. Incontinence and voiding difficulties associated with prolapse. J Urol 2004 Mar; 171(3): 1021-1028.

Mueller ER, Kenton K, Mahajan S, FitzGerald MP, Brubaker L. Urodynamic prolapse reduction alters urethral pressure but not filling or pressure flow parameters. J Urol 2007 Feb; 177(2): 600-603.

Nichols RL, Broido P, Condon RE, Gorbach SL, Nyhus LM. Effect of preoperative neomycin-erythromycin intestinal preparation on the incidence of infectious complications following colon surgery. Ann Surg 1973 October; 178(4): 453-462.

Nivatvongs S, Fang DT. The use of thumbtacks to stop massive presacral hemorrhage. Dis Colon Rectum 1986; 29(9): 589-590.

Olsen AL, Smith VJ, Bergstrom JO, et al. Epidemiology of surgically managed pelvic organ prolapse and urinary incontinence. *Obstet Gynecol.* 1997; 89(4): 501–506. doi: 10.1016/S0029-7844 (97) 00058-6.

Ostergard DR. Vaginal mesh grafts and the food and drug administration. Int Urogynecol J pelvic Floor Dysfunction 2010 October; 21(10): 1181-1183.

Persu C, Chapple CR, Cauni V, Gutue S, Geavlete P. Pelvic organ prolapse quantification system (POP-Q)- a new era in pelvic prolapse staging. J Med Life 2011 Jan-Mar; 4(1): 75-81.

Remzi, FH, Oncel M, Fazio VW. Muscle tamponade to control presacral venous bleeding: report of two cases. Dis Colon Rectum 2002; 45(8): 1109-1111.

Scali P, Blondon J, Bethoux A, Gerard M. Les operations de soutenement suspension par voie haute dans le traitement des prolapsus vaginaux. *J Gynecol Obstet Biol Reprod.* 1974; 3:365–378.

Shiozawa T, Huebner M, Hirt B, Wallwiener D, Reisenauer C. Nerve-preserving sacrocolpopexy: anatomical study and surgical approach. Eur J Obstst Gynecol Reprod Biol 2010 Sep; 152(1): 103-107.

Skala C, Renezeder K, Albrich S, Puhl A, Laterza RM, Naumann G, Koelbl H. The IUGA/ICS classification of complications of prosthesis and graft insertion: a comparative experience in incontinence and prolapse surgery. Int Urogynecol 2011 PMID 21789657.

Steensma AB, Oom DMJ, Burger CW, Schouten WR. Comparison of defecography and 3D/4D translabial ultrasound in patients with pelvic organ prolapse and/or evacuation disorders. Ultrasound in Ob/Gynecol 2007; 30:447.

Subak LL, Waetjen LE, Eeden S, et al. Cost of pelvic organ prolapse surgery in the United States.*Obstet Gynecol.* 2001; 98:646–651. Doi: 10.1016/S0029-7844 (01) 01472-7.

Tan-Kim J, Menefee SA, Luber KM, Nager CW, Lukacz ES. Prevalence and risk factors for mesh erosion after laparascopic –assisted sacrocolpopexy. Int Urogynecol J Pelvic Floor Dysfunct 2011 Feb; 22(2): 205-212.

Teleman P, Stenzelius K, Lorizzo L, Jakobsson U. Validation of the Swedish short forms of the pelvic floor impact questionnaire (PFIQ-7), pelvic floor distress inventory (PFDI-20) and pelvic organ prolapse/urinary incontinence sexual questionnaire (PISQ-12). Acta Obstetricia et Gynecologica Scan 2011; 90(5): 483-487.

20

Urinary Tract Injuries in Low-Resource Settings

Mathias Onsrud
Oslo University Hospital, Norway

1. Introduction

The purpose of this chapter is to elucidate some serious complications of hysterectomy when performed in low-resource countries. The main target is doctors intending to work under such conditions.

Urinary tract injuries are encountered in high-resource settings as well as in low-resource settings but comparative incidence data are lacking. Particular for low resource countries is the difficult situation under which the causative intervention was performed. Table 1 enumerates some general factors that can influence the risk of surgery. All of these factors may be present at the same time in the same place. Bleeding complications and postoperative infections are frequent. Conditions like HIV, tuberculosis and female genital schistosomiasis may intervene. A high prevalence of cervical cancer must be remembered. Factors relevant for the hysterectomy procedure in particular are: General anesthesia with muscle relaxation is seldom available; operations must be done in spinal anesthesia normally. Suitable instruments and equipment like suction and diathermia are often lacking. Minimal invasive procedures (laparoscopy, endoscopy) are seldom available.

Patient's nutritional status and co-morbidity
Disease stage and duration
Preoperative diagnosis and patient preparation
Laboratory facilities
Blood supply and antibiotics
Anesthesia
Surgeon's training and supervision
Instruments available
Postoperative service
Follow-up

Table 1. Factors influencing the operative risk in low-resource settings

2. Types of urinary tract injuries

Two main types of urinary tract injuries are encountered after hysterectomy: 1) bladder damage, with vesicovaginal fistula as the ultimate manifestation, and 2) ureteric damage, ranging from crushing to the most severe sequel, ureterovaginal fistulas. Probably, a large part of ureteric occlusions with hydronephrosis/renal damage pass undetected due to lack of awareness and diagnostic means.

1. Bladder damage

Incidental cystotomy most often occur during deliberation of the bladder from the uterus. Abnormal anatomy due to large uterine size and adhesions after pelvic inflammatory disease or cesarean sections can make dissection difficult. For benign hysterectomies, a 2.5% incidence of incidental cystotomies (34 of 1317 operations) has been reported (1) with a subsequent development of vesicovaginal fistula in 11.7% (4 out of 34 injuries). The main risk factor for this sequel is the extent of the injury, but large uterus, heavy blood loss and tobacco use may also be of importance (2).

2. Ureteric damage

For major gynecologic surgery, an average incidence of ureteric injuries of about 0.4% has been reported - 19 out of 4665 procedures (3). Data from low-resource countries are lacking, but the incidence is presumably higher there. Injuries are associated with both abdominal and vaginal hysterectomy, simple abdominal hysterectomy being most common. Operations on residual adnexae are at particular risk, as are those with large myomas, especially if located in the cervical part of uterus (4). The right ureter and the left ureter are equally affected. A common site of injury is near the pelvic brim, dorsal to the infundibulopelvic ligament. Injuries in the parametrial area are located at 1) the site where ureter crosses under the uterine artery, 2) in the tunnel towards the bladder ("tunnel of Wertheim"), or 3) in the intramural part of the bladder. These injuries are more difficult to detect and to handle. Lesions on the lateral pelvic sidewall are less frequent.

The severity of damage ranges from crushing, through ligation, transection, angulation to resection and fistula formation as late sequel (Table 2). Ischemic damage can appear if the ureter is dissected free from its adventitial sheath for several centimeters. It is remarkable though how well ureter can tolerate ischemia provided no postoperative radiation is added.

Crushing
Ligation
Angulation
Transection
Resection
Fistulation (late sequel)

Table 2. Types of operative ureteric injuries

3. Urogenital fistula

Urogenital fistula is the most important late sequel of an operative injury to the urinary tract. In developing countries the great majority of urogenital fistulas are obstetric ("the African fistula"). Long-standing, obstructed labor coupled with inadequate obstetric care is the main reason for this (5,6). In comparison, fistulas considered to be complications to hysterectomy are relatively few. In Nigeria, 96.5% of fistulas were related to delivery (7). This contrasts with the situation in developed countries where the majority of fistulas are due to pelvic surgery, malignancy and severe inflammatory conditions. A group of surgeons with experience both from Turkey and Niger found gynecologic surgery to be the main cause of fistula in the former country and obstetric complications in the latter (8). A change during the later decades from a mainly obstetric to a mainly iatrogenic etiology has been reported from some developing countries (9,10). The quality of obstetric care and surgical skills are important factors for this development.

3.1 Data from the Democratic Republic of Congo

Amongst 597 patients operated for urogenital fistulae at Panzi hospital from November 2005 till November 2007, 21 fistulas (3.5%) were related to a previous hysterectomy (11,12). Nine of these women (42.9%) had a ureterovaginal fistula compared to 27 out of 567 women (4.8%) in the obstructed labor group (OR 15, 95%CI 5.8-38.7) (Table 3). Twelve (57.1%) of the hysterectomy related fistulas were of the vesicovaginal type and located high up in the vagina, including one vesicocervical fistula after a subtotal hysterectomy. Vesicovaginal fistulas located in the lower part of vagina or involving urethra or its sphincter were not seen among the hysterectomy associated cases but were frequent in the obstructed labor group, 36.7% (208 of 567). None of the hysterectomy associated fistulas were surrounded by fibrosis or had a fistula size of more than 2 cm as compared to 64% with scar fibrosis and 34% with size more than 2 cm for those caused by obstructed labor. This indicates that the hysterectomy related fistulas had a "cleaner" origin.

Cause	All Fistulas		Type of urogenital fistula				
			VVF low	VVF high	VUF	UrVF	Combinations
	N	(%)	N	N	N	N	N
Obstructed labor	567	(95.0)	208	285	34	27	13
Hysterectomy							
Emergency peripartum	9	(1.5)		4	1*	4	
Abdominal, for benign gynecologic disease	9	(1.5)		5		4	
Vaginal, for benign gynecologic disease	3	(0.5)		2		1	
Sexual violence, infections	9	(1.5)	5	4			
Total	597	(100)	213	300	35	36	13
%			35.6	50.3	5.9	6.0	2.2

VVF vesicovaginal fistula, VUF vesicouterine fistula, UrVF ureterovaginal fistula
*vesicocervical fistula after subtotal hysterectomy

Table 3. Urogenital fistulas by cause and type. Panzi Hospital, Democratic Republic of Congo 2006-2007 (from ref.12)

Nine of the 21 postoperative fistulas (42.9%) appeared in women who had undergone an emergency peripartum hysterectomy. The indication for these hysterectomies is unknown. High median age (35 years) and the high median parity (8) make postpartum hemorrhage or poor uterine contractility probable, although uterine rupture cannot be excluded.

Nine women had undergone abdominal hysterectomy for uterine myomas and 3 had vaginal hysterectomy performed as part of an operation for pelvic organ prolapse. For these patients with a gynecologic reason for the hysterectomy, the median age was 40 years and median parity 5, as compared to 22 years and parity 1, respectively, for women with fistula caused by obstructed labor (Table 4).

Cause of fistula/type of operation	Median age (years)	Median parity
Obstructed labor - vaginal delivery (n=226)	22	1
Hysterectomy (n=21)		
Emergency, peripartum (n=9)	35	8
Abdominal or vaginal, non-obstetric indication (n=12)	40	5

Table 4. Median age and parity at time of fistula appearance by cause (derived from ref. 12)

3.2 Diagnosis

Vesicovaginal fistulas are normally visible high up in the vagina. Direct inspection for fistula is done after filling the bladder with diluted methylene blue. Dye will immediately be observed in the vagina or on a tampon left there ("tampon test"). Cystoscopy will confirm the fistula. Its localization in relation to the ureteric openings is of importance for planning of the operation. Sometimes, only sutures perforating the bladder mucosa or granulation tissue are observed.

Ureteric occlusion can be caused by inadvertent ligation giving ureteric stenosis and hydronephrosis. Symptomes can be flank pain or slow postoperative recovery only. This condition can pass undetected or be diagnosed late after permanent renal damage is induced. Sonography – an important diagnostic tool in low-resource countries - can be of great help. Intravenous pyelo-uretero-graphy and vesicography are available at some places whereas this is rarely the case for CT-scans and MRI.

Ureteric lacerations are generally detected early, about 50% of during operation and 50% during the first 2 weeks postoperatively. (3,4). Pain from uroplania or urine in the peritoneal cavity may appear, and sonography is then helpful. Urinary leakage through the vaginal top is more common. Creatinin measurement can be necessary to prove that the secretion really is urine. Dye inserted into the bladder will normally not leak to the vagina and cystoscopy is most often negative. Lack of urine secretion or intravenously infused dye from one of the ureteric openings is highly suggestive. Dye secretion to the vagina is confirmative. The ureterovaginal fistula is often not directly visible in the vagina.

3.3 Causative interventions and prevention

The types of hysterectomy covered in this chapter are those where urinary tract complications tend to occur most frequently: Emergency peripartum hysterectomy, abdominal hysterectomy and vaginal hysterectomy. Laparoscopic hysterectomy is seldom done under low-resource settings and will not be covered here.

1. Emergency peripartum hysterectomy

Injury to the urinary tract is a common complication to peripartum hysterectomy. The most important risk factors for emergency cesarean hysterectomy are reported to be: uterine rupture, postpartum hemorrhage, cervical tears, placenta accreta and placenta previa. Previous cesareans and multiparity (para >5) increase the risk by 6.9 and 3.4, respectively (13). The risk factors mentioned are all commonly encountered in developing countries.

Uterine rupture represents a serious health problem with high maternal and perinatal mortality. In the least developed countries, rates up to 1% have been reported (14). In developed countries, most cases are scar ruptures related to a previous cesarean section, whereas in Sub-Saharan Africa 75% are associated with an unscarred uterus (14). Here, the basis for rupture is mainly cephalopelvic disproportion. A typical scenario is that the first baby was delivered stillborn after a long-lasting, obstructed labor and the following pregnancy ends up with a uterine rupture. Other risk factors for rupture are abnormal presentations and multiparity (14). Populations with a high cesarean delivery rate - and thereby a high prevalence of scarred uterus - are at risk. The consequences for future pregnancies can be disastrous if these women are living in areas with poor access to emergency obstetric service. In areas with an increasing cesarean section rate, more uterine scar ruptures has been observed (15).

Obstructed labor is a common indication for cesarean section and few of the operations are planned. Cesarean delivery should protect against maternal mortality and morbidity and save the child. Nevertheless, 50% of women treated for fistula at Panzi hospital got their fistula despite a cesarean section was performed and 84% of the babies were stillborn. It is evident that in many cases, some form of assisted vaginal delivery would have been more appropriate. Unfortunately, the use of vacuum extraction has become rare and the cesarean delivery rate has increased in many areas (15,16). Fear of vertical HIV transmission is one factor for this development, lack of obstetrical training is another (12).

Most cases of uterine rupture are treated by hysterectomy. This major surgery is risky for patients in a bad general condition. Further, the loss of uterus and fertility has serious social consequences in many societies. Suturing, with or without sterilization, can be a safe alternative and has been used in more than 60% of cases in some reports (17,18). Additional ligature of the internal iliac arteries is sometimes necessary, and this technique should be known (19). A conservative approach necessarily implies that future pregnancies are strictly followed up of and a cesarean delivery performed in due time.

Postpartum hemorrhage accounts for 34% of maternal mortality in developing countries compared to 13% in developed countries (20) and is an important indication for emergency hysterectomy. The most common causes are uterine atony (80%), retained placental fragments, genital tract lacerations and uterine rupture. Risk factors include a history of post partum hemorrhage or retained placenta, placental abruption, placenta praevia, uterine fibroids, hydramnios, multiple pregnancies, prolonged labor and instrumental delivery. Although an assessment of risk factors is important, post partum hemorrhage typically occurs unpredicted and all parturients are at the risk. Prompt handling is essential. Peripartum hysterectomy - cesarean or postpartum - can be a life saving procedure, although difficult and risky. The cervical edges can be difficult to identify and damage to vagina, bladder and ureters often occur. A supracervical hysterectomy is much less dangerous and should be preferred. When removal of the cervix is necessary endocervical palpation will to help identify the cervical edges and avoid injuries.

Conservative management of postpartum hemorrhage should be tried before hysterectomy is considered. Access to uterotonics, *iv* fluids, blood transfusion and curettage is essential. Balloon tamponade of uterus has become an important conservative method (21). A simplified condom method is useful in low-resource settings (22). The B-Lynch suture technique (23) is a effective measure to obtain compression of an atonic uterus during cesarean delivery. Cervical tears detected postpartum should be explored and sutured by the vaginal approach. In case of high tears and extrauterine hemorrhage, hysterectomy can be necessary.

A cesarean section performed late - in the second stage of labor - when the lower uterine segment is stretched and the bladder lifted high up, can easily lead to lacerations of cervix and vagina due to difficult access to the presenting part. Bleeding and difficulties may entail inappropriate suturing that can affect both the bladder and ureters, or cause inadvertent lacerations of these organs. The reversed breech extraction procedure of an entrapped fetus is a method to diminish the risk of tears and the risk of peripartum hysterectomy (24).

2. Abdominal hysterectomy

The incidence of pelvic organ fistula after hysterectomy ranges from 0.1 to 4% in different studies (25,26). A higher incidence is reported after radical hysterectomy compared with hysterectomy on benign indications. In a nationwide cohort study of 182,641 hysterectomies from Sweden, 220 urogential fistulas (0.12%) were registered. Laparoscopic hysterectomy was associated with the highest rate of fistula surgery, and subtotal abdominal hysterectomy was associated with the lowest. Risk factors are age, adhesions and postoperative infections. Risk factors for urinary tract damage are basically the same in low-resource countries as in high-resource countries. Spinal anesthesia commonly used in developing countries, gives poor relaxation. Large myomas, a common indication for hysterectomy in those areas, make access to the pelvis particularly difficult, especially when the myomas are located in the cervical part. Dislocation of organs and difficulties in identification of the bladder and ureteres increase the risk of accidental damage.

Cervical cancer is also very common in the developing world, in many countries the most common malignancy in women. This disease is most often detected in an advanced and inoperable stage. Many cancer patients undergo, however, a hysterectomy trial which, due to parametrial involvement and bleeding, ends up with a urinary tract injury. Operable (stage Ib-IIa) patients should preferably have a radical hysterectomy (a.m. Wertheim) which include proper identification and dissection of the bladder and ureteres. If this operation method is not available, or operability cannot be assured, the treatment of choice is radiotherapy with concomitant chemotherapy whenever available. Radical vaginal trachelectomy as fertility sparing operation for early stage cervical cancer has the same risk of ureteric injury as radical hysterectomy although the rate of bladder injury is higher (27).

The risk of urinary tract damage highly depends on the indication and type of intervention performed. Operations for endometriosis and malignancy (with radical hysterectomy) run a higher risk. In many cases, no predisposing factor is identified. Attempt to obtain hemostasis is the most common activity leading to injury (27). Preoperative measures like *iv* pyelogram, computed tomography, prophylactic ureteric stint have not shown to be preventive. The best prevention is that the surgeon always is aware of where the ureters is and stay safely away from it and preserving its adventitial sheath. Ureter should be visualized, not only palpated. The surgeon should know well the retroperitoneal approach and use it in all difficult cases. Special care should be taken when thermocautery is used.

3. Vaginal hysterectomy

Most vaginal hysterectomies are performed as part of a treatment for genital organ prolapse. Bladder and ureter injuries related to vaginal operations occur in all parts of the world. Register data from Finland showed an incidence of 0.2 bladder injuries per 1000 vaginal hysterectomies and the same incidence for ureteric injuries (1). Sixty-five percent of the complications were fistulas. In a series from France urinary tract injury occurred in 1.7% of 3076 vaginal hysterectomies - 54 bladder lesions and 1 ureteric lesion (28). It is reason to believe that the incidence of injury is higher in low-resource countries. Some institutions tend to performed hysterectomy also in cases with less pronounced genital organ prolapse. High incidence of cervical cancer and contraceptive need may be reasons for a liberal attitude to hysterectomy. However, the Manchester technique with cervical amputation is a less risky procedure. Recurrence and vault prolapsed are best prevented by building up the posterior part of the pelvic floor.

Age, parity, body weight and mode of delivery are known risk factors (1.28) and are common for low-income and high-income countries. Multiparity, poor general condition and chronic infections are more prevalent in developing countries. High bacterial content in the vagina and particular inflammatory conditions like urogenital schistosomiasis and tuberculosis may be predisposing factors. Bladder damage should be avoided by careful dissection and ureters should be localized by palpation against a metal retractor in the paravesical space (27).

4. Treatment

Bladder injuries

Most bladder lesions are detected during the operation. The bladder wall should be closed in two layers with nonperforating, absorbable sutures and an indwelling urinary catheter for 5 days. The ureteric ostia should be located. When the lesion is in its proximity, temporary insertion of a ureteric stint is advisable. Normally, the lesion will be cured without sequel.

Vesicovaginal fistulas caused by abdominal hysterectomy are located high up in vagina (Table 3). The vaginal approach for repair may be possible even for high located fistulas. In developing countries, this way tends to be chosen for reasons of anesthesia and fear of postoperative intestinal problems. In the Panzi hospital material, 5 out of 11 vesicovaginal fistulas after hysterectomy were operated vaginally. The abdominal approach may be technically easier and safer, especially in cases of pelvic adhesions, and implies a possibility of interposing an omental flap between the closed bladder wall and the vaginal wall to reduce the risk of recurrence.

Some small, vesicovaginal fistulas can be managed conservatively by bladder drainage for some weeks. Fistula surgery can be a delicate procedure and every surgeon intending to start such activity should obtain adequate training at a fistula center. Valuable handbooks are available (27,29).

Certain principles for urogenital fistula surgery prevail: 1)The tissue operated on should be without necrosis or inflammation. If operation is not done within 5 days after the injury, it is better to wait 6 weeks or more until tissue reaction is resolved. 2) All scar tissue around the fistula is removed by deliberate dissection, 3) All sutures must be tension-free. For suture technique, see fig. 1. 4) The ureteric ostiae should be visualized during the operation and, especially when the vaginal approach is used, ureteric stints applied to protect the ureters against incidental ligation or injury. 5) Postoperatively, free urine drainage must be assured for at least 2 weeks using a urethric or a suprapubic catheter. 6) Before departure, complete fistula closure is asserted by vaginal inspection after insertion of dye in the bladder

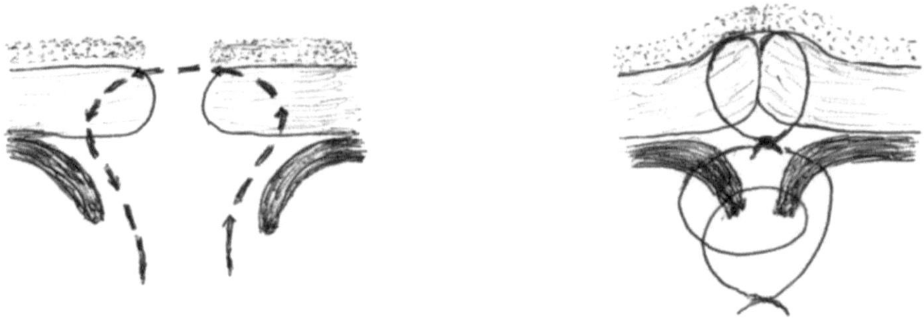

Fig. 1. Suture technique

Ureteric injuries

Ureteric occlusion should be diagnosed as early as possible before renal function is impaired. Time can be gained by temporary urinary deviation through percutaneous pyelostomy. This option is rarely available in low-resource settings. Immediate reoperation should be considered, provided the patient's general condition allows it and renal function is still possible to save. Any misplaced ligature or angulation should be removed, the viability of the ureter assessed and a stint placed through cystoscopy.

A partial transsection is repaired over a ureteral stint. Transection in upper or middle third is treated by uretero-ureterostomy over a ureteral stint. Some resection of the ureter ends can be necessary to assure viability, especially in cases of thermal injury. Spatulation of the ends is recommended to increase the lumen. The anastomosis must be completely tension free. Dissection must be done with care bearing in mind that blood supply to the ureter above the pelvic brim is coming from the medial side, below the prim from the lateral side. When the ureteric transsection took place less than 6 cm from the bladder vascularity is often impaired and primary anastomosis thereby risky. Transection of the lower third of the ureter is therefore most often treated by uretero-neocystostomy with Psoas hitch over a ureteric stint (27).

Once a ureterovaginal fistula has developed there is no longer an emergency situation. Renal function is normally not affected and a planned intervention can be performed. An abdominal, extraperitoneal approach is normally possible and preferable. The bladder is freed from its areolar attachment in the retropubic space and an extensive mobilization (almost 270 degrees) of its ventral surface performed. The bladder is elongated toward the Psoas tendon where it is fixed. The affected ureter is freed, transected as low as possible, and the stinted proximal end is anastomozed to the elongated bladder (27). All cases of ureterovaginal fistulas reported from Panzi Hospital (Table 3) were successfully treated by this method of uretero-neocystostomy.

All urogenital fistulas - iatrogenic as well as obstetric ones - should preferably be treated at a specialized fistula center. It is essential that the first operation is optimally performed. The chance of closure is greatly diminished after several attempts of repair (10).

5. Conclusions

Low-resource settings influence the risk of getting urinary tract injury as a complication to hysterectomy. Emergency peripartum hysterectomy is particularly risky and subtotal hysterectomy is a safer procedure. Postpartum hemorrhage should be managed conservatively whenever possible. Ureterovaginal and high located vesicovaginal fistulas are common sequels. These fistulas are smaller in size, have less scar tissue and appear in women with higher age and parity than the more common obstetric fistula. Repair is more often done through the abdominal route and should be performed at a specialized fistula center.

6. References

[1] Härkki-Sirén P, Sjöberg J, Tiitinen A. Urinary tract injuries after hysterectomy. Obstet Gynecol 1998;92(1):113-118.

[2] Duong TH, Gellasch TL, Adam RA. Risk factors for the development of vesicovaginal fistula after incidental cystotomy at the time of a benign hysterectomy. Am J Obstet Gynecol 2009;201(5):512.e1-4.

[3] Goodno JA, Powers TW, Harris VD. Ureteral injury in gynecologic surgery: A ten-year review in a community hospital. Am J Obstet Gynecol 1995;172(6):1817-1822.

[4] Preston JM. Iatrogenic ureteric injury: common medicolegal pitfalls. Brit J Urol Int 2000;86(3):313-317.

[5] Wall LL. Obstetric vesicovaginal fistula as an international public-health problem. Lancet 2006;368(9542):1201–1209.

[6] Muletta M, Rasmussen S, Kiserud T. Obstetric fistula in 14,928 Ethiopian women. Acta Obstet Gynecol Scand 2010;89(7):945-951.

[7] Wall LL, Karshima JA, Kirschner C, Arrowsmith SD. The obstetric vesicovaginal fistula: characteristics of 899 patients from Jos, Nigeria. Am J Obstet Gynecol 2004;190(4):1011-1019.

[8] Savan K, Ekin M, Kupelioglu L, Oral S. Surgical repair of genitourinary fistulae: comparison of experience at Turkey and Niger. Arch Gynecol Obstet 2010;282(6):649-653.

[9] El-Lamie IK. Urogenital fistulae: changing trends and personal experience of 46 cases. Int Urogynecol J Pelvic Floor Dysfunct 2008;19(2):267-272.

[10] Elkins T. Fistula surgery: past, present and future directions. Int Urogynecol J 1997;8(1):30-35.
[11] Sjøveian S, Vangen S, Mukwege D, Onsrud M. Surgery outcome of obstetric fistula: a retrospective analysis of 595 patients. Acta Obstet Gynecol Scand 2011;90(7):753-760.
[12] Onsrud M, Sjøveian S, Mukwege D. Cesarean delivery-related fistula in the Democratic Republic of Congo. Int J Gynecol Obstet 2011;114(1):10-14.
[13] Sheiner E, Levy A, Katz M, Mazor M. Identifying risk factors for peripartum cesarean hysterectomy. A population based study. J Reprod Med 2003;48:622-626.
[14] Hofmeyr GJ, Say L, Gülmezoglu AM. Systematic review: WHO systematic review of maternal mortality and morbidity. BJOG 2005;112(9):1221-1228.
[15] Onsrud M. Changed attitude to obstetrical delivery help in Eastern Congo (in Norwegian). Tidsskr Nor Legeforen 2008;128(9):1078-1080.
[16] Fauveau V. Is vacuum extraction still known, taught and practiced? A worldwide KAP survey. Int J Gynecol Obstet 2006;94(2):185-189.
[17] Sheth SS. Results of treatment of rupture of the uterus by suturing. BJOG 1968;75(1):55-58.
[18] Klungsøyr P, Kiserud T. Rupture of the uterus treated by suture. Acta Obset Gynecol Scand 189;68(1):1-2.
[19] Joshi V, Otiv S, Majumder R, Nikam Y, Shrivastava M. Internal iliac artery ligation for arresting postpartum haemorrhage. BJOG 2007;114:356–361.
[20] Khan KS, Wojdyla D, Say L, Gulmezoglu AM, Van Look PF. WHO analysis of causes of maternal death: a systematic review. Lancet 2006;367:1066–1074.
[21] Georgiou C. Baloon tamponade in the management of postpartum hemorrhage: a review. BJOG 2009;116(6):748-757.
[22] Akhtar S, Begum MR, Kabir Z, Rashid M, Laila TR, Zabeen F. Use of condom to control massive postpartum hemorrhage. MedGenMed 2003;5(3):38.
[23] Ferguson JE, Bourgeois FJ, Underwood PB. B-Lynch suture for postpartum hemorrhage. Obstet Gynecol 2000;95(6):1020-1022.
[24] Chopra S, Bagga R, Keepanasseril A, Jain V, Kalra J. Disengagement of the deeply engaged fetal head during cesarean section in advanced labor: Conventional method versus reverse breech extraction. Acta Obstet Gynecol Scand 2009;88(10):1163-1166.
[25] Forsgren C, Lundholm C, Johansson AL, Cnattingius S, Altman D. Hysterectomy for Benign Indications and Risk of Pelvic Organ Fistula Disease. Obstet Gynecol 2009;114(3):594-599.
[26] Forsgren C, Altman D. Risk of pelvic organ fistula in patients undergoing hysterectomy. Curr Opin Obstet Gynecol 2010;22(5):404-407.
[27] Montz FJ, Bristow RE, Del Carmen MG. Operative injuries to the ureter. In: Rock JA, Jones HW, eds. *Te Linde's Operative gynecology,* ninth edition. Philadelphia: Lippincott Williams & Wilkins, 2003:1081-1097. ISBN-10: 0781772346
[28] Mathevet P,Valencia P, Cousin C, Mellier G, Dargent D. Operative injuries during vaginal hysterectomy. Eur J Obstet Gynecol Reprod Biol 2001;97(1):71-75.
[29] *First steps in vesico-vaginal fistula repair.* Hancock B, ed. London: Royal Society of Medicine Press, 2005. ISBN 1-85315-611-6

Part 6

Hysterectomy: Multiple Aspects

21

Management of Pregnancy After Conization and Radical Trachelectomy

Keun-Young Lee and Ji-Eun Song
Division of Maternal-Fetal Medicine,
Department of Obstetrics and Gynecology, Hallym University,
Korea

1. Introduction

Cervical intraepithelial neoplasia (CIN) is commonly diagnosed in women of child-bearing age. (Castle et al., 2009) The excisional treatments of CIN include cold-knife conization, laser conization, loop electrosurgical excision procedure (LEEP), and large loop excision of the transformation zone (LLETZ). CIN is also treated by ablative procedures such as laser vaporization and cryotherapy. Recently, human papilloma virus (HPV) has led to the understanding of pathogenesis and management of cervical diseases. (Moscicki et al., 2004) The screening and subsequent treatment of CIN significantly reduces the risk of invasive cervical cancer, but the impact of excisional cervical treatment on subsequent pregnancy outcome must be evaluated.

Many women with a diagnosis of cervical cancer are child-bearing population, younger than 40 years. Fertility-sparing radical vaginal or abdominal trachelectomy is a safe and feasible procedure for the treatment of patients with early stage cervical cancer. (Plante et al., 2005; Roman, 2005; Hertel et al., 2006) The disease-free survival rates and overall survival rates of radical trachelectomy is comparable to those of radical hysterectomy (Rob et al., 2011) The proper waiting period after radical tracelectomy and before conception varies in the literature. Roy and Plante (Roy and Plante, 1998) recommend a 6 month follow-up, while Shlaerth *et al.* (Shlaerth et al., 2003) describe a period of 1 year. The issue of having a pregnancy and fetal viability must be addressed following radical trachelectomy.

This chapter will outline concerns and management options of pregnancy after cervical surgeries with conization and radical trachelectomy.

2. Pregnancy after conization and radical trachelectomy

The important issue following cervical surgery in child-bearing age is the fertility and pregnancy outcome. Excisional cervical surgery may contribute to decreased mechanical support of cervix, and increased susceptibility to ascending infection resulting from the loss of cervical mucus. Cervical surgery may alter reproductive function by cervical shortening, impairment of immunologic defence, and alteration of cervicovaginal bacterial flora, and thus expose those women to high risk of preterm birth. (Svare et al., 1992)

Early studies on the impact of conization on pregnancy are hindered by small study population, inadequately powered study design, and neglect of potential confounders such as socioeconomic status and previous preterm delivery. (Sadler et al., 2007)Recent well-designed studies with large sample sizes conclude that conization increases the risk of preterm birth and perinatal morbidities (Jakobsson et al., 2007; Sjoborg et al., 2007; Nohr et al., 2007) Jakobsson *et al.* (Jakobsson et al., 2007) found a significant increase of very preterm birth (28-31 weeks) and extremely preterm birth (< 28 weeks) following conization. [relative risk (RR) 1.99, 95% confidence interval (CI) 1.81-2.20; RR 2.86, 95% CI 1.30-2.32, respectively]. The study also showed a significant association of low birth weight (LBW) and conization.[RR 2.06, 95% CI 1.83-2.31] Other two meta-analyses also supported that excisional cervical treatments in CIN subsequently increase risk of preterm birth, and preterm premature rupture of membrane (PPROM) (Crane, 2003) Some studies reported the association between cone depth and higher risk of preterm birth, but the limited and conflicting data failed to demonstrate an accurate results. (Salder et al., 2004; Samson et al., 2005)

Because cervix is amputated below the cervical isthmus in radical trachelectomy, obstetric morbidity is higher than those of conization. The risk of preterm birth after radical trachelectomy increases two-fold than the general population. (Jolley et al., 2007; Martin et al., 2008) Boss *et al.* (Boss et al., 2005) reviewed obstetric outcomes of radical trachelectomy in the literature. A total of 335 cases of radical trachelectomy were analyzed. 153/355 (43%) patients attempted to become pregnant. About 30% of these women did not conceive. The causes of their infertility include anovulation, cervical factor such as cervical stenosis, and idiopathic factor. Other 70% of these women subsequently became pregnant. Of these, first and second trimester losses occurred in 47/161 (29%) pregnancies. 21% ended in the third trimester before 36 weeks of gestation. The causes of their preterm birth were attributed to cervical incompetence, ascending infection, and PPROM. (Boss et al., 2005)

2.1 Management options

It is clear that cervical surgeries attribute to increased risk of preterm birth (Kyrgiou et al., 2006; Plante et al., 2005; Samson et al., 2005; Sadler et al., 2004), but no specific rationale of pregnancy management after cervical surgeries exist. The management strategies for pregnancy after cervical surgeries should refer to those for women with short cervix who are at high risk for preterm birth.

2.1.1 Transvaginal ultrasound

It is well known that women with a short cervix in the mid-trimester have a higher risk for preterm birth. (Iam et al., 1996; To et al., 2001) Cervical length, as determined by vaginal sonography, has been shown to be sensitive, and reproducible than digital examination or transabdominal ultrasonogrphy in predicting the risk of preterm birth. (Berghella and Bega, 2008) Cervical length is measured from the internal os to the external os. When cervical funneling is visualized, cervical length is measurable form the functional internal os to the external os. Some researchers reported the effect of conization on subsequent cervical length. Gentry et al. (Gentry et al., 2000) found no difference in cervical length between before and after LEEP. Berghella et al.(Berghella et al., 2004) demonstrated that only 28% of patients showed cervical shortening following conization.

Between 14 and 22 weeks of gestation, the median cervical length is 35-40 mm. From 22 to 32 weeks, the 50th percentile for length is 35 mm, and the 10th percentile is 25 mm. (Iam, 2004) A cervical length cutoff level of < 25 mm was associated with a sensitivity of 69%, a specificity of 80%, and a positive predictive value of 55%. (Owen et al., 2001) The <25 mm cutoff level before 20 weeks of gestation predicted preterm birth at <35 weeks gestation [likelyhood ratio (LR) 4.31, 95% CI 30.8-6.01, n =2258] (Crane and Hutchens, 2008) Independent of baseline cervical length, dynamic cervical change (ie, millimeters per week) was significantly associated with higher risk for preterm birth. (Owen et al., 2001)

Funneling is defined as the opening of the internal os of cervix. The significance of funneling on pregnancy after conization has not been reported. Compared with a short cervix (<25mm) alone, The combination of short cervix (<25mm) and funneling increased the sensitivity of predicting preterm delivery from 61% to 74 %. (Berghella et al., 1999) However, the normal cervical length more than 25 mm plus funneling does not increase the prediction of preterm birth. (Berghella and Roman, 2005)

2.1.2 Nonsonographic methods

Fetal fibronectin (FFN) is a widely accepted predictor of preterm birth. The presence of FFN in cervicovaginal secretions is significantly associated with preterm birth. (Peaceman et al., 1997) Women with a positive FFN and a short cervix (<22mm) had a significantly shorter latency to delivery. (Rizzo et al., 1996)

The uterine electromyography, which detects the electrical activity of myometrium, may be used to diagnose preterm labor. (Lucovnik et al., 2011)

2.1.3 Infection

The presence of bacterial vaginosis increases the risk of preterm delivery, (Leitich and Kiss, 2007) but no data suggests the correlation between vaginal infection and pregnancy outcome after conization. Bacterial vaginosis is further attributable to preterm birth in women with short cervix (<25mm). (Rust et al., 2005) There is no study that reveals whether other infection such as Chlamydia, or gonorrhea contributes to preterm delivery and cervical length.

The lack of mechanical support of cervical mucus after radical trachelectomy may cause cervical incompetence and ascending infection. Shepherd et al (Shepherd et al., 2001) suggested the use of prophylactic antibiotics between 14 and 16 weeks of gestation following radical trachelectomy. Saling operation (complete cervicovaginal occlusion) which should be performed between 12 and 14 weeks of gestation may be the preventive strategy for reducing the risk of ascending infection and chorioamnionitis (Shlaerth et al., 2003; Gadducci et al., 2001)

2.1.4 Progesterone

Progesterone appears to prevent cervical ripening, (Word et al., 2007; Yellon et al., 2009) and anti-inflammatory properties. (Elovitz et al., 2008; Elovitz et al., 2005) The precise mechanisms of blockade of progesterone action against cervical changes are poorly understood.

Fonesca et al (Fonesca et al, 2007) specifically evaluated the impact of progesterone in women with a short cervix (<15mm) identified on transvaginal ultrasonography. Women were allocated to receive either 200 mg nightly intravaginal progesterone or placebo from 24 to 33 weeks of gestation. A total of 250 women were enrolled. Women administered progesterone less likely to have a spontaneous delivery before 34 weeks of gestation than placebo group. (19.2 % vs 34.4 %; relative risk [RR] = 0.56; 95% confidence interval [CI] = 0.36-0.86). There was a significant reduction in the risk of neonatal sepsis in women administered progesterone (274 infants, RR = 0.28, 95% CI 0.08 - 0.97). (Fonesca et al, 2007) A systematic meta-analysis by Dodd et al (Dodd et al., 2008) also demonstrated that vaginal progesterone significantly reduced preterm birth before 34 weeks of gestation in women with short cervix. Facchinetti et al (Facchinetti et al, 2007) reported a randomized clinical trial involving symptomatic women with preterm labor and intact membranes at 25- 34 weeks of gestation. For women administered intramuscular 341mg of 17-alpha-hydroxyprogesterone caproate (17P) twice a week until 36 weeks, when compared with observation group, there was a significant reduction in the risk of spontaneous delivery. (odds ratio [OR] = 0.15, 95% CI = 0.04-0.58) The subgroup analysis involving women with short cervix less than 25 mm at enrolment showed more significant difference between two groups. Women administered 17P had less cervical shortening at days 21 (1.38 ± 1.31 mm) compared to women who had not received 17P (day 21, 4.88 ± 3.14 mm, p = 0.0001) (Facchinetti et al, 2007) Future studies are needed to enlighten the association between prophylactic progesterone and pregnancy outcome after conization and radical trachelectomy.

2.1.5 Cerclage

There is considerable debate as to whether cerclage is efficient in pregnant women after conization. The exact mechanism of preterm birth after conization is unclear, and so the mechanisum of cervical shortening following conization is unclear.

Royal College of Obstetrics and Gynecology (RCOG, 1993) performed a trial of history-indicated cerclage (prophylactic cerclage). A total of 1292 women were enrolled and 138 women with a history of conization or cervical amputation were included among them. The subgroup analysis of those 138 women revealed no significant reduction in preterm birth or improvement in neonatal outcome. However, there was a significant reduction in delivery less than 32 weeks of gestataion in cerclage group with 3 or more second-trimester deliveries, and no histories of cervical surgeries. (RCOG, 1993) Other researchers also reported that a prophylactic cerclage was not beneficial for preventing preterm birth in women with prior conization. (Nam et al., 2010; Shin et al., 2010)

The transvaginal sonography of cervix enables obstetricians to detect cervical shortening or funneling in asymptomatic women. Ultrasound-indicated cerclage based on a short cervix has been proposed as a solution for preventing cervical incompetence and preterm birth. A meta-anaylsis (Berghella et al., 2005) including four randomized trials of ultrasound-indicated cerclage found that cerclage is beneficial in women with short cervix less than 25 mm before 24 weeks of gestation and index preterm birth. In these women, a relative risk reduction of preterm birth at < 35 weeks of gestation was enhanced. (RR, 0.61; 95% ci, 0.4-0.9) In the subgroup analysis, there was no beneficial effect of cerclage on women with prior conization. (Berghella et al., 2005) A short cervix in women with prior cervical surgery are predictive of preterm delivery, but the attributable risk is lower than in women with index preterm birth. More recently, the Vaginal Ultrasound Trail Consortium (Owen J,2008) demonstrated that the effect of cerclage for preventing preterm birth and prolonging gestation was identified only in women with a cervical length of less than 15 mm (RR 0.23, 95% CI 0.08 - 0.66). Zeisler et al (Zeisler et al., 1997) specifically evaluated the cerclage in women with prior conization, and concluded that prophylactic cerclage is not beneficial for preventing preterm birth. The combination of present cervical length, and prior histories of preterm birth and cervical surgeries is a pronounced risk factor of preterm delivery. Once the cervix is shortened, it is difficult to place satisfactory McDonald cerclage. Surgeons should avoid bladder or bowel injury during ultrasound-indicated cerclage.

Physical-examination based cerclage is placed in women with significant cervical dilatation (>1cm) and bulging membrane. It is referred to as a 'rescue' or 'emergency' cerclage, as it requires challenging skill to avoid a rupture of membrane during cerclage. Daskalakis et al. (Daskalakis et al., 2006) concluded that physical-examination cerclage reduced preterm delivery before 32 weeks of gestation and improved neonatal survival rate compared to bed rest group. Other researchers (Cockwell and Smith, 2005) also demonstrated that physical-examination cerclage prolonged pregnancy and improved neonatal outcome in women with dilated cervix and bulging membrane. Lee et al (Lee et al., 2004) reported that elevated interleukin-6 in amniotic fluid was adversely associated with interval between physical-examination cerclage and delivery. Weiner et al. (Weiner et al., 2005) found intrauterine inflammatory responses and decidual hemorrhage were correlated with adverse pregnancy outcome after physical-examination cerclage. A physical-examination cerclage could be considered in women with dilated cervix and bulging membrane after conization. In these women, the evaluation of subclinical inflammation may predict the prognosis of pregnancy.

Transabodminal cervico-isthmic cerclage (TCIC) is beneficial in women with cervix that is extremely short, congenital anomaly or markedly scarred due to previous vaginal cerclage. TCIC seems to be effective in women who are inadequate for vaginal cerclage. (Topping et al., 1995; Turnquest et al., 1999) The unrelenting complication during pregnancy following radical trachelectomy is late abortion and preterm delivery as cervix has markedly modified anatomy after radical trachelectomy. The prophylactic concomitant cerclage is usually placed at the time of radical trachelectomy. (Plante et al., 2005; Roman, 2005) When the cerclage placed too deeply within the cervical stroma, it can be expelled spontaneously. The success of pregnancy may depends on a stable maintenance of cerclage. (Plante et al., 2005) Transabdominal cervico-isthmic cerclage is an appreciable option for the pregnant women after radical trachelectomy because of lack of sufficient cervical tissue for vaginal cerclage. (Lee et al., 2007)

2.1.6 Multiple pregnancies

Preterm delivery in twin pregnancies is 5-10 time more frequent than that in singleton pregnancy. (Fuchs et al., 2004) There is no clear best cervical length for the prediction of preterm birth in multiple pregnancies. Nevertheless, the rate of delivery was inversely associated with cervical length in twin pregnancies, being 66% for 10 mm, 24% for 20 mm, 12% for 25 mm, and < 1% for 40 mm. (To et al, 2006).

Current evidence does not support prophylactic administration of progesterone in multiple pregnancies. Additional studies are needed to confirm the effect of progesterone supplementation in twin pregnancies.

There is no data that prophylactic cerclage should be performed in multiple pregnancies. Recent prospective non-randomized trial of prophylactic cerclage in asymptomatic twin pregnancies reported that cerclage is not beneficial. (Eskandar et al., 2007) Twin pregnancies following radical trachelectomy are at more increased risk for preterm birth compared to singleton pregnancies. (Plante et al., 2005) Lee et al (Lee et al., 2007) reported TCIC after radical trachelectomy in twin pregnancy improved the pregnancy outcome. Cerclage in twin pregnancy is effective in certain circumstances.

3. Conclusion

CIN is relatively common in women with child-bearing age. Several studies have reported that women undergoing conization are at increased risk for preterm delivery, a low birthweight neonate, and premature rupture of membrane. Recently, the conservative treatment of early cervical cancer to preserve fertility has improved. A cervix changes drastically after radical trachelectomy. In these women after conization or radical trachelectomy, obstetricians should consider the possible adverse effects on future pregnancies.

As noted earlier, there is no established rationale for the pregnancy management after conization and radical trachelectomy. There are several management options for preventing preterm birth in these women but none has been prove more effective than any other strategies: Transvaginal sonography is a sensitive and reproducible method to detect short cervix. The administration of progesterone is thought to have beneficial effect on prolonging pregnancy. History-indicated cerclage in women with previous conization seems to be inefficient in preventing preterm birth. Ultrasound-indicated cerclage could be beneficial in women with short cervix and a prior preterm birth history. Physical-examination cerclage could prevent preterm birth in women with dilated cervix and bulging membrane after cervical surgeries. TCIC is an acceptable option for pregnant women after radical trachelectomy and women with severely scarred cervix. The combination of above mentioned options and other adjunctive strategies such as detection of infection or inflammation, and antibiotics, etc. could reduce the rate of preterm birth in pregnancy after conization or radical trachelectomy.

Further studies are needed to assess an accurate measurement of cone tissue, and explore the relation between the amount of cone tissue and risk of deleterious pregnancy outcome.

Randomized clinical trials are needed to confirm the role of cerclage, and progesterone, and adjunctive therapies such as antibiotics, and in pregnant women with prior cervical surgeries.

4. Acknowledgments

We would like to thank all the members of the department of obstetrics and gynecology, Hallym University Medical Center.

5. References

Anonymous: Final report of the Medical Research Council/Royal College of Obstetrics and Gynecology multicenter randomized trial of cervical cerclage. Br J Obstet Gynecol 100:516-523,1993

Berghella V, Bega G: Ultrasound evaluation of ther cervix, in Callen PW (ed): Ultrasonography in Obstetrics and Gynecology (ed 5). Philadelphia, PA, Saunders Elsevier, 2008, pp 698-720

Berghella V, Dalsy SF, Tolosa JE, et al. Prediction of preterm delivery with tranvaginal ultrasonography of the cervix in patients with high-risk pregnancies: does cerclage prevent prematurity? Am J Obstet Gynecol 181:809-815,1999

Berghella V, Odibo AO, To MS, et al. Cerclage for short cervix on ultrasound:meta-analysis of trials using individual patient-level data. Obstet Gynecol 2005;106:181-189

Berghella V, Pereira L, GariepyA, Simonazzi G. Prior cone biopsy: prediction of preterm birth by cervical ultrasound. Am J Obstet Gynecol 2004;191:1393-1397

Berghella V, Roman A. Does funneling increase the incidence of preterm birth in women with normal cervical length? Am J Obstet Gynecol 193;S147,2005(abstr)

Boss EA, van Golde RJ, Beerendonk CC, Massuger LF. Pregnancy after radical trachelectomy: a real option. Gynecol Oncol 2005;99(Suppl 1):S152-6

Castle PE, Fetterman , Akhtar I, Husain M et al. Age-appropriate use of human papillomavirus vaccines in the U.S. Gynecol Oncol 2009;114(2):365-9

Cockwell HA, Smith GN.2005. Cervical incompetence and the role of emergency cerclage. Journal of Obstetrics and Gynecology Canada 27:123-129

Crane JMG: Pregnancy outcome after loop electrosurgical excision procedure: A systematic review. Obstet Gynecol 102 (2003) 1058

Crane JM, Hutchens D. Transvaginal sonogrpahic measurement of cervical length to predict preterm birth in astymptomatic women at increased risk: a systematic review. Ultrasound Obstet Gynecol 2008;31:579-587

Daskalakis G, Papantoniou N, Mesogitis S, Antasaklis A. 2006. Management of cervical insufficiency and bulging fetal membranes. Obstetrics and Gynecology 107:221-226

Dodd JM, Flenady VJ, Cincotta R: Progesterone for the prevention of preterm birth: a systematic review. Obstet Gynecol 112:127-134, 2008

Elovitz MA, Gonzalez J : Medroxyprogesterone acetate modulates the immune response in the uterus, cervix and placenta in a mouse model of preterm birth. J Matern Fetal Neonatal Med 21:223-230,2008

Elovitz MA, Mrinalini C Sammel MD: Can medroxyprogesterone acetate alter Toll-like receptor expression in a mouse model of intrauterine inflammation? Am J Obstet Gynecol 193:1149-1155, 2005

Eskandar M, Shafiq H, Almushait MA, et al. Cervical cerclage for prevention of preterm birth in women with twin pregnancy. Int Gynecol Obstet 2007;99:110-112

Facchinetti F, Paganelli S, Comitini G, et al: Cervical length changes during preterm cervical ripening: effects of 17-alpha-hydroxyprogesterone caproate. Am J Obstet Gynecol 196:453-54,2007

Fonesca EB, Celik E, Parra M, Singh M, Nicolaides KH, for the Fetal Medicine Foundation Second Trimster Screening Group. Progesterone and the risk of preterm birth among women with a short cervix. N Engl J Med 2007;357:462-9

Fuchs IB, Tsoi E, Herich W, et al; Sonographic measurement of cervical length in twin pregnancies in threatened preterm labor. Ultrasound Obstet Gynecol 23:42-45,2004

Gadducci A, Cosio S, Cionini L, Genazzani AR. Neoadjuvant chemotherapy and concurrent chemoradidation in the treatment of advanced cervical cancer. Anticancer Res 2001;21:3525-33

Gentry DJ, Baggish MS, Brady K, et al: The effects of loop excision of the transformation zone on cervical length: implications for pregnancy. Am J Obstet Gynecol 2000;182:516-20

Hertel H, Kohler C, Grund D, Hillemanns P,Possover M, Michels W, Schneider A. Radical vaginal trachelectomy (RVT) combined with laparoscopic pelvic lymphadenectomy: prospective multincenter study of 100 patients with early cervical cancer. Gynecol Oncol 2006;103:506-11

Iams JD, Goldenberg RL, Meis PJ, Mercer BM, Moawad A, Das A, Thom E, McNellis D, Copper RL, Johnson F, Roberts JM. The length of the cervix and the risk of spontaneous premature delivery. National Institute of Child Health and Human Development Maternal Fetal Medicine Unit Network. N Engl J Med 1996;334:567-572

Iam JD. 2004. Abnormal cervical competence. In: Creasy RK, Resnik R, Iams JD, editors. Maternal-fetal medicine: principals and practice. 5th ed. Philadelphia: W B Saunders. Pp 603-622.

Jakobsson M, Gissler M, Sainio S, et al. Preterm delivery after surgical treatment for cervical intraepithelial neoplaisa. Obstet Gynecol 2007;109:309-313

Jolley JA, Battista L, Wing DA. Management of pregnancy after radical trachelectomy: case reports and systematic review of the literature. Am J Perinatol 2007;24:531-540

Kyrgiou M, G Koliopoulos, P Marin-Hirsch, M Arbyn, W Prendiville, E Paraskevaidis: Obstetric outcomes after conservative treatment for intraepithelial or early invasive cervical lesions: systematic review and meta-analysis. Lancet 367(2006)489-98

Lee KY, Jun HA, Kim HB, Kang SW.2004. Interleukin-6, but not relaxin, predicts outcome of rescue cerclage in women with cervical incompetence. American Journal of Obsteterics and Gynecology 191:784-789

Lee KY, Jun HA, Roh JW, Song JE. Successful twin pregnancy after vaginal radical trachelectomy using trasabdominal cervicoisthmic cerclage. Am J Obstet Gynecol 2007;197(3):e5-6

Leitich H, Kiss H. Asymptomatic bacterial vaginosis and intermediate flora as risk factors for adverse pregnancy outcome. Best Pract Res Clin Obstet Gynaecol 2007; 21:375-390

Lucovnik M, KuonRJ, Chambliss LR, et al. Use of uterine electromyography to diagnose term and preterm labor. Acta Obstet Gynecol Scand. 2011;90(2):150-157

Martin JA, Kung HC, Mathews TJ, et al. Annual summary of vital statistics: 2006. Pediatrics 2008;121:788-801

MoscickiAB, S Shiboski, NK Hills, KJ Powell, N Jay, EN Hanson, S Miller, LK Canjura-Clayton, S Farhat, JM Broe ring TM Darragh: Regression of low-grade squamous intra-epitelial lesions in young women. Lacet 354 (2004) 1678

Nam KH, Kwon JY, Kim YH, Park YW. Pregnancy outcome after cervical conization: risk factors for preterm delivery and the efficacy of prophylactic cerclage. J Gynecol Oncol 2010;21:225-9

Nohr B, Tabor A, Fredericksen K, et al. Loop electrosurgical excision of the cervix and the subsequent risk of preterm delivery. Acta Obstet Gynecol Scand 2007;86:596-603

Owen J, Yost N, Berghella V, Thom E, Swain M, Dildy GA et al. Mid-trimester endogavinal sonography in women at high risk for spontaneous preterm birth. JAMA 2001;286:1340-8

Owen J for the vagnial ultrasound trial consortium: Multicenter randomized trial of cerclage for preterm birth prevention in high-risk women with shortened mid-trimester cervical length. Am J Obstet Gynecol 199;S3, 2008(6, suppl A)

Peaceman AM, Andrews WW, Thorp JM, et al: Fetal fibronectin as a predictor of PTB in patients with symptoms: a multicenter trial. Obstet Gynecol 177:13-18,1997

Plante M, Renaud MC, Hoskins IA, Roy M. Vaginal radical trachelectomy: a valuable fertility-preserving option in the management of early-stage cervical cancer. A series of 50 pregnancies and review of the literature. Gynecol Oncol 2005 Jul; 98:3-10

Rizzo G, Capponi A, Arduini D, et al: The value of fetal fibronectin in cervical and vaginal secretions and of ultrasonographic examination of the uterine cervix in predicting premature delivery for patients with preterm labor and intact membranes. Am J Obstet Gynecol 175:1146-1151, 1996

Rob L, Skapa P, Robova H. Fertility-sparing surgery in patients with cervical cancer. Lancet Oncol 2011;12:192-200

Roman LD. Pregnancy after radical vaginal tracelectomy: maybe not such a risky undertaking after all. Gynecol Oncol 2005 Jul; 98: 1-2

Roy M, Plante M. Pregnancies after radical vaginal tracelectomy for early-stage cervical cancer. Am J Obstet Gynecol 1998;179:1491-6

Rust OA, Atlas RO, Kimmel S, et al. Does the presence of a funnel increase the risk of adverse perinatal outcome in a patient with a short cervix? Am J Obstet Gynecol 192:1060-1066, 2005

Sadler L, Saftlas A. Cervical surgery and preterm birth. J Perinat Med 2007;35:5-9

Salder L, A Saftlas, W Wang, M Exeter, J Whittaker, L McCowan: Treatment for cervical intraepithelial neoplasia and risk of preterm delivery. J Am Med Assoc 29(2004) 2100-6

Samson SA, JR Bentley, TJ Fahey, DJ McKay, GH Gill: The effect of loop electrosurgical excision procedure on future pregnancy outcome. Obstet Gynecol 105(2005) 325-32

Shepherd JH, Mould T, Oram DH. Radical trachelectomy in early stage carcinoma of the cervix: outcomes as judged by recurrence and fertility rates. Br J Obstet Gynaecol 2001;108:882-5

Shin MY, Seo ES, Choi SJ, Oh SY, Kim BF, Bae DS, et al. The role of prophylactic cerclage in preventing preterm delivery after electrosurgical conization. J Gynecol Oncol 2010;21:230-6

Shlaerth JB, Spirtos NM, Shlaerth AC. Radical trachelectomy and pelvic lymphadenectomy with uterine preservation in the treatment of cervical cancer. Am J Obstet Gynecol 2003;188(1):29-34

Sjoborg KD, Vistad I, Myrh SS, et al. Preganancy outcome after cervical cone excision: a case-control study. Acta Obstet Gynecol Scand 2007;86:423-428

Svare JA, LF Anderson, J Langhoff-Roos, ET Jensen, B Bruun, I Lind, H Madsen: The relation ship between prior cervical conisation, cercial microbial colonization and preterm premature rupture of the membranes. Eur J Obstet Gynecol Repord Biol 47 (1992) 41

To MS, Fonseca EB, Molina FS, et al: Maternal characteristics and cervical length in the prediction of spontaneous early preterm delivery in twins. Am J Obstet Gynecol 194:1360-65,2006

To MS, Skentou C, Liao AW, Cacho A, Nicolaides KH. Cervical length and funneling at 23 weeks of gestation in the prediction of spontaneous early preterm delivery. Ultrasound Obstet Gynecol 2001;18:200-203

Topping J, Farquharson RG. Transabdominal cervical cerclage. Br J Hosp Med. 1995;54:510-12

Turnquest MA, Britton KA, Brown HL. Outcome of patients undergoing trasabdominal cerclage: a descriptive study. J Matern Fetal Med. 1999;9:225-227

Weiner CP, Lee KY, Buhimschi CS, Christner R, Buhimschi IA. 2005. Proteomic biomarkers that predict the clinical success of rescue cerclage. American Journal of Obstetrics and Gynecology.192:710-718

Word RA, Li XH, Hnat M, et al: Dynamics of cervical remodelling during pregnancy and parturition: mechanisms and current concepts. Sem Reprod Med 25:69-79,2007

Yellon SM, Ebner CA, Elovitz MA: Medroxyprogesterone acetate modulates remodelling, immune cell census, and nerve fibers in the cervix of a mouse model for inflammation-induced preterm birth. Reprod Sci 16:257-264,2009

Zeisler H, Journa EA, Bancher –Todesca D, et al. Prophylactic cerclage in pregnancy. Effect on women with a history of conization. J Reprod Med 1997;42:390-392

22

Know-How of the Hormonal Therapy and the Effect of the Male Hormone on Uterus in the Female to Male Transsexuals

Seok Kwun Kim[1] and Myoungseok Han[2]
[1]*Department of Plastic and Reconstructive Surgery,*
[2]*Department of Obstetrics and Gynecology,*
Dong-A University School of Medicine,
South Korea

1. Introduction

Management of the patient with gender identity disorder involves many different aspects of medical care. Transsexualism is a multidimensional phenomenon that requires a multidisciplinary approach in both the diagnostic and treatment phases. Endocrinologists have to work together with mental health professionals and surgeons to provide full counselling, confirm the diagnosis and avoid mistakes or regrets. Hormonal therapy not only has a therapeutic role but also an important diagnostic tool.

Trends in Europe are toward treatment of patients at early age if the diagnosis is appropriately established. This may begin with blocking agents that temporarily suppress pubertal transformation. Secondary sexual trait suppression allows much more successful gender transformation.

Hormonal therapy is used to suppress secondary sexual characteristic of the biological sex, to induce the secondary sex characteristics of the new sex. This therapy should continue lifelong[1].

2. Masculinizing effect in female to male hormonal therapy

Endocrinologic masculinization is achieved by the use of testosterone to induce male physical characteristics. Testosterone works primarily by direct stimulation of receptors in target tissues. It elevates serum testosterone level to a male reference range rather than a decrease in serum estradiol[2]. Testosterone also has antigonadotropic action in high doses.

Rapidity and degree of change from testosterone therapy depends on the agents used, dosage, and the patient's responsiveness to endocrine therapy. Typically, within the first 1-3 months patients experience oilier skin and acne, increased libido, increased muscle mass and upper body strength, and redistribution of the fat to a more masculine pattern[3, 12].

The voice changes to crack and deepen within the first 3-6 months, but it can take a year or more for the voice pitch to fully drop [13].

In 75% FTMs testosterone will cause voice pitch to drop to a level sufficient for passability as male even on the telephone [4].

The clitoral enlargement begins within the first few months of testosterone initiation and typically plateaus within the first year [14, 15]. The degree of enlargement is variable with studies reporting a range of 3.5 - 6 cm maximal when stretched [14, 15, 16]. Clitoral growth dose not appear to be enhanced by topical application of testosterone to the clitoris.

Long-term testosterone use causes vaginal and cervical atrophy [3, 17], with decreased vaginal secretion and difficult penetration [12].

In most cases, menses stop within 1 - 6 months [5-8, 14-16, 18, 19]. If after three months menses have not stopped, the dosage of testosterone may be increased until serum free testosterone is within upper quartile of the normal male range or menses stop. Despite endometrial atrophy, cessation of menses, and reduced fertility there is evidence of ovulation even after several years of testosterone administration [17].

There is gradual increased growth, coarseness, and thickness of hair on the torso and extremities in the first year [3, 4, 6, 7, 16]. Facial hair increases more slowly, typically taking 1 - 4 years to reach full growth. Some patients experience male pattern baldness during this later stage of masculinization [4, 6-8, 11, 20].

Voice change, facial hair growth and male pattern baldness are not reversible, which other changes are reversible if hormone is stopped. Clitoral growth and sterility may or may not reversible(Table 1).

Effect	Onset (months)	Maximum (yr)
Skin oiliness/acne	1-6	1-2
Facial/body hair growth	6-12	4-5
Scalp hair loss	6-12	
Increased muscle mass/strength	6-12	2-5
Fat redistribution	1-6	2-5
Cessation of menses	2-6	
Clitoral enlargement	3-6	1-2
Vaginal atrophy	3-6	1-2
Deepening of voice	6-12	1-2

Table 1. Masculinizing effects in FTM transsexual persons

3. Recommended masculinizing male hormone regimen

Most commonly used preparations are injectable testoterone esters (Jenatestoterone®) administration intramuscularly in dose 200 - 250 mg every two weeks [21]. Sometimes, masculinization effect is low or when patient wants to bring rapid masculinization testosterone esters administrated intramuscularly in dose 200 - 250 mg every week. Serum testosterone level is checked every 3 months for first year and then 1 - 2 times per year afterward for appropriate signs of feminization and for development of adverse reaction. Serum testosterone level should be maintained <55 ng/dl.

At least 12 months of treatment of testosterone can achieve the masculinization. After oophorectomy or achievement of masculinization, administration of testosterone will be reduced to every three or four weeks. Serum testosterone level should be needed to keep within the middle or lower-middle end of the male range. Long acting testosterone undecanoate 1000 mg is available and injections may leave a space at 10 - 12 weeks [22], but masculinizing effect is not certain. Transdermal gel and transdermal patch can be used and also provide good, steady-state testosterone level. AndroGel® is applied 5 - 10 g qd. Androderm® patch is also applied 5 – 10 g daily [23].

To preserve bone density following oophorectomy, testosterone supplementation should be maintained throughout life, and calcium and vitamine D supplementation is recommended [23].

4. Recommended monitoring following initial testosterone therapy

At minimum, patients should be seen every month after initiating treatment or while adjusting medication dosages, then every 3 months for the first year, then every six months thereafter. The primary focus of monitoring cross-sex hormone use is to assess the degree of masculinization and the possible presence of adverse effects of medication. However, as with monitoring of any long-term medication, monitoring should take place in the context of comprehensive care of all health concerns.

Mascullinization takes place gradually over a period of years. Observed changes to male pattern hair growth and voice should be noted, and the patient should be asked about changes to menstrual pattern, mood, clitoral growth, libido, and sexual function. Other changes should also be noted. To avoid a supraphysiological dose of testosterone, serum free testosterone should be checked 2 - 4 weeks after the starting dose or after a dose adjustment, and every 6 - 12 months thereafter.

All exams should include assessment of weight, cardiovascular risk, diabetes risk, and blood pressure. There are case reports of destabilization of bipolar disorder, schizophrenia, and schizoaffective disorder in non-transgender men with the use of testosterone. Mental health should be monitored carefully in FTMs with these condition for the duration of testosterone therapy.

At minimum, laboratory tests should include fasting blood glucose, hemoglobin, lipid profile, and liver enzymes. The fasting blood glucose should be checked 3 and 6 months after starting testosterone or after a dose adjustment, then annually increase frequency and monitor A1c if elevated lipids, significant weight gain, elevated fasting glucose levels, personal history of glucose intolerance, or family history of diabetes. Hemoglobin should be checked 3 and 6 months after starting testosterone or after a dose adjustment, then annually. Lipid profile is needed to evaluate 3 and 6 months after starting testosterone or after a dose adjustment, then annually. Liver enzymes also should be checked 3 and 6 months after starting testosterone or after dose increase, then annually.

5. Effect of the long-term treatment of testosterone on health

The goal of treatment in the FTM is to induce virilization, deepening of the voice, production of male-pattern body hair growth, and physical contours, and cessation of menses.

The principal hormonal treatment used to accomplish these goals is testosterone preparation. After reassignment surgery, which includes oophorectomy and hysterectomy, hormonal therapy must be continued. It is reasonable to assume that the principles of treatment are very similar to a person without their own gonadal hormone secretion.

An unresolved question is whether in the long term all functions of sex steroids of a subject are adequately covered by cross-sex hormones and whether the administration of cross-sex hormones is appropriate safe. Nearly all hormone related biochemical processes can be sex reversed by administration of cross-sex hormone.

The complication of cross-sex hormone therapy is underreported. Although complications occurring in the long term are seen in general practice, and these complication are only occasionally reported in the scientific literature.

Polycythemia and erythrocytosis were observed in testosterone administration as a rare complication[24, 25]. Relative contraindication (e.g. persons who smoke, have diabetes, have liver diseases,etc) to therapy have been published and should have an in-depth discussion with their physician to balance the risk and benefit of therapy[26]. The worrisome complication of water and sodium retention increased body weight, decreased insulin sensitivity, obstructive sleep apnea, acne, poor lipid profile, and an increase in hematocrit have raised the concern for cardiac and thromboembolytic events.

Cerebral vascular accidents have been reported for individuals with supraphysiological level of testosterone[27, 28]. Polycystic ovarian disease is a risk factor for endometrial cancer[27] As the association between polycystic ovarian disease and risk of endometrial and ovarian malignancy are not entirely clear and seen in greater numbers in transsexual people before androgen therapy than in the general population[28, 29]. Mild endometrial hyperplasia has been appreciated on removal of the uterus[30]. A case reported in 2 transsexuals with ovarian cancer[31]. Recommendation for hysterectomy and bilatel salpingoooporectomy, generally carried out around 15 months after the start of testosterore treatment in the male to female transsexuals, has yet to be fully justified, at least on the grounds of enhanced risk of malignancy.

Total hysterectomy after 2 years of testosterone therapy, followed by 50% reduction in hormone man be a way to avoid these risks[32, 33](Table 2).

1. Water and sodium retention
2. Increased erythropoiesis
3. Decreased carbohydrate tolerance
4. Decreased serum high-density lipoprotein (HDL) cholesterol
5. Elevated liver enzymes
6. Weight increase >10%
7. Emotional or psychiatric problems
8. Sleep apnea
9. Acne
10. Endometrial hyperplasia
11. Aggression and hypersexuality
12. Decreased insulin sensitivity
13. Increased IGF
14. Decreased bone mineral density after gonadectomy
15. Ovarian cancer

Table 2. Side Effects of Androgen Therapy in F-T-M Transsexuals

6. The effect of the testosterone on uterus and ovary

Human endometrium is a steroid-hormone-dependent tissue whose growth and remodeling respond to estrogen and progesterone secreted from ovary. Increasing circulating estradiol (E2) levels, a consequence of ovarian follicular growth named as 'follicular' phase of the cycle, promote endometrial cellular proliferation and tissue thickness, from approximately 2 mm after the postmenstrual repair phase, to 10–12 mm in the periovulatory period. [34] Although myometrial tissues are also influenced by estrogen stimulation for the growth and remodeling, they do not show such dramatic change as much as endometrium.

Testosterone treatments to the female to male transsexuals are a usual method to induce masculinization. Testosterone is one of the potent circulating androgens which are produced from testis and ovary. Ovary and adrenal gland in women produce not only female sex hormones and mineralcorticoid, but also androgens, such as testosterone, androstenedione and dehydroepiandrostenedione or its sulfate. Several studies have shown that high plasma androgen levels are associated with adverse reproductive outcome, including infertility and increased incidence of miscarriage.[35, 36] Those clinical features imply that androgens have a potency to affect the endometrial cellular function and promote histological changes.

Polycystic ovary syndrome (PCOS), which is characterized by high circulating testosterone and androstenedione level, expresses different endometrial pattern, such as endometrial hyperplasia or cancer, compared to women with normal androgen level.[37] Those pathologic changes in PCOS patients are attributed to estrogen stimulation to the endometrium, which is aromatized from circulating androgens. Hyperandrogenic symptoms like acne or hirsutism are found in some PCOS patients.

However, it is rarely reported what effect on the uterus would be observed after long term exogenous testosterone treatment among FTM patients. Although it is easily acceptable that there are no definite gross changes of uterus and ovary, interesting histological features are expressed in a few articles. In 1986, Miller et al. reported histologic characteristics of uterus extirpated from FTMs. In the study, severe atrophied uterine cervix was found and variable degrees of atrophic change of endometrium were observed as well.[38] Such changes have been also observed in our previous histologic study on the extirpated uterus from 16 FTMs.(Fig.1, Fig.2) These changes are comparable with proliferative change of endometrium in PCOS. This means that androgen action on endometrium in FTMs is much higher than that of PCOS patients. Meanwhile, we also found that ovarian histologic changes in FTMs were polycystic appearance similar to those of PCOS.[39](Fig. 3) It is thought that the polycystic change of ovary might be due to multiple follicle recruitment action caused by androgen, which is thought to be the pathophysiologic theory about PCOS.

Finally, it is concluded that the histolgic changes of endometrium and ovary are atrophic and polycystic appearance according to the duration of testosterone treatments. Molecular mechanisms on those changes would be clarified in the future.

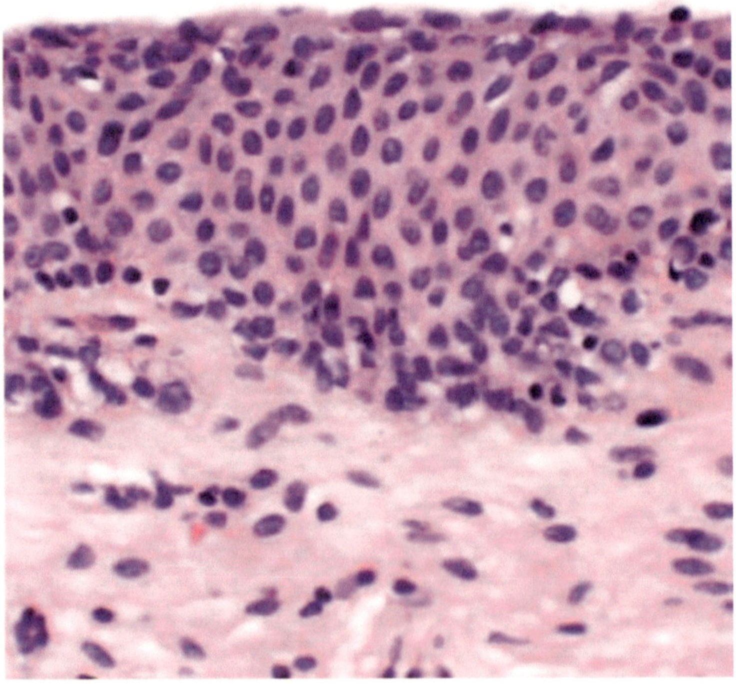

Fig. 1. Atrophied epithelium of exocervix (H-E, X400) (Kor J Fertil Steril 2005;32:325-330)

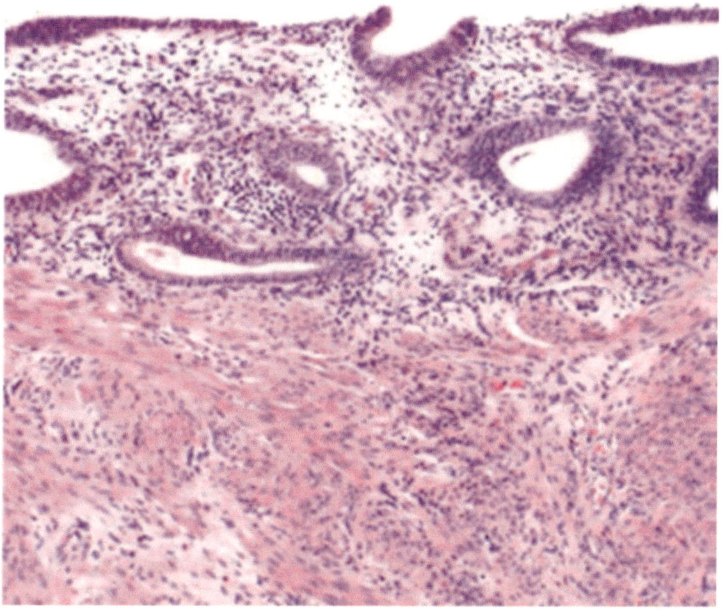

Fig. 2. Atrophy of endometrium (H-E, x200). (Kor J Fertil Steril 2005;32:325-330)

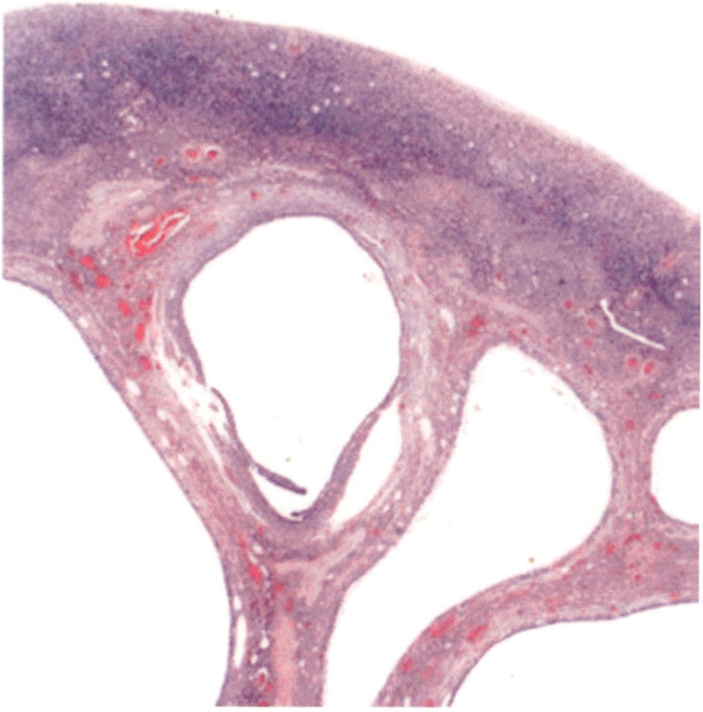

Fig. 3. Multiple cystic follicles in the ovarian cortex (H-E, X10) (Kor J Fertil Steril 2005;32:325-330)

7. Conclusions

The use of hormonal therapy in transsexualism is associated with appropriate physical change. Side effects in carefully monitored patients are usually few but are more likely to cause serious complications when therapy is too aggressive. This is particularly true in the FTM transsexual patients who are likely candidates for complications of dyslipoproteinemia which include premature atherogenesis, diabetes mellitus, hypertension, increased insulin resistance, and obesity. Investigators propose that initial treatment with androgen therapy which must be supraphysiological to suppress gonadotropins and virilize the patient should be kept to maximum of no more than 2 years. Following sex reassignment surgery, the dosage should be reduced by half in most patients.

It is likely to reduce not only the duration of large dosage androgen therapy but also the potential risk of endometrial hyperplasia and uterine carcinoma. The role of the concerned physician is to be fully aware of potential risk of this therapy so as to adjust treatment and minimize potential complications.

8. References

[1] Kaufman, D., & Maasdam, J. V. (2006). Surgery for gender identity disorder, Plastic surgery, 2nd ed. Philadelphia, PA: Sounders., 1305-1316.

[2] Moore, E., Wisniewski, A., & Dobs, A. (2003). Endocrine treatment of transsexual people: a review of treatment regimens, outcomes, and adverse effects. Journal of Clinical Endocrinology & Metabolism, 88, 3467-3473.

[3] Schlatterer, K., von Werder, K., & Stalla, G. K. (1996). Multistep treatment concept of transsexual patients. Experimental and Clinical Endocrinology and Diabetes, 104, 413-9.

[4] Kirk, S., & Rothblatt, M. (1995). Medical, legal and workplace issues for the transsexual. Watertown, MA: Together Lifeworks.

[5] Steinbeck, A. (1997). Hormonal medication for transsexuals. Venereology: Interdisciplinary, International Journal of Sexual Health, 10, 175-177.

[6] Tangpricha, V., Ducharme, S. H., Barber, T. W., & Chipkin, S. R. (2003). Endocrinologic treatment of gender identity disorders. Endocrine Practice, 9, 12-21.

[7] Bromham, D. & Pearson, R. (1996). The pharmacological treatment of transsexuals. British Journal of Sexual Medicine, 23(5) [no page numbers in file copy].

[8] Flaherty, C., Franicevich, J., Freeman, M., Klein, P., Kohler, L., Lusardi, C., Martinez, L., Monihan, M., Vormohr, J., & Zevin, B. (2001). Protocols for hormonal reassignment of gender. San Francisco: San Francisco Department of Public Health. Retrieved January 1, 2005, from http://www.dph.sf.ca.us/chn/HlthCtrs/HlthCtrDocs/TransGendprotocols.pdf

[9] Elbers, J. M. H., Asscheman, H., Seidell, J. C., & Gooren, L. J. G. (1999). Effects of sex steroid hormones on regional fat depots as assessed by magnetic resonance imaging in transsexuals. American Journal of Physiology, 276, E317-E325.

[10] Slabbekoorn, D., Van Goozen, S. H. M., Gooren, L. J. G., & Cohen-Kettenis, P. T. (2001). Effects of cross-sex hormone treatment on emotionality in transsexuals. International Journal of Transgenderism, 5. Retrieved January 1, 2005, from http://www.symposion.com/ijt/ijtvo05no03_02.htm

[11] Dimensions (2003). Informed consent for testostorone therapy for female-to-male transition. San Francisco, CA: Castro-Mission Health Center, San Francisco Department of Public Health. Retrieved January 1, 2005, from http://tghealth-critiques.tripod.com /consen2.htm
[12] The Gender Centre Inc. (2001). Testosterone hormone information II. Sydney, Australia: The Gender Centre Inc. Retrieved January 1, 2005, from http://www.gendercentre.org.au/testosterone_2.htm
[13] Van Borsel, J., De Cuypere, G., Rubens, R., & Destaerke, B. (2000). Voice problems in female-to-male transsexuals. International Journal of Language & Communication Disorders, 35, 427-442.
[14] Gooren, L. J. G. (n.d.). Transsexualism: Introduction and general aspects of treatment. Retrieved January 1, 2005, from http://www.xs4all.nl/~txtbreed/gender/gooren.html
[15] Meyer, W. J., III, Webb, A., Stuart, C. A., Finkelstein, J. W., Lawrence, B., & Walker, P. A. (1986). Physical and hormonal evaluation of transsexual patients: a longitudinal study. Archives of Sexual Behavior, 15, 121-138.
[16] Meyer, W. J., III, Finkelstein, J. W., Stuart, C. A., Webb, A., Smith, E. R., Payer, A. F., & Walker, P. A. (1981). Physical and hormonal evaluation of transsexual patients during hormonal therapy. Archives of Sexual Behavior, 10, 347-56.
[17] Miller, N., Bedard, Y. C., Cooter, N. B., & Shaul, D. L. (1986). Histological changes in the genital tract in transsexual women following androgen therapy. Histopathology, 10, 661-669.
[18] Futterweit, W. (1998). Endocrine therapy of transsexualism and potential complications of long-term treatment. Archives of Sexual Behavior, 27, 209-226.
[19] Israel, G. E, & Tarver, D. E. I. (1997). Transgender care: Recommended guidelines, practical information, and personal accounts. Philadephia, PA: Temple University Press.
[20] Feldman, J. & Bockting, W. O. (2003). Transgender health. Minnesota Medicine, 86, 25-32.
[21] Louis, J. G., Erik J. G., & Mathijs, C. B. (2008). Long-Term Treatment of Transsexuals with Cross-Sex Hormones: Extensive Personal Experience. J Clin Endocrinol Metab, 93, 19-25.
[22] Louis, G. (2005). Hormone Treatment of the Adult Transsexual Patient. Horm Res, 64(2), 31-36
[23] Vancouver Coastal Health, Transcend Transgender Support & Education Society, and the Canadian Rainbow Health Coalition. (2006). Endocrine therapy for transgender adults in British Columbia: Suggested guidelines. from http://transhealth.vch.ca
[24] Wilson, J., & Griffin, J. (1980). The use and misuse of androgens. Metabolism, 29, 1278–1295.
[25] Ammus, S. (1989) The role of androgens in the treatment of hematologic disorders. Adv Intern Med, 34, 191–208
[26] Nagelberg, S., Laue, L., Loriaux, L., Liu, L., & Sherins, R. (1986) Cerebrovascular accident associated with testosterone therapy in a 21-year-old hypogonadal man. N Engl J Med, 314, 649–650
[27] Futterweit, W. (1984) Clinical features of polycystic ovarian disease. In: Polycystic ovarian disease. New York: Springer-Verlag; 83–95

[28] Futterweit, W., Weiss, R., & Fagerstrom. (1986) Endocrine evaluation of forty female-to-male transsexual people: increased frequency of polycystic ovarian disease in female transsexualism. Arch Sex Behav, 15, 69–78.
[29] Balen. A., Schachter. M., Montgomery, D., Reid, R., & Jacobs, H. (1993) Polycystic ovaries are a common finding in untreated female to male transsexual people. Clin Endocrinol (Oxf) 38, 325–329.
[30] Futterweit. W., & Deligdisch, L. (1986) Histopathological effects of exogenously administered testosterone in 19 female to male transsexual people. J Clin Endocrinol Metab, 62, 16–21.
[31] Hage, J., Dekker, J., Karim. R., Verheijen, R., & Bloemena, Em. (2000) Ovarian cancer in female-to-male transsexual people: report of two cases. Gynecol Oncology, 76, 413–415.
[32] Michel, A., Mormont, C., & Legros, J. (2001). A psycho-endocrinological overview of transsexualism. Eur J Endocrinol, 145, 365–376.
[33] Leiter, E., Futterweit, W,, & Brown, G. (1993). In: Webster G, Kirby R, King L, Goldwasser B, eds. Reconstructive urology. Boston: Blackwell Scientific Publications; 23, 921–932
[34] Giudice LC. Elucidating endometrial function in the post-genomic era. Human Reproduction Update 2003;9: 223–235.
[35] Okon MA, Laird SM, Tuckerman EM, Li TC. Serum androgen levels in women who suffer recurrent miscarriage and their correlation with markers of endometrial function. Fertil Steril 1998;69:682–90.
[36] Tulppala M, Stenman UH, Cacciatore B, Ylikorkala O. Polycystic ovaries and levels of gonadotrophins and androgens in recurrent miscarriage: prospective study in 50 women. Br J Obstet Gynaecol 1993;100:348 –52.
[37] Cheung AP. Ultrasound and menstrual history in predicting endometrial hyperplasia in polycystic ovary syndrome. Obstetrics and Gynecology 2001; 98: 325–331.
[38] Miller N, Bedard YC, Cooter NB, Shaul DL. Histological changes in the genital tract in transsexual women following androgen therapy. Histopathology 1986; 10: 661-9.
[39] Byun JC, Kwak BG, Shin JH, Cha MS, Han MS, Rha SH, Kim SK. The Histologic Features of the Uterus and Adnexa Extirpated from Gender Identity Disorder Patients with Depot Androgen Injection. Kor J Fertil Steril 2005;32:325-330.

23

The Role of Prophylactic Oophorectomy in the Management of Hereditary Breast & Ovarian Cancer Syndrome

A.J. Lowery and K.J. Sweeney
Department of Surgery, National University of Ireland Galway, Ireland

1. Introduction

1.1 Historical perspective of prophylactic-oophorectomy in ovarian and breast cancers before the era of BRCA1/BRCA2 testing

Prophylactic salpingo-oophorectomy (PO) entails removal of the ovaries prior to the clinical occurrence of cancer. Prophylactic removal of the ovaries, during hysterectomy or other abdominal surgery, to prevent ovarian cancer in postmenopausal women was popularised in the 1940s by Crossen, who stated *"the involuting ovaries have fulfilled their reproductive and endocrine function. They are....vestigial structures which carry a special tendency to cancer"* (Crossen, 1942). The first report of prophylactic oophorectomy for familial ovarian cancer was in 1950 when A.M Liber described a family of five sisters and their mother, all with histologically confirmed papillary adenocarcinoma of the ovary; it was recommended that family members should undergo frequent gynaecologic screening, and that prophylactic oophorectomy should be considered (Liber, 1950)

The role of oophorectomy in the management of breast cancer dates further back to 1889 when it was first proposed by Albert Schinzinger (Schinzinger, 1889); he observed that the prognosis for breast cancer appeared better in older women than younger women and postulated that oophorectomy would initiate atrophy of the breast and any cancer within the breast. Shinzinger suggested oophorectomy both as therapy for advanced breast cancer and prophylaxis against local recurrence, but he never actually performed the surgery; it was George Thomas Beatson who first performed a bilateral oophorectomy on a patient with metastatic breast cancer in 1895 , this was reported in the Lancet in 1896 (Beatson, 1896). A subsequent report detailed that this patient experienced remission of her disease and lived another four years. Beatson hypothesized that oophorectomy caused fatty degeneration of the malignant cells accounting for its beneficial effect in breast cancer (Beatson, 1896; Thomson, 1902). An English surgeon, Stanley Boyd performed the first oophorectomy as adjuvant breast cancer therapy in 1897 (Boyd, 1897). He commented "my working hypothesis is that internal secretion of the ovaries in some cases favors the growth of the cancer" and subsequently reported that that one third of breast cancer patients benefited from oophorectomy as adjuvant therapy (Boyd, 1900), in this way the rationale for hormonal treatment of breast cancer was first implied. In 1968 Feinleib observed that premenopausal oophorectomy decreased the rate of subsequent breast cancer (Feinleib, 1968) however it was a further twenty years before Brinton proposed the potential of oophorectomy as a breast cancer *prevention* strategy, reporting that women, with a family history of breast cancer, who underwent oophorectomy before the age of 40 years had a 45% reduction in breast cancer risk compared with women who underwent natural menopause (Brinton et al, 1988). Meijer and van Lindert similarly reported that surgery performed before the age of natural menopause significantly reduced breast cancer risk (Meijer & van Lindert, 1992). These studies commented on patients with a family history of breast cancer, introducing the role of prophylactic salpingo-oophorectomy (PSO) as a risk reducing strategy in hereditary breast cancer. At this time the genetic etiologic association between breast and ovarian cancer was also being investigated; first put forward by Henry Lynch who collected pedigrees and samples from high risk breast and/or ovarian cancer families showing autosomal dominant inheritance patterns for breast cancer in the late 1960s (Lynch et al, 1972), and identifying HBOC families long before the discovery of breast cancer susceptibility genes. In the past two decades however, since the identification of increased genetic susceptibility to breast and ovarian cancer, in particular the BRCA1 and BRCA2 genetic mutations, the role of prophylactic oophorectomy has become more clearly defined, particularly in the setting of HBOC.

2. Identification of HBOC associated mutations and risks of breast and ovarian cancer

In the early nineties, the first breast cancer susceptibility gene – BRCA1 (Miki et al, 1994) and the second BRCA2 (Wooster et al, 1995) were identified as the cause of genetic predisposition in hereditary breast and ovarian cancer. This milestone in breast and ovarian cancer research was one of the most significant cancer discoveries of the twentieth century, both in terms of scientific impact and public interest. These breakthroughs were the culmination of five years of focused work based on the report in 1990 by Marie Claire King's group who undertook segregation analyses on breast cancer pedigrees and mapped a predisposing gene for both breast and ovarian cancer to chromosome 17q (Hall et al, 1990). Following this report a collaboration of international groups, termed "The Breast Cancer Linkage Consortium" further specified the site of the BRCA1 locus by linkage analysis (Easton et al, 1993). The 1994 report from Miki *et al* outlined the exact structure of the BRCA1 gene which had been determined by a team of scientists at the University of Utah using positional cloning techniques (Miki et al, 1994). The second predisposition gene, BRCA2 was mapped to chromosome 13 and reported by Wooster *et al* in the UK (Wooster et al, 1994; 1995).

At a molecular level, BRCA1 is a 100kb gene located on chromosome 17q21.1. It consists of 24 exons, 22 of which encode for a 1863 amino-acid nucleoprotein. BRCA2 is an even larger gene composed of 27 exons distributed over 70kb of genomic DNA on chromosome 13q12–q13, and enocoding for a protein of 3418 amino acids. The complete repertoire of function of the BRCA1 and BRCA2 proteins has not yet been determined, however several functions have been uncovered; both proteins are integral to the DNA damage response pathway and facilitate DNA damage repair through homologous recombination. BRCA1 also plays a role in cell-cycle control, gene expression control, protein ubiquination and chromatin remodelling (Aiyar et al, 2007; Foulkes 2010; Huen et al, 2010; Ma et al, 2010). In cells which are deficient in BRCA1 or BRCA2, double-strand breaks may be repaired in an erroneous manner (non-homologous end-joining), which may lead to chromosomal rearrangements. The resultant chromosomal instability is a key feature of carcinogenesis. BRCA1 and BRCA2 are classified as tumour suppressor genes, and since their discovery, hundreds of different mutations have been reported in these genes. The prevalence of BRCA mutations in most European and North American countries is reported as 0.06 - 0.24% (Malone et al, 2006; Whittemore et al, 1997 & 2004). However there are specific populations in which the frequency of mutations are higher due to strong founder effect; these include ethnic and geographic populations worldwide including those of Norwegian, Dutch and Icelandic descent (Neuhausen et al, 2009). The Ashkenazi Jewish population is perhaps the best characterised example; three specific mutations; 185delAG and 5382insC in the BRCA1 gene, and 6174delT in BRCA2 are the most common mutations in this population and have been found to occur with frequencies of 2-2.5% which is at least five times that of the general population (Ferla et al, 2007; Neuhausen et al, 2009; Struewing et al, 1997; Warner et al, 1999), thus endowing this population with a significantly increased risk of breast and ovarian cancer.

The risk of breast and ovarian cancer in the general population is 10-13% and 1.7% respectively. This risk is significantly elevated in women carrying mutations of the BRCA1 or BRCA2 genes. BRCA1 and BRCA2 mutation carriers have a 54-85% and 45% lifetime risk of developing breast cancer, respectively and an 18-60% and 11-27% lifetime risk of developing ovarian cancer (Antoniou et al, 2003; Easton et al, 1995; King et al, 2003). Furthermore, BRCA1 mutation carriers are at increased risk for fallopian tube carcinoma (Paley et al, 2001; Zweemer et al, 2000), primary peritoneal carcinoma (Levine et al, 2003; Olivier et al, 2004), and uterine serous papillary carcinoma (Biron-shental et al, 2006). BRCA2 mutations are also associated with increased risk for a variety of other cancers including melanoma, pancreas, bone, hepatobiliary and pharyngeal cancer (Breast Cancer Linkage Consortium, 1999). Both BRCA1 and BRCA2 are associated with an increased risk of male breast cancer (Tai et al, 2007) and early onset prostate cancer (Agalliu et al, 2009; Mitra et al, 2008).

It is important to note that the breast and ovarian cancers in patients with a BRCA mutation exhibit phenotypic characteristics that are distinct from sporadic cancers, a fact that may have implications for local and systemic treatment. The ovarian cancers in families with BRCA mutations are predominantly histologically serous adenocarcinomas frequently exhibiting papillary changes; epithelial ovarian adenocarcinomas that occur in patients with transmitted germ-line BRCA1 mutations are characteristically high-grade with underpresentation of mucinous or borderline tumours (Kurian et al, 2005; Chiaffarino et al, 2007). Hereditary breast cancers due to BRCA mutations occur at a much younger age than sporadic cancers, and are more likely to be multi-focal and bilateral. BRCA 1 and BRCA2 related breast cancers however, have a distinct morphologic and molecular signature (Bane et al, 2007; Foulkes et al, 2003). The breast cancers that develop in BRCA2 gene mutation carriers are similar to sporadic breast cancers, they are more likely to exhibit the luminal phenotype of breast cancer and express the oestrogen receptor. Conversely, the breast cancers associated with BRCA1 mutation usually exhibit a distinct basal phenotype (Foulkes et al, 2003) characterised by lack of estrogen, progesterone and HER2/neu receptors and abundant expression of basal-type cytokeratins. The basal subtype of breast cancer is an aggressive form of tumour associated with increased metastatic potential and decreased overall survival (Billar et al, 2010; Dent et al, 2007) ; the poor prognosis and high recurrence rate of these tumours has raised the question of whether BRCA1 breast cancers have a poorer outcome than sporadic breast cancers. The evidence supports an increased risk for contralateral breast cancer, but the data assessing local recurrence are inconsistent and overall survival appears to be similar (Liebens et al, 2007; Brekelmans et al, 2007). Breast conserving therapy should be employed with caution in women with hereditary BRCA related breast cancer in view of the increased likelihood of multicentricity and contralateral breast cancer.

3. Risk reducing effect of PSO on ovarian & breast cancer

Prophylactic salpingo-oophorectomy has been shown to decrease the risk of both breast cancer and ovarian cancer in BRCA1 and BRCA 2 mutation carriers (Domchek et al, 2006, 2010 ; Eisen et al, 2005; Finch et al, 2006; Kauff et al, 2002, 2008 ; Kramer et al, 2005; Rebbeck et al, 1999, 2002, 2009 ; Rutter et al, 2003) This evidence is predominantly based on the results of observational case control and cohort studies. There are no randomised clinical trials of PSO and these may not be feasible or ethically appropriate (Klaren et al, 2003). Rebbeck and colleagues were among the first to provide evidence of the risk reducing effect of PSO in BRCA mutation carriers; in 1999 they reported a 47% decreased risk of breast cancer in a series of 43 women with a BRCA1 mutation who underwent PSO compared to 79 matched controls who did not undergo PSO (Rebbeck et al, 1999). The findings from this relatively small series were enough to trigger a number of larger series, investigating health outcomes following PSO in patients with known BRCA mutations, in an effort to establish whether this risk-reducing effect was significant enough to incorporate PSO into routine clinical practice as a cancer prevention strategy.

3.1 Ovarian cancer reduction

In 2002, Rebbeck reported ovarian cancer incidence in a larger series of 551 BRCA mutation carriers, 259 who underwent PSO and 292 who did not (Rebbeck et al, 2002). After 8 years follow-up the risk of coelomic epithelial cancer was significantly reduced by 96% in the patients who had undergone prophylactic oophorectomy (HR=0.04, 95% CI 0.01-0.16). In the same issue of the New England Journal of Medicine, Kauff et al published their results from the first prospective series of 173 BRCA mutation carriers, of whom 101 underwent PSO (Kauff et al, 2002). In this series, PSO was associated with an 85% reduction in subsequent ovarian cancer. These findings have been substantiated in a number of subsequent series; in a prospective study of 1828 BRCA mutation carriers Finch *et al* reported a significantly lower ovarian cancer risk after PSO (HR 0.2, 95% CI 0.07-0.58) (Finch et al, 2006). A prospective multicentre study of 1079 BRCA mutation carriers demonstrated that PSO significantly reduced the risk of BRCA1 associated gynaecologic cancer risk (HR 0.15, 95% CI 0.04-0.56), however this reduction was not observed in patients with a BRCA2 mutation (Kauff et al, 2008). In 2009 a meta-analysis of the published literature, including 10 studies, was performed to assess the magnitude of the risk reduction effect (Rebbeck et al, 2009), the results of which showed an 80% reduction in ovarian/fallopian tube cancer risk associated with PSO in women carrying a BRCA1 or BRCA2 mutation.

The efficacy of prophylactic oophorectomy for reduction of ovarian cancer risk is somewhat compromised by the residual risk of papillary serous carcinoma of the peritoneum; this refers to diffuse involvement of the peritoneal surfaces with a neoplasm bearing all the histological characteristics of papillary serous carcinoma of the ovary which can occur even after oophorectomy. This phenomenon was initially reported by Tobacman who reported an adenocacinoma indistinguishable from ovarian cancer after oophorectomy in women with a strong family history of ovarian cancer (Tobacman et al, 1982). The source of this extra-ovarian malignancy may be any of the following; microscopic foci of residual ovary, pre-existing carcinomatosis not detected at the time of prophylactic surgery, or multifocal origin of peritoneal tissue which shares a common embryonic origin with mullerian duct epithelium. The reported incidence of papillary serous adenocarcinoma in BRCA mutation carriers following PSO is 4.3% (Finch et al, 2006) and women should be counselled regarding this risk when making a decision regarding PSO.

3.2 Breast cancer reduction

The reduction in breast cancer risk associated with PSO in BRCA mutation carriers is approximately 50%. In the 2002 report from Rebbeck et al the incidence of breast cancer in patients who underwent PSO was 21.1% compared to 42.3 % in those who did not (Rebbeck et al, 2002). Kauff et al reported an even greater risk reduction of 68% in subsequent breast cancer for BRCA mutation carriers who underwent PSO (Kauff et al, 2002), they subsequently reported a 72% reduction in BRCA2 associated breast cancer risk following PSO, but no statistically significant reduction in BRCA1 associated breast cancer (Kauff et al, 2008). In a case control study of over 3,000 patients, Eisen et al reported a reduction in breast cancer risk of 56% in the BRCA1 mutation carriers, and 46% in the BRCA2 mutation carriers who underwent PSO (n=166) (Eisen et al, 2005). Kramer et al prospectively evaluated the risk of breast cancer in 98 patients with, and 353 without BRCA1 mutations, and found that among BRCA1 mutation carriers oophorectomy was associated with a 62% reduction in breast cancer risk (Kramer et al, 2005). In the 2009 meta-analysis performed by Rebbeck et al, PSO was associated with a statistically significant reduction in breast cancer risk of approximately 50% for both BRCA1 (HR 0.47, 95% CI 0.35-0.64) and BRCA2 (HR 0.47, 95% CI 0.26-0.84) mutation carriers (Rebbeck et al, 2009). Some of the prospective studies included in this meta-analysis had suggested that there may be a difference in risk reduction between BRCA1 and BRCA2 carriers depending on the specific mutation (Kramer et al, 2005, Kauff et al, 2008), however the data in retrospective series was inconsistent and insufficient to provide any definitive evidence in this regard. Thus, it was confirmed that there is a reduction in both ovarian and breast cancer risk following PSO in BRCA mutation carriers, but questions regarding the differential magnitude of risk reduction according to clinical variables such as the specific BRCA mutation (i.e. BRCA1 or BRCA2), or other factors in the patients clinical history.

It was with these questions in mind that Domcheck and colleagues prospectively analysed the largest cohort to date of BRCA mutation carriers, reporting risk reduction after PSO considering a number of different scenarios (Domcheck, 2010). The authors prospectively followed 2, 482 women with BRCA mutations identified between 1974 and 2008. The median follow up for patients who underwent prophylactic surgery was 3.65 years, and 4.29 years in those who did not opt for prophylactic surgery. A total of 993 women underwent PSO; of these 1.1% were subsequently diagnosed with ovarian cancer, 11.4% were subsequently diagnosed with breast cancer and the all cause mortality was 3%. This represents a significant reduction when compared with women who did not undergo PSO, of whom 5.8% were diagnosed with ovarian cancer, 19.2% were diagnosed with breast cancer, and all cause mortality was 9.8%. These findings again confirmed the risk reducing effect of PSO in both breast and ovarian cancer. In this series, however a previous diagnosis of breast cancer was accounted for and it was found that the risk of ovarian cancer was reduced in BRCA mutation carriers with and without a history of breast cancer. However, the risk of breast cancer was reduced following PSO in those without prior breast cancer, but PSO had no effect on the risk of developing a second primary breast cancer in patients who had a previous breast cancer diagnosis. This is an interesting finding and may relate to the fact that patients who have previously been treated for breast cancer with cytotoxic chemotherapeutic agents inducing a menopausal state derive no further benefit from oophorectomy. Unfortunately this series was limited by insufficient adjuvant therapy data and this question may be further addressed in future prospective series. Another interesting finding in this series was the difference in breast cancer risk reduction following PSO in BRCA2 mutation carriers (64%) compared to BRCA1 mutation carriers (37%), which had previously been reported in smaller prospective studies (Kauff et al, 2008). It is possible that this difference relates to the distinction in breast cancer phenotype exhibited in BRCA1 and BRCA2 mutation carriers. In the BRCA2 cohort there is a high proportion of ER-positive breast tumours and it has been hypothesized that PSO may actually "treat" subclinical breast tumours present at the time of oophorectomy (Rebbeck et al, 2009). Such a treatment effect would not be evident in BRCA1 tumours which are predominantly ER-negative. The "protective" effect of PSO may take longer to become evident, thus a longer follow up time in addition to mechanistic studies may be required to definitively answer this question.

In conclusion, PSO has been proven to be associated with a reduction in ovarian cancer risk of approximately 80% and a reduction in breast cancer risk of approximately 50%, with the most recent analyses suggesting that the risk reducing effect may be more pronounced in BRCA2 mutation carriers (Domchek, 2010). Despite the uncertainties that remain to be addressed regarding the extent of risk reduction according to specific clinical variables, the evidence has sufficiently demonstrated a reduction in breast and ovarian cancer risk following PSO in patients with BRCA1 and BRCA2 mutations, that the National Comprehensive Cancer Network (NCCN) has incorporated this strategy into guidelines for recommended management of individuals carrying a BRCA mutation. These guidelines are as follows:

- Self-breast examination monthly starting at age 18 years
- Clinical breast examination semi-annually starting at age 25 years
- Annual mammogram and breast MRI starting at age 25 years or based on earliest age of onset in family
- Prophylactic oopherectomy between ages 35 and 40 years or upon completion of childbearing
- For individuals not electing a prophylactic oophorectomy, concurrent transvaginal ultrasound and CA125 levels semi-annually starting at age 35 years or 5-10 earlier than the first diagnosed case of ovarian cancer in the family
- Consider chemoprevention options (e.g tamoxifen)
- Consider research studies testing investigational imaging and screening options.

Clearly, such recommendations are meant to lower the woman's risk or identify a cancer as early as possible in the development of the disease. While PSO is an acceptable risk reduction strategy for many BRCA1/BRCA2 mutation carriers, the decision to undergo prophylactic surgery is a complex one, and there are a number of considerations which should be taken into account and discussed with patients during the decision making process.

4. Practical considerations: Timing & approach to surgery

4.1 Timing of PSO

As evidence supporting a risk reducing role for PSO in BRCA1 and BRCA2 mutation carriers accumulates, the clinical management of cancer risk in these patients remains complex and multifactorial; one issue that remains incompletely resolved is the optimum timing of PSO. Eisen *et al* reported improved risk reduction in BRCA mutation carriers who underwent PSO before the age of 50 years compared to those older than 50 years at the time of surgery (Eisen et al, 2005). These findings are supported by results from Domchek's series in which there was a reduction in breast cancer risk in patients who underwent PSO before the age of 50 years, but no significant reduction in women over 50 years of age. These studies are limited by small numbers in subgroup analyses and a limited follow-up time, leaving this question incompletely addressed by the currently available data. As outlined above, the current recommendations from the NCCN is that prophylactic oophorectomy should be offered to patients between the ages of 35 and 40 years, or when the woman has finished childbearing. The risk-reduction benefit of oophorectomy must be balanced against the side effects and potential morbidity associated with early menopause. This is highlighted by evidence suggesting that PSO in women under the age of 45 years is associated with increased mortality, particularly in patients who do not receive hormone replacement therapy (HRT) (Rocca et al, 2006). Women with a BRCA mutation have a unique risk and benefit profile which must be considered when making recommendations regarding the use of HRT following PSO in the premenopausal age-group. HRT is the most effective strategy for the management of postmenopausal symptoms and sequelae such as osteoporosis and cardiovascular risk in young females undergoing abrupt menopause through PSO. However, its use in patients with an increased risk of breast cancer has been questioned since the publication of Women's Health Initiative studies which provided evidence of a breast cancer risk associated with combined oestrogen and progestin hormone replacement therapy (Beral et al, 2003; Rossouw et al, 2002).

The PROSE study group in a prospective multicentre study of 462 patients with BRCA mutation found that the breast cancer risk reduction/protective effect attained following PSO was not significantly changed by the use of HRT (Rebbeck et al, 2005). Similarly, Eisen et al observed no increased risk of breast cancer associated with HRT use in patients following PSO (Eisen et al, 2005). Armstrong et al developed a Markov decision analytical model to calculate the impact of prophylactic oophorectomy and HRT use on breast and ovarian cancer risk, cardiac disease, osteoporosis and venous thrombosis (Armstrong et al, 2004). This model predicted that BRCA mutation carriers undergoing PSO between the ages of 30 and 40 years would obtain a significant gain in life expectancy irrespective of HRT use. However, this gain in life is predicted to decrease as the age at time of PSO increases. The short term use of HRT does not appear to increase breast cancer risk, and should be considered in young patients to alleviate menopausal symptoms which may interfere with quality of life. In high-risk patients carrying a BRCA mutation, estrogen-only HRT is preferable.

4.2 Surgical approach

The extent of gynaecologic surgery in patients with BRCA1/2 mutations has been the subject of debate in view of the risk of proximal fallopian tube malignancy and subsequent peritoneal cancer of ovarian origin in patients post oophorectomy. For risk-reducing surgery to be successful all of the "at risk" tissue should be removed. It is essential that the fallopian tube is resected as close as possible to the uterine cornua to prevent the occurrence of proximal fallopian tube malignancy. Indeed the risk of proximal fallopian tube malignancy in the uterine fundus and the low risk of uterine papillary carcinoma in BRCA1/BRCA2 mutation carriers raises the question of whether these patients should undergo concomitant hysterectomy as part of risk reducing surgery (Biron-Shental et al, 2006; Hornreich et al, 1999; Paley et al, 2001). Removal of the entire fallopian tube can be optimally accomplished by performing a hysterectomy but the majority (92%) of fallopian tube malignancies occur in the mid and distal portions of the tube (Alvarado-Cabrero et al, 1999) thus there is little evidence to support systematic hysterectomy at the time of PSO on this basis. However there are other factors which may influence decisions regarding whether hysterectomy is performed at the time of salpingo-oophorectomy in BRCA1/2 mutation carriers:

HRT use: Post-PSO HRT does not appear to increase the risk of cancer in premenopausal women who undergo PSO (Rebbeck et al, 2005). However, unopposed oestrogen does pose a substantial risk of uterine cancer while combined HRT has been shown in the Women's Health Initiative studies to increase the risk of breast cancer (Beral et al, 2003; Grady et al, 1995; Rossouw et al, 2002). Hysterectomy at the time of PSO would negate the uterine cancer risk facilitating the use of unopposed oestrogen as HRT in these patients.

Tamoxifen chemoprevention: Tamoxifen is a selective oestrogen receptor modulator (SERM) which is routinely used as adjuvant therapy in women with estrogen receptor positive breast cancer to prevent the development of cancer in the contralateral breast and to prolong disease free survival (Osborne, 1998). Tamoxifen has also been shown to reduce the risk of developing cancer in high risk women without prior breast cancer and can be used as a chemoprevention strategy in these patients to reduce the risk of invasive ER positive breast cancer (Visvanathan et al, 2009). Regarding BRCA1/BRCA2 mutation carriers specifically, tamoxifen use has been shown to reduce the incidence of contralateral breast cancer in BRCA mutation carriers with a prior history of breast cancer (Metcalfe et al, 2004; Narod et al, 2000). The protective effect of tamoxifen in BRCA mutation carriers without prior breast cancer has been less well defined and the available evidence is extrapolated from subset analyses of large randomised trials evaluating the efficacy of chemoprevention for breast cancer in the general population. A subgroup analysis of the NSABP-P1 data (King et al, 2001) was performed; only 19 of the 288 women who developed breast cancer had BRCA1 or BRCA2 mutations, and tamoxifen use did not appear to have a significant effect on breast cancer risk in these patients. In a review of the evidence regarding Tamoxifen use as chemoprevention in patients with a BRCA mutation, the ASCO panel concluded that the "limited evidence precludes reliable evidence of Tamoxifen effects in this setting". However as it has a proven risk reduction benefit in BRCA patients with a history of breast cancer and in women with an increased risk of breast cancer, Tamoxifen is frequently offered as chemoprevention to BRCA mutation carriers who do not choose to undergo prophylactic mastectomy (Eisen & Weber, 2001). Risks and side effects must be considered when proposing Tamoxifen as a chemopreventive strategy, and consist predominantly of vascular, thromboembolic and neoplastic events. Tamoxifen use has been shown to be associated with an increased risk of uterine malignancy, including early stage adenocarcinomas , endometriod, mucinous, clear cell and uterine sarcomas. A meta-analysis of the breast cancer prevention trials reported more than doubling of uterine cancer with tamoxifen use (Cuzick et al, 2003). This is a risk of malignancy that would be negated if the patient underwent concomitant hysterectomy at the time of PSO.

Surgical Approach: Laparoscopy has become the most commonly used approach to PSO as it offers many advantages in improved visualisation of the pelvic peritoneum, avoidance of a large abdominal incision, shorter hospital stay, decreased post-operative pain and a rapid recovery time (Hidlebaugh et al, 1996; Leetanaporn & Tintara, 1996). Traditionally, a total abdominal hysterectomy (TAH) and PSO has been associated with a higher morbidity and longer recovery time when compared with laparoscopic PSO, a factor which may influence the decision to undergo concomitant hysterectomy. However, the last decade has seen an increase in the laparoscopic approach to hysterectomy which has been successfully employed for endometrial and cervical malignancy with comparable surgical and oncologic outcomes to laparotomy (Cho et al, 2007; Eltabbakh et al, 2000). Laparoscopic vaginal hysterectomy combined with laparoscopic PSO is a feasible minimally invasive approach to risk reducing surgery in patients with BRCA1/2 mutations (Casey et al, 1998; Eltabbakh et al, 1999). Recent advances have seen the development of an even less invasive approach to laparoscopic surgery known as laparoendoscopic single-site surgery (LESS). This approach uses a single port which accommodates the camera and operating instruments, needing only a single incision (Canes et al, 2008). This approach to gynaecologic surgery has been pioneered by Escobar and colleagues in the Cleveland Clinic who have reported its use in benign and malignant gynaecologic conditions (Escobar et al, 2009 & 2010; Fader et al, 2009). This group have recently reported on a retrospective series of 58 patients at high risk for breast/ovarian cancer who underwent LESS PSO with (n=13) and without (n=45) hysterectomy (Escobar et al, 2010). All cases were performed successfully with LESS in a mean operative time of 38 minutes (35minutes without hysterectomy and 42 minutes with hysterectomy), and there were no surgical complications. The majority of patients had this procedure performed as day case surgery. Although larger prospective studies are required to validate these results, this single - port laparoscopic approach represents an advance in minimally invasive gynaecologic surgery that may become an attractive option for BRCA mutation carriers and breast cancer patients due to the favourable cosmetic outcome and rapid recovery time.

As outlined, there are a number of considerations which must be taken into account when planning and counselling a patient for PSO. The timing of surgery, surgical approach, use of HRT and the risks and benefits of hysterectomy at the time of PSO should all be discussed with patients on an individual basis to aid the decision making process.

5. Morbidity associated with prophylactic oophorectomy and issues of regret

Despite the lack of evidence that ovarian cancer screening is effective in reducing the risk of developing ovarian cancer or in reducing the risk of death from ovarian cancer (Stirling et al, 2005; Olivier et al, 2006), the uptake of PSO in BRCA1/2 mutation carriers is variable across published datasets.

Patients considering PSO are faced with complex information regarding cancer risk and the risk/benefit profile of prophylactic surgery including factors such as surgical risk, hormonal deprivation and residual cancer risk. It is important that patients are supported in processing this information in order to help them make the best individual decision. Numerous variables have been identified as factors in this decision making process. Demographically older women, women with children and married women are more likely to opt for PSO (Madalinska et al, 2007; Miller et al, 2010), an association which is not unsurprising as this cohort of women may have completed their childbearing and may not have to deal with the sudden severe menopausal symptoms that are associated with surgical menopause in younger women. Interestingly, a lower level of education is also associated with an increased likelihood to opt for PSO. Proposed explanations for this are that such patients may be more inclined to follow a gynaecologists recommendation for surgery without seeking alternative options, or that they may prefer a more definitive solution (surgery) to regain a sense of control (Hallowell et al, 2004; Madalinska et al, 2007; Miller et al, 2010). Clinical predictors of PSO include a family history of ovarian cancer and a personal history of breast cancer (Miller et al, 2010). The most consistent psychosocial predictor of PSO uptake is the patients perception of their own health and the risk of ovarian cancer; patients who perceive their own health as poor, patients who overestimate their ovarian cancer risk and those who view ovarian cancer as an incurable disease are more likely to opt for PSO as a risk reducing strategy (Miller et al, 2010). Importantly, a physician/gynaecologists recommendation is a powerful determinant of PSO uptake (Madalinska et al, 2007) and it has been reported that failure to discuss this option with the patient may be perceived as a recommendation against this strategy (Madalinska et al, 2007; Tiller et al, 2002). Ideally, all patients with a BRCA1/2 mutation should be offered comprehensive counselling regarding the risks of breast and ovarian cancer and the surveillance and risk-reducing strategies which may be undertaken.

In the course of such counselling, it is also important that the side-effects and potential outcomes of risk reducing surgery be discussed; surgical risk, residual cancer risk and the effects of hormonal deprivation should all be clearly explained to every patient considering risk reducing surgery. It is crucial to consider the impact of this surgery on premenopausal women in particular; the effect of menopausal symptoms, cognitive changes, loss of fertility, osteoporosis, heart disease, vasomotor symptoms, urogenital symptoms and the effect on sexuality and body image are all important factors that the patient should be aware of prior to surgery (Taylor, 2001). Qualitiative studies indicate that post surgery, the majority of women are satisfied with their decision to undergo PSO (Miller et al, 2010). There are a number of positive quality of life changes reported following PSO including a reduced perception of ovarian cancer risk, reduced anxiety levels and an increased sense of control over ones' health (Elit et al, 2001; Miller et al, 2010; Robson et al, 2003; Tiller et al, 2002). The majority of patients do report side effects related to hormonal deprivation, including hot flushes, vaginal dryness, decreased sexual interest and decreased sexual pleasure. These symptoms are most common in younger women (Miller et al, 2010; Robson et al, 2003). There is conflicting evidence regarding the level of patients satisfaction with pre-operative counselling with some women reporting that they were fully informed and others feeling that they could have been provided with more information, particularly regarding the option to use HRT post PSO (Hallowell et al, 2004; Miller et al, 2010). Campfield-Bonadies et al recently reported the results of a questionnaire based study of BRCA carriers who had undergone PSO regarding their post-operative symptoms, their recollection of pre-operative counselling, and what information they would have found helpful to have prior to surgery (Campfield-Bonadies et al, 2011). It was found that most patients were counselled pre-operatively regarding the impact of PSO on ovarian and breast cancer risk, the pros and cons of surgical approaches and the impact of surgery on menopause, however the most common surgical symptoms were vaginal dryness, changes in libido and sleep disturbances and the majority of women would have found it helpful to have more information regarding the impact of PSO on their sex life, the availability of sex counselling and the risk of coronary heart disease, which were not commonly discussed during pre-operative counselling. Despite this, the overall satisfaction with PSO remains high in this cohort of patients (Miller et al, 2010)

6. Alternatives to surgery – Surveillance & chemoprevention

Not all women who are diagnosed with a BRCA1/2 mutation will opt for PSO. Younger women who have not completed childbearing and wish to maintain fertility may seek alternative strategies to minimise risk or expedite diagnosis of a potential ovarian or breast cancer to improve survival.

The alternative options to risk reducing surgery for these women are: surveillance or chemoprevention.

6.1 Surveillance

Breast cancer surveillance

The goal of surveillance is early detection of cancer. In the case of breast cancer, this involves:

- Regular (monthly) self breast examination from age 18 years
- Annual or semi-annual clinical breast examination
- Annual mammography beginning at age 30 years
- Annual breast MRI beginning at age 30 years (Robson & Offit, 2007; Saslow et al, 2007)

The sensitivity of mammography to detect malignancy in women with a genetic predisposition to breast cancer is approximately 33%, MRI increases this to approximately 80%. Surveillance with alternating mammography and MRI six monthly has a sensitivity of 95% for the detection of breast cancer (Warner et al, 2001 & 2004).

Ovarian cancer surveillance

Screening for the early detection of ovarian cancer involves:

- Annual or semi-annual transvaginal pelvic ultrasonography from age 35 years or at 5 years younger than the earliest ovarian cancer diagnosis in the family
- Annual CA-125 testing (NCCN, 2007)

The advantages of surveillance are the fact that it is non-invasive, has no effect on fertility or childbearing, and leaves the other options for risk reduction available to the patient should she choose them at any time (eg. when finished childbearing). However there are disadvantages, the most obvious being that there is no reduction in cancer risk for these patients, and in the case of ovarian cancer, there is no evidence that the recommended surveillance strategies even reduce cancer-related mortality. Furthermore, there is an inherent level of anxiety associated with surveillance and both breast MRI and pelvic USS can yield false positives which increase this anxiety (Spiegel et al, 2011). It has been recommended that women opting for surveillance should be provided with professional psychosocial support when necessary (Warner, 2011).

6.2 Chemoprevention

The development of effective prevention strategies for breast and ovarian cancers is predominantly based on hormonal responsiveness. As discussed above, selective oestrogen receptor modulators (SERMS) have emerged as the first class of therapeutic agents in breast cancer chemoprevention trials (Fisher et al, 1998; Vogel et al, 2010). However, their efficacy in reducing breast cancer risk in BRCA1/2 mutation carriers is unclear, and questionable in BRCA1 carriers in whom breast cancers are predominantly ER negative. The potential of the aromatase inhibitor exemestane as a chemopreventive agent has been evaluated in a randomized, placebo-controlled, double-blind trial in 4560 women at high risk of breast cancer (Goss et al, 2011). There was a with a 65% relative reduction in the annual incidence of invasive breast cancer in the exemestane group indicating that this agent may have a role to play in breast cancer chemoprevention. There is no data to date regarding the protective effect of aromatase inhibitors in patients with BRCA1/2 mutations, but again it is doubtful that there will be a significant benefit in BRCA1 patients at risk of developing ER negative breast cancers. In the event that SERMs or aromatase inhibitors are deemed effective as chemoprevention for BRCA1/2 mutation carriers their benefit must be weighed against the side effect profiles including an increased risk of endometrial cancer with tamoxifen and the potential for thromboembolic events.

The oral contraceptive pill (OCP) has been shown to be effective in reducing epithelial ovarian cancer risk by 40-50% (McLaughlin et al, 2007; Narod et al, 2001). This strategy is well tolerated and inexpensive however OCP use also increases the risk of thromboembolic events and is associated with a slightly increased risk of breast cancer in BRCA mutation carriers if used for more than 5 years (Milne et al, 2005).

Translational research in breast cancer is largely focused on the development of targeted therapy. In addition to targeting the oestrogen pathway, researchers are continually investigating novel approaches to preventive therapy for breast cancer. Agents which have shown promise in breast cancer risk reduction include: non-steroidal anti-inflammatory drugs (NSAIDS) (Harris et al, 2003), bisphosphonates (Chlebowski et al, 2010; Rennert et al, 2010) and metformin (Bodmer et al, 2010; Bosco et al, 2011). The data to date however is all observational and prospective trials are underway to confirm a protective effect before these agents can be considered or recommended for clinical use (Cuzick et al, 2011). In the context of BRCA mutation carriers, the investigation of novel strategies to target ER negative breast cancers is most likely to yield a potentially effective agent. Perhaps the most promising agents under investigation at present are the poly-ADP ribose polymerase (PARP) inhibitors which induce synthetic lethality in homozygous BRCA-deficient cells. Recent reports of phase II trials have shown efficacy and tolerability for PARPs, or poly ADP (adenosine diphosphate)-ribose polymerase inhibitors, in BRCA mutation carriers with advanced breast and ovarian cancers (Audeh et al, 2010; Tutt et al, 2010), and BRCA1/2 mutation status is the best predictor of clinical response to PARP inhibitor treatment in patients with breast or ovarian cancer, highlighting the potential for these agents as therapeutic and future preventive agents in this cohort of patients.

7. Conclusions

Prophylactic oophorectomy is proven to be an effective risk-reducing strategy in hereditary breast and ovarian cancer. In women diagnosed with a BRCA1/2 mutation the decision of whether to undergo risk reducing surgery is a complex one. Adequate consideration must be given to the risks and benefits of surgery, particularly in relation to timing of surgery, fertility, reduction in cancer risk, the need for hysterectomy and the symptoms of early menopause. Patients should be adequately counseled by regarding the options available to them including surveillance and risk reducing strategies.

8. References

Agalliu I, Gern R, Leanza S, et al. (2009) Associations of high-grade prostate cancer with BRCA1 and BRCA2 founder mutations. *Clin Cancer Res,* 15: 1112-1120.

Aiyar SE, Blair AL, Hopkinson DA, et al. (2007) Regulation of clustered gene expression by cofactor of BRCA1 (COBRA1) in breast cancer cells. *Oncogene,* 26: 2543–2553

Alvarado-Cabrero I, Young RH, Vamvakas EC & Scully RE (1999). Carcinoma ofthe fallopian tube: a clinicopathological study of 105 cases withobservations onstaging and prognostic factors. *Gynecol Oncol,* 72:367–379.

Antoniou A, Pharoah PD, Narod S, et al. (2003). Average risks of breast and ovarian cancer associated with BRCA1 or BRCA2 mutations detected in case series unselected for family history: a combined analysis of 22 studies. *Am J Hum Genet,* 72:1117–1130

Armstrong K, Schwartz JS, Randall T, Rubin SC, Weber B (2004). Hormone replacement therapy and life expectancy after prophylactic oophorectomy in women with BRCA1/2 mutations: a decision analysis. *J Clin Oncol,* 22:1045–1054.

Audeh MW, Carmichael J, Penson RT, et al (2010) Oral poly(ADP-ribose) polymerase inhibitor olaparib in patients with BRCA1 or BRCA2 mutations and recurrent ovarian cancer: a proof-of-concept trial. *Lancet,* 24(376):245–251

Bane AL, Beck JC, Bleiweiss I, et al (2007). BRCA2 mutation-associated breast cancers exhibit a distinguishing phenotype based on morphology and molecular profiles from tissue microarrays. *Am J Surg Pathol* 2007;31:121- 128.

Beatson GT (1896). On the treatment of inoperable cases of carcinoma of the mamma. Suggestions for a new method of treatment with illustrative cases. *Lancet,* II(104-7):162-5.

Beral V; Million Women Study Collaborators (2003). Breast cancer and hormone replacement therapy in the Million Women Study. *Lancet,* 362:419–427.

Billar JA, Dueck AC, Stucky CC, et al (2010) Triple-negative breast cancers: unique clinicalpresentations and outcomes. *Ann Surg Oncol,* 17: 384-90,(Suppl 3)

Biron-Shental T, Drucker L, Altaras M, Bernheim J & Fishman A (2006). High incidence of BRCA1-2 germline mutations, previous breast cancer and familial cancer history in

Jewish patients with uterine serous papillary carcinoma. *Eur J Surg Oncol,* 32:1097–1100.

Bodmer M, Meier C, Krahenbuhl S, Jick SS & Meier CR (2010)Long-term metformin use is associated with decreased risk of breast cancer, *Diabetes Care*, 33: 1304–1308.

Bosco JL, Antonsen S, Sørensen HT, Pedersen L & Lash TL (2011). Metformin and incident breastcancer among diabetic women: a population-based case control study in Denmark. *Cancer Epidemiol Biomarkers Prev* 20: 101–111.

Boyd S (1897) On oophorectomy in the treatment of cancer. *BMJ,* 2:890–6.

Boyd S (1900) On oophorectomy in cancer of the breast. *BMJ,* 2:1161–7.

Brekelmans CT, Tilanus-Linthorst MM, Seynaeve C, et al (2007). Tumour characteristics, survival and prognostic factors of hereditary breast cancer from BRCA2-, BRCA1- and non-BRCA1/2 families as compared to sporadic breast cancer cases. *Eur J Cancer,* 43: 867–876

Brinton LA, Schairer C, Hoover RN, & Fraumeni JF Jr. (1988) Menstrual factors andrisk of breast cancer. *Cancer Invest.,* 6:245-254.

The Breast Cancer Linkage Consortium (1999). Cancer risks in BRCA2 mutationcarriers. *J Natl Cancer Inst,* 91: 1310–1316

Campfield-Bonadies D, Moyer A & Matloff ET (2011). What I wish I'd known before surgery: BRCA carriers' perspectives after bilateral salpingo- oophorectomy. *Fam Cancer,* 10(1):79-85

Canes D, Desai M.M, Aron M, et al (2008), Transumbilical single-port surgery: evolution and current status. *Eur. Urol.* 54 (5): 1020–1029

Casey M, Garcia-Padial J, Hakert D et al (1998) Changing trends in surgical approaches to hysterectomy: an analysis of the use of laparoscopic assisted vaginal hysterectomies in clinicpractice. *J Gynecol Surg* 14:15–24

Chiaffarino, F, Parazzini, F, Bosetti, C et al. (2007). Risk factors for ovarian cancer histotypes. *Eur JCancer,* 43:1208–1213

Chlebowski RT, Chen Z, Cauley JA et al. (2010) Oral bisphosphonate use and breast cancer incidence in postmenopausal women, *J Clin Oncol* 28: 3582-3590

Cho Y.H, Kim D.Y, Kim J.H, Kim Y.M, Kim Y.T & Nam J.H.(2007) Laparoscopic management of early uterine cancer: 10-year experience in Asan Medical Center, *Gynecol. Oncol.* 106:585–590

Crossen H S (1942). The menace of "silent" ovarian carcinoma. *JAMA* 1191485–1489

Cuzick J, Powles T, Veronesi U, et al (2003). Overview of the main outcomes in breast-cancer prevention trials. *Lancet* 361:296-300

Cuzick J, DeCensi A, Arun B, et al. (2011). Preventive therapy for breast cancer: aconsensus statement. *Lancet Oncol.,* 12(5):496-503

Dent R, Trudeau M, Pritchard KI, et al (2007). Triple-negative breast cancer: clinicalfeatures and patterns of recurrence. *Clin Cancer Res,* 13: 4429-34.

Domchek SM, Friebel TM, Neuhausen SL, et al (2006). Mortality after bilateralsalpingo oophorectomy in BRCA1 and BRCA2 mutation carriers: aprospective cohort study. *LancetOncol,* 7:223–229.

Domchek SM, Friebel TM, Singer CF, et al. (2010). Association of risk-reducingsurgery in BRCA1 or BRCA2 mutation carriers with cancer risk andmortality. *JAMA,* 304(9):967-75.

Easton DF, Bishop DT, Ford D, Crockford GP (1993). The Breast Cancer LinkageConsortium. Genetic linkage analysis in familial breast and ovariancancers: Results from 214 families. *Am. J.Human Genetics,* 52: 678–701

Easton DF, Ford D, Bishop DT (1995). Breast and ovarian cancer incidence inBRCA1-mutation carriers. Breast Cancer Linkage Consortium. *Am J HumGenet,* 56:265–271.

Eisen A, Weber BL (2001). Prophylactic mastectomy for women withBRCA1 and BRCA2 mutations - facts and controversy. *N Engl J Med*345:207-208, 2001.

Eisen A, Lubinski J, Klijn J, et al (2005). Breast cancer risk following bilateraloophorectomy in BRCA1 and BRCA2 mutation carriers: an internationalcase-control study. *J Clin Oncol,* 23(30):7491-7496

Elit L, Esplen MJ, Butler K, Narod S (2001). Quality of life and psychosexualadjustment after prophylactic oophorectomy for a family history ofovarian cancer. *Fam Cancer,* 1:149–56.

Eltabbakh G, Piver M, Hempling R et al (1999) Laparoscopic management ofwomen with a family history of ovarian cancer. *J Surg Oncol* 72:9–13.

Eltabbakh G.H, Shamonki M.I, Moody J.M. & Garafano L.L (2000). Hysterectomyfor obese women with endometrial cancer: laparoscopy or laparotomy?,*Gynecol. Oncol.,* 78:329–335.

Escobar P.F, Fader A.N, Paraiso M.F, Kaouk J.H & Falcone T.(2009) Roboticassisted laparoendoscopic single-site surgery in gynecology: initial reportand technique, *J. Minim. Invasive Gynecol.* 16 (5): 589–591

Escobar P.F, Bedaiwy M.A, Fader A.N & Falcone T (2010). Laparoendoscopicsingle-site (LESS) surgery in patients with benign adnexal disease, *FertilSteril.,* 93(6):2074e7-2074e10

Escobar P.F, Starks D.C, Fader A.N, Barber M & Rojas-Espalliat L (2010). .Singleport risk-reducing salpingo-oophorectomy with and withouthysterectomy: surgical outcomes and learning curve analysis. *GynecolOncol.,* 119(1):43-7.

Fader A.N, Escobar P.F.(2009). Laparoendoscopic single-site surgery (LESS) ingynecologic oncology: technique and initial report, *Gynecol. Oncol.* 114 (2):157–161

Feinleib M. Breast cancer and artificial menopause: a cohort study(1968). *J Natl CancerInst,* 41:315-329.

Ferla R, Calò V, Cascio S, et al. (2007) Founder mutations in BRCA1 and BRCA2genes. *Ann Oncol* 18:vi93–vi98

Finch A, Beiner M, Lubinski J, et al (2006). Hereditary Ovarian Cancer ClinicalStudy Group. Salpingooophorectomy and the risk of ovarian, fallopiantube, and peritoneal cancers in women with a BRCA1 or BRCA2 mutation.*JAMA,* 296:185–192.

Fisher B, Costatino JP, Redman CK, et al (1994). Endometrial cancer in tamoxifentreated patients:Findings from the National Surgical Adjuvant Breast andBowel Project (NSABP) B-14. *J Natl Cancer Inst* 86:527-537. .

Fisher B, Constantino JP, Lawrence-Wickerman D, et al (1998). Tamoxifen forprevention of breast cancer: report of the National Surgical AdjuvantBreast and Bowel Project P-1 Study. *J Natl Cancer Inst,* 90:1371–88.

Foulkes WD, Stefansson IM, Chappuis PO, et al. (2003). Germline BRCA1mutations and a basal epithelial phenotype in breast cancer. *J Natl CancerInst,* 95:1482–1485.

Foulkes WD (2010). Traffic control for BRCA1. *N Engl J Med,* 362: 755–756 Goss PE, Ingle JN, Alés-Martínez JE, et al (2011). NCIC CTG MAP.3 Study Investigators. Exemestane for breast-cancer prevention in postmenopausal women.*N Engl J Med,* 23;364(25):2381-91

Grady D, Gebretsadik T, Kerlikowske K et al (1995) Hormone replacement therapy and endometrial cancer risk: a meta-analysis. *Obstet Gynecol* 85:304–313. Hall JM, Lee MK, Morrow J et al (1990). Linkage analysis of early onset familial breast cancer tochromosome 17q21. *Science,* 250: 1684–9

Hallowell N, Mackay J, Richards M, Gore M & Jacobs I (2004). High-risk premenopausal women's experiences of undergoing prophylacticoophorectomy: a descriptive study. *Genet Test,* 8:148–56.

Harris RE, Chlebowski RT, Jackson RD, et al (2003). Women's Health Initiative.Breast Cancer and nonsteroidal anti-inflammatory drugs: prospectiveresults from the Women's Health Initiative. *Cancer Res,* 63(18):6096-101

Hidlebaugh DA, Vulgaropulos S & Orr R (1996) Trends in oophorectomy bylaparoscopic versus open techniques. *J Am Assoc Gynecol Laparosc* 3:S17S18.

Hornreich G, Beller U, Lavie O, et al (1999). Is uterine serous papillary carcinoma aBRCA1-related disease? Case report and review of the literature. *GynecolOncol,* 75:300–304.

Huen MS, Sy SM, & Chen J (2010). BRCA1 and its toolbox for the maintenance ofgenome integrity. *Nat Rev Mol Cell Biol* , 11: 138–148

Kauff ND, Satagopan JM, Robson ME, et al (2002). Risk reducing salpingooophorectomy in women with a BRCA1 or BRCA2 mutation. *N Engl J Med,*346:1609– 1615.

Kauff ND, Domchek SM, Friebel TM, et al (2008). Risk-reducing salpingooophorectomy for the prevention of BRCA1 and BRCA2 associated breastand gynaecologic cancer: a multi-center, prospective study. *J Clin Oncol,*26:1331–1337.

King MC, Wieand S, Hale K, et al (2001). Tamoxifen and breast cancer incidenceamong women with inherited mutations in BRCA1 and BRCA2: NationalSurgical Adjuvant Breast and Bowel Project (NSABP-P1) breast cancerprevention trial. *JAMA,* 286:2251-225

King MC, Marks JH, Mandell JB (2003). New York Breast Cancer Study Group.Breast and ovarian cancer risks due to inherited mutations in BRCA1 andBRCA2. *Science,* 302:643–646

Klaren HM, van't Veer LJ, van Leeuwen FE & Rookus MA (2003). Potential for biasin studies on efficacy of prophylactic surgery for BRCA1 and BRCA2mutation. *J Natl Cancer Inst.,* 95(13):941–947

Kramer JL, Velazquez IA, Chen BE, et al (2005). Prophylactic oophorectomyreduces breast cancer penetrance during prospective, longterm follow-upof BRCA1 mutation carriers. *J Clin Oncol.,*23:8629–8635.

Kurian AW, Balise RR, McGuire V, & Whittemore AS (2005). Histologic types ofepithelial ovarian cancer: have they different risk factors? *GynecologicOncology, 96*: 520–530

Leetanaporn R & Tintara H (1996) A comparative study of outcome of laparoscopicsalpingo-oophorectomy versus open salpingo-oophorectomy. *J ObstetGynaecol Res* 22:79–83

Levine DA, Argenta PA, Yee CJ, et al (2003). Fallopian tube and primary peritonealcarcinomas associated with BRCA mutations. *J Clin Oncol,* 21: 4222–4227.

Liber AM (1950). Ovarian cancer in a mother and five daughters. *Arch Pathol.,*49:280–290

Liebens FP, Carly B, Pastijn A, et al.(2007) Management of BRCA1/2 associatedbreast cancer: Asystematic qualitative review of the state of knowledge in2006. *Eur J Cancer* , 43: 238–257.

Lynch HT, Krush AJ, Lemon HM, et al. (1972). Tumor variation in families withbreast cancer. *JAMA,* 222: 1631–1635

Ma Y, Fan S, Hu C, et al (2010). BRCA1 regulates acetylation and ubiquitination ofestrogen receptor alpha. *Mol Endocrinol,* 24: 76–90

Madalinska JB, van Beurden M, Bleiker EM, et al (2007). Predictors of prophylacticbilateral salpingo-oophorectomy compared with gynecologic screening usein BRCA1/2 mutation carriers. *JClin Oncol.,* 25(3):301-7

Malone KE, Daling JR, Doody DR, et al. (2006) Prevalence and predictors of BRCA1and BRCA2 mutations in a population-based study of breast cancer inwhite and black American women, ages 35 to 64 years. *Cancer Res* 66:82978308

McLaughlin JR, Risch HA, Lubinski J, et al (2007). Hereditary Ovarian CancerClinical Study Group. Reproductive risk factors for ovarian cancer incarriers of *BRCA1* or *BRCA2* mutations: a case control study. *Lancet Oncol.,*8(1):26-34.

Metcalfe K, Lynch HT, Ghadirian P, et al (2004). Contralateral breast cancer inBRCA1 and BRCA2 mutation carriers. *J Clin Oncol* 22:2328- 2335

Meijer WJ & van Lindert AC (1992). Prophylactic oophorectomy. *Eur J ObstetGynecol Reprod Biol* 47:59-65

Miki Y, Swensen J, Shattuck-Eidens D, et al (1994). A strong candidate for thebreast and ovarian cancer susceptibility gene BRCA1. *Science,* 266(5182):6671.

Miller SM, Roussi P, Daly MB & Scarpato J (2010). New strategies in ovariancancer: uptake and experience of women at high risk of ovarian cancerwho are considering risk-reducing salpingo-oophorectomy.*Clin CancerRes.,* 16(21):5094-106.

Milne RL, Knight JA, John EM, et al (2005). Oral contraceptive use and risk ofearly-onset breast cancer in carriers and noncarriers of *BRCA1* and *BRCA2*mutations. *Cancer Epidemiol Biomarkers Prev.,* 14(2):350-356.

Mitra A, Fisher C, Foster CS, et al (2008). Prostate cancer in male BRCA1 andBRCA2 mutation carriers has a more aggressive phenotype. *Br J Cancer,* 98:502–507

Narod SA, Brunet JS, Ghardirian P, et al (2000). Tamoxifen and risk of contralateralbreast cancer in BRCA1 and BRCA2 mutation carriers: a case-control study.*Lancet,* 356:1876-1881

Narod SA, Sun P, & Risch HA (2001). Ovarian cancer, oral contraceptives, andBRCA mutations. *N Engl J Med,* 345:1706–1707.

National Comprehensive Cancer Network. NCCN & Clinical Resources Web site.NCCN clinicalpractice guidelines in oncology (NCCN Guidelines).Genetic/familial high-risk assessment: breast and ovarian. Hereditarybreast and/or ovarian cancer. Version 1.2010.2010. http://www.nccn.org/professionals/physician_gls/f_guidelines.asp. Accessed August 21, 2010.

Neuhausen SL, Ozcelik H, Southey MC, et al. (2009). BRCA1 and BRCA2 mutationcarriers in the Breast Cancer Family Registry: an open resource forcollaborative research. Breast Cancer Family Registry. *Breast Cancer ResTreat,* 116:379-386

Olivier RI, van Beurden M, Lubsen MA, et al (2004). Clinical outcome ofprophylactic oophorectomy in BRCA1/BRCA2 mutation carriers andevents during follow-up. *Br J Cancer,* 90: 1492–1497.

Olivier RI, Lubsen-Brandsma MA, Verhoef S, et al (2006). CA125 and transvaginalultrasound monitoring in high-risk women cannot prevent the diagnosis ofadvanced ovarian cancer. *Gynecol Oncol*, 100:20-26

Osborne CK (1998) Tamoxifen in the treatment of breast cancer. *N Engl J Med*,339(22):1609-18.

Paley PJ, Swisher EM, Garcia RL, et al (2001). Occult cancer of the fallopian tube inBRCA-1 germline mutation carriers at prophylactic oophorectomy: a casefor recommending hysterectomy at surgical prophylaxis. *Gynecol Oncol*,80:176–180.

Rebbeck TR, Levin AM, Eisen A, et al (1999). Breast cancer risk after bilateralprophylactic oophorectomy in BRCA1 mutation carriers. *J Natl Cancer Inst* ,91:1475–1479

Rebbeck TR, Lynch HT, Neuhausen SL, et al (2002). Prevention and Observation ofSurgical End Points Study Group. Prophylactic oophorectomy in carriersof BRCA1 or BRCA2 mutations.*N Engl J Med*, 346: 1616–1622.

Rebbeck TR, Friebel T, Wagner T, et al (2005). PROSE Study Group. Effect of shortterm hormonereplacement therapy on breast cancer risk reduction afterbilateral prophylactic oophorectomy in BRCA1 and BRCA2 mutationcarriers: the PROSE Study Group. *J ClinOncol*, 23:7804–7810.

Rebbeck TR, Kauff ND, Domchek SM (2009). Meta-analysis of Risk ReductionEstimates Associated With Risk-Reducing Salpingo-oophorectomy in*BRCA1* or *BRCA2* Mutation Carriers. *J Natl Cancer Inst.*, 101(2): 80–87.

Rennert G, Pinchev M, & Rennert HS (2010). Use of bisphosphonates and risk ofpostmenopausal breast cancer, *J Clin Oncol*, 28: 3577–3581

Robson M, Hensley M, Barakat R, et al (2003). Quality of life in women at risk forovarian cancer who have undergone risk-reducing oophorectomy. *GynecolOncol*, 89:281–7.

Robson M & Offit K (2007). Clinical practice: management of an inheritedpredisposition to breastcancer. *N Engl J Med*, 357(2):154-162.

Rocca WA, Grossardt BR, de Andrade M, Malkasian GD & Melton LJ (2006).Survival patterns after oophorectomy in premenopausal women: apopulation-based cohort study. *Lancet Oncol*, 7(10):821–828.

Rossouw JE, Anderson GL, Prentice RL, et al (2002). Writing Group for theWomen's Health Initiative Investigators. Risks and benefits of estrogenplus progestin in healthy postmenopausal women : principal results fromthe Women's Health Initiative randomized controlled trial. *JAMA*,288:321–333.

Rutter JL, Wacholder S, Chetrit A et al (2003). Gynecologic surgeries and risk ofovarian cancer in women with BRCA1 and BRCA2 Ashkenazi foundermutations: an Israeli population-based case-control study. *J Natl CancerInst*, 95:1072–1078.

Saslow D, Boetes C, Burke W, et al. (2007). American Cancer Society Breast CancerAdvisory Group. American Cancer Society guidelines for breast screeningwith MRI as an adjunct to mammograph *CA Cancer J Clin*, 57(2):75-89.

Schinzinger A (1889). Ueber Carcinoma Mammae. Verhandlungen der DeutschenGesellschaft furChirurgie. 18th Kongress, Berlin, Apr 24–27, Berlin, Germany: Hirschwald; 1889:28[abstract]

Spiegel TN, Esplen MJ, Hill KA, Wong J, Causer PA & Warner E (2011). Psychological impact of recall on women with BRCA mutationundergoing MRI surveillance. Breast. 2011 May 23[Epub ahead of print]

Stirling D, Evans DG, Pichert G, et al (2005). Screening for familial ovarian cancer:Failure of current protocols to detect ovarian cancer at an early stageaccording to the International Federation of Gynecology and ObstetricsSystem. *J Clin Oncol*, 23: 5588-5596

Struewing JP, Hartge P, Wacholder S, et al (1997). The risk of cancer associatedwith specific mutations of BRCA1 and BRCA2 among Ashkenazi Jews. *NEngl J Med*, 336(20):1401-1408

Tai YC, Domchek S, Parmigiani G, et al (2007). Breast cancer risk among maleBRCA1 and BRCA2 mutation carriers. *J Natl Cancer Inst*, 99: 1811-1814.

Taylor M (2001) Psychological consequences of surgical menopause. *J Reprod Med*,46:317-324

Thomson A (1902). Analysis of cases in which oophorectomy was performed forinoperable carcinoma of the breast. *BMJ*, 2:1538-41.

Tiller K, Meiser B, Butow P, et al (2002). Psychological impact of prophylacticoophorectomy in women at increased risk of developing ovarian cancer: Aprospective study. *Gynecol Oncol*, 86:212-219,

Tobacman JK, Greene MH, Tucker MA, Costa J, Kase R & Fraumeni JF Jr (1982).Intraabdominalabdominal carcinomatosis after prophylacticoophorectomy in ovarian-cancer-prone families. *Lancet*, 2:795-797.

Tutt A, Robson M, Garber JE, et al (2010). Oral poly(ADP-ribose) polymeraseinhibitor olaparib in patients with BRCA1 or BRCA2 mutations andadvanced breast cancer: a proof-of-concept trial. *Lancet*, 24(376):235-244.

Visvanathan K, Chlebowski RT, Hurley P et al (2009). American Society of ClinicalOncology Clinical Practice Guideline Update on the Use of PharmacologicInterventions Including Tamoxifen, Raloxifene, and Aromatase Inhibitionfor Breast Cancer Risk Reduction. *J Clin Oncol*, 27(19); 3235-3258

Vogel VG, Costantino JP, Wickerham DL, et al (2010). National Surgical AdjuvantBreast and Bowel Project. Update of the National Surgical Adjuvant Breastand Bowel Project Study of Tamoxifen and Raloxifene (STAR) P-2 Trial:Preventing breast cancer. *Cancer Prev Res (Phila)*,3(6):696-706.

Warner E, Foulkes W, Goodwin P, et al (1999) Prevalence and penetrance ofBRCA1 and BRCA2 gene mutations in unselected Ashkenazi Jewishwomen with breast cancer. *J Natl Canc Inst*,91(14):1241-1247.

Warner E, Plewes DB, Shumak RS, et al (2001). Comparison of breast magneticresonance imaging, mammography, and ultrasound for surveillance ofwomen at high risk for hereditary breastcancer. *J Clin Oncol*, 19(15):35243531.

Warner E, Plewes DB, Hill KA, et al (2004). Surveillance of *BRCA1* and *BRCA2*mutation carriers with magnetic resonance imaging, ultrasound,mammography, and clinical breast examination.*JAMA*, 292:1317-1325

Warner E (2011). Impact of MRI surveillance and breast cancer detection in youngwomen with BRCA mutations. *Ann Oncol*, 22 Suppl 1:i44-9

Whittemore AS, Gong G, Itnyre J (1997) Prevalence and contribution of BRCA1mutations in breast cancer and ovarian cancer: results from three U.S.population-based case-control studies ofovarian cancer. *Am J Hum Genet*60:496-504

Whittemore AS, Gong G, John EM, et al. (2004) Prevalence of BRCA1 mutationcarriers among U.S. non-Hispanic Whites. *Cancer Epidemiol Biomark Prev*13:2078-2083

Wooster R, Neuhausen SL, Mangion J et al (1994). Localization of a breast cancersusceptibility gene, *BRCA2*, to chromosome 13q 12–13. *Science*, 265: 2088-90

Wooster R, Bignell G, Lancaster J, et al (1995). Identification of the breast cancersusceptibility gene BRCA2. *Nature*, 378(6559):789-92.

Zweemer RP, van Diest PJ, Verheijen RH, et al (2000). Molecular evidence linkingprimary cancer of the fallopian tube to BRCA1 germline mutations.*Gynecol Oncol*, 7:45–50.

24

Psychological Aspects of Hysterectomy & Postoperative Care

Amitabha Majumdar and Sepeedeh Saleh
East Lancashire Hospitals NHS Trust,
United Kingdom

1. Introduction

Hysterectomy is one of the commonest gynaecological procedures undertaken in the UK and in the USA. (Gupta & Manyonda, 2011) It is carried out both for benign indications (namely abnormal uterine bleeding and pelvic pain) and for malignancies of the female genital tract. In some cases there are multiple indications for hysterectomy, for example, menorrhagia and dysmenorrhoea (Williams & Clark, 2000) and chronic pelvic pain can accompany a variety of other gynaecological diagnoses. Bilateral salpingo-oophrectomy is often carried out concurrently and this may be followed by postoperative commencement of hormone replacement therapy (HRT).

Subgroups of patients undergoing hysterectomy have the procedure undertaken via the vaginal route, which may also be laparoscopically-assisted. These procedures are less invasive than abdominal hysterectomies and may therefore have better recovery profiles. (Nieboer et al., 2009) Hysterectomies have been extensively studied because of the large numbers of the operations performed annually.

As with any major surgical procedure the postoperative phase of a hysterectomy is complex and multimodal. Measures of postoperative recovery tend to focus on physical aspects, often overlooking the equally important psychological elements of recovery. (Gath et al., 1982) The impact of hysterectomy on sexual function is a major cause of preoperative anxiety which unfortunately is seldom articulated by patients or explored routinely by clinicians. Reports regarding the impact of hysterectomy on sexual function draw conflicting conclusions.

In exploring the psychological aspects of post-hysterectomy recovery we must first take into account preoperative factors. Levels of psychiatric morbidity in hysterectomy patients preoperatively have been found to be high in comparison to women in the general population. (Khastgir & Studd, 1998) This could be explained by a variety of factors including depression in response to the ongoing physical symptoms for which hysterectomy is planned and anxiety regarding the upcoming surgery. Other hypotheses include that of physical symptoms occurring as psychophysiological correlates to psychological disorders and the theory that a proportion of women are listed for major surgery (in this case hysterectomy) having repeatedly presented with physical complaints of nonorganic origin. (Stockman, as cited in O'Hara et al., 1995; Thornton et al., 1997)

Patients with pre-existing psychological disorders or those currently displaying psychopathological symptoms are also at increased risk of postoperative psychological disorders. These women with increased preoperative psychiatric morbidity are, almost by definition, at higher risk of further psychological disturbances in the event of protracted recovery or complications of surgery. More recent research has also identified increased risk of psychological morbidity in response to hysterectomy in women with a past history of sexual abuse and assault. (Swales & Sheikh, 1992; Wukasch, 1996)

It may be that certain pre-surgical risk factors antedate the problems and increase the likelihood of post-surgical psychological problems. The most common issues which have been highlighted in this capacity are chronic anxiety and depression, disorders of body image, problems in relationships with a partner and chronic pain.

Hysterectomy may be performed in response to a subjective assessment of physical symptoms rather than an objective assessment of gynaecological abnormality, for example in conditions such as dysfunctional uterine bleeding. Patients are likely to benefit from increased awareness of the global nature of their individual problems by all healthcare professionals in their care. Tools such as questionnaires which measure subjective aspects of the patients' symptoms may be helpful in these cases; highlighting potential psychological issues of concern and guiding clinicians to alter treatment options if necessary or even to seek further referral for behavioural therapies, counselling, etc. prior to surgery. Studies have shown that, although hysterectomy may significantly reduce negative mood status, clinical levels of anxiety are found in a majority of women undergoing the procedure. Preoperative mood status has been found to be inversely related to an intrapersonal dimension of 'dispositional resilience' and to 'family cohesiveness'. It is suggested that monitoring of preoperative mood, family cohesiveness and dispositional resilience may provide a useful adjunctive measure in attempting to identify women at risk of reporting an unsatisfactory surgical outcome. (Thornton et al., 1997)

There are three broad subsets of psychological symptoms referred to in the literature. These are: anxiety and depression attributed to the operation, sexual dysfunction (presenting as diminished libido, pain, dyspareunia or anxiety surrounding sexual activity) and reactions related to perceptions of feminity and low self-esteem. (Kinsey & McFarlane, as cited in Broome & Wallace, 1984)

Female sexual dysfunction is a multifactorial phenomenon comprising physiological, psychological and social components. The main physiological requirements for sexual function include an operational system of sex steroids, autonomic and somatic nerves and blood supply to the genital organs. (Nappi et al., 2005) Although data are sparse, it has been claimed there is pathophysiological involvement of abnormal sex steroid levels, damage to blood supply and nerve supply in women with problems of sexual desire, arousal or orgasm. (Mokate et al., 2006) The psychological aspects of sexual dysfunction are complex. The traditional 4-stage model first characterized by Masters and Johnson in 1966 (Masters & Johnson, 1966) was later modified by Kaplan (Kaplan, 1974). Basson, in 2001, proposed a new model called the sexual response cycle which was different from the traditional model and involved physical, emotional and cognitive feedback. (Basson, 2001) Interestingly, elements of this new model corresponded to the sexual difficulties arising before and after hysterectomy.

As alluded to earlier, women undergoing hysterectomy for pelvic organ prolapse and chronic pelvic pain constitute an interesting group in which preoperative expectations of the surgical procedure and outcomes have a marked impact on postoperative psychological wellbeing. This is more relevant in women undergoing hysterectomy for chronic pelvic pain. (Melzack, 1982) In these groups problems with anxiety, depression or reduced libido may already exist preoperatively, only to come to the fore if patients' expectations of the surgical procedure are not fulfilled.

Work has been done to compare differing types and routes of hysterectomy and to examine whether this has any impact on postoperative psychological status. In general, no significant differences have been identified between postoperative psychological morbidity relating to the various routes and types of hysterectomy. (Strauss et al., 1996)

Studies have also looked into more conservative approaches to the management of menorrhagia such as endometrial ablation, in terms of their comparative psychological impact. It has been concluded that it may be reasonable, in this subgroup of women, to offer conservative treatment after a psychomotor evaluation. (Alexander et al., 1996)

In many cases (for example, surgery to correct pelvic organ prolapse), the impact of surgery on the preoperative symptoms, particularly in terms of quality of life, may prove to have the most discernible effect on psychological status. In these cases it is usually subjective rather than objective outcome measures which are the most relevant to positive postoperative results. (Helström & Nilsson, 2005)

In this chapter, the authors reviewed the literature on the psychological and sexual impact of hysterectomy. The question of psychological and sexual morbidity following hysterectomy is multifaceted and a broad area is covered. Perhaps due to the popularity of work on hysterectomy, literature searches yielded a multitude of articles. It was, however, soon realised that, where themes such as relevance of route of surgery to psychological morbidity were commonly investigated in the recent literature, recent work on issues such as a history of sexual abuse was not so abundant. A distinct shift in the understanding of psychological aspects of hysterectomy was also noticed, from the older literature which used mostly retrospective and observational methods to arrive at conclusions to the newer studies which strived to prospectively study women's attitudes towards hysterectomy. It came as no surprise, therefore, that very different conclusions were reached by the two styles of research.

Ideally, double-blind randomised controlled trials would be performed to assess the psychological and sexual effects of hysterectomy. As women and surgeons often have strong opinions regarding surgical treatment of gynaecological problems, however, randomised trials are difficult to orchestrate and rarely performed. With regard to blinding, although this may be done for some aspects of surgical management, in many cases it is not possible; hence, most evidence on this topic is based on observational studies.

2. Hysterectomy and sexual functioning: The Maryland Women's Health Study

Before proceeding to a more detailed discussion we briefly consider, individually, the Maryland Women's Health Study as it holds a central place in our current discussion. (Rhodes et al., 1999) The study was a large, prospective two-year study which aimed to investigate changes in sexual functioning in women between the ages of 35 and 49 undergoing hysterectomy for benign disease. The main outcome measures studied were frequency of sexual relations, dyspareunia, orgasm, vaginal dryness and sexual desire. A total of 1299 women were interviewed, 84.8% of whom completed the study and provided information about their sexual functioning. Data was collected prior to hysterectomy and at 6, 12, 18 and 24 months after hysterectomy.

The percentage of women engaging in sexual relations increased significantly from 70.5% before hysterectomy to 77.6% and 76.7% at 12 and 24 months after hysterectomy. The rate of frequent dyspareunia dropped significantly (from 18.6% before hysterectomy to 4.3% and 3.6% at 12 and 24 months after hysterectomy) as did the rates of not experiencing orgasm (from 10.4% before hysterectomy to 6.3% and 6.2% at 12 and 24 months after hysterectomy). The proportion of women who had not reported vaginal dryness in the past month improved significantly from 37.3% before hysterectomy to 46.8% and 46.7% at 12 and 24 months after hysterectomy. Pre-hysterectomy depression was found to be associated with dyspareunia, vaginal dryness, low libido, and not experiencing orgasm after hysterectomy.

In probably the largest case series reported on this topic, Rhodes et al. concluded that women may simply feel better after hysterectomy and that sexual functioning improves along with overall health status and quality of life. The women in this study were highly symptomatic before their hysterectomies and reported improvements in both sexual functioning and in other aspects of their health. It was suggested that freedom from vaginal bleeding and fear of pregnancy may be amongst the reasons for this. What the authors did point out, however, was that a majority of women studied had identifiable gynaecological pathologies and that the symptomatic improvements seen could be secondary to this. The same improvements in sexual functioning would not, therefore, be seen in women with no pelvic pathology.

Apart from the Maryland Women's Health Study various smaller analyses have been performed to explore the factors affecting the presence of postoperative sexual problems. Shifren and Avis found, interestingly, that suffering from depression before hysterectomy was associated with not experiencing orgasms after the surgery. (Shifren & Avis, 2007) Additionally, for each sexual problem encountered in the postoperative period, experiencing the problem preoperatively was found to be the single most important predictor for suffering from the same problem postoperatively.

3. Discussion

3.1 Route and type of surgery

Although hysterectomy has been performed for many years and is the most commonly performed operation both in the UK (Department of Health, 1999) and in the US (Lepine et al., 1997), an area of persistent conflict has been the conservation of cervix. There have been suggestions in the past that the cervix could be important in preserving sexual function and gynaecologists were pilloried for performing total hysterectomies and thereby destroying women's sexual function. (Masters & Johnson, 1966) Whilst earlier research may have quoted adverse psychological effects of hysterectomy, this has been refuted in recent research and it has also been suggested that either no benefit or even improvements in quality of life and psychological outcomes might be achieved by hysterectomy.

3.1.1 Total versus subtotal hysterectomy

Thakar et al., in a prospective, randomized, double-blind study on two hundred and seventy-nine women undergoing hysterectomy for benign disease randomly allocated the women to either total hysterectomy or subtotal hysterectomy. (Thakar et al., 2004) The women and the investigator were blinded to the type of operation for one year. Health status and quality of life was assessed using the SF-36 questionnaire (McHorney et al., 1994 & Jenkinson et al., 1995) which looked mainly at health perceptions, mental health, energy, physical function, role limitation, emotional factors, social functioning and pain. The GHQ-28 questionnaire (Goldberg, 1972) was used to assess psychological symptoms. This questionnaire is a valuable tool in detecting current psychiatric disorders and looks specifically at depression, anxiety, social dysfunction and somatic symptoms. The study was claimed to be the first trial to compare the impact of total versus subtotal hysterectomy on quality of life and psychological symptoms with a 12-month postoperative follow up period.

An improvement was found in quality of life after hysterectomy in six of the eight domains. There was no significant difference between the two groups in any outcome apart from that of emotions, which showed greater improvements from baseline at 12 months after subtotal hysterectomy. When this difference was examined further by looking at the change in the GHQ subscales, there was no significant difference at 12 months between the total and subtotal hysterectomy groups in the degree of change from baseline in anxiety, depression, somatic symptoms or social dysfunction. All women showed improvements in psychological symptoms following both operations.

It was found that, although quality of life improved, the scores for all domains were lower than normal at 6 and 12 months postoperatively, reported energy/vitality remained unchanged and pain scores were worse. The authors found this difficult to explain but suggested that full recovery from hysterectomy may take longer than is currently appreciated. Physical recovery and relief of symptoms could explain initial improvements in quality of life but it was felt that the delay in complete recovery of quality of life may be explained by the nature of the procedure, constituting both major surgery and removal of an organ central to concept of womanhood. The worsening postoperative pain scores could not be fully accounted for and did not agree with findings from other similar studies. The authors plan to further examine these findings by following up the same group of women with quality of life scores at 5 and 10 years.

Kuppermann et al. compared sexual functioning and health related quality of life outcomes between women undergoing abdominal hysterectomy and supracervical hysterectomy for benign conditions as part of the 'Total Or Supracervical Hysterectomy' (TOSH) study. (Kuppermann et al., 2005) One hundred and thirty five women scheduled to undergo abdominal hysterectomy were randomly assigned to either a total or supracervical procedure. The primary outcome considered was sexual functioning at two years, as assessed by the Sexual Problems Scale of the Medical Outcomes Study (MOS), looking at mainly four problems: lack of sexual interest, inability to relax and enjoy orgasm, difficulties in arousal, and orgasm. A scale value contributed to analysis only if the participant reported sexual activity. To measure specific aspects of sexual functioning in more detail, four new scales were developed using a combination of items from the MOS Sexual Problems Scale. The factors included pelvic problems interfering with sex, sexual desire, orgasm frequency and quality and satisfaction with sex. These were measured at six months and two years after hysterectomy.

Sexual problems improved dramatically in both randomised groups during the first six months and plateaued at one year postoperatively. Health related quality of life also improved in both groups. At two years both groups reported few problems. This study failed to demonstrate any difference between outcomes after total and supracervical hysterectomy. The authors concluded that the analysis confirms and extends findings from other similar studies in the field, implying that clinicians should be provided with more information to assist in appropriate decision-making.

Persson et al. looked at whether day-by-day postoperative recovery differed between women undergoing subtotal and total hysterectomy for benign disease and analysed various related factors. (Persson et al., 2010a) They measured general wellbeing on a visual analogue score (VAS), starting one week before surgery and continuing daily until day 35 postoperatively. Psychometric assessments of psychological and general wellbeing, depression and anxiety including the Psychological General Well-Being Schedule (PGWB-S), Women's Health Questionnaire (WHQ), State-Trait Anxiety Inventory (STAI) and Beck's Depression Inventory (BDI) were undertaken preoperatively and at five weeks and six months postoperatively.

The study found no difference in day-to-day recovery between the two operating methods. The level of psychological wellbeing preoperatively was found to be strongly associated with day-to-day general wellbeing.

Persson et al. then followed up the same group of women from the previous trial at five weeks, six months and 12 months using the same four tools: PGWB-S, WHQ, STAI and BDI. (Persson et al., 2010b) In addition, they also measured the serum concentration of sex hormones in the patients. The authors failed to find any significant differences between the two groups in any of the psychometric tests. Both surgical methods were associated with significantly higher degrees of psychological wellbeing at 6 and 12 months postoperatively compared with preoperative levels. No association was found between psychological wellbeing and serum sex hormone concentration.

3.1.2 Abdominal versus laparoscopic hysterectomy

Persson et al. compared the psychological wellbeing of women undergoing laparoscopic surgery with those undergoing total abdominal hysterectomy for benign disease in a prospective randomized multi-centre study. (Persson et al., 2006) Psychological functioning was measured one week preoperatively (baseline), then at five weeks and at six months postoperatively with psychometric tests. The PGWB-S and WHQ were used to assess general psychological wellbeing and the STAI and BDI were used to measure anxiety and depression levels.

No significant differences were observed between the scores of patients undergoing laparoscopic assisted hysterectomy and those of abdominal hysterectomy patients in any of the four psychometric tests. Both surgical methods were associated with a significantly higher degree of psychological wellbeing five weeks postoperatively than preoperatively and this improvement persisted at six months postoperatively in both groups.

Ellström et al. evaluated changes in psychological wellbeing and sexuality 1 year after laparoscopic and abdominal hysterectomy. (Ellström et al., 2003) Seventy four women reportedly unsuitable for vaginal hysterectomy and undergoing hysterectomy for benign disease were randomly allocated to either abdominal or laparoscopic hysterectomy. Psychological wellbeing was evaluated using the PGWB-S and the McCoy scale was used to evaluate changes in sexuality. The effect of hysterectomy on sexuality tends to be less well defined than that of psychology with studies showing differing results. The authors in this study recognised the importance of sexuality as a key factor in quality of life measures. In using the McCoy scale to analyse sexuality, identifying sexual cognition rather than sexual behaviour, the authors aim to highlight the socioemotional aspects of sexuality which are at least as important as quantitative variables such as frequency of coitus in considering the whole concept of sexuality. The two main parameters were examined prior to surgery and one year after surgery and comparisons were made, both between individuals and also within and between the two patient groups.

The authors could not demonstrate any significant differences between the two groups with respect to psychological differences or sexuality after one year. Psychological wellbeing did improve after surgery in both groups, as reported elsewhere in the literature, but was unaffected by mode of surgical approach.

3.1.3 Vaginal versus abdominal hysterectomy

Gütl et al. investigated the impact of vaginal and abdominal hysterectomy on women's sexual behaviour, sexual dysfunction, body image and satisfaction with surgery in a prospective study involving 90 women. (Gütl et al., 2002) Data was collected at three points: one day before surgery, three months after surgery and two years after surgery. The questionnaires used were self-reported and included the Tübinger scale for sexual therapy (TSST), the self-developed sexual dysfunction scale (SDS), the relationship assessment scale (RAS German version) and the body image questionnaire (FBK).

The results showed significant differences in women's sexual behaviour and sexual dysfunction before and after hysterectomy which were independent of the surgical procedure performed. Women in both groups reported improvements in sexual desire, sexual activity and sexual intercourse three months and two years after surgery. Sexual dysfunction, dyspareunia, vaginismus, lack of orgasm and loss of sexual interest diminished significantly after surgery. Regression analysis revealed that postmenopausal status, severity of preoperative gynaecological complaints and frequency of sexual intercourse were the most important factors in improved sexual outcomes. Women in the abdominal hysterectomy group were dissatisfied with their body image because of the abdominal scars. They also tended to experience more pain and had longer recovery periods from surgery compared to women in the vaginal hysterectomy group. These results demonstrate that sexual behaviour alone is not a significant factor in choosing vaginal or abdominal surgery. Sexual behaviour is, however, an important element to consider when evaluating outcomes after any type of hysterectomy.

In conclusion, it seems that hysterectomy has traditionally been thought to be associated with adverse psychiatric sequelae but studies coming to such conclusions have often been found to be methodologically flawed, many being retrospective analyses lacking conceptual clarity. With the use of more modern tools, entirely different conclusions have been reached. Unless women embark on hysterectomy with preoperative depression, in which case they are at increased risk of depression, psychiatric symptoms have been shown to be reduced following hysterectomy. This is consistent with findings of the Maryland Study (discussed above): the largest prospective study on the subject to date, which reported a substantial reduction in depression and anxiety levels after hysterectomy. (Rhodes et al., 1999)

3.2 Preoperative psychiatric morbidity

Psychiatric symptoms can arise as a result of physical illness but may also themselves influence both manifestation and outcome of the illness. The effects of hysterectomy provide a perfect example of this.

Gath et al. in their paper published in 1982 reported a prospective case series on one hundred and fifty six women undergoing hysterectomy for benign disease. (Gath et al., 1982) Psychiatric and social assessments were made at initial interview and four weeks before hysterectomy. Comparable follow-up interviews were then done at six months and again at 18 months postoperatively. The main standardised measure used was the Present State Examination or PSE. (Wing et al., 1974) Marriage and social adjustments were measured with the interview schedule devised by Brown and Rutter (1996) and elaborated by Quinton et al. (1976). Two self-explanatory questionnaires were used: the Eysenck Personality Inventory or EPI (Eysenck HJ & Eysenck SB, 1964) and the Profile Of Mood States or POMS (McNair & Lorr, 1964).

There were three main findings reported by the author. The first was that levels of psychiatric morbidity fell significantly after hysterectomy as evidenced by PSE scores with similar postoperative improvements seen in mental state (measured using the POMS). Virtually all improvements were noted in the first six months after surgery. The second finding was that hysterectomy itself rarely, if ever, led to psychiatric disorders. The third finding was that levels of psychiatric morbidity, both before and after hysterectomy, were much higher than in the general population of women, though lower than in psychiatric patients.

Gath et al. in their paper published in 1995, compared the findings of three studies carried out at intervals over the years 1975-1990. (Gath et al., 1995) The study was designed to answer two main questions. The first of these was whether levels of psychiatric morbidity had changed since their previous two studies of women undergoing hysterectomy for benign disease. Secondly, they aimed to examine the observed changes, if any, in levels of psychiatric morbidity were associated with demographic and social characteristics, duration and severity of menstrual symptoms, treatment with anti-menorrhagic medication, past psychiatric illnesses and women's understanding and expectations. The three studies considered looked at different issues but each examined psychiatric issues among women undergoing hysterectomy for menorrhagia of benign origin. In all three studies level of psychiatric morbidity were measured before the operation and six months after the operation by means of the PSE and the EPI.

Levels of psychiatric morbidity were found to have fallen significantly across the three studies with Study one reporting reductions from 58% to 26%, Study two also reporting reductions from 28% to 7% and with further reductions from 9% to 4% seen in Study three. This decline in psychiatric morbidity was independent of demographic and social characteristics, previous psychiatric history, family history of psychiatric illness, nature of menstrual complaints and the women's understanding and expectations of the operation.

The authors concluded by reporting that levels of psychiatric morbidity have continued to fall in recent years. The last study in the series showed a doubling in the frequency of prescription of antimenorrhagic drugs compared with the first two studies, although this could be due to increased availability of these drugs. However, this increase in prescribing does not seem to explain the reduced psychiatric morbidity from hysterectomy procedures. The authors did not offer any positive explanation for the reduction but attributed it to a change in referral practices by general practitioners and gynaecologists. It may have been assumed that clinicians are less inclined to opt for hysterectomy in patients with psychological problems.

3.3 Concomitant oophorectomy

We propose to outline a little of the physiology regarding endocrine changes and resulting symptomatology after oophorectomy in premenopausal women as an appreciation of these mechanisms is central to understanding the potential for psychological and sexual as well as physical effects following bilateral oophorectomy before commenting on findings in the literature.

In younger women during a normal menstrual cycle the ovaries produce oestradiol, testosterone and progesterone in a cyclical pattern under the control of Follicle Stimulating Hormone (FSH) and Luteinising Hormone (LH), both produced by the pituitary gland. Blood oestradiol levels remain well-preserved throughout a woman's reproductive life. They may increase slightly in the approach to the menopause but are, in general, fairly stable until at least the late perimenopause. This increase is presumed to be in response to elevated FSH levels. However, the menopause transition is characterized by marked, and often dramatic, variations in FSH and oestradiol levels, and because of this, measurements of these hormones are *not* considered to be reliable guides to a woman's exact menopausal status.

Menopause occurs due to a natural or surgical cessation of oestradiol and progesterone production by the ovaries, which are a key part of the endocrine system. These hormones are responsible for reproduction and also influence sexual behaviour. After menopause, oestrogen continues to be produced in other tissues, notably the ovaries but also in bone, blood vessels and even in the brain. The dramatic fall in circulating oestradiol levels at the time of menopause, however, impacts many tissues from brain to skin.

In contrast to the sudden fall in oestradiol during menopause, the levels of total and free testosterone, as well as dehydroepiandrosterone sulfate (DHEAS) and androstenedione appear to decline fairly steadily with age. No effect of natural menopause on circulating androgen levels has been observed thus specific tissue effects of natural menopause cannot be attributed to loss of androgenic hormone production. Women who have had the ovaries surgically removed, damaged by chemotherapy or radiotherapy or who have undergone ovarian suppression with gonadotropins, however, do have loss of ovarian androgen production as a result.

The decline of adrenal Dehydroepiandrosterone (DHEA) and DHEAS with age has been described by Labrie et al. and Ferrari et al. but the mechanism underlying this reduction is unclear. (Labrie et al., 1997; Ferrari et al., 2001) An alteration in adrenal zonation leaving the zona reticularis with lesser mass with advancing age has been described as a possible factor. (Parker et al., 1997)

The perimenopausal years in a woman's life involve a gradual change in ovarian function, leading to decreased fertility, a marked reduction in steroidogenesis, the menopause and the subsequent involuntary changes due to oestrogen deficiency. In gynaecological practice, both ovaries may be removed at the time of hysterectomy or at other points for various reasons such as cancer, endometriosis and pelvic inflammatory disease. Ovaries are sometimes removed on the presumption that they have ceased to perform and could become the seat of neoplastic changes. Women undergoing this operation experience almost immediate endocrinological effects and are at risk of the consequent symptoms.

If oophorectomy is performed before the menopause has occurred, the circulating levels of oestradiol will quickly fall to levels similar to those seen in postmenopausal women. Serum levels of FSH and LH start to rise and reach peak values six to eight weeks after surgery. These findings have been confirmed by studies looking at urinary excretion of gonadotrophins and oestrogens. The appearance of vasomotor symptoms is one of the first clinical indicators of reduced serum oestradiol levels and may occur within the first week of surgery. After the ovaries are removed the main source of oestradiol remaining is the adrenal cortex- principally through the secretion of androstenedione and the aromatization of this steroid in peripheral and growth-responsive tissue. A significant reduction is seen in levels of testosterone immediately after oophorectomy, but within five years of surgery or menopause the difference is minimal. (Shifren & Avis, 2007)

With this background, we now move on to the recent literature regarding oophorectomy and psychological wellbeing after hysterectomy.

By comparing the effects of hysterectomy alone with those of hysterectomy and bilateral salpingo-oophorectomy (BSO) it is possible to study the effects of oophorectomy on psychological wellbeing. Nathorst-Boos et al. published a small retrospective observational cohort study comparing oophorectomised women receiving oestrogen replacement therapy, oophrectomised women not receiving oestrogen replacement and women whose ovaries were conserved. (Nathorst-Boos et al., 1993) This was a Swedish study including all the women aged 47 to 55 years who had undergone total abdominal hysterectomy for benign disease in a single centre between 1984 and 1988. Approximately 100 women participated in the trial, doing so 3 years, on average, after surgery. On the basis of the Psychological General Well-Being Schedule (PGWB-S) women in the hysterectomy with BSO category reported significantly more anxiety and depression and less positive wellbeing than women whose ovaries had been preserved. As the investigators did not perform an assessment prior to surgery, they could not control for presurgical differences among the groups of women and this constituted the major limitation of the study.

A prospective observational study by Aziz et al. in 2005 again compared psychological wellbeing in women following hysterectomy alone versus hysterectomy with BSO. (Aziz et al., 2005a)This was done in a group of perimenopausal women aged 45 to 55 years, who were scheduled to undergo the surgery for benign disease at a Swedish hospital. All women in the group were sexually active and free from psychiatric disease preoperatively. Of the 362 women initially enrolled in the study, 106 underwent concurrent BSO and 89% of these went on to complete the one-year study.

Postoperatively, all oophorectomised women and those who had undergone hysterectomy only but were experiencing climacteric symptoms were recommended to commence oestrogen replacement therapy. The McCoy Sexual Rating Scale and the PGWB-S were administered and hormone levels were measured both 2 months before and one year after surgery. The general wellbeing of the two groups did not differ, either before surgery or at one-year follow-up. Postoperatively, both groups displayed increased wellbeing in terms of mood, general health and total wellbeing scores. The hysterectomy-only group had increased vitality and the hysterectomy plus oophorectomy group showed increased positive wellbeing and decreased anxiety.

Farquhar et al. carried out a prospective study comparing women 46 years or younger who had conservation of at least one ovary with women who had hysterectomy and BSO. (Farquhar et al., 2006) Using the Center for Epidemiological Studies-Depression (CES-D) scale, they found decreased levels of depression in both groups after surgery compared with preoperative levels. The rate of depression amongst women who underwent BSO was found to be significantly higher than that for women in whom at least one ovary was conserved (67% compared with 43%). This difference persisted even after three years (50% compared with 27%).

These differences between the findings of Farquhar et al. and those of Aziz et al. earlier could have a few explanations. Firstly, the later study involved women of a younger age group and secondly, the presurgical assessments were completed two to three months prior to surgery in the first study but only one week before surgery in the study by Farquhar et al. Neither studies randomly assigned women to treatment, which makes comparisons difficult. Farquhar et al. also reported that women who underwent BSO were often nulliparous, more likely to have an abdominal hysterectomy, and more likely to have abdominal pain. This again highlights the limitations of observational studies in which patients choose their treatment and may help to explain the disparity in results.

Before moving on to analyse the effects of concomitant oophorectomy on sexuality it is interesting to note that traditional views of women's sexual response and desire have in recent years been questioned. Sexual desire, being primarily an emotion, is a psychological entity but also incorporates biological elements. It is expected that gynaecologists accept sexual difficulties as a legitimate women's health issue and are able to address them accordingly. This includes open discussion of potential effects of any planned surgery on the patient's sexual life.

The Maryland Women's Health Study examined women's sexual function after bilateral salpingo-oophorectomy (BSO) and compared this with sexual function in the women who had opted to keep their ovaries. (Rhodes et al., 1999) Removal of the ovaries generally results in a 50% reduction in circulating androgen levels. As testosterone plays a key role in sexuality and is an important hormone in the physiology of sexual desire, comparing libido and sexual response after hysterectomy with and without concurrent BSO is useful in assessing the part of testosterone in female sexual function. In considering the effects of hysterectomy and BSO on sexual function Rhodes et al. concluded that, after adjusting for age and for patients who had not been experiencing orgasms before surgery, only preoperative depression and BSO were associated with anorgasmia after hysterectomy.

Nathorst-Boos et al. found no significant difference in the frequency of intercourse or orgasm, dyspareunia, arousal, or partner satisfaction between women after hysterectomy with or without BSO. (Nathorst-Boos et al., 1993) There was, however, a difference in libido between the groups, with women retaining their ovaries significantly more likely to report either the same or better libido. Conversely, women were significantly more likely to report a worsening in libido after BSO in comparison to women who retained their ovaries. This worsening was seen even in women who were using oestrogen replacement therapy after their surgery.

In an earlier retrospective observational study by the same authors, worsening was seen in the sexual lives of women who had undergone BSO. (Nathorst-Boos et al., 1992) The authors failed to find any correlations in this study between levels of total testosterone, androstenedione, or DHEAS and any of the psychological or sexual variables examined.

Aziz et al. also compared sexual function in women after hysterectomy with function after hysterectomy with BSO in another study done in 2005. (Aziz et al. 2005b) Due to the prospective nature of this trial, the investigators were able to assess baseline sexual function before hysterectomy as well as after the surgery. Interestingly, women who opted to retain their ovaries had significantly higher preoperative scores on most measures of sexual function and this advantage continued when assessed one year after hysterectomy. Measures considered included sexual arousal, satisfaction, enjoyment, and orgasmic frequency.

When differences between preoperative and postoperative scores were calculated and compared for the two groups, however, the hysterectomy only group scored significantly less than the group who had also undergone concurrent BSO. It is possible, given these findings, that the earlier reported poorer sexual function after hysterectomy with concurrent BSO compared with hysterectomy alone may be explained by a confounding selection bias, with women with poorer baseline sexual function being more likely to opt for BSO at the time of hysterectomy. No correlations were found between changes in androgen levels postoperatively and measures of psychological wellbeing or sexuality.

Bellerose conducted as part of his PhD thesis a study on five groups of women with ages between 35 and 55 years. (Bellerose & Binik, 1993) The groups included a nonsurgical control group, a hysterectomy only group, and three hysterectomy plus BSO groups: women untreated postoperatively, women on oestrogen replacement therapy postoperatively, and women on combined androgen-oestrogen replacement therapy postoperatively. The study comprised two separate sessions: an interview/questionnaire session and a sexual arousal session. The interview/questionnaire session assessed mood, body image and sexual functioning. In a second session completed by 45% of subjects a vaginal photoplethysmograph, (Sintchak & Geer, 1975) an instrument used to indirectly measure sexual arousal, measured vaginal blood flow in response to an erotic stimulus while subjects concurrently monitored subjective arousal. Overall, the groups of women who had undergone hysterectomy with BSO, both with no postoperative treatment and with postoperative oestrogen replacement had significantly lower self-reported desire and arousal than the remaining three groups. Body image was significantly poorer in the untreated hysterectomy plus BSO group. Furthermore, a third of the control group reported positive changes in body image and sexuality in the previous five years. This effect was attenuated in the hysterectomy only group, the hysterectomy and combined therapy group, and the hysterectomy and oestrogen replacement group. No significant differences were reported in mood, vaginal blood flow and subjective arousal to an erotic stimulus.

A majority of studies demonstrate improvements in sexual functioning after hysterectomy for benign disease. Several studies have suggested that concurrent BSO does not have any effect on sexual functioning but others have refuted these claims postulating that adverse effects of BSO on libido and orgasmic response are caused by the postoperative decline in circulating androgens levels. The reasons behind this apparent lack of consensus have been alluded to earlier and are perhaps rooted in the deficiency in randomised controlled trials in this field. Women should therefore be informed that although the majority of studies into oophorectomy have not demonstrated any adverse effects on sexuality, some women may suffer from the sudden and significant decline in ovarian hormones. Although many forms of hormone replacement therapy are available to treat hot flushes, sleep deprivation and vaginal dryness, only testosterone has been shown to be effective in the treatment of hypoactive sexual disorders.

Preoperative counselling is essential in enabling women to make well-informed decisions regarding postoperative hormone replacement bearing in mind the recommendations of the Women's Health Initiative Study. Women should also be informed that the majority of women undergoing hysterectomy for benign disease will experience improved psychological wellbeing and improvements in sexual function postoperatively. Women with preoperatively depression or sexual problems have an increased risk of worsening mood, libido and sexual response after the surgery. Additionally, it may be worth discussing the fact that psychologically healthy women without sexual problems can usually maintain a similar or perhaps even better quality of life post-hysterectomy than that which they enjoyed prior to the surgery.

3.4 Sexual abuse

Hendricks-Matthews reported a case in 1991 of a 33-year-old attorney scheduled for a vaginal hysterectomy who presented to hospital with panic attacks. (Hendricks-Matthews, 1991) She experienced feeling numb as she looked around at other women in a store. She also spoke of feeling very isolated and different from other women around her and kept pondering the upcoming loss of her womb. She later confessed to having the same feelings of being different and isolated from other women when she was raped at knifepoint at the age of 21.

During her counselling sessions she was embarrassed by her "crazy thoughts" as she realised her fears about her upcoming surgery, yet she felt unable to calm herself. Her fears and anxiety were compounded by the fact that she would be under a general anaesthetic during the procedure and would not have any control over what would be done to her body.

This woman had had no prior counselling regarding her sexual abuse. She had been relatively successful in trying to forget her past experiences until the reality of her upcoming hysterectomy made it almost impossible for her to repress the thoughts of the trauma.

Depression and sexual dysfunction are two of the most widely recognized consequences of sexual assualt. (Briere & Runtz, 1988; Finkelhor, 1990; Kroll 1988; Lowery, 1987) Being sexually active does not necessarily mean that the survivor has resolved a sexually traumatic experience. (Mackey et al., 1992) In fact, Karasu has warned that such problems, being unrevealed, are also likely to be unresolved. (Karasu, 1990)

Medical literature had previously been divided on whether women experience psychological disturbance after hysterectomy. Whereas with the introduction of prospective studies this controversy seems to have subsided, there is no controversy regarding the fact that women with pre-existing psychological problems will have poorer outcomes post-hysterectomy. The violence associated with rape and sexual abuse is a cause of major health and social problems in the modern world and the incidence of these events is sadly rising. There is consequently a requirement for healthcare providers to identify women who may be at risk of such postoperative psychological sequelae.

Hendricks-Matthews, in reporting the above case, emphasises this fact, highlighting the increased needs of women with unresolved sexual abuse issues as surgery may re-evoke negative feelings which had previously been suppressed.

This issue was also discussed by Briere and Runtz who stated that that it is not uncommon for survivors of abuse to dissociate themselves from the experience until a triggering event occurs, of which hysterectomy is a prime example. (Briere & Runtz, 1988) It is therefore understandable in such cases that patients have not only to cope with the stress of surgery but also with the burden of all the negative memories associated with the abusive experience.

Hendricks-Matthews also draws parallels between hysterectomy and sexual abuse in terms of violation of bodily boundaries, loss of control, disruption of sexual identity, society viewing a woman differently from how she was before and, in vaginal hysterectomy, the similarity of vaginal pain afterwards. It is suggested that women's previous defences of repression, minimisation, and denial may crumble during the crisis of surgery and bring buried effects flooding through, usually in the form of symptom formation, psychological distress, or both.

Ruth Wukasch, in 1996, conducted a cross-sectional study to examine the impact of a history of rape and/or incest on the post-hysterectomy experience stating that, where many events in women's lives influence their psychological response to medical interventions. (Wukasch, 1996) A special subgroup of women with negative sexual experiences was identified from a larger study looking at women's post-hysterectomy experiences. The decision to explore this subgroup was the result of the finding that a large number of women in the group had been subjected to negative sexual experiences.

In the retrospective cross-sectional study, participants were interviewed at 6, 12, 18, and 24 months after their elective hysterectomies, with a grace period of 4 weeks on either side of these time intervals. The time intervals were selected after a review of several studies examining various time periods in the measurement of sexual and emotional adjustment to a hysterectomy. (Gath et al., 1981; Polivy, 1974; Richards, 1978, Travis, 1988) Polivy suggested that it was during the period of 12-24 months after a hysterectomy that a woman might experience the most distress.

The post-hysterectomy questionnaire developed and used by the author was a three-part questionnaire which took the form of a semi-structured interview with some open-ended questions and prompts and some exploration of fixed categories. Part one determined which surgical procedures were undertaken and looked at recovery and the impact such surgery might have on her sexual functioning preoperatively and during hospitalization. Part two focused on the impact the hysterectomy had on the patient's sexuality and part three elicited demographic details.

The personal reflections on the 'My Hysterectomy Experience' scale, devised by the author specifically for this study, focused on four perceptions of experience: body image, effects of the hysterectomy, the decision to have a hysterectomy and feelings about physicians. The CES-D scale, also used in this study, measured the current levels of depression.

Another standardised, self-evaluation questionnaire used was the The Derogatis Sexual Functioning Inventory (DSFI) which looks at levels of sexual functioning and global sexual satisfaction as well as psychological symptoms and affects related to sexual functioning.(Derogatis, 1975) The main areas this tool assesses are 1) general sexual knowledge, 2) types of sexual behaviour experienced, 3) drive for and real and ideal frequency of various sexual behaviours, 4) sexual attitudes, 5) psychological symptoms, 6) affect, both positive and negative, 7) gender role, 8) sexual fantasies, 9) body image, 10) degree of satisfaction with one's current sexual relationship.

There were no significant differences in sexual functioning or satisfaction with the decision to have a hysterectomy between the abused and the non-abused women. Significantly higher levels of depression were seen in women with a history of abusive sexual experiences compared with non-abused women. Importantly, there was a significant relationship between the two time-interval groups and levels of depression: the abused women were more depressed in the first year after hysterectomy than were women who had not been sexually abused. However, in the second year there were no significant differences in depression level between the two groups.

The first finding, that abused women were more depressed than non-abused women and had more negative affective symptoms, supports findings by Hendricks-Matthews that sexual assault could precipitate post-hysterectomy psychological sequelae. In view of the current high incidence of sexual abuse in the female population, it is important to consider the additional burden faced by such women when undergoing hysterectomy.

Wukasch emphasises the need to ask patients specifically about a history of negative sexual experiences prior to planning for hysterectomy as this information, being sensitive, is unlikely to be volunteered. On uncovering a positive history of sexual abuse specific preoperative counselling regarding the woman's thoughts, fears and fantasies about the forthcoming surgery should be undertaken.

In conclusion, hysterectomy is one of the most commonly performed gynaecological operations worldwide and has unique emotional, medical, social, and sexual significance for many women. All health care professionals must understand the consequences for women (particularly women with the additional burden of negative sexual experience) and develop ways to provide valid information, education and affirmation to these women before and after a hysterectomy. Family physicians have an important role in the perioperative journey, eliciting any history of sexual abuse, offering counselling and support throughout and coordinating further multidisciplinary support as required.

3.5 Comparison between alternative forms of treatment for menorrhagia

One of the major limitations of research in the field of quality of life assessment and sexual dysfunction is the over-reliance on observational studies. Randomized controlled trials in this field are difficult to perform, but in spite of the challenges a few trials have been conducted and reported comparing outcomes in women randomly assigned to either hysterectomy or medical treatment for menorrhagia.

One such reported study has been conducted by Kupperman et al., who randomly assigned 63 premenopausal women (aged between 30 and 50 years) with abnormal uterine bleeding for a median of four years to hysterectomy or expanded medical treatment with oestrogen and/or progesterone and/or a prostaglandin synthetase inhibitor. (Kupperman et al., 2004) The primary outcome was mental health, measured by the Mental Component Summary (MCS) of the RAND 36-Item Short-Form Health Survey (SF-36). Secondary outcomes included physical health, measured by the Physical Component Summary (PCS), symptom resolution and satisfaction, body image, and sexual functioning, as well as other aspects of mental health and general health perceptions. At six months, women in the hysterectomy group had greater improvement in MCS scores than women in the medicinal management group. They also had greater improvements in symptom resolution, symptom satisfaction, interference with sex, sexual desire, health distress, sleep problems, overall health, and satisfaction with health. By the end of the study, 53% of the women in the medicine group had requested and received hysterectomy and these women reported improvements in quality of life outcomes during the two years which were similar to those reported by women randomised to the hysterectomy group. Women who continued medical treatment also reported some improvements with the result that most differences between randomised groups at the end of the study were no longer statistically significant in the intention-to-treat analysis.

Hurskainen et al. randomly assigned two hundred and thirty six women complaining of menorrhagia to hysterectomy or treatment with a levonorgestrel intrauterine system releasing 20 micrograms of levonorgestrel on a daily basis and monitored all the women for five years. (Hurskainen et al., 2004) Health-related quality of life (HRQL), as measured by the 5-Dimensional EuroQol and other measures of psychosocial well-being (anxiety, depression, and sexual function) measured by the SF-36, were assessed in all the women. After five years of follow-up, both groups showed improved quality of life scores as well as decreases in anxiety and depression. There were no significant differences in these measures between the two groups, although 42% of women in the levonorgestrel intrauterine system group eventually underwent hysterectomy. Sub-analysis revealed that women in the levonorgestrel intrauterine system group had poorer baseline measurements in many of the considered factors.

Alexander et al., in a prospective randomised controlled trial, compared in psychiatric and psychological terms the outcome of endometrial ablation and hysterectomy for the treatment of dysfunctional uterine bleeding. (Alexander et al., 1996) Two hundred and four women with dysfunctional uterine bleeding who would otherwise have all undergone hysterectomy were randomised to either hysterectomy or endometrial ablation, which was carried out either by transcervical resection or by laser ablation of the endometrium. The main outcome measures considered were mental state, marital relationship, psychosocial and sexual adjustment in assessments conducted before the operation and one month, six months, and 12 months postoperatively. The four questionnaires that were used included the Eysenck personality questionnaire, the Hospital Anxiety and Depression Scale, the Psychosocial Adjustment to Illness Scale, and the Golombok Rust Inventory of Marital State. (Eysenck & Eysenck, 1964; Zigmond & Snaith, 1983; Derogatis, 1986; Rust et al., 1986)

Both treatments for dysfunctional uterine bleeding significantly reduced anxiety and depression present before the operation and there were no differences in mental health between the groups at 12 months. There were no links between hysterectomy and postoperative psychiatric illness. In terms of sexual interest, 46 out of a total of 185 women studied (25%) reported a loss of sexual interest with 50 out of 185 (27%) reporting increased sexual interest. There was no difference in postoperative level of sexual interest between the two procedures. Marital relationships were found to be unaffected by surgery. Personality and duration of dysfunctional uterine bleeding played no significant part in determining treatment outcome.

3.6 Hysterectomy in malignant disease

A large amount of research has been undertaken on the psychological and sexual aspects of hysterectomy for benign disease. This has, in most cases, found hysterectomy to have positive effects on psychological, sexual and quality of life indices. Discussion of hysterectomy is not complete without discussing hysterectomy for malignant disease. The existing literature on hysterectomy due to cervical or endometrial cancer tends to depict more negative postoperative outcomes than those seen thus far. In further analysing the various factors involved, however, we realise that these findings may not necessarily solely reflect the effects of hysterectomy per se.

Sexuality is central to quality of life and wellbeing, during the disease-free stage of the illness at least. Psychological function is clearly affected by gynaecological cancer and its treatment in concert with the physical sequelae. Threats to sexual identity and self-esteem, personal control over body functions, intimacy, relationship stability and the potential termination of reproductive capacity have all been implicated in negative effects on sexual function after cancer and its treatment. In many cases these effects could be more salient to women than the effect of the surgery itself. Additionally, changes in emotional wellbeing, for example the experiences of depression, anxiety, anger, and fatigue relating both to the fact of diagnosis as well as the physical illness symptoms can affect sexuality indirectly.

Research on appropriate interventions targeting these acquired sexual arousal complaints is sparse. There is little or no evidence for physical interventions aimed at addressing sexual issues and, in any case, such interventions would rarely address the significant psychological concerns emerging from cancer surgery. Postoperative counselling and support for cancer is extensively available but education about sexual physiology and about potential physical and psychological changes pertaining to sexuality in the disease is still limited, if available at all. Women are generally dissatisfied with the lack of attention given to such concerns. (Butler et al., 1998)

Capone et al. has reported that psychoeducation, combining education and information with elements of psychological therapy, significantly improves frequency of coital activity. (Capone et al., 1980) Robinson et al. also found that psychoeducation enhances compliance with sexual rehabilitation, reduce fear about intercourse, and improve sexual knowledge among early stage cancer patients.

Brotto et al. studied the efficacy of psychoeducational intervention to evoke sexual awareness, teach arousal-enhancing techniques, and facilitate capacity for change in various sexual functions. (Brotto et al., 2008) The primary endpoint of the study was sexual arousal and secondary endpoints were orgasm, sexual desire, sexual distress, relationship satisfaction, depressive symptoms and quality of life. The authors also compared women with cervical cancer with those with endometrial cancer to assess possible differential effects.

A brief, three-session psychoeducational intervention targeting female sexual arousal disorder in women with early stage gynaecological cancer was first developed and pilot tested. Twenty-two women participated in the total of four sessions. The intervention consisted of three one-hour sessions combining elements of cognitive and behavioural therapy with education and mindfulness training. Women completed questionnaires and underwent physiological measurement of genital arousal pre- and post-intervention (sessions one and four) and participated in a semi-structured interview (session four) during which their feedback was elicited. Significant positive effects were seen in terms of sexual desire, arousal, orgasm, satisfaction, sexual distress, depression and overall wellbeing and trends towards improved physiological genital arousal and perceived genital arousal were also displayed. These findings suggest that a brief three-session intervention can significantly improve aspects of sexual response, mood, and quality of life in gynaecological cancer patients. It also carries implications for establishing the components of the program for women with female sexual arousal disorders.

We now move on to looking specifically at hysterectomy carried out for malignant disease. This analysis, as we discussed previously, reveals the negative psychological and sexual impact of such surgery in contrast to positive outcomes seen with hysterectomy for other indications. When compared with a control group of women undergoing surgery for benign disease, radical hysterectomy for cervical cancer has been seen to produce significantly more lubrication problems, decreases in postoperative sexual activity, impairment in all phases of the sexual response cycle and an increase in diagnosable sexual dysfunctions. (Grumann et al., 2001; Kylstra et al., 1999)

Both physical and physiological mechanisms are involved in these negative effects. In a comparative study followed up over one year looking at women undergoing radical hysterectomy versus a healthy control group the cancer patients experienced significant impairment in genital arousal and negative genital sensations despite no differences in frequency of intercourse. The genital problems reported in these studies included lubrication difficulties, reduced vaginal length and elasticity and more importantly and distressingly, absence of genital swelling in more than half of sexual encounters. Impaired vaginal blood flow in response to sexual stimuli following radical hysterectomy has been quantified using a vaginal photoplethysmograph (Maas et al., 2002): these changes have been linked to autonomic nerve damage. (Butler-Manuel et al., 2000, 2002)

The radical trachelectomy, a fertility preserving surgery, has increasingly been used as a safe alternative to radical hysterectomy with similar recurrence rates for early stage cervical cancer in women of childbearing age. Radical trachelectomy offers hope for future child bearing with promising obstetric outcomes. These hopes and concerns are obviously associated with significant psychological and quality of life issues, the impacts of which are not fully understood. Carter et al. prospectively assessed and described the emotional, sexual and quality of life concerns of women with early-stage cervical cancer undergoing surgery. (Carter et al., 2010) A group of 71 women, consented for either radical trachelectomy or radical hysterectomy were enrolled for the study preoperatively in this two-year study. Participants completed a preoperative survey addressing sexual functioning, mood, distress, quality of life, and issues of fertility and treatment choice, which were explored by qualitative means. Follow-up questionnaires were completed at approximately 3, 6, 12, 18 and 24 months post-surgery.

The surveys used included the Functional Assessment of Cancer Therapy (FACT) scale, the Center for Epidemiological Studies Depression Scale (CES-D), the Impact of Event Scale (IES), the Female Sexual Function Index (FSFI) and background/medical information forms.

At preoperative assessment, women opting for radical hysterectomy reported greater concern about cancer recurrence than those undergoing radical trachelectomy. Of the women undergoing radical hysterectomy 48% reported having had adequate time to complete childbearing compared to 8.6% of those undergoing radical trachelectomy. Both groups preoperatively demonstrated scores suggestive of depression and distress in CES-D and IES scales respectively. Over time, however, CES-D and IES scores generally improved. Scores on the FSFI for the total sample were below the population mean, suggesting sexual dysfunction. These also continued to improve, however, both at 12 and then at 24 months. Overall, scores generally improved during the first year, reaching a plateau between year one and year two, which could reflect a new level of functioning in survivorship. The study concluded that measurements of mood, distress, sexual function and quality of life did not differ significantly with surgical type, and instead reflected the challenges faced by the young cervical cancer patients.

Grumann et al. noticed that despite extensive research on sexual dysfunction after gynaecological cancers, there is persisting uncertainty regarding its extent and nature. (Grumann et al., 2001) A trial was therefore carried out to determine whether radical hysterectomy for stage IB cervical cancer without adjuvant treatment leads to short and/or long-term sexual dysfunction. The authors prospectively studied 20 patients undergoing radical hysterectomy for stage IB cervical cancer, 18 women undergoing hysterectomy for benign disease, and 20 healthy women. Data was collected preoperatively and at four and eight months postoperatively using standardised questionnaires and specifically developed scales. Preoperatively, the cancer patients interestingly exhibited slightly better sexual functioning than women in the other two groups but this deteriorated slightly over time. Conversely, sexual functioning improved consistently over time in the women undergoing hysterectomy for benign disease.

Although the actual number of patients in this study was small, leading the authors to urge caution in interpreting the results, most studies addressing these issues have reported similar, significant disruptions in sexual function following surgery for cancer. (Schover et al., 1989; Wejmar Schultz et al., 1992; Anderson et al.,1989; Wejmar Schultz et al., 1991) Furthermore, adjuvant therapy for cancer following surgery is usually found to be associated with far greater sexual dysfunction. (Schover et al., 1989 and Wejmar Schultz et al., 1991)

In a similar study to the one described above, Serati et al. evaluated sexual functioning in a group of women undergoing radical hysterectomy for stage IB cervical cancer, again comparing them with a control group. (Serati et al., 2009) They also compared the same group of patients with a group undergoing laparoscopic assisted radical hysterectomy for the same indication. This was done using a validated questionnaire (FSFI) to assess the possible differences between laparoscopic radical hysterectomy and abdominal hysterectomy in terms of their impact on sexuality. The FSFI measures six domains of female sexuality: desire, arousal, lubrication, orgasm, satisfaction and pain. The authors recruited thirty-eight consecutive sexually active women due to undergo radical hysterectomy for the treatment of early stage cervical cancer and divided them into two groups according to the surgical approach. These patients were all asked to complete the FSFI at their follow-up appointment six months after surgery. Comparisons were made between the women undergoing radical hysterectomy and those undergoing laparoscopic radical hysterectomy. Further comparisons were made between the women undergoing laparotomic radical hysterectomy and a group of thirty-five healthy women (as controls) who were seen in the gynaecology clinic for routine gynaecologic evaluation.

Somewhat predictably, the FSFI scores were significantly higher in the healthy controls than in the abdominal radical hysterectomy group. Again as expected, the total score and scores in all the individual domains of the FSFI were lower in the laparoscopic radical hysterectomy group compared with healthy controls. There were no significant differences between laparotomic and laparoscopic surgery despite the minimally invasive nature of laparoscopic surgery.

The authors of this study concluded that it is important to inform women due to undergo radical hysterectomy of the commonly inevitable negative effects on sexuality. These effects may be minimised by open discussion prior to surgery and by commencing rehabilitation as soon as is feasible postoperatively.

Jongipipan examined prospectively the effect of radical hysterectomy on postoperative sexual function in South-East Asian women with early stage cervical cancer. (Jongpipan & Charoenkwan, 2007) The authors feel that sexual dysfunction is the leading cause of symptom-induced distress after surgery for early-stage cervical cancer. Thirty patients were recruited and interviewed at preoperative admission and at three and six months after surgery. Seven aspects of sexual function were assessed using visual analogue scores. These features included overall satisfaction with sexual intercourse, sexual desire, vaginal lubrication, vaginal elasticity, orgasmic satisfaction, patient-perceived partner satisfaction and associated anxiety. The authors in this study could not demonstrate any significant short-term negative impacts of radical hysterectomy on sexual function. As this was an observational study, however, without a comparison group and taking into account the small sample size, it is difficult to relate these results to the general population.

3.7 Vaginal surgery for prolapse and incontinence

Helström and Nilsson, in a prospective comparative cohort study, examined the effects of vaginal surgery for urinary incontinence and genital prolapse on sexual function and quality of life. (Helström and Nilsson, 2005) A total of 118 women, of whom 41 were undergoing surgery for urinary incontinence and 77 for genital prolapse, completed a questionnaire looking at uterovaginal symptoms, quality of life and sexuality one week prior to surgery. One year later, 101 women, of whom 88 were sexually active, accepted to complete the same questionnaire by mail. The women reported improvement in quality of life on two different scales and no difference was found between scores in women undergoing surgery for genital prolapse and those having surgery for urinary stress incontinence. The total score for sexual variables and the mean frequency of sexual intercourse had both reduced at this point. Amongst women with genital prolapse, 14% experienced more urinary incontinence and 13% experienced more dyspareunia after the operation.

Although pelvic floor disorders are known to impair sexual function, there was no improvement in sexuality after surgery for urinary incontinence or genital prolapse. On the contrary, it seemed from this study that sexual function and dyspareunia may both have deteriorated after vaginal surgery. The explanation for this could lie in the vulnerability of the vaginal nerves and vaginal wall blood supply to disturbance during surgery resulting in impaired sexual arousal and lubrication.

Depending on age it has been estimated that up to 40% of women have complaints of sexual problems, including decreased libido, vaginal dryness, pain with intercourse, decreased genital sensation and difficulty or inability to achieve orgasm. In a review by Tunuguntla et al (2006) the etiologies and incidence, evaluation and treatment of female sexual dysfunction following vaginal surgery for indications such as stress urinary incontinence and pelvic organ prolapse; anterior and or posterior colporrhaphy, perineoplasty and vaginal vault prolapse was studied. Literature on the mechanisms by which vaginal surgery affects female sexual function was discussed along with related pathophysiology to potential causes. The anatomy, neurovascular supply of the clitoris and introitus, and intrapelvic nerve supply were discussed in relation to vaginal surgery. Techniques to avoid neurovascular damage during pelvic floor surgery were corroborated by supporting literature and female sexual dysfunction following other procedures, such as vaginal hysterectomy, Martius flap interposition, and vesicovaginal and rectovaginal fistula repair were also discussed. Current literature did not support an association between vaginal length following vaginal surgery and sexual function. The proportion of women who were sexually active was not affected by vaginal surgery. Sling surgery for urinary incontinence did not appear to adversely affect overall sexual function, although individual parameters of sexual function scores may vary. Some patients experienced improved overall sexual function due to complete relief from coital incontinence. Symptomatic vaginal narrowing was rare even in women undergoing simultaneous posterior repair. Overall sexual satisfaction appeared to be independent of therapy for urinary incontinence or prolapse and defect specific posterior colporrhaphy with the avoidance of levator ani plication might improve sexual function. The authors concluded that possible etiological factors for sexual dysfunction following vaginal surgery deserve further investigations.

3.8 Hysterectomy for chronic pelvic pain

Chronic pelvic pain is a common symptom which affects about 15% of women in the United States. (Mathias et al., 1996) It remains poorly understood and there is no clear consensus on whether it should be classed as a diagnosis or a symptom. Zondervan et al. carried out a postal questionnaire study looking into chronic pelvic pain in women. (Zondervan et al., 2001) The population prevalence of the condition was found in this study to be about 24% with pain in one third of these cases apparently lasting for more than five years. The most troublesome aspects of the symptoms reportedly included pain severity, use of healthcare, effects on physical and mental health, sleep quality and pain-related absence from work. High levels of symptom-related anxiety were also identified in this group of women.

Despite the poor understanding of the condition by clinicians various treatment options, both medical (including various types of analgesia) and surgical (such as complete and partial resection of pelvic organs and neuroablative procedures) have been discussed. (Howard, FM. 2003) Of all the hysterectomies performed in the US 12% quote pelvic pain as the primary indication making hysterectomy one of the main treatment modalities for chronic pelvic pain even though 70% of aetiologies attributed to the development of chronic pelvic pain are not gynaecological in origin. (Lee et al., 1984; Wu et al., 2007; Lamvu et al., 2006; Zondervan et al., 1999; Zondervan et al., 2001) The role of hysterectomy in treating chronic pelvic pain therefore remains controversial.

A literature search on chronic pelvic pain and hysterectomy revealed a paucity of relevant evidence. Stovall et al. published long term outcomes from 99 women undergoing hysterectomy for idiopathic chronic pelvic pain. (Stovall et al., 1990) Most of these women had histories of failed medical or surgical treatments for chronic pelvic pain. Hysterectomies were undertaken in these subjects in the belief that the uterus was the origin of the chronic pelvic pain. It was found, however, that 22% of the women complained of continued chronic pelvic pain 12 to 64 months after hysterectomy. The authors were surprised at these findings, particularly as a proportion of the women complaining of continued pelvic pain post-hysterectomy were those in which histology results had confirmed uterine disease.

Hillis et al. confirmed these findings when a similar cohort of 308 women with chronic pelvic pain was studied undergoing hysterectomy. (Hillis et al., 1995) Of this sample 21% reported continued but decreased pain and another 5% reported unchanged or increased pain after hysterectomy. Interestingly, the authors found that women who were younger than 30 years of age, uninsured, without identifiable pathology at the time of surgery and with a history of pelvic inflammatory disease were at increased risk of non-resolving pain. Stovall et al. concluded that, particularly in these groups, hysterectomy might ameliorate the pain but was unable to cure it.

Both of the above studies were limited by the relatively small numbers of participants, absence of control groups and by the fact that they did not consider confounding factors such as histories of psychological illness and abuse in the patients studied. Moreover, the studies did not identify and evaluate quality of life markers, activity levels and sexual functions.

The relationships between hysterectomy, quality of life and pelvic pain were explored by Hartmann et al. in a study which aimed to evaluate differences in quality of life and sexual function after hysterectomy in 1249 women, a proportion of whom suffered from preoperative pain and depression. (Hartmann et al., 2004) Preoperative pain was assessed and defined in terms of its duration, character and intensity. The women were monitored for up to 24 months in outcome measures including physical function, social function, health perception, continued pain, sexual frequency, dyspareunia and satisfaction with surgery. Subjects were divided into three groups: women with preoperative pain, women with preoperative depression and women with both pain and depression. They were also compared against a healthy control group. All of the variables were studied at 6, 12 and 24 months for each study group.

The authors found that women with preoperative pain, depression or with both conditions improved substantially above baseline, with improvement in pain sustained throughout the study period. However, when compared with the control group women with pre-existing pain and depression were three to five times more likely to suffer impairments in quality of life and to experience pelvic pain and dyspareunia 24 months after hysterectomy. This study had a few limitations in terms of methodology. Firstly, the patients' initial diagnoses of pelvic pain and depression were self-reported. In addition, the indications for undergoing hysterectomy were varied and psychiatric comorbidities such as anxiety and partner interactions were not considered.

The Maine Women's Health Study, a prospective cohort study of 418 women undergoing hysterectomy for non-malignant conditions, interviewed women at the time of surgery and at 3,6, and 12 months postoperatively. (Carlson et al., 1994) The main outcome measures considered were symptom relief, changes in quality of life and the development of new symptoms during the year following surgery. Chronic pelvic pain was found to be the primary indication for hysterectomy in 18% of the women studied. It was noted that hysterectomy had positive effects on pelvic pain, psychological symptoms, and sexual dysfunction, although it was not specified whether these figures pertained specifically to women undergoing hysterectomy for chronic pain. If these results relate to all hysterectomies considered in the study, this must be borne in mind during interpretation in the knowledge that such outcomes are likely to vary according to indication for hysterectomy.

4. Conclusion

Hysterectomy is one of the commonest operations performed in the UK and in the US, carried out in most cases for benign disease. Most studies revealed significant improvements in general wellbeing, psychological measures and sexuality following hysterectomy which were unrelated to route and type of surgery. Concomitant oophorectomy also yielded similar benefits. The only exceptions to this rule were hysterectomies undertaken for malignant disease: cases which are often complicated by other major factors relating to the disease. Psychological and sexual outcomes of surgery were found to be even poorer in cases requiring adjuvant therapy for the cancer. When hysterectomy is carried out on a background of long-term morbidity including depression, anxiety and chronic pain the results in terms of postoperative psychological and sexual functioning may again be less favourable. In these cases preoperative assessment and counselling is a key to optimising postoperative psychological and sexual outcomes.

5. References

Alexander DA, Naji AA, Pinion SB, Mollison J, Kitchener HC, Parkin DE, Abramovich DR & Russell IT. (1996) Randomised trial comparing hysterectomy with endometrial ablation for dysfunctional uterine bleeding: psychiatric and psychosocial aspects. *BMJ.* 312(7026): 280-4

Anderson BL, Anderson B & deProsse C. (1989) Controlled prospective longitudinal study of women with cancer: I. Sexual functioning outcomes. *Journal of Consulting and Clinical Psychology.* 57(6):683-691

Aziz A, Brännström M, Bergquist C & Silfverstolpe G. (2005a) Perimenopausal androgen decline after oophorectomy does not influence sexuality or psychological well-being. *Fertility and Sterility*. 83: 1021-1028

Aziz A, Bergquist C, Nordholm L, Moller A & Silfverstolpe G. (2005b) Prophylactic oophorectomy at elective hysterectomy: Effects on psychological well-being at 1 year follow up and its correlation to sexuality. *Maturitas, the European Menopause journal*. 51: 349-357

Basson, R. (2001) Human sex-response cycles. *Journal of Sex & Marital Therapy*. 27: 33-43

Bellerose, SB & Binik, YM. (1993) Body image and sexuality in oophrectomised women. *Archives of Sexual Behaviour*. 22: 435-457

Briere J & Runtz M. (1988) Symptomatology associated with childhood sexual victimization in a nonclinical adult sample. *Child abuse and neglect*. 12, 51-59

Broome A & Wallace L, eds. (1984). *Psychology and Gynecological Problems*. Tavistock Publications, London.

Brotto LA, Heiman JR, Goff B, Greer B, Lentz GM, Swisher E, Tamimi H & Van Blaricom A. (2008) A psychoeducational intervention for sexual dysfunction in women with gynecologic cancer. *Archives of Sexual Behavior*. 37(2): 317- 329

Butler L, Banfield V, Sveinson T & Allen K (1998) Conceptualizing sexual health in cancer care. *Western Journal of Nursing Research*. 20(6):683-705

Butler-Manuel SA, Buttery LD, A'Hern RP, Polak JM & Barton DP. (2000). Pelvic nerve plexus trauma at radical hysterectomy and simple hysterectomy: The nerve content of the uterine supporting ligaments. *Cancer*. 89: 834-841

Butler-Manuel SA, Buttery LD, A'Hern RP, Polak JM & Barton DP. (2002) Pelvic nerve plexus trauma at radical hysterectomy and simple hysterectomy: A quantitative study of nerve types in the uterine supporting ligaments. *Journal of the Society for Gynecologic Investigation*. 9: 47-5.

Capone MA, Good RS, Westie KS & Jacobson AF. (1980) Psychosocial rehabilitation of gynecologic oncology patients. *Archives of Physical Medicine and Rehabilitation*. 61(3):128–132

Carlson KJ, Miller BA & Fowler FJ Jr. (1994) The Maine Women's Health Study: I. Outcomes of hysterectomy. *Obstetrics and Gynecology*. 83(4):556-65

Carter J, Sonoda Y, Baser RE, Raviv L, Chi DS, Barakat RR, Iasonos A, Brown CL & Abu-Rustum NR. (2010) A 2-year prospective study assessing the emotional, sexual and quality of life concerns of women undergoing radical hysterectomy versus radical trachelectomy for treatment of early-stage cervical cancer. *Gynaecologic Oncology*. 119: 358-365

Department of Health (1989-1999) Hospital Episode Statistics. Elephant & Castle, London SE1 6TE.

Derogatis LR. (1975). Derogatis Sexual Functioning Inventory (DSFI): Preliminary Scoring Manual. *Clinical Psychometric Research*. Baltimore, MD.

Derogatis LR. (1986) The psychosocial adjustment to illness scale (PAIS). *Journal of Psychosomatic Research* 30(1):77-91

Domingo S & Pellicer A. (2009) Overview of Current Trends in Hysterectomy: Indications for Hysterectomy, *Medscape*, 07/08/2011, Available from: <http://www.medscape.com/viewarticle/712569_2>

Ellström MA, Astrom M, Moller A, Olsson JH & Hahlin M. (2003) A randomized trial comparing changes in psychological well-being and sexuality after laparoscopic and abdominal hysterectomy. *Acta Obstetricia et Gynecologica Scandinavica*. 82: 871-875

Eysenck HJ & Eysenck SB. (1964) *Manual of the Eysenck Personality Inventory*. London University Press, London.

Farquhar CM, Harvey SA, Yu Y, Sadler L & Stewart AW. (2006) A prospective study of 3 years of outcomes after hysterectomy with and without oophorectomy. *American journal of obstetrics and gynecology*. 194: 711-717

Ferrari E, Casarotti D, Muzzoni B, Albertelli N, Cravello L, Fioravanti M, Solerte SB & Magri F. (2001) Age-related changes of the adrenal secretory pattern: possible role in pathological brain aging. *Brain Research Reviews*. 37:294 –300

Finkelhor, D. (1990) Early and long-term effects of child sexual abuse: An update. *Professional Psychology: Research and Practice*. 21(5): 325-330

Gath D, Cooper P, Bond A & Edmonds, G. (1981) Hysterectomy and psychiatric disorder: II. Demographic psychiatric and physical factors in relation to psychiatric outcome. *British Journal of Psychiatry*. 143:1293-1296

Gath, D. Cooper, P. Day, A. (1982) Hysterectomy and psychiatric disorder: I. Levels of psychiatric morbidity before and after hysterectomy. *The British Journal of Psychiatry*. 140: 335-342

Gath D, Rose N, Bond A, Day A, Garrod A & Hodges S. (1995) Hysterectomy and psychiatric disorder: are the levels of psychiatric morbidity falling? *Psychological medicine*. 25(2):277-283

Goldberg, DP. (1972) *The Detection of Psychiatric Illness by Questionnaire*. Oxford University Press, New York. (Moudsley Monograph No 21.)

Grumann M, Robertson R, Hacker NF & Sommer G. (2001) Sexual functioning in patients following radical hysterectomy for stage IB cancer of the cervix. *International Journal of Gynecological Cancer*. 11(5): 372-380

Gupta S & Manyonda I. (2011) Total and subtotal abdominal hysterectomy for benign gynaecological disease *Obstetrics, Gynaecology and Reproductive Medicine*. 21(2):36-40

Gütl P, Greimel ER, Roth R & Winter R. (2002) Women's sexual behavior, body image and satisfaction with surgical outcomes after hysterectomy: a comparison of vaginal and abdominal surgery. *Journal of Psychosomatic Obstetrics and Gynecology*. 23(1):51-59

Hartmann KE, Ma C, Lamvu GM, Langenberg PW, Steege JF & Kjerulff KH.(2004) Quality of life and sexual function after hysterectomy in women with preoperative pain and depression. *Obstetrics and Gynecology*. 104(4):701-9

Helström L & Nilsson B. (2005) Impact of vaginal surgery on sexuality and quality of life in women with urinary incontinence or genital descensus. *Acta Obstetricia et Gynecologica Scandinavica*. 84(1):79-84

Hendricks-Matthews, MK. (1991) The importance of Assessing a Woman's History of sexual abuse before hysterectomy. *The Journal of Family Practice*. 32(6): 631-632

Hillis SD, Marchbanks PA & Peterson HB. (1995) The effectiveness of hysterectomy for chronic pelvic pain. *Obstetrics and Gynecology*. 86(6):941-5

Howard FM. (2003) Chronic pelvic pain. *Obstetrics and Gynaecology*. 101(3):594-611

Hurskainen R, Teperi J, Rissanen P, Aalto AM, Grenman S, Kivelä A, Kujansuu E, Vuorma S, Yliskoski M & Paavonen J. (2004) Clinical outcomes and costs with the levonorgestrel-releasing intrauterine system or hysterectomy for treatment of menorrhagia: randomized trial 5-year follow-up. *JAMA*. 291(12): 1456-63

Jenkinson C, Lawrence K, McWhinnie D & Gordon J. (1995) Sensitivity to change of health status measures in a randomized controlled trial: comparison of the COOP charts and the SF-36. *Quality of Life Research*. 4(1):47-52

Jongpipan J & Charoenkwan K. (2007) Sexual function after radical hysterectomy for early-stage cervical cancer. *Journal of Sexual Medicine*. 4(6):1659-1665

Kaplan HS. (1974) *The New Sex Therapy: Active Treatment of Sexual Disorders*. Balliere Tindall, London.

Karasu TB. (1990) Toward a clinical model of psychotherapy for depression, I: Sytematic comparison of three psychotherapies. *American Journal of Psychiatry*. 147(2):133-147

Khastgir G & Studd J. (1998) Hysterectomy, ovarian failure, and depression. *Menopause*. 5(2):113-122

Kroll J. (1988) *The challenge of the borderline patient: Competency in diagnosis and treatment*. W.W. Norton, New York.

Kuppermann M, Summitt RL Jr, Varner RE, McNeeley SG, Goodman-Gruen D, Learman LA, Ireland CC, Vittinghoff E, Lin F, Richter HE, Showstack J, Hulley SB & Washington AE; Total or Supracervical Hysterectomy Research Group.(2005) Sexual functioning after total compared with supracervical hysterectomy: a randomized trial. *Obstetrics and Gynecology*. 105(6):1309-18

Kuppermann M, Varner RE, Summitt RL Jr, Learman LA, Ireland C, Vittinghoff E, Stewart AL, Lin F, Richter HE, Showstack J, Hulley SB & Washington AE; Ms Research Group. (2004) Effect of hysterectomy vs medical treatment on health-related quality of life and sexual functioning: the medicine or surgery (Ms) randomized trial. *JAMA*. 291(12):1447-1455

Kylstra WA, Leenhouts GH, Everaerd W, Panneman MJ, Hahn DE, Weijmar Schultz WC, Van De Wiel HB & Heintz AP. (1999) Sexual outcomes following treatment for early stage gynaecological cancer: a prospective multicentre study. *International Journal of Gynaecological Cancer*. 9(5):387-395

Labrie F, Bélanger A, Cusan L, Gomez JL & Candas B. (1997) Marked decline in serum concentrations of adrenal C19 sex steroid precursors and conjugated androgen metabolites during aging. *The Journal of Clinical Endocrinology & Metabolism*. 82(8):2396–2402

Lamvu G, Williams R, Zolnoun D, Wechter ME, Shortliffe A, Fulton G & Steege JF. (2006) Long-term outcomes after surgical and non-surgical management of chronic pelvic pain: one-year after evaluation in a pelvic pain speciality clinic. *AJOG*. 195(2): 591-8

Lee NC, Dicker RC, Rubin GL & Ory HW. (1984) Confirmation of the preoperative diagnoses of hysterectomy. *AJOG*. 150(3):283-7

Lepine LA, Hillis SD, Marchbanks PA, Koonin LM, Morrow B, Kieke BA & Wilcox LS. (1997) Hysterectomy surveillance - United States, 1980- 1993. Morbidity and Mortality Weekly Report (MMWR) CDC Surveillance Summaries. 46(4):1-14

Lowery M. (1987) Adult survivors of childhood incest. *Journal of Psycholosocial Nursing and Mental Health Services*. 25(1):27-31

Maas CP, ter Kuile M, Tuynman C, Laan E, Weyenborg P, Trimbos JB, et al. (2002). Disturbance of sexual response after radical hysterectomy: A psychophysiologic study. *International Journal of Gynecologic Cancer*, 12:613-614

Mackey T, Sereika SM, Weissfeld LA, Hacker SS, Zender JF & Heard SL. (1992) Factors associated with long-term depressive symptoms of sexual assault victims. *Archives of Psychaitric Nursing*. 6(1):10-25

Masters WH & Johnson VE. (1966) *Human Sexual response*. Little, Brown Co. 117, Boston, MA.

Mathias SD, Kuppermann M, Liberman RF, Lipschutz R & Steege JF. (1996) Chronic pelvic pain: prevalence, health-related quality of life, and economic correlates. *Obstetrics and Gynecology*. 87(3): 321-7

McHorney CA, Ware JE Jr, Lu JF & Sherbourne CD. (1994) The MOS 36-item short-term health status survey (SF-36) III: Tests of data quality, scaling assumptions, and reliability across diverse patient groups. *Medical Care*. 32(1):40-66

McNair D M & Lorr M. (1964) An analysis of mood in neurotics. *I. Journal of Abnormal Psychology*. 69:620-7

Melzack R. (1982) *The Challenge of Pain*. Harmondsworth: Penguin.

Mokate T, Wright C & Mander T. (2006) Hysterectomy and sexual function. *Journal of British Menopause Society*. 12(4):153-157

Nappi R, Salonia A, Traish AM, van Lunsen RH, Vardi Y, Kodiglu A & Goldstein I (2005) Clinical biologic pathophysiologies of women's sexual dysfunction. *The Journal of Sexual Medicine*. 2(1):4-25

Nathörst-Boos J & von Schoultz B. (1992) Psychological reactions and sexual life after hysterectomy with and without oophorectomy. *Gynecologic and Obstetric Investigation*. 34(2):97-101

Nathörst-Boos J, von Schoultz B & Carlström K. (1993) Elective ovarian removal and estrogen replacement therapy--effects on sexual life, psychological well-being and androgen status. *Journal of Psychosomatic Obstetrics and Gynecology*. 14(4):283-293

Nieboer TE, Johnson N, Lethaby A, Tavender E. Curr E, Garry R, van Voorst S, Mol BWJ & Kluivers KB. (2009) Surgical approach to hysterectomy for benign gynaecological disease. *Cochrane Database of Systematic Reviews*. 25;(1):CD003677

O'Hara MW, Reiter RC, Johnson SR, Milburn A & Engeldinger J. (eds). (1995) *Psychological Aspects of Women's Reproductive Health*. Springer Publishing Company, New York

Parker CR Jr, Mixon RL, Brissie RM & Grizzle WE. (1997) Aging alters zonation in the adrenal cortex of men. *The Journal of Clinical Endocrinology & Metabolism*. 82(11):3898–3901

Persson P, Brynhildsen J & Kjølhede P; Hysterectomy Multicentre Study Group in South-East Sweden. (2010a) Short-term recovery after subtotal and total abdominal hysterectomy--a randomised clinical trial. *BJOG*. 117(4):469-478

Persson P, Brynhildsen J & Kjølhede P; Hysterectomy Multicentre Study Group in South-East Sweden. (2010b) A 1-year follow-up of psychological wellbeing after subtotal and total abdominal hysterectomy--a randomised study. *BJOG*. 117(4): 479-487

Persson P, Wijma K, Hammar M & Kjølhede P. (2006) Psychological wellbeing after laparoscopic and abdominal hysterectomy--a randomised controlled multicentre study. *BJOG*. 113(9):1023- 1030

Polivy, J. (1974) Psychological reactions to hysterectomy: A critical review. *AJOG*. 118(3):417-426

Rannestad, T. Eikeland, O. Helland, H. Quarnstorm, U. (2001) The quality of women suffering from gynaecological disorders is improved by means of hysterectomy. *Acta Obstet Gynaecol Scand* 80: 46-51

Rhodes JC, Kjerulff KH, Lagenberg PW & Guzinski GM. (1999) Hysterctomy and sexual functioning. *JAMA*. 282(20):1934-41

Rust J, Bennum I, Crowe M & Golombok S. (1986) The construction and validation of the Golombok Rust inventory of marital state. *Sexual and Marital Therapy*.1:34-40

Schover LR, Fife M & Gershenson DM. (1989) Sexual dysfunction and treatment for early stage cervical cancer. Cancer. 63(1):204-12

Serati M, Salvatore S, Uccella S, Laterza RM, Cromi A, Ghezzi F & Bolis P. (2009) Sexual dysfunction after radical hysterectomy for early stage cervical cancer: is there a difference between laparoscopy and laparotomy? *Journal of Sexual Medicine.* 6(9):2516-2522

Shifren JL & Avis, N. (2007) Surgical menopause: effects on psychological well-being and sexuality. *Menopause.* 14 (3):586-91

Sintchak G & Geer JH. (1975) A vaginal plethysmograph system. *Psychophysiology.* 12(1):113-115

Stovall TG, Ling FW & Crawford DA. (1990) Hysterectomy for chronic pelvic pain of presumed uterine etiology. *Obstetrics and Gynecology.* 75(4):676-9

Strauss B, Jäkel I, Koch-Dörfler M, Lehmann-Willenbrock E, Giese KP & Semm K. (1996) [Psychiatric and sexual sequelae of hysterectomy--a comparison of different surgical methods] *Geburtshilfe Frauenheilkd.* 56(9):473-81.

Swales PJ & Sheikh JI. (1992) Hysterectomy in patients with panic disorder. *The American Journal of Psychiatry.* 149(6): 846-7.

Thakar R, Ayers S, Georgakapolou A, Clarkson P, Stanton S & Manyonda I, (2004) Hysterectomy improves quality of life and decreases psychiatric symptoms: a prospective and randomied comparison of total versus subtotal hysterectomy. *BJOG* 111(10):1115-1120.

Thornton EW, McQueen C, Rosser R, Kneale T & Dixon K. (1997) A prospective study of changes in negative mood states of women undergoing surgical hysterectomy: the relationship to cognitive predisposition and familial support. *Journal of Psychosomatic Obstetrics & Gynecology.* 18(1):22-30

Tunuguntla, H.S.G.R. Gousse, A.E. (2006) Female sexual dysfunction following vaginal surgery: A review. *Journal of Urology.* 175: 439-446.

Weijmar Schultz WCM, Van de Weil HBM & Bouma J. (1991) Psychosexual functioning after treatment for cancer of the cervix: a comparative and longitudinal study. *International Journal of Gynecological Cancer.* 1(1):37-46

Weijmar Schultz WCM, Bransfield DD, Van de Weil HB & Bouma J. (1992) Sexual outcomes following female genital cancer treatment: a critical review of methods of investigation and results. *Sexual & Marital Therapy.* 7(1):29-64

Williams RD & Clark, AJ. (2000) A qualitative study of women's hysterectomy experience. *Journal of Women's Health & Gender-Based Medicine.* 9 Suppl 2:S15-25.

Wing JK, Cooper JE & Sartorius N. (1974) *The measurement and classification of psychiatric symptoms.* Cambridge University Press, London.

Wu J, Wechter M, Geller E, Nguyen T & Visco A. (2007) Hysterectomy rates in the United States.*Obstetrics and Gynecology.* 110:1091-5

Wukasch RN. (1996) The impact of a history rape and incest on the post-hysterectomy experience. *Healthcare for Women International.* 17(1):47-55

Zondervan KT, Yudkin PL, Vessey MP, Dawes MG, Barlow DH, Kennedy SH. (1999) Patterns of diagnosis and referral in women consulting for chronic pelvic pain in UK primary care. *BJOG.* 106(11):1156-61

Zondervan KT, Yudkin PL, Vessey MP, Jenkinson CP, Dawes MG, Barlow DH, Kennedy SH. (2001) Chronic pelvic pain in the community – symptoms, investigations, and diagnosis. *AJOG.* 184(6):1149-55

Zigmond AS & Snaith RP. (1983) The hospital anxiety and depression scale. *Acta Psychiatrica Scandinavica.* 67(6):361-70

What Do We Know About Hysterectomy?

Karolina Chmaj-Wierzchowska[1], Marcin Wierzchowski[2],
Beata Pięta[1], Joanna Buks[1] and Tomasz Opala[1]
[1]*University of Medical Sciences, Department of Mother's and Child's Health Poznan,*
[2]*University of Medical Sciences,*
Chair and Department of Chemical Technology of Drugs Poznan,
Poland

1. Introduction

A total hysterectomy is the most common type of gynecologic surgery and may be performed to treat many diseases that affect the uterus including: abnormal uterine bleeding, uterine fibroids, endometriosis and chronic pelvic pain, anatomic uterine defects, uterine prolapse and cancer (Reich, 2003). Based on German studies from 2005 and 2006 (overall 305 015 hysterectomies performed during the study period) the hysterectomy rate for benign diseases of the genital tract among women aged 20 or older (3.6 out of 1000 women) was higher than in Sweden but lower than in the US or Australia (Gupta, 2006, Stang 2011). The United States still has the highest incidence of hysterectomy, with about 550 000 women undergoing this operation annually, at a cost of more than $5 billion. The rate of this procedure in the USA is 5.4/1000 women, whereas in Italy it is 3.7/1000 and in Norway only 1.2/1000 women (Manyonda, 2003).

The hysterectomy can be done in different ways. These procedures can be performed using one of three main approaches: laparoscopic hysterectomy (LH), abdominal hysterectomy (AH) and vaginal hysterectomy (VH) (Clayton 2006). In laparoscopic, abdominal and vaginal hysterectomy can we removal of the uterus and cervix with/or without removal of ovaries. Table 1 show three main procedures of hysterectomy and surgery extension of female organs (tab.1).

Laparoscopic hysterectomy	**Abdominal hysterectomy**	**Vaginal hysterectomy**
Complete removal of the uterus and with/or without cervix with/or without removal of ovaries. Lymph nodes, ovaries and fallopian tubes can also be removed in this situation.	Removal of the uterus, cervix, upper vagina, and parametrium. Lymph nodes, ovaries and fallopian tubes can also be removed in this situation.	Removal of the uterus, cervix with/or without removal of ovaries

Table 1. Three main procedures of hysterectomy

The type of hysterectomy depends on the reason for the surgery and other factors for example age or general health condition and main disease and expertise, as the indications for each technique overlap. VH is probably the preferred route because it is quicker and cheaper than LH, with no other clear differences in outcome measures. LH has a number of advantages over AH like specifically, shorter hospital stay and quicker return to normal activities; complication rates, however, appear to be greater (Clayton 2006). In gynecological practice in the UK and the USA, 60–80% of all hysterectomies are performed by the abdominal route. In one of the German studies for all performed hysterectomies only 6% were laparoscopically assisted vaginal hysterectomies and 5% laparoscopic hysterectomies. 10% of laparoscopical hysterectomies and 1% of vaginal hysterectomies necessitated a conversion to an abdominal hysterectomy (Stang 2011).

There are three basic types of hysterectomy: total hysterectomy, supracervical also called subtotal or partial hysterectomy and radical hysterectomy. All these procedures can be conducted with or without the removal of the ovaries and the fallopian tubes on one or both sides (Tab. 2).

Total hysterectomy	Subtotal hysterectomy	Radical hysterectomy
Complete removal of the uterus and cervix with/or without removal of fallopian tubes and ovaries	Removal of the uterus, leaving the cervix with/or without removal of fallopian tubes and ovaries	Removal of the uterus, cervix, upper vagina, and parametrium. Lymph nodes, ovaries and fallopian tubes are also usually removed in this situation.

Table 2. Three basic types of hysterectomy

The ACOG (American Congress of Obstetricians and Gynecologists) has suggested that concomitant bilateral oophorectomy should be performed during the hysterectomy for benign uterine diseases in peri- and postmenopausal women. Strong consideration should be made for retaining normal ovaries in premenopausal women who are not at increased genetic risk of ovarian cancer. In Germany, 4% and 26% of all hysterectomies for benign diseases of the genital tract included bilateral oophorectomy among peri- and postmenopausal women respectively. The highest hysterectomy rates were among women aged 40–49 years (9.9 per 1,000 women) (Stang 2011). Twenty-six percent of hysterectomies for benign diseases among women aged 50 or older were bilateral oophorectomy. Another study conducted in the USA showed that 37% of hysterectomies among women with benign diseases of the genital tract aged 15–44 years were accompanied by bilateral oophorectomy.

2. Abdominal hysterectomy procedures

2.1 General information on abdominal hysterectomy procedures

A hysterectomy (from Greek ὑστέρα hystera "womb" and εκτομία ektomia "a cutting out of") is the surgical removal of the uterus. Hysterectomy is the second most commonly performed surgical procedure in the United States after cesarean delivery (Falcone, 2008). Hysterectomy is a common procedure in Australia; approximately 1 in 5 Australian women undergoing a hysterectomy by the age of 50 for indications such as fibroids, disorders of menstruation (including excessive or irregular menstrual bleeding), and endometriosis (Graham, 2008).

In the management of early-stage cancer a radical hysterectomy can be performed (Panici, 2011). The most commonly used definition was proposed by Pivera, Rytledge'a and Smitha (tab.3). Five classes (class I–V) of extended hysterectomy were described. Class II and Class III are the most commonly employed (Piver 1974; Clayton 2006).

Type of surgery	Scope of procedure
Class 1	Outer facial surgical excision of the uterus. As a master of fact it is not a radical hysterectomy, it comprises only pushing the ureters away laterally without their preparation, which allows to clamp the vagina. The uterus is removed with an additional margin of the parametrium and the vagina.
Class 2	Excision of the uterus along with the primary ligament which is intersected centrally in relation to the ureter. Excision of the sacro-uterine ligaments in the middle of their length and 1/3 of the upper vagina.
Class 3	It assumes the intersection of the primary ligaments laterally from the ureter by the pelvic wall and the intersection of the sacro-uterine ligaments as close to the sacrum as possible, i.e. hysterectomy with the removal of the entire broad and sacro-uterine ligaments as well as 1/2 of the vagina.
Class 4	Excision of the uterus and the periuretal tissue, resection of the upper vesical artery 3/4 of the vagina
Class 5	Excision of the urinary bladder with distal ureteral segments.

Table 3. Types of operations according to Piver, Rytledge and Smith (Piver 1974)

Laparotomy is still considered the standard approach for radical hysterectomy; however, the total extraperitoneal abdominal radical hysterectomy (TEARH) has been described as a valid alternative for pelvic lymphadenectomy, with shorter operative time, shorter ileus and reduced postoperative pain and hospitalization (Panici, 2011).

2.2 Indications and contraindications

2.2.1 General indications for abdominal hysterectomy

General, noncancer indications for the abdominal surgeries of the removal of the uterus include: uterus "too big" or vagina "too narrow" (pubic arch < 90 degrees, bituberous diameter < 8.0 cm), uterus "too high" or "will not come down" also intra-abdominal conditions contraindicate vaginal approach (adhesions, endometriosis, adnexal disease, previous pelvic surgery, chronic pelvic pain, previous cesarean delivery) (Kovac, 2004; Learman, 2011). The indications for AH or VH in 2005 have changed little over the last decade, with uterine leiomyomata (33%) and being the most common, followed by prolapse (13%) and endometriosis (9%) (NIS 2007; Falcone 2008) . One should not forget that one of the indications for hysterectomy is sex reassignment. The predictors of hysterectomy is also performs as a treatment for menstrual problems (Graham, 2008).

Indications for radical surgeries depend on the severity and type of tumour show the table (tab.4).

Type of surgery	Indications
Class 1	Preinvasive carcinoma, early invasion
Class 2	Neoplastic invasion greater than in class 1.
Class 3	Clinical severity 1b, 2a
Class 4	Neoplastic process involving the bladder and distal ureteral segments
Class 5	Neoplastic process involving the bladder and distal ureteral segments

Table 4. Types of surgeries

2.2.2 Obstetrical hysterectomy

Perinatal hysterectomy is the removal of the uterus immediately after delivery or caesarean section or up to 24 hours after delivery or cesarean section. It is a difficult procedure, performed rarely usually due to emergency indications, burdened with a high risk of postoperative complications. It is often a consequence of previously performed caesarean section and accompanying complications such as uterine rupture in the scar or bleeding from the villi of the placenta located on the front wall of the uterus, which grow into the scar (Poręba, 2007).

Flood et al. (Flood et all, 2009) was performed a retrospective cohort study from 1966-2005 of patients who had peripartum hysterectomy (PH). There were 872,379 deliveries during the study period, among which 358 women underwent PH (0.4/1000 deliveries). In a comparison of the study decades 1966-1975 with 1996-2005, peripartum hysterectomy decreased from 0.9 per 1000 deliveries to 0.2 of 1000 deliveries. Although the overall cesarean delivery rate has increased from 6-19% during these 2 decades, the percentage of peripartum hysterectomy that occurs in the setting of a previous cesarean delivery has increased from 27-57% ($P < .00001$). According to the authors, main indications for PH had changed significantly in this time period, with "uterine rupture" as the indication for peripatum hysterectomy decreasing from 40.5-9.3% ($P < .0001$) and placenta accreta as the indication increasing significantly from 5.4-46.5% ($P < .00001$) (Flood et all, 2009). Poręba et all. (Poręba et all,) had analysed 63 232 labours between 1980-2005. 10 317 deliveries were eventually managed by caesarean section, and the emergency peripartum hysterectomy was necessary in 39 cases after labour in Department of Gynecology and Obstetrics Medical University of Silesia in Poland. In the opinion of the researchers, peripartum and intraoperational haemorrhage being a result of uterine atony was the most frequent cause of emergency peripartum hysterectomy (Poręba et all,). Shellhaas et all (Shellhaas, 2009) were described a total of 186 cesarean hysterectomies (0.5%) which were performed from a cohort of 39,244 women who underwent cesarean delivery. The leading indications for hysterectomy were placenta accreta (38%) and uterine atony (34%). Of the hysterectomy cases with a diagnosis recorded as accreta, 18% accompanied a primary cesarean delivery while 82% had a prior procedure ($p<0.001$). Of the hysterectomy cases with atony recorded as a diagnosis, 59% complicated primary cesarean delivery whereas 41% had a prior cesarean ($p< 0.001$). Major maternal complications of cesarean hysterectomy included transfusion of red blood cells (84%) and other blood products (34%), fever (11%), subsequent laparotomy (4%), ureteral injury (3%), and death (1.6%). Accreta hysterectomy cases were more likely than atony hysterectomy cases to require ureteral stents (14% versus 3%, $p=0.03$) and to instill sterile milk into the bladder (23% versus 8%, $p=0.02$) (Shellhaas, 2009). Peripatum hemorrhage remains a cause of significant maternal morbidity and mortality. Accurate diagnosis and appropriate management of obstetric hemorrhage can reduce maternal morbidity and mortality worldwide (Kuczkowski, 2009).

2.3 Complications of hysterectomy and the quality of life

Hysterectomy is one of the safest surgical procedures. Overall mortality rate is 0,5-2/1000. The complications are most common in women treated for uterine fibroids, within the group on which hysterectomy performed for benign gynecological indications and overall rate decreases with age (Manyonda, 2003).

The advantages of abdominal hysterectomy are: good access into the peritoneal cavity, wide access to the site of operation and easier technique to remove appendages. At the same time, this traditional method of hysterectomy has many disadvantages associated with abdominal incision and greater operational trauma (Barwijuk 2005).

The complications of hysterectomy may occur during the operation or a few days, weeks, or even years after the surgery. Intraoperative complications include: bladder and urethra injury, bowel injury and also vascular injury with bleeding that requires transfusion. Short-term complications are connected with vaginal and sometimes urinary infection. Long-term side effects of hysterectomy are fistula and bladder dysfunction or prolapse. Many women complain of chronic pain. These complications are more common after an abdominal hysterectomy.

One of the long-term complications of gynecological surgeries is urinary incontinence. The aim of the study conducted by Jędrzejczyk et al. (Jędrzejczyk, 2008) was to assess the prevalence of urinary incontinence after some gynecological-obstetrical surgeries and to specify the type of incontinence, depending on the type of surgery and its access, in groups of premenopausal and postmenopausal patients. It appears that abdominal and vaginal accesses equally predispose to stress urinary incontinence (SUI). After abdominal hysterectomy the most common is SUI, while after caesarean section mixed urinary incontinence (MUI). Urgent UI is more common after vaginal plastic surgeries than after abdominal surgeries (Jędrzejczyk, 2008). However, the proportion of patients with urinary incontinence is lower by 50% in patients after over cervical amputation than after hysterectomy, and thus it should be a reason to consider the possibility of limiting the scope of the surgery in postmenopausal patients in order to prevent urinary incontinence. Obviously, it requires providing thorough information about the prevention of cervical cancer and further regular cytological testing (Jędrzejczyk, 2008). Forsgren et al. (Forsgren, 2009) observed that the pelvic organ fistula surgery was four times more common in women after hysterectomy compared with women not having the procedure. The highest fistula rates were observed the first year after surgery (Forsgren, 2009).

In case of patients who cannot be operated in a preserving way due to their serious diseases, a new technique of radical hysterectomy which saves the vegetative nervous system (RHOUW) should be considered. *Nerve - sparing technique* reduces the number of side effects from the urinary tract, and enables to perform the surgery with the same extent as in traditional nerve-sparing radical hysterectomy, giving identical oncological results (Maas, 2005; Raspagliesi, 2003; Sakuragi, 2005; Fujii, 2007; Kalemli, 2005). A comparative study of Sakuragi et al. (Sakuragi, 2005) analyzing a group of patients who have had RHOUW and a group in which an attempt to perform this surgery failed, clearly shows that after one year of observation urinary incontinence and reduced sensation in the bladder has not occurred in the group after RHOUW, and appeared in 100% of patients after classic radical hysterectomy (Sakuragi, 2005). In addition, Sasaki et al (Sasaki, 1982) reported that radical hysterectomy was followed by the reduction of maximum urethral closure pressure, which was probably related to the damage of the abdominal nerve (Sasaki, 1982). A paper by Morgan et al. (Morgan, 2000) showing the relationship of the radical hysterectomy with urethral sphincter insufficiency (ISD) on the basis of leek point pressure (LPP) in the urodynamic study would confirm these findings (Morgan, 2000).

3. Laparoscopic hysterectomy

3.1 General information on laparoscopic hysterectomy procedures

Laparoscopic hysterectomy includes both vaginal excision of the uterus, where the endoscopic part of the surgery consists in releasing adhesions or intersecting some ligaments and uterine vessels, as well as a radical removal of the uterus with the parametrium, vaginal cuff, and the lymph nodes, where all operations are performed laparoscopically, and the extraction of the uterus takes place not through the vagina (Barwijuk, 2005; Lee, 2002).

The type of laparoscopic hysterectomy is usually defined by the extent of laparoscopic dissection performed during the procedure (LAVH, LH, TLH, Robot-assisted laparoscopic hysterectomy). Table 5 show the type of surgical technique on laparoscopic hysterectomy procedures.

The concept of laparoscopic hysterectomy is therefore not so wide. Each procedure in which the uterus is extracted from the abdominal cavity through the vagina is in fact a laparoscopically assisted vaginal hysterectomy - as in LAVH, or a laparoscopically assisted total vaginal hysterectomy - as in LATVH, or a laparoscopically assisted radical vaginal hysterectomy - as in LAVRH. Only LSH and LTH are laparoscopic hysterectomy surgeries, and in both cases the uterus is extracted by means of a laparoscopic morcellation.

3.2 Indications and contraindications for laparoscopic hysterectomy

The development of laparoscopy has made it an essential and irreplaceable element in modern gynaecology, both in the diagnostic and therapeutic process. Currently, the scope of laparoscopic surgeries is wide and includes almost all procedures performed by laparotomy, thus eliminating the consequences such as extensive postoperative scars (Malinowski, 2009). Nevertheless, the indications for different types of laparoscopic hysterectomy are different. Indications for various laparoscopic surgeries show table 6.

Type of surgical technique	Detailed scope of procedure
Laparoscopic Supracervical Hysterectomy	The technique of the procedure is based on cutting off ligamentum teres uteri and infundibulo-pelvicum or ovarian ligaments, intersection of both plaques of the broad ligament of the uterus, closure of the lumen of both uterine arteries, and cutting off the uterine body from the cervix. In the next stage, the uterine body is extracted from the peritoneal cavity using morcellator.
Laparoscopically Assisted Vaginal Hysterectomy	The technique of the operation is based on cutting off primary ligaments and uterosacral ligaments from the laparoscopic access and cutting off the uterus from the vaginal vault from the vaginal access.
Laparoscopic Total Hysterectomy	The uterus is cut off from the vaginal vault, the vaginal stump is stitched up and the preparation is extracted from the abdominal cavity by a morcellator.
Laparoscopic Total Radical Hysterectomy and Pelvic Lymphadenectomy	After removal of all levels of the pelvic lymph nodes, the next step is to remove the uterus through the abdominal wall.
Laparoscopically Asissted Total Vaginal Hysterectomy	All stages of the operation with cutting off the uterus from the vaginal vault are performed laparoscopically. The extraction of the preparation and stitching of the vaginal stump is conducted from the vaginal access.
Laparoscopically Assisted Radical Vaginal Hysterectomy	After removal of all levels of the lymph nodes, the next step of LARVH is to remove the uterus through the vagina. 2 types of operations are performed, depending on the extent: either like in type 2 according to Piver and Rutledge, or in a more radical way according to Schaut-Amreich. It is similar to hysterectomy conducted from the abdominal access, classified as type 3 according to Piver and Rutledge.

Table 5. Types of hysterectomy procedures using a laparoscope (Chapron, 1996; Parker, 2000; Dargent, 2001; Barwijuk, 2005; Lee, 2002, Vizza, 2011).

Kruijdenberg et al. (Kruijdenberg, 2011) reviewed current literature on total laparoscopic (TLRH) and robot assisted radical hysterectomy (RRH) with pelvic lymphadenectomy in the treatment of early stage cervical cancer. He analyzed 27 studies comprising 342 RRH patients and 914 TLRH patients. There was no statistical difference between the methods in terms of age, BMI or prior abdominal surgery. Estimated mean operative time, blood loss and number of lymph nodes retrieved did not statistically differ between the RRH and TLRH method. Less blood transfusions were needed in patients treated by RRH versus TLRH (5.4% vs 9.7%, $p<0.05$). Both methods were similar in respect to adjuvant chemo- or (chemo) radiation and recurrence rate. When complications were prioritized in severity, major post-operative complications where more frequent in RRH patients than in TLRH patients (9.6% vs 5.5%, $p<0.05$). The length of hospital stay was significantly shorter in RRH compared to TLRH treatment (3.3 versus 6.2 days respectively; $p=0.04$). According to the authors, robot-assisted and total laparoscopic radical hysterectomy appears to be equally adequate and feasible. RRH studies had small patient populations and further experience

Laparoscopic surgeries procedures	Indications for various laparoscopic surgeries
LSH	Symptomatic myomas of the uterus, overgrowth of the uterine mucosa, heavy uterine bleeding resistant to pharmacotherapy, adenomiosis and endometriosis, and pelvic pain syndrome
LAVH	Symptomatic myomas of the uterus, overgrowth of the uterine mucosa, heavy uterine bleeding resistant to pharmacotherapy, adenomiosis and endometriosis, and pelvic pain syndrome. Alternatively additionally extended by cervical pathologies, such as e.g. dysplasia and early neoplasia
LTH	Symptomatic myomas of the uterus, overgrowth of the uterine mucosa, heavy uterine bleeding resistant to pharmacotherapy, adenomiosis and endometriosis, and pelvic pain syndrome, alternatively additionally extended by cervical pathologies, such as e.g. dysplasia and early neoplasia. Patients who did not give birth and who have been diagnosed with uterine myomas with a diameter larger than 5 cm by ultrasonography, with the uterus weighing more than 300 g and with non-malignant lesions in appendages which accompany uterine pathology.
LATVH	Pelvic organ prolapse accompanying a main disease, requiring surgery and perineal laceration repair.
LARVH	It is performed exclusively in oncological indications, i.e. in the early stages of ovarian cancer, cervical cancer and endometrial cancer. Ovarian cancer is a controversial indication and many clinicians are of the opinion that in this case laparoscopy should be replaced with a radical abdominal surgery.
LRH	Can be performed in stage Ia2–Ib1 or less advanced node negative cervical cancer patients without compromising survival. The feasibility of LRH for more advanced patients needs further investigations.
TLRH	Can be safely performed in patients with stage IB2-IIB carcinoma of cervix after NACT, with advantages of minimal blood loss and morbidity (can be performed in stage IB2-IIB with complete clinical response after 3 courses of NACT with paclitaxel 175 mg/m2, ifosfamide 5 g/m2 and cisplatin 75 mg/m2.

Table. 6. Indications for various laparoscopic surgeries (Malinowski, 2009; El-Mowafi, 2004; Chapron, 1996; Parker, 2000; Reich, 1990 & 2003; Childers, 1992; Querleu, 1991; Skręt, 2003; Vizza, 2011; Yan, 2011).

beyond the learning curve phase may improve operative time and complication rate (Kruijdenberg, 2011). Yan et all (Yan, 2011) presented Twelve-year experience with laparoscopic radical hysterectomy and pelvic lymphadenectomy in the study of the morbidity, oncological outcome, and prognostic factors of cervical cancer patients treated with LRH. According to FIGO stage, the number of patients with stage Ia2, Ib1, Ib2, IIa, and

IIb was 2, 163, 34, 35, and 6, respectively. The authors suggests that the short-term follow-up in this study was not allow to draw a definitive conclusion on the impact of laparoscopic technique on the outcome. More multicenter studies and longterm follow-up were required to identify the oncologic outcomes of this procedure (Yan, 2011).

3.3 Complications of hysterectomy and the quality of life

A retrospective analysis Davies et all. (Davies, 2002) of 1000 consecutive hysterectomies showed that the overall complication rates were 34, 24 and 21% for abdominal, vaginal and laparoscopic hysterectomy, respectively. The results show that women undergoing hysterectomy for benign indications have a 1:3 to 1:5 chance of developing an operative or postoperative complication, most likely of minor nature (Davies, 2002).

Labrador et all. (Labrador, 2008) analyzed retrospective review of the medical records of 716 women who had a hysterectomy. Of the 716 hysterectomies, the abdominal (60.34%) route was the most common, followed by total laparoscopic hysterectomy (25.84%), vaginal hysterectomy (8.38%), Laparoscopic supracervical hysterectomy (3.77%), laparoscopically assisted vaginal hysterectomy (1.26%) and Subtotal abdominal hysterectomy (0.42%) routes. Patients were an average of 44 years. The 94.97% had benign indications and 5.03% have not benign indications. Mean operating time was 112 minutes for total abdominal hysterectomy, 113.13 minutes for Subtotal abdominal hysterectomy, 131.1 minutes for total laparoscopic hysterectomy, 103.73 minutes for Laparoscopic supracervical hysterectomy, 92.41 minutes for vaginal hysterectomy and 138.88 minutes for laparoscopically assisted vaginal hysterectomy. Blood loss was fewer in vaginal hysterectomies. They found that Laparoscopic supracervical hysterectomy and vaginal hysterectomy required less operative time and was associated with less blood loss. There were 7 conversions of surgery, 6 intraoperative bleeding, and 4 urinary tract injuries for total abdominal hysterectomy. For total laparoscopic hysterectomy there were 6 urinary tract injuries, and 5 conversion of surgery and 1 patient with intraoperative bleeding. Also, 1 patient had a bowel injury for vaginal hysterectomy. Blood loss was fewer in vaginal hysterectomies. They found that the most important complication was conversion of burgery (Labrador, 2008).

On the other hand the laparoscopic hysterectomy involves smaller incisions and is less painful. Moreover, the hospital stay after laparoscopic surgery may be shorter and the risk of infection is lower. Laparoscopic hysterectomy is also a feasible alternative to abdominal hysterectomy in obese patients weighing over 100 kg with low morbidity and fast recovery and short hospital stay. TLH is associated with significantly longer operative time and shorter hospital stay than VH. There is a trend towards more intraoperative and postoperative complications in the TLH group than in the VH group (McMaster-Fay, 2004).

The laparoscopic hysterectomy is associated with an increased risk of the urinary tract and bladder injury and of complications due to general anesthesia. In this retrospective cohort, body mass index does not affect surgical outcomes or increase complications during laparoscopic assisted hysterectomy. The complications of LAVH performed after prior laparotomy includes: damage of the urinary bladder, ureter, intestines and large blood vessels, bladder-vaginal and uretero-vaginal fistulas, bleeding from the vaginal stump, postoperative ileus and empyemas of the pelvis. The incidence of these complications is estimated at 1.3-12%. Nevertheless, the efficacy of laparoscopy in patients with previous surgeries in the peritoneal cavity can amount to even up to 96.9% (Shen, 2003; Ballesta, 2003).

It is now widely recognized that in clinical research it is not sufficient to simply measure the outcome of a clinical intervention in terms of morbidity and mortality. Recent research presents compelling evidence that hysterectomy improves the quality of life. The study comparing abdominal or vaginal hysterectomy to endometrial ablative techniques has shown consistently higher quality of life scores for hysterectomy. On the other hand, retrospective studies suggest that abdominal and particularly vaginal hysterectomy may predispose to vault prolapse and the quality of life was lower in these patients compared to women after laparoscopic hysterectomy.

4. General information on vaginal hysterectomy procedures

4.1 Vaginal hysterectomy

The vaginal route of hysterectomy is considered as a first choice of all benign indications as the post-operative rates of morbidity and complications are lower than abdominal open hysterectomies according to the Society of Obstetricians and Gynaecologists of Canada (SOGC) clinical guidelines (Lefebvre 2002, Stang 2011). Abdominal hysterectomy involves removal of the uterus through an incision on the lower abdomen. Vaginal hysterectomy involves removal of the uterus via the vagina, with no abdominal incision. Vaginal hysterectomy should be performed in preference to abdominal hysterectomy, where possible. The ratio of vaginal hysterectomy (VH) to abdominal hysterectomy (AH) varies from 1:3 to 1:4 or less, depending on the country and surgeons' technique. This review found that vaginal hysterectomy meant quicker return to normal activities, fewer infections and episodes of raised temperature after surgery, and a shorter stay in hospital compared to abdominal hysterectomy (Nieboer, 2009; Sheth 2005).

4.2 Indications and contraindications for vaginal hysterectomy

There are well-defined indications for both VH. Table 7 present indications and contraindications for vaginal hysterectomy.

Although currently a standard surgery for endometrial cancer is abdominal hysterectomy with the excision of appendages and maintenance of oncological sterility, when the possibility of abdominal approach is limited (due to severe obesity or internal complications), vaginal hysterectomy can be recommended. However, it must be borne in mind that it limits the possibility of assessing the actual tumour stage (inability to remove the lymph nodes, palpate the small pelvic area and the abdominal cavity and to collect cytological smears or washings) (Łapińska-Szumczyk, 2009). A decision to resign from lymphadenectomy can be made provided that the patient is qualified into a group of low-risk recurrence of the disease: histological form of adenocarcinoma endometriale G1 or G2, in a situation when the carcinoma is present only in the endometrium or the depth of the infiltration does not exceed 50% of the uterine muscularis (Carey, 1995; Mariani, 2000).

Indications for vaginal hysterectomy	Contraindications for vaginal hysterectomy
1. Menorrhagia 2. Uterine fibroids 3. Genital and uterine prolapse 4. Neoplasia - Very early invasive cervical cancer - Carcinoma-in-situ of the cervix - Endometrial cancer 5. Endometrial complex hyperplasia with atypia 6. Recurrent postmenopausal bleeding 7. Chronic pelvic pain 8. Special indications - ventral scar hernioplasty - morbid obesity - high risk—e.g. interstitial lung disease which markedly restricts pulmonary function, poor cardiac status, obesity, diabetes, and hypertension - tuberculous abdomen - keloids 9. common - uterus 12 weeks or less in size or uterine volume 300 cm3 or less; - uterus is freely mobile; and - normal adnexa	1. Common - uterus more than 12 weeks' size or uterine volume more than 300 cm3 - restriction of uterine mobility - adnexal pathology. 2. Uncommon - cervix flush with the vagina - past Fothergill's operation - inaccessible cervix: uncommonly, after repeated uterine surgery, particularly past caesarean section, adhesions there are dense adhesions between the uterocervical surface, the bladder and the lower abdominal wall which makes the cervix inaccessible to an approach by the vaginal route - vesicovaginal and/or rectovaginal fistula repair - invasive cancer of the cervix.

Table. 7. Indications and contraindications for vaginal hysterectomy (Sheth, 2005)

4.3 Complications of hysterectomy and the quality of life

Nieboer et all (Nieboer, 2009) were included 34 studies with 4495 women. The benefits of VH versus AH were speedier return to normal activities (mean difference (MD) 9.5 days), fewer febrile episodes or unspecified infections (odds ratio (OR) 0.42), and shorter duration of hospital stay (MD 1.1 days). There was no evidence of benefits of LH versus VH and the operation time (MD 39.3 minutes) as well as substantial bleeding (OR 2.76) was increased in LH. For some important outcomes, the analyses were underpowered to detect important differences or they were simply not reported in trials (Nieboer, 2009).

Meta-analysis of these procedures shows that vaginal hysterectomy results in fewer complications than the other types of hysterectomy and is a very safe way to remove the uterus. VH is also associated with shorter hospital stay and faster return to normal activities than abdominal hysterectomy.

In another analysis, randomized, non-blinded, three-arm, controlled study it was revealed that the length of hospital stay was shorter by 0,9 day for vaginal hysterectomy and by 0,6 day for laparoscopic assisted vaginal hysterectomy in comparison with total abdominal hysterectomy. However the duration of the surgery was longer on average by 13 min for VH and 34 min for LAVH (Ottosen, 2000). Ottosen et all. suggested that LAVH might carry a higher risk of conversion to abdominal hysterectomy than vaginal hysterectomy. But in opinion Summitt (Summitt, 2002) the relatively small numbers of subjects within each surgical group did not allow this conclusion to be made.

5. Economic analysis

Economic aspect can be difficult to assess because of the nature of healthcare systems in various countries.

6. Alternatives to hysterectomy

6.1 The levonorgestrel – Releasing intrauterine system (Mirena, LNG-IUS)

Conservative alternatives including the Mirena IUS. The levonorgestrel- releasing intrauterine system (Mirena, LNG-IUS) is effective in reducing menstrual blood loss and should be considered as an alternative to surgical treatment. Surgery, especially hysterectomy, reduces menstrual bleeding more than medical treatments at one year but LNG-IUS may be comparable in improving quality of life. The evidence for longer-term comparisons is weak and inconsistent. Oral medication suits a minority of women long term. Randomised controlled trials (RCTs) comparing conservative surgery or hysterectomy versus medical therapy (oral or intrauterine) for HMB. Twelve parallel-group RCTs that included 1049 women met the inclusion criteria. In comparisons of oral medication versus surgery, 58% of the women randomised to medical treatment had received surgery by two years. Compared to oral medication, endometrial resection was significantly more effective in controlling bleeding (at four months: RR 2.66 (95% CI 1.94 to 3.64); NNT = 2 (95% CI 2 to 3), one study) and hysterectomy resulted in significantly greater improvements in mental health (at six months: P = 0.04, one study). In comparisons of LNG-IUS versus conservative surgery or hysterectomy, at one year there was no statistically significant difference in satisfaction rates nor in most measures of quality of life, though adverse effects were significantly less likely with conservative surgery (RR 0.51 (95% CI 0.36 to 0.74); NNT = 4 (95% CI 3 to 7), three studies). Conservative surgery was significantly more effective than LNG-IUS in controlling bleeding at one year (RR 1.19 (95% CI 1.07 to 1.32); NNT = 7 (95% CI 5 to 19), five studies). Two small studies with longer follow up found no difference or favoured LNG-IUS, but both of these studies had skewed data and there were high losses to follow up. Hysterectomy stopped all bleeding but caused serious complications for some women (Marjoribanks, 2006).

6.2 Uterine artery embolization

Uterine artery embolization is also effective for fibroids and endometrial ablative techniques may be an effective therapy for menorrhagia. Uterine artery embolization (UAE) is helpful for uterine fibroids that cause symptoms such as heavy bleeding, pain, pressure symptoms and subfertility. The two main surgical approaches are myomectomy (hysteroscopic or abdominal approach) to remove the fibroids or hysterectomy where the uterus is removed: both are associated with complications. There were two randomized controlled trials (RCT) comparing UAE with hysterectomy and another comparing UAE with myomectomy. Two of these trials had a minimum of six months follow-up and the other is a peri- and postprocedural complications report for up to 6 weeks follow-up only. There was no evidence of benefit of UAE compared to surgery (hysterectomy / myomectomy) for satisfaction. There were more minor complications, more unscheduled visits and readmission rates after discharge in the UAE group compared to hysterectomy. However, there were no differences between major complication rates and UAE is associated with shorter hospital stay and return to work. Further research was awaited with long term follow up. Women with symptomatic fibroids may be offered UAE as a treatment option but more research with a longer follow up is needed (Gupta, 2006).

6.3 Endometrial hyperplasia can sometimes be treated medically with progestins or destruction of endometrial tissue by either TCRE

Destruction of endometrial tissue by either TCRE (transcervical resection) or ablation is an effective alternative to hysterectomy for heavy menstrual bleeding (sometimes defined as a loss of 80mls or more of blood per menstrual cycle). Hysterectomy is effective in stopping HMB permanently, but also ends fertility and has all the risks of major surgery including infection and blood loss. Endometrial resection and other methods of ablation are less invasive methods of surgery that aim to remove the entire thickness of the endometrium (lining of the uterus). The Cochrane review of trials found TCRE or ablation is an effective and possibly cheaper alternative to hysterectomy with faster recovery although re-treatment is sometimes needed. There was a significant advantage in favour of hysterectomy in the improvement in HMB (OR=0.04, 0.01 to 0.2 at one year) and satisfaction rates (up to four years post surgery) (OR=0.5, 0.3 to 0.8 at 2 years) compared with endometrial ablation. Duration of surgery, hospital stay and recovery time were all shorter following TCRE or endometrial ablation, although these outcomes varied between trials. Most adverse events, both major and minor, were significantly more likely after hysterectomy and before discharge from hospital. After discharge from hospital, the only difference that was reported for this group was a higher rate of infection (OR=0.2, 0.1 to 0.5). Repeat surgery because of failure of the initial treatment, either endometrial ablation or hysterectomy, was more likely after endometrial ablation than hysterectomy (OR=16.7, 5.8 to 48.6). The total cost of endometrial destruction was significantly lower than the cost of hysterectomy but the difference between the two procedures narrowed over time because of the high cost of re-treatment in the endometrial destruction group (Lethaby, 1999).

7. Conclusions

- laparoscopic hysterectomy should be considered as an alternative to abdominal hysterectomy
- uterine fibroids are the most common indication for hysterectomy
- the decision to perform oophorectomy should be individualized
- subtotal hysterectomy has no advantage over total hysterectomy and might result in persistent cyclic bleeding
- conservative alternatives include the Mirena IUS and uterine artery embolization for fibroids and endometrial ablative techniques

8. References

American College of Obstetricians and Gynecologists (ACOG). Elective and risk-reducing salpingo-ophorectomy. Washington (DC): *American College of Obstetricians and Gynecologists (ACOG)*; 2008 Jan. 11 p. (ACOG practice bulletin; no. 89).

Ballesta Lopez, C., Ruggerio, R., Poves, I., et al. 2003). Laparoscopic procedures in patients who have previously undergone laparotomic operations. *Minerva Chir*. Vol. 58, pp. 53-56.

Barwijuk, A., & Szymczyk, G. (2005). Co oznacza termin – histerektomia laparoskopowa? *Prz Menopauz* Vol. 4, pp.14–16

Carey, M. et all. (1995). Good outcome associated with a standardized treatment protocol using selective postoperative radiation in patients with clinical stage I adenocarcinoma of the endometrium. *Gynecol Oncol,* Vol. 57, pp.138-144

Chapron, C, Dubuisson, JB, Ansquer, Y. (1996). Hysterectomy for patients without previous vaginal delivery: results and modalities of laparoscopic surgery. *Human Reprod* Vol. 11, pp.2122-6.

Childers, JM., Surwit, EA. (1992). Combined laparoscopic and vaginal surgery for the management of two cases of stage I endometrial cancer. *Gynecol Oncol* Vol. 45, pp. 486-71.

Clayton, R.D. (2006). Hysterectomy. *Best Practice & Research Clinical Obstetrics and Gynaecology*. Vol. 20, No. 1, pp. 73–87

Dargent, D. (2001). Laparoscopic surgery in gynecologic oncology. *Surg Clin North Am* Vol. 81, No. 4, pp. 949-64.

Davies, A. et all. (2002). Hysterectomy: surgical route and complications. *European Journal of Obstetrics & Gynecology and Reproductive Biology*. Vol.104, pp. 148–151

El-Mowafi, D., Madkour, W., Lall, C., et al. (2004). Laparoscopic Supracervical Hysterectomy versus Laparoscopic-Assisted Vaginal Hysterectomy. *J Am Assoc Gynecol Laparosc* Vol. 11, No. 2, pp. 175-80.

Falcone, T & Walters,M. (2008). Hysterectomy for Benign Disease. *Obstet Gynecol* Vol. 111, pp.753–67

Flood, K., et all. (2009). Changing trends in peripartum hysterectomy over the last 4 decades. *Am J Obstet Gynecol,* Vol. 200, pp. 632.e1-632.e6

Forsgren,C. et all. (2009). Hysterectomy for Benign Indications and Risk of Pelvic Organ Fistula Disease. *Obstet Gynecol*, Vol. 113, pp. 601–608

Fujii, S. et all. (2007). Precise anatomy of the vesico-uterine ligament for radical hysterectomy. *Gynecol Oncol*, Vol. 104, pp.186-91

Graham, M., James, E., Keleher, H. (2008). Predictors of hysterectomy as a treatment for menstrual symptoms. *Women's Health Issues* Vol. 18, pp. 319–327

Gupta, JK., Sinha, A., Lumsden, MA., Hickey, M. (2006). Uterine artery embolization for symptomatic uterine fibroids. Cochrane Database of Systematic Reviews 2006, Issue 1. Art. No.: CD005073. DOI: 10.1002/14651858.CD005073.pub2

Gupta, S, & Manyonda, I. (2006). Hysterectomy for benign gynaecological disease. *Current Obstetrics & Gynaecology,* Vol. 16, pp. 147–153

Jędrzejczyk, S. et all. (2008). Effects of selected obstetric-gynaecological surgery on female urinary incontinence in pre- and postmenopausal patient. *Przegląd Menopauzalny,* Vol. 2, pp.91–95

Kalemli, M. et all. (2005). Urodynamic evaluation of lower urinary tract function in relation to total abdominal hysterectomy. *Patophysiology,* Vol. 12, pp. 121-4.

Kovac, R. (2004). Clinical opinion: Guidelines for hysterectomy. *American Journal of Obstetrics and Gynecology,* Vol. 191, pp.635-640

Kruijdenberg, C.B.M., van den Inden, L.C.G., Hendricks, J.C.M., Zusterzeel, P.L.M., Bekkers, R.L.M. (2011). Robot-assisted versus total laparoscopic radical hysterectomy in early cervical cancer, a review. *Gynecologic Oncology* Vol. 120, pp. 334–339

Kuczkowski, K. (2009). Cesarean hysterectomy in the parturient with abnormal placentation: evidence based strategy. *Anestezjologia i Ratownictwo,* Vol. 3, pp. 296-303

Labrador, A. et all. (2008). Retrospective Review of 716 Women Who Underwent Different Types of Hysterectomy. *Journal of Minimally Invasive Gynecology,* Vol. 15, pp. S1e-S159

Łapińska-Szumczyk, S. et all. (2009). Vaginal hysterectomy as a method of treatment of endometrial cancer. *Curr. Gynecol. Oncol,* Vol.7, No.3, pp. 206-216

Learman, LA., Gregorich, SE., Schembri, M., et al. (2011). Symptom resolution after hysterectomy and alternative treatments for chronic pelvic pain: does depression make a difference? *Am J Obstet Gynecol* Vol. 204, pp. 269.e1-9.

Lee, CL., & Huang, KG. (2002). Total laparoscopic radical hysterectomy using Lee-Huang portal and McCartney transvaginal tube. *J Am Assoc Gynecol Laparosc* Vol. 9, No. 4, pp. 536-54

Lefebvre, G., Allaire, C., Jeffrey, J., Vilos, G., Arneja, J., Birch, C. (2002). SOGC clinical guidelines. Hysterectomy. *J Obstet Gynaecol Can. Vol.* 24, No. 1, pp.37–61

Lethaby A, Shepperd S, Farquhar C, Cooke I. (1999). Endometrial resection and ablation versus hysterectomy for heavy menstrual bleeding. Cochrane Database of Systematic Reviews 1999, Issue 2. Art. No.: CD000329. DOI: 10.1002/14651858.CD000329

Maas, C., et all. (2005) Anatomical basis for nerve-sparing radical hysterectomy: immunohistochemical study of pelvic autonomic nerves. *Acta Obstet Gynecol Scand* Vol. 84, pp.868-74

Malinowski, A., Wiecka-Płusa, M., Molas, J. (2009). Laparoscopic-assisted vaginal hysterectomy after multiple abdominal surgeries - case study. *Ginekol Pol.* Vol. 80, pp. 865-869

Manyonda, I. (2003). Hysterectomy for benign gynaecological disease. *Current Obstetrics & Gynaecology,* Vol. 13, pp. 159—165

Mariani, A. et all. (2000). Low-risk corpus cancer: is lymphadenectomy or radiotherapy necessary? *Am.J. Obstet. Gynecol.* Vol. 182, pp.1506-1519

Marjoribanks, J., Lethaby A., Farquhar C. (2006). Surgery versus medical therapy for heavy menstrual bleeding. Cochrane Database of Systematic Reviews 2006, Issue 2. Art. No.: CD003855. DOI: 10.1002/14651858.CD003855.pub2

McMaster-Fay, R. (2004). Laparoscopic hysterectomy in patients weighing 100 kg or more:a 7-year experience. *Gynecol Surg* Vol. 1, pp. 233–235

Morgan, J. (2000). Is intrinsic sphincter deficiency a complication of simple hysterectomy? *J Urol* Vol. 164, No 3 Pt 1, pp. 767-9.

Nationwide Inpatient Sample (NIS) of the Healthcare Cost and Utilization Project (HCUP). (2007).Available at: www.hcupnet.ahrq.gov. Retrieved December 28, 2007.

Nieboer, T. et all. (2009). Surgical approach to hysterectomy for benign gynaecological disease. *Cochrane Database of Systematic Reviews,* Issue 3. Art. No.: CD003677. DOI: 10.1002/14651858.CD003677.pub4.

Ottosen, C., Lingman, G., Ottosen, L. (2000). Compared to total abdominal hysterectomy, hospital stay was shorter with vaginal or laparoscopic assisted vaginal hysterectomy. *Br J Obstet Gynaecol* Vol. 107. pp. 1380-1385

Panici, P. et all. (2011). Feasibility and safety of type C2 total extraperitoneal abdominal radical hysterectomy (TEARH) for locally advanced cervical cancer. *Gynecologic Oncology*, Vol. 120, pp. 423–429

Parker, W. (2000). Total laparoscopic hysterectomy. *Obstet Gynecol Clin North Am.* Vol. 27, pp. 431-40.

Piver, M.S, Rutledge, F., Smith, J.P. (1974). Five classes of extended hysterectomy for women with cervical cancer. *Obstet Gynecol* Vol. 44, No. 2, pp. 265–272

Poręba, R., Jastrzębski, A. & Obcowska-Lech, M (2007). Peripartum hysterectomy in emergency obstetrical cases. *Kliniczna Perinatologia i ginekologia,* Vol. 43, No. 4, pp. 29-31

Querleu, D., Leblanc, E., Castelain, B. (1991). Laparoscopic pelvic lymphadenectomy in the staging of early carcinoma of the cervix. *Am J Obstet Gynecol* Vol. 164, pp.579-81.

Raspagliesi, F. et all. (2003). Nerve-sparing radical hysterectomy: a pilot study. *Tumori* Vol.89, pp.497-501

Reich H & Roberts L. (2003). Laparoscopic hysterectomy in current gynaecological practice. *Rev Gynaecol Pract.* Vol. 3, pp. 32–40.

Reich, H., McGlynn, F., Wilkie, W. (1990). Laparoscopic management of stage I ovarian cancer: a case report. *J Reprod Med* No. 35, pp. 601-604.

Rosenberg, D. (2002). A randomised comparison and economic evaluation in laparoscopic assisted hysterectomy and abdominal hysterectomy. Comment on. BJOG. December Vol. 109, No, 12, pp. 1429

Sakuragi, N. et all. (2005). A systematic nerve-sparing radical hysterectomy technique in invasive cervical cancer for preserving postsurgical bladder function. *Int J Gynecol Cancer* Vol. 15, pp. 389-97

Sasaki, H. et all. (1982). Urethral pressure profiles following radical hysterectomy. *Obstet Gynecol,* Vol.59, pp.101-104

Shellhaas, C., et all. (2009) The Frequency and Complication Rates of Hysterectomy Accompanying Cesarean Delivery. *Obstet Gynecol,* Vol. 114, pp. 224-229

Shellhaas, C., et all. (2009). The Frequency and Complication Rates of Hysterectomy Accompanying Cesarean Delivery. *Obstet Gynecol.* August, Vol. 114, pp.224–229.

Shen, C., Wu, M., Kung, F., et al. (2003). Major complications associated with laparoscopic-assisted vaginal hysterectomy: ten-year experience. *J Am Assoc Gynecol Laparosc.* Vol.10, pp. 147-153.

Sheth, S. (2005). Vaginal hysterectomy. *Best Practice & Research Clinical Obstetrics and Gynaecology.* Vol. 19, No. 3, pp. 307–332, 2005

Skręt, A., Obrzut, B., Kluz, T., et all. (2003). Laparoskopowo-pochwowa histerektomia radykalna w leczeniu raka szyjki macicy. *Gin Pol No.* 5, pp. 377-83

Stang, A., Merrill, R.A., Kuss, O. (2011). Nationwide rates of conversion from laparoscopic or vaginal hysterectomy to open abdominal hysterectomy in Germany. *Eur J Epidemiol* Vol.26, pp.125–133

Vizza, E., Pellegrino, A., Milani, R., Fruscio, R., Baiocco, E et all. (2011). Total laparoscopic radical hysterectomy and pelvic lymphadenectomy in locally advanced stage IB2-IIB cervical cancer patients after neoadjuvant chemotherapy. EJSO Vol. 37, pp. 364-369

Yan, X, Li, G., Shang, H., Wang, G., Han, Y., Lin, T., Zheng, F. (2011). Twelve-year experience with laparoscopic radical hysterectomy and pelvic lymphadenectomy in cervical cancer. Gynecologic Oncology Vol. 120, pp. 362–367

26

Predictive Value of Cellular Immune Response and Tumor Biomarkers in Patients Surgically Treated for Cervical Cancer in Relation to Clinical Outcomes

E. Ancuta[1], Codrina Ancuta[2] and D. Sofroni[3]

[1]*Research Department, "Cuza-Voda" Hospital Iasi,*
[2]*"Gr.T.Popa" University of Medicine and Pharmacy Iasi,*
[3]*Institute of Oncology, Chisinau,*
[1,2]*Romania*
[3]*Moldova*

1. Introduction

Cervical carcinoma remains a leading cause of death among women in developing countries. Because recent advances in the immune pathways of gynaecologic cancers have been achieved, this field has become important in the current practice of modern oncologists.

Contemporary investigations have focused on tumor infiltrating lymphocytes, reflecting the status of the cellular immune system in different types of cervical carcinoma.

Despite complex management of cervical cancer according to the risk stratification for recurrence and local guidelines (radical hysterectomy, meaning the removal of the uterus and cervix, one third of the vagina, the parametrial tissue at the pelvic sidewall and ligature of utero-sacrals with or without lymphadenectomy, followed by adjuvant radio and chemotherapy), up to 40% of patients still develop relapse of their cancer.

Since the immune response towards cervical cancer is thought to be important in either clearing or controlling the viral infection, the evaluation of local cellular immune response seems to be critical for the classification of patients according to their risk for the therapeutic decision and also may potentially indicate new adjuvant treatment strategies including immunotherapy. Moreover, new predictive biomarkers (including tumor proliferation and tumor invasion markers) are essential to identify patients with high risk of relapse and to optimize disease management.

Research on both intra- and peritumoral infiltration of immune cells has lead to a better understanding and management of cervical cancer, especially in recognition of new predictive biomarkers. Also, the evaluation of local cellular immune response in cervical cancer with or without relapse may indicate new strategies in order to improve survival.

Nowadays, promising vaccines to prevent the development of *Human Papillomavirus* (HPV)-induced cervical carcinoma are already distributed all over the world.

In addition to the scientific world interest in understanding the mechanisms of mucosal HPV carcinogenesis in the less susceptible organs, the findings indicate that HPV type 16 and 18 vaccines could also potentially protect HPV-vaccinated persons against cancers, including the following: anus, vagina, vulva, penis, oral cavity and oropharynx.

There has been recently a great interest in understanding the role of host's immune response in the natural history of HPV and in particular anti-viral cell mediated immunity. Several studies have shown that altered cell mediated immunity is strongly associated with increased HPV infection and cervical cancer. Persistent infection with HPV oncogenic types is the most important event in the progression to cervical precancerous lesions and cervical cancer.

Several immune cells subtypes are strongly involved in the cellular immune response after exposure to a non-self antigen including mononuclear phagocytes, natural killer (NK) cells, polymorph nuclear leukocytes and biochemical factors such as complement system.

Immune effector system involves essential processes as innate or adaptive that occurs in sequences after the exposure to a non-self antigen. After antigen ingestion, activation of NK cells allows the recognition of the processed by specific T-cells which play a central role in cellular immune response. On the other hand, B-cells control and regulate the humoral immune response.

It is now widely accepted that disease is caused by infection with high risk HPV types which may or may not be associated with clinically apparent lesion. Woman who cannot clear the viral infection became persistent HPV carriers and constitute the high risk group for progression to cervical cancer.

Current studies have suggested that immunological defects are associated with higher prevalence and persistence of HPV infection, especially in individuals with *Human Immunodeficience Virus* (HIV) infection. In addition, some evidences have found that other mechanisms than immunosuppression such as interactions between HIV and HPV viral genes may influence the increased risk of neoplasia and invasive cancer (Moscicki, 2000; Scott, 2000).

The anti-viral effects of cellular immunity have been hampered by several factors including (i) gene transcription patterns of HPV, (ii) inadequate interpretation, (iii) assessment of HPV type specificity.

Conversely, the lesions caused by HPV infection are generally localized to squamous epithelial sites. HPV has learned to evade the host's immunity through years of co-evolution, with the consequence that the immune response induced by HPV after natural infection, aiming to clear or control an incident infection with oncogenic HPV types, is, therefore, attenuated (Goncalves & Donadi, 2004; Hatch, 1999; Piersma, 2007; Scott, 2001; Stoler, 2010).

2. Epidemiology

The leading cause for human cervical cancer is still represented by HPV infection, a common sexually transmitted disease. While the risk for acquiring HPV infection is directly linked to the number and behavior of sexual partners, most infections have a benign clinical course and resolve spontaneously. However, up to 10% of women became persistent HPV carriers and constitute the high risk group for progression to cervical carcinoma (Goncalves & Donadi, 2004; Scott, 2001).

It is widely recognized that HPV types with specific oncogenic risk include HPV type 16, HPV type 18, HPV type 31, HPV type 33, HPV type 35, HPV type 45, HPV type 51, HPV type 52, HPV type 58, HPV type 59, 66 and 68.

Based on its rarity, recurrent respiratory papillomatosis (RRP) recognized as one potential manifestation of HPV infection in the airways, gives only unsatisfactory reports.

Of notice is that for some locations the cases are in men (penile cancer) or both in men or women (anal cancer and cancers of the oropharynx and oral cavity) needs to be further examined.

3. Screening and diagnosis

The most common screening method used to detect high grade squamous intraepithelial lesions (HSIL) is conventional cervical cytology, followed by colposcopy and directed biopsy. Furthermore, the PAP-test continues to have an unclear meaning.

Thus, approximately 1/1000 of women will develop cervical carcinoma.

The findings gained during the last years on persistent high risk HPV types in women developing cervical carcinoma have provided the basis for evaluation of the clinical utility of testing for cancer-associated HPV types (Ancuta, 2009; Goncalves & Donadi, 2004; Scott, 2001).

International guidelines recommend screening in women aged 25-50 years every three years and in women aged 51-60 years every five years. Women older than 60 years of age are not the subject for screening.

Women who are both vaccinated and test negative for HPV are typically characterized by a low risk for emergent cervical disease. In addition, they can be safely reassured for a long time prior to their next screening assessment. In contrast, women who are HPV positive could undergo cytological testing and follow well-established protocols for clinical assessment.

It is widely accepted that the evaluation of cervical cancer should include a clinical staging system, as well as an imaging and biological assessment. Chest X-ray, intravenous urography, cystoscopy and proctoscopy, lymphangiography, CT scan, CT directed lymph node aspiration, magnetic resonance imaging (MRI), positive emission tomography (PET) scan, blood count, serum chemistry profile and urine analysis are allowable techniques for documenting the extent of tumor spread (Goncalves & Donadi, 2004; Scott, 2001).

4. Management

The case for beginning to introduce HPV testing as the primary screening test for women aged over 30 years is now overwhelming. Different cross-sectional studies have already demonstrated a far higher sensitivity for detecting cervical intraepithelial neoplasia grade 2 (CIN2) or grade 3 (CIN3) than cytology (HPV sensitivity over 95%, cytology sensitivity between 55% and 75%), even if a lower specificity was proposed.

The variables that can potentially interfere with HPV infection comprise the following (Stoler, 2010):

- Cervical anatomy and the location of the squamo-columnar junction;
- The nature and size of the biopsy specimen;
- The location of the biopsy;
- The number of biopsies;
- The colposcopic appearance;
- The orientation on embedding;
- The depth and the quality of the histologic sections;
- The criteria used for interpretation;
- The inter-observer variation amongs pathologists.

Colposcopy has the sensitivity for the detection of neoplastic disease in the range of 60 to 70% in the management of women presenting with abnormal cervical cytology and those with lesions of intraepithelial disease. However, its sensitivity may be increased into range of more than 90% when employed together with exfoliative cytology or HPV-DNA testing or both. Therefore, all HPV positive women should be referred for colposcopic evaluation.

HPV-testing strategy is the preferred management option for women with an equivocal cytology derived from a liquid-based PAP sample.

Women who are ASC-US HPV positive are best managed by colposcopic technique.

Treatment options classically include surgery, radiotherapy and chemotherapy, while modern approach is also based on immunotherapy.

Immunotherapy represents the manipulation of immunologic processes, namely biologic therapy, or the application of biologic response modifiers (BRMs). It is nowadays widely recognized that the biologic therapy may have immunologic effects and can act through multiple mechanisms such as:

- to increase the number of effector cells;
- to decrease host's suppressor immunologic mechanisms;
- to make the tumor cells more susceptible to damage by immunologic activity;
- to improve the host's tolerance to radiotherapy or chemotherapy (Goncalves & Donadi, 2004; Nedergaard, 2007; Nedergaard, 2008; Scott, 2001).

4.1 Passive immunotherapy

Passive immunotherapy techniques have been used in some melanoma and renal carcinoma patients resulting in objective responses. Because the lymphokine-activated killer cells (LAK) plus interleukin-2 (IL-2) technique is associated with significant toxicity, variations of these methods need further studied (Monie, 2007; Scott,, 1997; Scott, 2001; Wang, 1999).

4.2 Passive humoral immunotherapy

The passive humoral immunotherapy technique allows *in vitro* detection of monoclonal anti-tumor antibodies directed against a variety of human cancers (Goncalves & Donadi, 2004; Monie, 2007; Scott, 2001).

4.3 Active specific immunotherapy

Active specific immunotherapy has been used to induce therapeutic cellular immunity by using intact tumor cells, defined tumor antigens, and immunostimulants. Moreover, autochtonous tumor cells genetically modified to produce immunostimulatory molecules are being evaluated in clinical trials (Monie, 2007; Norris, 1990; Scott, 2001).

Granulocyte-macrophage colony stimulating factor (GM-CSF) or interleukin-2 co-stimulatory molecules such as B7-1 and allogeneic class I MHC molecules are commonly used (Monie, 2007; Scott, 2001).

4.4 Allogeneic tumor cells

This procedure may be performed in patients with acute lymohoblastic and acute myeloblastic leukemia. Irradiated allogeneic tumor cells and bacille Calmette-Guerin vaccine (BCG) are used (Monie, 2007; Scott, 2001).

4.5 Defined tumor antigen based vaccines

More recently, approaches using defined tumor antigen based vaccines are among the most promising techniques. Prolonged remissions have been observed because a defined end-point is available. There is enough evidence that antigens derived from genes that have mutated during tumor development and antigens that have a normal sequence but are not expressed in the tumor have been demonstrated as a target of specific T-cells grown from cervical cancer patients (Monie, 2007; Norris, 1990; Scott, 2001).

5. Immunological aspects in cervical cancer

Immunological aspects of cervical cancer are still of interest, tumor specific immune response being one of the most promising fields in cervical cancer research. As HPV is the etiological agent of a family of diseases that cause more cancer death in women worldwide than any other form of cancer, the goal of the newer trials is to identify novel strategies for cervical cancer immunotherapy (Monie, 2007; Scott, 2001).

HPV types 16 and 18 represent probably the most prevalent oncogenic types found in cancerous cervical tissues, accounting for up to 80% of the cervical cancer cases. Moreover, the risk of progression to cervical carcinoma is higher for HPV types 16 and 18 than for other known types of HPV (Ancuta, 2009; Goncalves & Donadi, 2004; Scott, 2001).

However, most adult women will completely recover from their HPV infection, with a reported clearance rate of 30% at 6 months and 50% at 12 months. Therefore, a persistent infection with HPV may be defined as the continued detection of viral DNA of the same HPV type for at least 12 months.

After transmission by sexual contact, it has been demonstrated that the virus does not cause viraemia or systemic infection and remains located in the epithelial cells of cervical mucosa.

It is well known that the virus adaptation to the differentiation of the superficial cells is an essential process to evade the host's immunity. Besides, HPV by itself is not cytolytic for the keratinocytes. The squamous epithelium undergoes a programmed cell death and descuamation. HPV infects basal layer of the epithelium that mature vertically to the superficial surface of it; therefore, the viruses are released only in the most superficial layers of the squamous epithelium into the cervical lumen (Goncalves & Donadi, 2004; Scott, 2001).

Usually, the entire process from infection to viral release is less than three weeks. The natural keratinocytes death is not accompanied by inflammation and, therefore, viral proteins are not visible to the host immune system.

Most of women with early invasive cervical cancer are asymptomatic. In such cases, cervical smears may be effective in detecting early stage disease. On the other hand, advanced cervical cancer displays two primary pathways of extension: (i) local expansion and (ii) lymphatic or hematogenous dissemination.

It is actually known that mononuclear cells commonly infiltrate cervical tissue in different types of carcinoma, particularly in intra-tumoral sites, supporting the immune response against tumor. Previous studies have already shown the importance of local immune cell response in patient stratification according to the risk of disease recurrence after treatment. Moreover, three different cell subsets including TCD3+, BCD20+ and CD45+ leucocytes have been extensively studied among women with or without recurrence of their cancer after the surgery (Ancuta, 2009). Higher densities infiltrates are thought to be associated with a better clinical outcome. In addition, it seems that there is a relationship between different types of immune cells and survival: high density of cells is frequently observed in connection with free survival (Ancuta, 2009). The strongest discriminatory potential was attributed to densities of CD3+ in both intra- and peritumoral tissue; besides, according to a multiple regression model, CD3+ seems to be considered a potent prognostic factor for relapse (Ancuta, 2009). Nevertheless, no predictive biomarker is still validated for the use in clinical practice (Ancuta, 2009).

5.1 The innate immune system

The innate immune system generates non-specific protection against non-self antigens and does not intensify following repetitive infection events, while the aim of adaptive immunity is to induce cell mediated immune response by providing pathogen specific immunological memory.

Inflammation is a complex process that involves the recruitment of macrophages, neutrophils, dendritic cells and the release of cytokines and complement components. Dendritic cells activated by local cell injuries take up and process microbial agents while migrating to the draining lymph nodes, where they become antigen presenting cells and interact with T helper lymphocytes. Moreover, they are able to activated differentiation of T cytotoxic lymphocytes that allows rapid and strong response directed against the pathogen infected cells able to kill the pathogen (effector T-cells) and a fraction of the T cytotoxic and T helper cells becomes T memory cells (Arany, 1995; Arany & Tyring, 1996; de Gruijl, 1998; Goncalves & Donadi, 2004; Scott, 2001; Moscicki, 2000).

On the other hand, T helper lymphocytes activate the humoral immune response, which results in the production of specific antibodies against viral infection. In addition, these cells activate the differentiation of B lymphocytes into plasma cells that will neutralize the virus by binding to the viral capside proteins and other plasma cells that are able to synthetize and to secrete antibodies which maintain a protective level of antibodies long time after the first contact with the virus (al-Saleh, 1998; Bell, 1995; de Gruijl, 1998; Goncalves & Donadi, 2004; Scott, 2001).

B memory cells will provide rapid and amplified antibody response after re-infection with the same pathogen.

HPV is a double stranded DNA virus that contains 8000 base pairs. There is strong evidence that two key regions have been described in HPV:

- the early region which contains eight genes (E1 to E8), involved in the viral DNA replication function (E1 and E8), transcription control (E2 and E8) and cellular transformation (E5, E6 and E7);
- the late region, with two genes (L1-L2), which code for the capsid proteins.

Viral DNA replication remains located mainly in the basal cells of the epithelium's proliferative cells, whereby most individuals eliminate the HPV 12 to 24 months after the diagnosis.

On the other hand, the oncogenic viral types are associated with high grade squamous intraepithelial lesions and it is known that the host's humoral and cellular immune system can explain the latency of HPV infection. Also, the responses to cytokine action during carcinogenic and non-carcinogenic processes are evidence of the role of immunological control in tumoral progression or progress of lesions associated with HPV infection (Ancuta, 2009; Bethwaite, 1996; Crowley-Nowick , 2000; Scott, 2001).

The interaction between these mechanisms is responsible for malignant transformation in women with HPV infection:

- one of these involves a modification of the AP1 transcription factor, endogenous synthesis of anti-viral interferon beta;
- the other involves the interaction between INK4A and transforming activity of E6.

Modern data support the fact that epithelial cells appear to play much more complex roles in cell mediated immune response than a mechanical barrier.

Cervical keratinocytes constitutively secrete pro-inflammatory cytokines, growth factors and chemokines. Main cytokines which promote anti-viral effects are represented by transforming growth factor beta (TGF-β), tumor necrosis factor alpha (TNF-α) and beta (TNF-β) and interferon (IFN), respectively. Several cytokines such as IFN-α, IFN-β, TNF-α and TGF-β which are essentially produced by epithelial cells, display significant anti-viral and anti-proliferative effects.

Additionally, a promising mechanism by which TGF-β, TNF-α and the IFNs are able to inhibit the *in vitro* proliferation of both HPV-transformed keratinocytes and expression of HPV genes including the early genes E6 and E7 has been advanced (Crowley-Nowick, 2000; Scott, 2001).

It has been demonstrated that E7 interacts with the tumor suppressing retinoblastoma gene protein, while E6 has been shown to be critical in cancer development by enhancing protein p53 degradation through ubiquitin-mediated proteolysis via a mechanism requiring E6-

associated protein. Thus, all these data highlighted once more the notion that E6 and E7 proteins appear to have essential role in malignancy (Youde, 2000; Scott, 2001).

Varied results of the potential for HPV-infected cells to escape immune response, accompanied by the growth inhibitory effects of cytokines, are highly depending on experimental findings.

TGF-β1 provides a good example of growth inhibitory effect in either HPV type 16 or HPV 18 transformed cells. Studies investigating the role of exogenous effects of TGF-β1 showed that the TGF-β1 induce growth inhibition in HPV 16 immortalized human keratinocyte cell line may be accompanied by suppression of steady-state levels of RNA down-regulation of the genes c-*myc*, suggesting a mechanistic association between TGF-β up-regulation and HPV-infected cells. The same researches also reported that over-expression of TGF-β1 treatment of HPV 16 immortalized cells results in proliferation enhancing bcl-2 and NFkB genes (Goncalves & Donadi, 2004; Scott, 2001).

HPV infected cells are grown in a medium that stimulates early stages of tumor progression; therefore, TGF-β appears to stimulate cells growth. The effect is seen only in HPV infected cells, but not in HPV negative ones, favoring increased expression of epidermal growth factor receptor and its ligand. These examples suggest that HPV infected cells may escape early, even before malignant transformations occurs.

The evaluation of the growth inhibitory effects of TNF-α in HPV infected cells has revealed that TNF-α appears to have an anti-proliferative effect on HPV 16 infected cells. The characterization of this growth inhibitory effect has lead to the suggestion that it involves growth arrest in G0-G1 phase.

As recently reviewed by certain authors, a growth-stimulatory effect involving an amphiregulin-mediated autocrine loop has been demonstrated for both IL-10 and TNF-α in some HPV 16 or 18 infected epithelial cells. They finally concluded that it could provide an early escape from growth inhibition in HPV-immortalized cells. In addition to the anti-proliferative effect, IFNs have also been investigated.

It seems that IFN-α inhibits the proliferation of HPV 16 infected cells at lower dose as compared to those needed to inhibit the growth of normal keratinocytes. It has also been shown that IFN-α inhibits E7 protein expression without interfering with transcription, suggesting that the inhibition of proliferation is mediated through E7 protein but not E6 protein expression. Moreover, the authors have concluded that IFNs may be virus-type specific or cell-line specific. A direct potential anti-viral role for IFNs in HPV-infected cells was therefore identified (Hatch & Fu, 1999; Nakagawa, 2000; Scott, 2001; Wang, 1999).

Interestingly, neither IFN-α and IFN-γ have been shown to reduce the transcription of E6 and E7 genes in a HPV 16 transformed keratinocyte line (HPK-1A) (Kleine, 1995; Lee, 1999; Scott, 2001). More recent work indicates that IFN-β reduces the transcription of both E6 and E7 genes in HPV 16 transfected keratinocyte-line (HPK-1A). Besides, there is actually strong evidence that malignant transformation is accompanied by the loss of responsiveness to the inhibitory properties of cytokines. TGF-β, for example, may play roles in checking the HPV gene transcription in non-tumorigenic HPV 16 immortalized cell type lines and malignant transformation could involve partial resistance to it (Nakagawa, 2000; Scott, M, 2001; Stoler, 2010).

The hypothesis that the resistance to the growth-inhibitory effects of several cytokines may occur in HPV-immortalized cells even prior to malignancy is actually proposed. The authors suggested that chronic inflammation has led to a selective advantage for abnormal cells *in vivo* by synthesis of pro-inflammatory cytokines. They concluded that a possible escape of cytokine mediated growth inhibition in HPV infected cells was identified.

The studies described above suggest the possibility that HPV infected cells may evade the growth inhibitory effects of cytokines by modulating the production of cytokines and other mechanisms. For example, they have more recently demonstrated that a correlation between increased tumorigenicity, significantly decreased expression of TNFα receptors and resistance to TNF-mediated inhibition of proliferation was observed. The studies concluded that type I and type II receptors levels in serum of patients with HPV 16 or 18 cervical carcinoma were significantly increased (Bontkes, 1999; Scott, 2001).

The characterization of this effect has led to the suggestion that soluble type I and type II TNF-α receptors may facilitate the growth of lesions in the HPV infected epithelium. As a further example, a possible mechanism by which HPV infected cells may escape the anti-proliferative cytokines effect, that conversion of non-tumorigenic He La fibroblast hybrids to malignant cells is accompanied by the ability of TNF-α to suppress HPV 18 gene transcription, suggesting a mechanistic association between loss of TNF-α sensitivity and alterations in the composition of the activator protein 1 complex.

HPV 16 E7 inactivates the induction of the IFN-α inductible genes by blocking the translocation of p48, the DNA binding part of the IFN stimulated gene factor 3 transcription complex, to the molecules upon IFN-α stimulation. The characterization of this cytokines role, except IFN-γ, in keratinocyte growth regulation in HPV infected cells has led to the observation that these may play autocrine roles in HPV infection (Goncalves & Donadi, 2004; Kleine, 1995; Lee, 1999; Norris, 1990; Scott, 2001; Symington & Santos, 1990).

5.2 Adaptive cell mediated immunity

The findings provide preliminary evidence for an association between two phases (recognition and effector), focusing on the cells involved and membrane bound molecules that mediate the immune response.

5.2.1 Recognition phase

Several studies have addressed the potential role of Langerhans cells in HPV lesions which may contribute to persistence of the infection. For example, S100+cells (antibodies) are significantly reduced in SIL compared to normal cervical epithelium, whereas CD1+ (antibodies) cells are not. As recently reviewed, cytokines with some contribution from Langerhans cells appear to be crucial mediators of the recognition phase. It seems that IL-1β, IL-1α, TNF-α and IL-10 are involved in Langerhans cells migration, acting as promoters or inhibitors of these cells.

Several investigators have described a possible association between HPV infection and deficits in production of these cytokines, based on findings of reduced IL-1α, IL-1β, TNF-α and GM-CSF and cervical carcinoma lines.

Besides, there is a relationship between diminished production of certain cytokines and persistent HPV infection. For example, TNF-α expression was highly expressed in low-grade squamous intraepithelial lesions (LSIL) biopsy specimens as compared to HSIL specimens. These abnormalities may contribute, along with local other immune processes, to an altered antigen-presentation to T cells in pre-invasive cervical lesions. Thus, abnormal immune responses suggest the possibility that HPV may evade immune-surveillance (Bethwaite, 1996; Goncalves & Donadi, 2004; Scott, 2001).

5.2.2 Effector phase

5.2.2.1 T-cell responses to HPV infection

Different analyses have suggested the potential role of T helper lymphocytes in providing protection against the persistence of HPV infection by measuring T-cell proliferative responses (Ancuta, 2009). It seems that more frequent responses to HPV 16 antigens E6 and E7 gene products were observed in subjects who had developed SIL compared to those who were cytologically normal, indicating that these antigens are important in SIL prevention.

In a similar study focused on HPV 16 proteins other than E6 and E7 (HPV 16 E2, HPV 16 E5, HPV 16 L1), T-cell proliferative responses to HPV 16 showed no association with disease outcome.

Moreover, results from certain trials have been equally confused by several factors including differences in subject populations, antigens (making the interpretation of T-cell helper response to HPV infection difficult) and the activities of T helper cells themselves (these are involved in production of auto-antibodies by B lymphocytes).

Other researchers have shown that responses to HPV 16 E5 proteins are more frequently observed in subjects with progressing LSIL than subjects without LSIL and those with HSIL. The results revealed that these responses may be correlated with clearance of HPV infection than with resolution of SIL.

Since T helper lymphocytes have important roles in aiding the development of cytotoxic lymphocytes, a possible association between these cells and clearance of virus may not be accurate reflections of a correlation between T helper cells responses and the HPV infection (Arany, 1995; Bethwaite, 1996; Dolei, 1999; Goncalves & Donadi, 2004; Nakagawa, 2000; Scott, 2001).

5.2.2.2 Research on CTL-mediated killing

Few studies have demonstrated the presence of activated CTL in SIL. CD8+CTL are known to be responsible for recognizing and killing HPV infection and SIL. One such study has reported that subjects with positive responses to E6 or E7 peptide can lead to the regression of tumors expressing E6 or E7; additionally, this regression is mediated by TCD8+, MHC class-I-CTL. Also, HPV E6 and/or E7 specific CTL were observed in patients with cervical carcinoma. Moreover, it has been demonstrated that CTLs were not only be capable of leasing HLA-matched, but also identified HPV specific CTL in lymph nodes and cervical cancer. Across sectional analysis of HPV16 E6 and/or E7-specific CTL showed that these were lower in women with HPV 16 infection who have developed SIL than in women with HPV 16 infection who had not developed SIL.

Lack of CTL response to the HPV 16 E6 protein is more frequently observed in subjects with persistent HPV infection, suggesting that CTL response to E6 was correlated with viral clearance. However, additional studies are necessary for defining the role of CTL in the regression of SIL.

Some researchers reported positive tetramer responses to HPV 16 E7 by isolating T lymphocytes specific for HPV, but the interpretation is difficult since the development of cervical cancer was not prevented (Bethwaite, 1996; Nakagawa, 2000; Scott, 2001; Sheu, 1999).

5.2.2.3 Studies of antigenic epitopes in HPV infection

There is little information about antigenic epitopes of HPV using mouse model systems and human systems, respectively. Nevertheless, certain research papers focusing on CTL epitopes of HPV 16 E6 and E7 proteins have identified five common HLA types; also, the immunological response of nine of these potential epitopes for HLA-2.1 was demonstrated. For example, E6 (29-38), E7 (11-20), E7 (82-90) and E7 (86-93) were identified using HLA-2.1. Immunogenicity of three of the four peptides [E7 (11-20), E7 (82-90) and E7 (86-93)] was confirmed by using CTL induction of peripheral blood mononuclear cells (PBMCs) from humans *in vitro*. The fourth of these peptides (CTL4) has been observed in SIL and cervical cancer (de Gruijl , 1998; Youde, 2000; Scott, 1999; Scott, 2001; Wang, 1999).

5.2.2.4 MHC class II restricted antigen presentation in the effector phase

A couple of recent studies have concluded that transcription of class II MHC molecules may be due to interferon gamma treatment of HPV 16 or 18 immortalized keratinocytes. They have demonstrated that HLA-DR epithelial cells, T-cells and Langerhans cells may participate in immune reactions by down-regulating HLA-DR due to interferon gamma secretion by activated T cells.

The hypothesis that up-regulation of HLA-DR expression was absent in cutaneous warts was suggested based on differences between cutaneous and mucosal anti-HPV immune responses. Also, other authors have reported that expression of HLA-DR is associated with HSIL and HPV may evade immune responses by blocking up-regulation of MHC class II expression. In addition, impaired up-regulation of this antigen in patients with genital condylomas responded to interferon treatment compared to those who did not; a possible causal link between high E7 expression in the non-responders and the lower inducibility of HLA-DR expression was identified (Crowley-Nowick, 2000; de Gruijl, 1998; Goncalves & Donadi, 2004; Youde, 2000; Scott, 2001; Wang, 1999).

5.2.2.5 MHC class I restricted antigen presentation in the effector phase

While normal keratinocytes constitutively express MHC class I molecules, HPV-infected tissues also commonly express high MHC class I levels as suggested by one report. Besides, these keratinocytes are susceptible to class I mediated lysis by alloantigen-primed CTL.

In a recent analysis, loss of MHC class I expression have been reported in cutaneous warts, although only partial loss of expression was seen in condylomas. In addition, studies using specimens from cervical cancers biopsies have reported a drastic reduction in MHC class I expression.

Finally, many investigators have described a possible correlation between loss of MHC class I in cervical cancer biopsy specimens and tumor type, disease stage and HPV 16 or 18 types. They concluded that loss or down-regulation if MHC class I expression is associated with more frequent disease recurrences.

Another research group has demonstrated that expression of the transporter associated with antigen presentation (TAP-1) is also associated with recurrence of the disease, suggesting that HPV may evade immune-surveillance by down-regulating TAP-1. As well, loss or down–regulation of MHC class I expression is critical for CTL-mediated killing (Bethwaite, 1996; Crowley-Nowick, 2000; de Gruijl, 1998; Youde, 2000; Scott, 2001; Wang, 1999).

5.3 Regulation of T cell immune responses

5.3.1 Chemokines and adhesion molecules

Another area of interest is the recruitment of activated lymphocytes at the sites of inflammation, defining immune processes that involve both chemokines and membrane bound adhesion molecules.

Several studies have described a close association between IL-8 production and the recruitment of neutrophils and T cells, while other have reported that malignant transformation of cervical keratinocytes is associated with higher IL-8 levels, especially when stimulated by IL-1 or TNF-α. In addition, T cells synthesis and secretion of IFN-γ may be accompanied by high IL-8 levels, stimulating, in turn, cellular immune responses.

Certain novel papers on malignant transformation have also mentioned higher IL-8 levels in women with histologic evidence of HPV infection, whereas the levels of RANTES (Regulated on Activation Normal T Expressed Secreted Factor) and MIP-1α (Macrophage Inflammatory Protein-1 alpha) are confounded. On the other hand, some approaches suggest that IL-8 synthesis in HPV 16 or 18 immortalized cell lines was significantly diminished.

Cervical keratinocytes are capable of producing MCP-1 (Macrophage Chemo-attractant Protein 1) and HPV 18+ HeLa cells transfected without the vector containing cDNA for MCP-1 lead to rapidly growing tumors. Some recent data suggest that ICAM-1 (Intercellular Adhesion Molecule-1) and its ligand, LFA-1 (Leukocyte Function Associated Antigen 1), seems to be important in adhesion processes by involving specific antigen recognition and CTL mediated killing.

Advanced researches have proposed the hypothesis that the adhesion process is accompanied by increased expression of ICAM-1 as a result of TNF-α and IFN-γ contribution. In addition, small clusters of LFA-1 positive T cells were found in the lower half of the epithelium surrounding ICAM-1 positive keratinocytes. Furthermore, the communication between T cells and keratinocytes is believed to be supported by the ICAM-1 overlapped with HLA-DR expression as bystanders of the adhesion process.

Whereas old data support the observation that impaired expression may play a role in the progression of the malignant process, the role of adhesion molecules in cervical cancer was recently up-dated (Bethwaite, 1996; Bell, 1995; Dolei, 1999; Monnier-Benoit, 2006; Scott, 2001; Wang, 1999).

5.3.2 Cytokines regulating T-cell responses

In the last years, many articles have reviewed the classification of activated T-helper cells aiming to understand humoral and cellular immune responses in cervical cancer (Ancuta, 2009).

A larger number of cells with particular focus on Th1 and Th2 cytokines production may play a role in local immune response. The classification include IFN-γ, TNF-α and IL-2 producing T helper type 1 cells which stimulate cellular immune response and IL-4, IL-5, IL-10 and IL-13 producing T helper type 2 cells, which in turn stimulate humoral immune response.

The observation that Th1-Th2 paradigm may play a role in HPV infection has support from several studies. Th1 cytokines such as IFN-γ and IL-2 may also be important in the natural history of HPV infection (Mosmann & Sad; 1996; Scott, 1999; Scott, 2001).

Moreover, immunohistochemmical analysis has been proposed by many researchers to study cervical cancer biopsy specimens; they compared immunohistological studies of cervical carcinoma with results from normal cervical epithelium demonstrating fewer Th1 cells (IL-2+) and higher density of Th2 cells (IL-4+).

The authors have suggested that the IL-2 synthesis may be related to HPV type 16 *in vitro* stimulation. For example, the lowest IL-2 levels were demonstrated in women with cervical cancer, while the highest levels of IL-2 were reported in cytologically normal HPV women. Besides, there is strong evidence that MHC class I and/or MHC class II molecules down-regulation may decrease immune recognition of HPV-associated tumors through modulating IL-10 production (Bethwaite, 1996; Dolei, 1999; Goncalves & Donadi, 2004; Monnier-Benoit, 2006; Wang, 1999).

5.4 Clearance of HPV infection and clinical implications

As emphasize by some authors, HPV may evade local immune response by limiting the extent of viral antigens to immunologic recognition.

Three potential mechanisms for HPV immune-surveillance were actually proposed, including:

- E7 protein may inhibit local immune response by blocking the antigen presenting function of dendritic cells from the epithelium in cervical tissue;
- an effective immune response against the HPV infected cells in the basal epithelium, where the E6 and E7 early genes are expressed; capsid encoding genes delayed expression may be the consequence of the inhibition promoted by a codon usage still remain exploratory, but this scenario is still exploratory;
- lack of CTL response to the HPV infected cells: keratinocytes may be less susceptible to class I mediated lysis by alloantigen-primed CTL (Bethwaite, 1996; Dolei, 1999; Goncalves & Donadi, 2004; Palefsky, 1999; Scott, 2001; Wang, 1999)

6. Prophylactic HPV vaccines

Multiple studies indicate there are several challenges and uncertainties that need to be resolved before HPV vaccination. In addition, socio-cultural factors will affect the acceptability of the HPV vaccine in high risk developing countries. Patients must acquire more information for accepting HPV vaccination. After considering the evidence, the clinicians come to a unanimous decision that such information might include the need for prevention and applicable information concerning where to acquire and how to fund HPV vaccination.

Two prophylactic HPV vaccines, namely Cervarix^R and Gardasil^R (Silgard), have been already approved; they are directed against and contain virus-like particles (VLPs) specific for two of the most important oncogenic HPV types 16 and 18. In addition, Gardasil^R is a quadrivalent vaccine that also includes VLPs for HPV 6 and 11, the most common HPV types found in up to 90% of genital warts (Harper, 2009; Kitcher, 2008). These vaccines offer protection for 70% of cancers, but also for about 90% of HPV type 16/18 associated CIN (Kitcher, 2008).

Although the immunogenic properties of the prophylactic HPV vaccines give the possibility of long term protection for women in a wide range of years, the vaccination seems to be most advantageous in preadolescent girl (Kitcher, 2008). It is widely recognized that the above mentioned prophylactic vaccines are able to induce high titers of neutralizing antibodies; however, Cervarix^R is responsible for significantly higher titers of antibodies than Gardasil^R (Harper, 2009).

With regard to baseline seropositivity, increased memory B cell response is commonly reported in women who were both seronegative and PCR negative for oncogenic HPV types 16 and 18 at the time of vaccination (Harper, 2009). Also, several studies showed that adolescents mounted an antibody response that was significantly higher compared to the seronegative old women (Harper, 2009). Because the meaning of loss of antibody titers is unclear, long term studies are necessary to prove the efficacy for the HPV vaccines.

In general, both Gardasil^R and Cervarix^R are safe for the majority subjects who received vaccines. The most commonly reported adverse events were pain, erythema, swelling, myalgias, arthralgias, headaches and gastrointestinal symptoms. In the mean time, no serious adverse events (hospitalization, disability, death) have been reported (Harper, 2009).

Special consideration should be made about vaccine administration in pregnancy; three therapeutic scenarios are defined, as follows:

- the vaccination during pregnancy is not allowed;
- if one dose of vaccine has been received before pregnancy, all three administration should be taken after delivery;
- if two doses have been received before pregnancy, the last dose could be administrated in postpartum period (Harper, 2009).

No scientific evidence supports the interruption of a pregnancy because of the partial vaccine administration; additionally, there is no formal contraindication to vaccination during lactation (Harper, 2009).

7. Conclusions

Developments in the technology of measuring HPV antibody response in serum specimens would facilitate directions for further research in the prevention, control and management in cervical cancer and might encourage additional clinical trials research on HPV infection and cervical carcinoma that need to be widely disseminated to the clinicians and women by updating screening and management protocol.

The current perception of HPV persistency is not fully understand by many physicians and researchers. Therefore, viral persistency will be taken into account in an organized context in screening programs.

Because of the very high efficacy shown by HPV vaccines, the cytology-based screening programs will be less efficient and potentially rates of over-diagnosis and over-treatment of indefinite lesions will multiply.

Transition time to redefine screening protocols including a later age at the beginning and less frequent screening visits is thus essential.

In addition to HPV-based screening programs, many issues are not fully comprehend, requiring a lot of educations: triage of cytological pre-invasive lesions, follow-up after treatment of SIL, detection of p16, detection of HPV mRNA, prophylactic vaccination against HPV infection.

Baseline assessment of women with cervical carcinoma with and without relapse is critical in order to identify association with classical negative prognostic factors including tumor size and grading, histological type, clinical stage FIGO and lymph node invasion.

The assessment of local cellular immune response seem to be critical for stratifying patients according to their risk, for the therapeutic option; moreover, understanding of local immune response in cervical carcinoma may potentially guide new adjuvant treatment strategies including immunotherapy.

Several studies have already demonstrated that tumor-infiltrating lymphocytes (composition, distribution, cell count) reflect the status of the cellular immune system in patients with cervical cancer. Different immune cell subsets, especially T-cells subpopulation, were assessed in tissue specimens from different types of cervical carcinoma; despite some controversial data, the majority of researchers have indicated that tumor infiltration by immune cells are associated with improved clinical outcome in cancer patients, especially in cervical cancer.

To identify the immune cells of interest, the specific antigens expressed on cell surface could be detected by immunohistochemistry, using corresponding antibodies. There is some evidence that immunohistochemistry assessment in women experiencing recurrence of their cervical cancers has revealed low densities of immune cells infiltrating the tumor.

There is actually enough evidence to promote the hypothesis that local cellular immune response is essential for guiding further cancer evolution and prognosis. However, larger cohort studies based on extended analysis of several immune cells are critical for the validation of prognostic biomarkers in cervical cancer.

8. References

al-Saleh, W.; Giannini, L.M, Jacobs, N., Moutschen, M., Doyen, J., Boniver, J., Delvenne, P. (1998). Correlation of T-helper secretory differentiation and types of antigen-presenting cells in squamous intraepithelial lesions of the uterine cervix. *J. Pathol.*, Vol. 184, pp.283–290, ISSN: 1096-9896

Arany, I.; Goel, A., Tyring, S.K. (1995). Interferon response depends on viral transcription in human papillomavirus-containing lesions. *Anticancer Res,* Vol. 15, pp.2865–2869, ISSN: 0250-7005

Arany, I. & Tyring, S.K. (1996). Activation of local cell-mediated immunity in interferon-responsive patients with human papillomavirus-associated lesions. *J. Interferon Cytokine Res*. Vol. 16, pp. 453–460, ISSN: 1079-9907

Ancuta, E.; Ancuta, C., Zugun-Eloae, F., Iordache, C., Chirieac, R., Carasevici, E. (2009). Predictive value of cellular immune response in cervical cancer, *RJME*, Vol. 50, No. 4, pp.651–655, ISSN, 1220-0522

Bethwaite, P.B.; Holloway, L.J.; Thornton, A.; Delahunt, B. (1996). Infiltration by immunocompetent cells in early stage invasive carcinoma of the uterine cervix: a prognostic study, *Pathology*, Vol. 28, No. 4, pp. 321–327, ISSN: 09728074

Bell, M.C.; Edwards, R.P.; Partrige, E.E., Kuykendall, K.; Conner, W.; Gore, H.; Turbat-Herrara, E.; Crowleynowick, P.A. (1995). CD8+ T lymphocytes are recruited to neoplastic cervix, *J Clin Immunol*, Vol. 15, No. 3, pp. 130–136., ISSN: 1573-2592

Bontkes, H. J.; de Gruijl, T.D., Bijl, A., Verheijen, R.H., Meijer, C.J., Scheper, R.J., Stern, P.L., Burns, J.E., Maitland, N.J., Walboomers, J.M. (1999). Human papillomavirus type 16 E2-specific T-helper lymphocyte responses in patients with cervical intraepithelial neoplasia. *J. Gen. Virol.* Vol. 80, pp.2453–2459, ISSN: 0022-1317

Chao, H.T.; Wang, P.H., Tseng, L.Y., Lai, C.R., Chiang, S.C., Yuan, C.C. (1999). Lymphocyte-infiltrated FIGO Stage IIB squamous cell carcinoma of the cervix is a prominent factor for disease-free survival, *Eur J Gynaecol Oncol*, Vol. 20, No. 2, pp.136–40. ISSN: 0392-2936.

Crowley-Nowick, P.A.; Ellenberg, J.H., Vermund, S.H., Douglas, S.D., Holland, C.A., Moscicki, A.B. (2000). Cytokine profile in genital tract secretions from female adolescents: impact of human immunodeficiency virus, human papillomavirus, and other sexually transmitted pathogens. *J. Infect. Dis*, Vol. 181, pp.939–945, ISSN:0022-1899

de Gruijl, T. D.; Bontkes, H.J., Walboomers, J.M., Stukart, J., Doekhie, F.S., Remmink, A.J., Helmerhorst, J., Verheijen, R.H., Duggan-Keen, M.H., Stern, P.L., Meijer, P., Scheper, R.J. (1998). Differential T helper cell responses to human papillomavirus type 16 E7 related to viral clearance or persistence in patients with cervical neoplasia: a longitudinal study. *Cancer Res*, Vol. 58, pp.1700–1706, ISSN: 0008-5472.

Dolei, A.; Curreli, S., Marongiu, P., Pierangeli, A., Gomes, E., Bucci, M., Serra, C., Degener, A.M. (1999). Human immunodeficiency virus infection in vitro activates naturally integrated human papillomavirus type 18 and induces synthesis of the L1 capsid protein. J. *Gen. Virol*, Vol. 80, pp.2937–2944, ISSN: 0022-1317

Goncalves, M.A.G. & Donadi, E.A. (2004). Immune cellular response to HPV: current concepts, *Braz Journal Infect Dis*, Vol. 8, No. 1, pp.1–9., ISSN 1413-8670

Hatch, D.K. & Fu, Y.S. (1999). Cervical and vaginal cancer. In: *Novak's Gynecology*, Berek, J.S. Callisto Medical Press, Turkey, 1111–55.

Harper,D.M. (2009). HPV vaccines. In: *Textbook of Gynaecological Oncology*, Ayhan, A.; Gultekin, M. & Dursun, P. (Eds), Gunes Publishing.

Youde, S. J.; Dunbar, P.R., Evans, E.M., Fiander, A.N., Borysiewicz, L.K., Cerundolo, V., Man, S. (2000). Use of fluorogenic histocompatibility leukocyte antigen-Ap0201/HPV 16 E7 peptide complexes to isolate rare human cytotoxic T-lymphocyte-recognizing endogenous human papillomavirus antigens. *Cancer Res.* Vol. 60, pp.365–371, ISSN: 0008-5472.

Kitchener, H.C. (2008). Prophylactic HPV vaccination: current status. In: *Vaccines for the prevention of cervical cancer,* Stern, L.P. & Kitchener, H.C. (Eds), Oxford University press; ISBN; 978-0-19-954345.

Kleine, K.; Konig, G., Kreuzer, J., Komitowski, D., Zur Hausen, H., Rosl, F. (1995). The effect of the JE (MCP-1) gene, which encodes monocyte chemoattractant protein-1, on the growth of HeLa cells and derived somatic- cell hybrids in nude mice. *Mol. Carcinog.* Vol. 4, pp.179–189, ISSN: 0899-1987.

Lee, B.N.; Follen, M., Tortolero-Luna, M., Eriksen, N., Helfgott, A., Hammill, A., Shearer, W.T., Reuben, J.M. (1999). Synthesis of IFN-gamma by CD8(1) T cells is preserved in HIV-infected women with HPV-related cervical squamous intraepithelial lesions. *Gynecol. Oncol,* Vol. 75, pp.379–386, ISSN 0090-8258.

Monie, A.; Hung, C.F.; Wu, T.C. (2007). Preventive and therapeutic HPV vaccines, *Curr Opin Invest Drugs,* Vol.8, No.12, pp.1038–50, ISSN: 1472-4472

Monnier-Benoit, S.; Mauny, F., Riethmuller, D., Guerrini, J.S., Capilna, M., Felix, S., Seilles, E., Mougin, C., Pretet, J.L. (2006). Immunohistochemical analysis of CD4+ and CD8+ T-cells subsets in high risk human papillomavirusassociated pre-malignant and malignant lesions of the uterine cervix, *Gynecol Oncol,* Vol. 102, No. 1, pp.22–31, ISSN 0090-8258

Moscicki, A.B.; Ellenberg, J.H., Vermund, S.H., Holland, C.A., Darragh, T., Crowley-Nowick, A., Levin, L., Wilson, C.M. (2000). Prevalence of and risks for cervical human papillomavirus infection and squamous intraepithelial lesions in adolescent girls: impact of infection with human immunodeficiency virus. *Arch. Pediatr. Adolesc. Med,* Vol. 154, pp.127–134, ISSN 1072-4710.

Mosmann, T.R. & Sad, S. (1996). The expanding universe of T-cell subsets: Th1, Th2 and more. *Immunol. Today,* Vol. 17, pp.138–146, ISSN: 0167-4919

Nakagawa, M.; Stites, D.P., Patel, S., Farhat, S., Scott, M., Hills, N.K., Palefsky, J.M., Moscicki, A.B. (2000). Persistence of human papillomavirus type 16 infection is associated with lack of cytotoxic T lymphocyte response to the E6 antigens. *J. Infect. Dis.* Vol. 182, pp.595–598, ISSN:0022-1899

Nedergaard, B.S.; Ladekarl, M., Thomsen, H.F., Nyegaard, J.R., Nielsen, K. (2007). Low density of CD3+, CD4+ and CD8+ cells is associated with increased risk of relapse in squamous cell cervical cancer, *Br J Cancer,* Vol. 97, No. 8, pp. 1135–1138, ISSN:0007-0920

Nedergaard, B.S.; Ladekarl, M., Nyegaard, J.R., Nielsen, K. (2008). A comparative study of cellular immune response in patients with stage IB cervical squamous cell carcinoma. Low number of several immune cell subtypes are strongly associated with relapse of disease within 5 years, *Gynecol Oncol,* Vol. 108, No. 1, pp.106–111, ISSN 0090-8258

Norris, D.A. (1990). Cytokine modulation of adhesion molecules in the regulation of immunologic cytotoxicity of epidermal targets. *J. Investig. Dermatol.* Vol. 95, pp.111S–120S, ISSN: 0022-202X

Palefsky, J.M.; Minkoff, H., Kalish, L.A., Levine, A.L., Sacks, S., Garcia, P., Young, M., Melnick, S., Miotti, P., Burk, R. (1999). Cervicovaginal human papillomavirus infection in human immunodeficiency virus-1 (HIV)-positive and high-risk HIV-negative women. *J. Natl. Cancer Inst.* Vol. 91, pp.226–236, ISSN 0027-8874

Piersma, S.J.; Jordanova, E.S., van Poelgeest, M.I.E., Kwappenberg, K.M.C., van der Hulst, J.M., Drijfhout, J.W., Melief, C.J.M., Kenter, G.G., Fleuren, G.J., Offriga, R., van der Burg, S.H. (2007). High number of intraepithelial CD8+ tumor-infiltrating lymphocytes is associated with the absence of lymph node metastases in patients with large early-stage cervical cancer, *Cancer Res*, Vol. 67, No. 1, pp.354–361, ISSN: 0008-5472

Scott, M.; Stites, D.P., Moscicki, A.B. (1999). Th1 cytokine patterns in cervical human papillomavirus infection. *Clin. Diagn. Lab. Immunol.* Vol. 6, pp. 751–755. ISSN (printed): 1071-412X

Scott, M.; Nakagawa, M., Moscicki, A.B. (2001). Cell-Mediated Immune Response to Human Papillomavirus Infection, *Clin Diagn Lab Immunol*, pp. 209–220, ISSN (printed): 1071-412X

Symington, F.W. & Santos, E.B. (1990). Recognition of keratinocytes by cytotoxic T cells specific for conventional HLA class-I alloantigen. J. *Investig. Dermatol.* Vol. 95, pp.224–228, ISSN: 0022-202X

Sheu, B.C.; Hsu, S.M., Ho, H.N., Lin, R.H., Torng, P.L., Huang, S.C. (1999). Reversed CD4/CD8 ration of tumor-infiltrating lymphocytes are correlated with the progression of human cervical carcinoma, *Cancer*, Vol. 86, No.8, pp.1537–1543, ISSN: 1097-0142

Stoler, M.H. (2010). HPV in screening and triage. It is more complicated than you think: doctor, which HPV type cause that lesion, *Newsletter on HPV*, No.20, pp. 4-6

Wang, B.; Amerio, P., Sauder, D.N. (1999). Role of cytokines in epidermal Langerhans cell migration. *J. Leukoc. Biol.* Vol. 66, pp.33–39, ISSN: 0741-5400